William M. Warfel

NURSING MANAGEMENT DESK REFERENCE

CONCEPTS, SKILLS & STRATEGIES

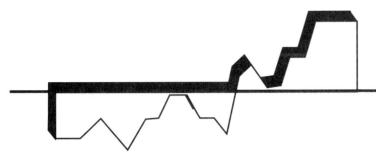

NURSING MANAGEMENT DESK REFERENCE

CONCEPTS, SKILLS & STRATEGIES

Roxane Spitzer-Lehmann, *PhD, MBA, RN, FAAN, CHE, CNAA*

Adjunct Associate Professor, University of Southern California Department of Nursing and University of California, Los Angeles, School of Nursing, Los Angeles, California; Visiting Professor, University of Colorado School of Business, Denver, Colorado; National Advisor, MEDICUS Systems; Chief Executive Officer, S/L Associates, San Diego, California

W.B. SAUNDERS COMPANY

A Division of Harcourt Brace & Company

Philadelphia   London   Toronto   Montreal   Sydney   Tokyo

W. B. Saunders Company
A Division of
Harcourt Brace & Company
The Curtis Center
Independence Square West
Philadelphia, PA 19106

Library of Congress Cataloging-in-Publication Data

Nursing management desk reference   :   concepts, skills & strategies   /
  [edited by] Roxane Spitzer-Lehmann.—1st ed.
      p.   cm.
   ISBN 0-7216-4346-9
   1. Nursing services—Administration.   I. Spitzer-Lehmann, Roxane.
   [DNLM: 1. Nurse Administrators.   2. Nursing Service, Hospital—
organization & administration.   3. Nursing Staff, Hospital—
organization & administration.   WY 105 N97477 1994]
   RT89.N797 1994
   362.1′73′068—dc20
   DNLM/DLC   93-35928

NURSING MANAGEMENT DESK REFERENCE   ISBN 0-7216-4346-9
Concepts, Skills & Strategies

Printed in United States of America

Last digit is the print number: 9   8   7   6   5   4   3   2   1

CONTRIBUTORS • • • • • •

Rhonda Anderson, RN, MPA, CNAA, FAAN
President, American Organization of Nurse Executives; Vice President of Patient Operations, Hartford Hospital, Hartford, Connecticut
Managing in a Managed Care Environment

Sue Barrett, RN, MS
Doctoral Candidate, University of Illinois, Chicago, Illinois
Policies, Politics, and Legislation

Janet Barron, RN, MS
Chief Executive Officer, PolyOptimum, Inc., San Francisco, California
Productivity and Cost Per Unit of Service

Marjorie Beyers, RN, PhD, FAAN
Adjunct Faculty, University of Michigan School of Nursing, Ann Arbor, Michigan; Associate Vice President, Mercy Health Services, Farmington Hills, Michigan
Management Problem Solving and Decision Making

Olive Y. Burner, RN, PhD
Professor Emeritus, University of California, Los Angeles, School of Nursing, Los Angeles, California
Developing a Framework for Nursing Management Practice

Dixie Cornell, RN, MEd
Principal, The Cornell Group, Eau Claire, Wisconsin
Effective Communication and Nurse Manager Success

Susan H. Cummings, MN, RN
President, Cummings Associates, San Diego, California
Staff Development and Mentoring

Maryann Davivier, PhD, CHT
President, Davivier Associates, Ojai, California
DRGs: Their Impact on Nursing Management

Karen S. Ehrat, RN, PhD
Senior Vice President/Chief Operating Officer, St. Joseph's Mercy Hospital and Health Centers, Clinton Township, Michigan
Mission Statement, Goals, and Values

Sally Everson-Bates, RN, DNSc

Director, Change Management, University of Arkansas Medical Sciences, Medical Center, Little Rock, Arkansas
Becoming a Manager

Janine Fiesta, BSN, JD

Vice President of Legal Services and Risk Management, Lehigh Valley Hospital, Allentown, Pennsylvania
Labor Relations and the Law

Steven A. Finkler, PhD, CPA

Professor of Health Administration, Accounting, and Financial Management, Robert F. Wagner Graduate School of Public Service, New York University, New York, New York
Marketing for Nurse Managers

Maryann F. Fralic, RN, DrPH, FAAN

Vice President for Nursing, The Johns Hopkins Hospital, Baltimore, Maryland
Quality Management in the Hospital Setting: New Horizons

Shirley Frederiksen, MS, RN

Research Coordinator, St. Joseph Mercy Hospital, Ann Arbor, Michigan
Wages and Salaries

Susan Gadbois, RN, BSN

President, Staff Nurses Association, Santa Rosa Memorial Hospital, Santa Rosa, California
Collaborative Practice in a Union Environment

Paul L. Grimaldi, PhD

Contributing Editor, *Nursing Management*, Cincinnati, Ohio
Cost: Concepts and Measurement

Robin Hagenstad, BS, RN

Executive Director, Nursing Service, Santa Rosa Memorial Hospital, Santa Rosa, California
Collaborative Practice in a Union Environment

Barbara Marion Hill, MSN, RN, CNAA

Adjunct Lecturer, University of Michigan School of Nursing; Nonresident Lecturer, University of Michigan School of Public Health; Vice President, Nursing and Emergency Services, St. Joseph Mercy Hospital, Catherine McAuley Health System, Ann Arbor, Michigan
Wages and Salaries

Christeen A. Holdwick, MA, RN

Director, Behavioral Services Operations, St. Joseph Mercy Hospital, Ann Arbor, Michigan
Wages and Salaries

Linda Jenkins, RN, BSN, MBA

Patient Care Services Leader, University of California, San Diego, Medical Center, Thornton Hospital, San Diego, California
Becoming a Manager

Judith E. Johnson, MS, RN

Vice President for Patient Care, St. Joseph's Hospital, Lancaster, Pennsylvania
Wages and Salaries

Katherine R. Jones, RN, PhD, FAAN

Associate Professor, School of Nursing, University of Michigan; Adjunct Nursing Administrator, University of Michigan Hospitals, Ann Arbor, Michigan
Budgeting Practices

Beth R. Keely, MSN, PhD, RN

Lecturer, California State University, Domingues Hills California, Carson, California
Orienting and Training of the New Nurse

Karlene M. Kerfoot, RN, PhD, CNAA, FAAN

Executive Vice President, Patient Care, and Chief Nursing Officer, St. Luke's Episcopal Hospital, Houston, Texas
Leaders: Yesterday, Today, and Tomorrow

Karin T. Kirchhoff, PhD, RN, FAAN

Professor, College of Nursing, University of Utah; Director of Nursing Research, University Hospital, Salt Lake City, Utah
Responsibilities of Nurse Executives in Conducting and Using Research in the Practice Setting

JoEllen Koerner, RN, PhD, FAAN

Adjunct Faculty, South Dakota State University, Brookings, South Dakota, and Augustana College; Vice President, Patient Services, Sioux Valley Hospital, Sioux Falls, South Dakota
Managing the Nurse–Physician Link

Christine T. Kovner, PhD, RN, FAAN

Associate Professor, Division of Nursing, School of Education, New York University, New York, New York
Marketing for Nurse Managers

David M. Lehmann, PhD, BSME, MBA

Vice President and General Manager Manufacturing, Solar Turbines Incorporated, San Diego, California
Innovation, Change, and Continuity

Leslie L. McCombs, PhD, RN, CNAA

Assistant Professor, University of California, Los Angeles, Los Angeles, California
Developing a Framework for Nursing Management Practice

Kathryn J. McDonagh, MSN, RN, CNAA

President, Saint Joseph's Hospital; Senior Vice President, Saint Joseph's Health System, Atlanta, Georgia
Resource Allocation and Material Management: Purchase of Supplies and Minor Equipment and Capital Acquisition Process

Michael L. Moore, CPA

Comptroller, Francis O. Day Company, Inc., Rockville, Maryland
Cost: Concepts and Measurement

Becky Nelson, RN, MS

Nursing Administrator for Critical Care Services, Sioux Valley Hospital, Sioux Falls, South Dakota
Managing the Nurse–Physician Link

Jane Fairbanks Neubauer, MS, RN

Visiting Fellow, King's Fund College, London, England
Building Your Team

Jim O'Malley, MSN, RN

Adjunct Faculty, Duquesne University and University of Pittsburgh; Vice President, Nursing Services, Allegheny General Hospital, Pittsburgh, Pennsylvania
Executive Self-Development

Carol A. Orme, RN, MSN

Director of Clinical Operations, San Francisco Bay Area, HSSI Home Care, San Francisco, California
Job Satisfaction and Retention

Sue E. Parks

President/Chief Executive Officer, HELP Management Group, Phoenix, Arizona
Risk Management

Linda J. Pierog, RN, MBA, CCRN

Associate Professor, California State University, Long Beach, California; Executive Director, Nursing Case Management and Service Line Development, Saint Joseph Hospital, Orange, California
Discharge Planning and Case Management

Jane Englebright Pollock, MS, RN

Doctoral Candidate, Texas Woman's University, Denton, Texas
Controlling Drug Distribution and Abuse

Tim Porter-O'Grady, EdD, RN, CS, CNAA, FAAN

Assistant Professor, Emory University; Senior Partner, Tim Porter-O'Grady Associates, Inc.; Senior Consultant, Affiliated Dynamics, Inc., Atlanta, Georgia
Entrepreneurialism in a Time of Great Change

Barbara Klug Redman, PhD, RN, FAAN

Professor and M. Adelaide Nutting Chair, The Johns Hopkins University School of Nursing, Baltimore, Maryland
Management of Patient Education

Karen Kohrt Ringl, MSN, RN

Faculty, Undergraduate and Graduate Colleges of Nursing, University of Southern California, Los Angeles, California; Vice President, Patient Care Services, San Gabriel Valley Medical Center, San Gabriel, California
Patient Care Delivery Systems

Nancy E. Royal, RN, MS, CPHQ

Administrative Director, Quality Management Services, Robert Wood Johnson University Hospital, New Brunswick, New Jersey
Quality Management in the Hospital Setting: New Horizons

Harry J. Schuler, PhD

Vice Provost of Lifelong Learning and Director of Health Science Division, Chapman University, Orange, California
Quality Management

Janet A. Secatore, RN, MS

Program Director, Institute for Clinical Management and Leadership, Beth Israel Hospital, Boston, Massachusetts
In Search of the Perfect Match

Roy L. Simpson, RN, C

Executive Director, Nursing Affairs, HBO & Company, Atlanta, Georgia
Information Management and Computer Technology

Marie Smith, MSN

Vice President, Client Services, PolyOptimum, Inc., San Francisco, California

Staffing and Scheduling: A Systems Approach

Roxane Spitzer-Lehmann, PhD, MBA, RN, FAAN

Adjunct Associate Professor, University of Southern California, Department of Nursing, and University of California, Los Angeles, School of Nursing, Los Angeles, California; Visiting Professor, University of Colorado School of Business, Denver, Colorado; National Advisor, MEDICUS Systems; Chief Executive Officer, S/L Associates, San Diego, California

Organizational Structures for Effective Patient Care Delivery
DRGs: Their Impact on Nursing Management

Nancy Steiger, MSN, RN

Assistant Clinical Professor, Department of Physiological Nursing, University of California, San Francisco, San Francisco, California; Vice President, Patient Care Service, Santa Rosa Memorial Hospital, Santa Rosa, California

Collaborative Practice in a Union Environment

Susan Sumner Stengrevics, RN, MSN

Nurse Manager, Beth Israel Hospital, Boston, Massachusetts

In Search of the Perfect Match

Joanne Marky Supples, RN, PhD

Assistant Professor, University of Colorado Health Sciences Center School of Nursing, Denver, Colorado; Clinical Director, University of Colorado Nursing Clinic, Littleton, Colorado

Managing Chemical Dependency in the Workplace

Marita G. Titler, PhD, RN

Adjunct Assistant Professor, College of Nursing, and Associate Director of Nursing Research, University of Iowa Hospitals and Clinics, Iowa City, Iowa

Responsibilities of Nurse Executives in Conducting and Using Research in the Practice Setting

Margaret Murphy Vosburgh, RN, MS, MBA

Adjunct Faculty, University of California, Los Angeles, University of Southern California, and California State, Los Angeles, California; Medical Executive Committee, Hospital Board of Directors, Medical Care Improvement Committee, Nursing Administrators Council, Work Redesign Committee, and Hospital Administrative Planning Committee, Hoag Memorial Hospital, Los Angeles, California

Managing the Difficult Employee

William M. Warfel, PhD, RN, CNAA

Adjunct Faculty, School of Nursing, LaSalle University; Adjunct Lecturer, School of Nursing, University of Pennsylvania; Associate General Director, Albert Einstein Medical Center, Philadelphia, Pennsylvania
Strategic Planning

Susan Chamberlain Williams, RN, MS

Consultant, Special Projects, Medical University of South Carolina, Charleston, South Carolina; Member, Board of Trustees, Beaufort Memorial Hospital, Beaufort, South Carolina
Managing Nursing's Future: Challenging the Profession

Gail A. Wolf, RN, BSN, MSN, DNS

Vice President, Nursing and Patient Care, Shadyside Hospital, Pittsburgh, Pennsylvania
Job Satisfaction and Retention

Barbara J. Youngberg, JD, MSW, BSN

Lecturer at Law, Health Law Institute, Loyola University College of Law; Assistant Professor, Health Sciences, University of Chicago Medical School; Vice President, Insurance, Risk, and Quality Management, University Hospital Consortium, Chicago, Illinois
Ethical Issues in Nursing Practice

PREFACE •   •   •   •   •   •

Change is a way of life in today's culture and in the health care system. Nurse managers, the audience for this book, must develop skills to work with that change. These skills are applied not only in the external environment—finance and delivery systems in particular—but also in the internal environment of our organizations. The nurse manager cannot manage change without knowing the strengths and capabilities of the organization in which she or he works.

The purpose of this book is to provide nurse managers with the skills that are used on a daily basis. Thus emphasis is placed on those cognitive skills related to issues of finance, business management, technology, and the process inherent in change management. The art of management is often intuitive as well: Understanding the business we are in, who the clients are, and what processes we use to meet their needs is essential to the work we do as managers. A significant element in the art of management is the ability to develop the skills and potential of others. We do this to achieve both organizational and unit-based success as well as personal fulfillment. The cognitive and analytic aspects of management share equal weight with the intuitive, and both dimensions are vital to the effective application of the principles and concepts underlying why we do (or should do) what we do.

The framework of this book is announced in the subtitle, *Concepts, Skills and Strategies*. Throughout we have presented the art and science of implementing both those concepts that remain tried and true despite changing organizations and those concepts that have yet to be fully proven in health care. Whether we are exploiting innovative methods and concepts for achieving managerial success or relying on traditional practices and procedures, we need to make sure that we are asking the right questions and not seeking solutions to the wrong problems. We have heard it many times: Doing the right thing, as distinct from doing the thing right. Excellent nurse managers and leaders build their experience, knowledge, and insight on a foundation of concepts, whether consciously or not. These concepts (Part One) give rise to the skills (Part Two) necessary to "make it happen" and to the strategies that direct these skills toward the achievement of specific outcomes (Part Three).

Part One, Concepts, establishes the basis for management in health care, with the opening chapter describing a framework for nursing management (Burner and McCombs). The importance of leadership (Kerfoot), a strong sense of direction expressed through mission, goals, and values (Ehrat), and the organizational structures designed to achieve that mission (Spitzer-Lehmann) are all spelled out with practical yet theory-based models and concepts. Part One also describes the excitement and complexity of becoming a manager (Everson-Bates and Jenkins) and includes critical elements in problem solving and decision making (Beyers). These chapters will help the nurse manager develop the vision necessary to managerial excellence.

Part Two details the skills necessary to make the vision work and provides the front line manager with the necessary tools to be successful. The critical application of information science and computers (Simpson), team building (Neubauer), the importance of self-development (O'Malley), and effective communication (Cornell) are discussed. Skill attainment is hard work; it is not inborn. It is an acquired ability and requires practice, thought, and perseverance. Formal education may enhance skill attainment; certainly training in the art and science of nursing management—including reading, listening, and practicing—is essential. The wise nurse manager will seek guidance, however, not only from the nursing management literature but also from the principles and tenets of general business management.

The bulk of this book is devoted to strategies. It may not always be clear how some of the strategies are distinguished from the practical skill sets, but the underlying assumption is that strategy is a continuous process that shapes the success of present ventures and, more importantly, lays the groundwork for directing the future shape and functioning of the organization. Strategies can thus be seen as focused application of the more general skills directed toward specific outcomes. In presenting this content our intention was not only to provide our readers with strategies for today but also to begin the process of a paradigm shift. Simply stated, we want the reader to see things the way others see them and yet to see them differently, thereby providing a proactive vision that is desperately needed in health care today.

Planning is critical in the strategic process. Planning mandates a flexibility in the nurse manager, since the ability to change plans is essential to meeting the challenges and opportunities that arise continuously in the internal and external environments of health care management.

Whereas concepts provide the framework and skills provide the means, strategies engender the impetus to question, challenge, understand, create, and—most importantly—innovate. "Imagination is more important than knowledge," as Einstein reminds us. Part Three, Strategies, which is subdivided into four subsections, transforms the plain old daily management tasks into leadership challenges that often require as much imagination as the familiar skills. The four subsections of the strategy section address the four primary domains where contemporary nurse managers must demonstrate their competence: human resources, material resources, quality, and change.

Managing Human Resources. In the strategic arena of managing human resources we recognize that successes are often dependent on "finding the perfect match" (Secatore and Stengrevics) while focusing on the basics of staffing and scheduling (Smith) and incorporating the wisdom inherent in assuring job satisfaction and retention (Wolf and Orme). Wages and salaries are discussed (Frederiksen et al.), while the importance of appropriate orientation and training for the new nurse (Keely) and the necessity of staff development and mentoring (Cummings) are stressed. A more realistic way to measure productivity that meets unit-sensitive needs helps the nurse manager use alternatives to the traditional full-time equivalents per adjusted occupied bed (FTE/AOB) formula

(Barron). Managing the difficult employee (Vosburgh), the difficulties inherent in the labor relations environment (Fiesta), and the alternatives to an adversary relationship with unionized professionals (Steiger et al.) provide a succinct framework for learning about management-labor relationships. A discussion of the real life practical problems of chemical dependency (Supples) will help the nurse manager deal with this dangerous problem. Critical applications for the future include a discussion of the nurse-physician link (Koerner).

Managing Material Resources. Each of the chapters on managing material resources is presented in concrete fashion ready for application in any setting. The chapter on managed care (Anderson) is further developed in the chapter on DRGs (Spitzer-Lehmann and Davivier), which lays the foundation for understanding the importance of managing material resources. Budgeting practices (Jones) and cost concepts and measurements (Grimaldi and Moore) establish the framework for the analytic side of management, whereas materials management (McDonagh) and principles and practices in drug distribution (Pollock) offer the reader effective tactics to deal with concrete problems.

Managing Quality. Managing quality sounds easier than it is. This subsection focuses on more than just words; it addresses the *actions* necessary to achieve quality-driven goals. Beginning with a comprehensive overview of quality management (Schuler) and specific applications in the workplace (Royal and Fralic), the broad concept of quality is discussed in all its facets and contexts, including ethical dilemmas (Youngberg), various hospital-based delivery systems designed to enhance and maintain quality (Ringl), patient education (Redman), and discharge planning and case management (Pierog). The importance of risk management as a preventive measure is emphasized in a discussion of this important strategy to avoid hazards and diminish errors (Parks). The research chapter (Kirchhoff and Titler) reveals the many opportunities nurse managers have to validate concepts and investigate new phenomena. The marketing chapter (Finkler and Kovner) emphasizes the exercise of creativity while showing the nurse manager how to provide nursing services that meet real consumer needs.

Managing Change. The reader may find this last subsection the most challenging and thus the most exciting. The authors ask us to expand our perspectives and shift from the paradigm of what is to what could be. The discussion of innovation, change, and continuity (Lehmann) provides a method for realizing our dreams. Strategic planning (Warfel) and politics (Barrett) help us imagine what the future world of health care might look like. The description of entrepreneurialism (Porter-O'Grady) challenges us to take risks. Finally, being proactive about the challenge of the future (Williams) completes the path we started with a nursing management model similar to the concept of moving from novice to expert in clinical practice that was developed by Patricia Benner.

Although it would have been impossible to cover all there is to know about front line nursing management, we believe we have created a reference manual that offers our readers the concepts, skills, and strategies that will assure—at the very least—that we ask the right questions instead of solving the wrong problems.

ACKNOWLEDGMENTS • • • • • •

Upon completion of a book of this magnitude, it is difficult to know where to begin in acknowledging the many people who played a significant part in its design and completion. First, special thanks are due to the many wonderful contributors who wrote the chapters in this book. All are gifted people in their areas of expertise who will continue to make invaluable contributions to the fields of general and nursing management. I would also like to thank Thomas Eoyang of W. B. Saunders Company for coming up with the idea for the book and for believing in my ability to put together a comprehensive manual for a critical resource for the future of health care: the front line nurse manager. Robin Richman, also of Saunders, helped greatly in putting the manuscript into final form. A personal note of thanks goes to my colleague Maryann Davivier, who assisted me in organizing the content into the broad framework of the book. Sue Cummings played a critical role in follow-up and in helping to assure completion of the chapters.

I also need to acknowledge a special mentor, Dr. Peter Drucker, who has given me the license and the tools to think futuristically and the support and encouragement to keep me facing ahead. Kudos also to the chair of my dissertation committee, Dr. Paul Albrecht, who exemplifies all that ethical professional management is about.

Many thanks also to my daughter, Deborah, my sons, David and Michael, my husband, Dave, and my sister, Susan, all of whom have always believed in me.

ROXANE SPITZER-LEHMANN

CONTENTS   •   •   •   •   •   •

PART ONE   •   •   •   •

CONCEPTS OF NURSING MANAGEMENT

> "**N**ursing's ability to secure and maintain a role as a key player in developing health care policy will depend on having highly qualified nurse executives available to function as top decision makers in the health care system. In such positions, they will have the power to affect the way health care is delivered and financed in this country."
>
> OLIVE Y. BURNER AND LESLIE L. McCOMBS

CHAPTER 1

DEVELOPING A FRAMEWORK FOR NURSING MANAGEMENT PRACTICE

OLIVE Y. BURNER
LESLIE L. MCCOMBS

EXECUTIVE SUMMARY

A manager deals with people; people differ in their abilities, traits, and motives. Although you cannot directly motivate someone, you can attempt to tap into what does. Groups have their good points, but dysfunctional groups can be quite damaging to productivity, creativity, and morale. Conflict may not always be pleasant, but it's not always something to be avoided. The organization has a life and a life cycle. When considering the organization perspective, keep in mind structure, technology, and environment. There probably is no one right way to deal with all individuals, all organizations, under all circumstances. Probably the closest you might come to a quasi-universal law of management is "The answer is . . . it all depends."

Koontz (1961, 1980) capsulized nicely the plethora of theories, models, and approaches used by managers and those who study management. The most practically significant contributions that nurse managers (and all managers, for that matter) can make to management theory are to lay to rest once and for all the models that do not work in the real world, and apply and promulgate the ones that do. Nurse managers should avoid adding to Koontz's "management theory jungle" (1980) and, instead, review existing models and develop approaches that work for them in their particular environment. Finally, to aid other nurse managers, they should share with their colleagues their failures as well as their successes as we all strive for newer and more efficient methods of management practice.

M any nurse academicians are suggesting that it is time to develop more clearly defined nursing management theory. At the risk of sounding heretical, we should resist the urge to reinvent the wheel and put aside any attempts to craft a theory of nursing administration. Instead, nurse managers should acknowledge the existence of management and organizational theories applicable and appropriate within a nursing management frame of reference.

Sensing that the typical (if we may be so bold!) reader of this book is quite likely an eminently practical person, with little time to waste and relatively little interest (at least at this time) in being a theorist or an organizational behaviorist, the purpose of this chapter is to provide the reader, as painlessly as possible, with a thumbnail sketch of selected theoretical foundations relevant to nursing management. More specifically, this chapter is intended to expose the nurse manager to an eclectic variety of managerial concepts and theories, some tried and true, some not—but worthy of mention for that very reason.

The nature of management is to get work done—to achieve goals and objectives—through others. Generally, where there is a need for a manager, there coexists an organization, with a structure, entwined with technologies and constrained by environment(s). There are theories of the management of human resources and organizations. If nursing management is viewed as a variation on the management theme, an efficient use of very valuable nursing management time is to accept, adapt, test, or reject existing management theories rather than to add to what Koontz (1961, 1980) so aptly described as the "management theory jungle."

Conceptual managerial models are time and energy savers. They are the shortcuts known and valued by seasoned managers and, more often than not, are derived from applied theory. Theory provides a rational, reasonable approach to predict or explain phenomena. A good theory consists of concepts, definitions, and patterns of association. It is both comprehensive and practical and is verifiable and disconfirmable. Applied theory refers to the processes and outcomes of testing, accepting, revising, or abandoning theories or models.

The beauty of applied, theory-driven research lies in what is provided to the practitioner. One is handed the assumptions, limitations, and caveats of the investigation and findings, as well as definitions, plausible alternative explanations, and rival hypotheses (if the investigator has the ego strength to report disconfirming findings!). Applying managerial or organizational theories to practice does not require that one become a cold, number-crunching manager. Actually, the use of theories, models, and heuristics provides a sound foundation for critical thinking, more timely problem identification, and, most importantly, more effective problem resolution.

Nursing is confronting an era of increasing challenges. The pressures on the profession are enormous and far-reaching. In this environment, nurse managers at every level will be influential in shaping what the profession will look like in the years ahead. Nursing's ability to secure and maintain a role as a key player in developing health care policy will depend on having highly qualified nurse executives available to function as top decision makers in the health care system. In such positions, they will have the power to affect the way health care is delivered and financed in this country.

To cope with all the pressures confronting them, nurse managers need outstanding skills in managing resources of people, capital, and equipment efficiently and effectively. They also need expertise in sophisticated budget analysis, strategic planning, personnel management, and systems design and evaluation. In addition, nurse managers must maintain a sound knowledge of clinical issues so they can understand and interpret and make appropriate decisions about the systems and structures supporting the safe, competent delivery of nursing services. Essentially, they must understand the critical dimensions of the art and science of nursing and its relationship to the business-oriented elements of the health care system. Nurse managers should review specific management-related theory from the standpoint of "Will it help me analyze and solve problems encountered in my everyday work life?" It is critical for those who want to apply theory to their practice to evaluate each relevant theory individually and determine if it is applicable and pragmatic for their purposes.

Gaining these skills is critical to those making the transition from the nurse practice role to the perspective of the nurse manager. This text covers the major areas of importance to those who have made or are contemplating making that transition at any level of the management hierarchy. The purpose of this chapter is to assist managers at any level to refine the framework guiding their administrative practice.

Because of the numerous conflicting demands on the managerial role in health care organizations, many consider management in health care systems to be very different from management in other fields of endeavor. This perception underestimates the complexity of managing human and financial resources in other kinds of organizations. In discussing this issue, Shortell et al. (1988) note: "It is the confluence of professional, technological and task attributes that make the management of health care organizations particularly challenging" (p. 14). Those who manage other complex service organizations (e.g., welfare, fire and police departments) would suggest that such confluence also affects managerial functioning in their speciality areas. Thus, nurse managers have more commonalities than differences with managers in other disciplines. This leads us to the question of what can assist the manager in functioning effectively in complex organizations, most specifically, health care organizations.

For the nurse manager, the nursing process of assessing a patient's needs, developing a plan of care to meet those needs, implementing the plan, and evaluating its effectiveness can be an effective model for management functioning. It is a concrete way of looking at a situation, assessing the dimensions involved, and arriving at a decision to deal with it in the most efficient manner possible.

It helps to have basic guidelines to follow and the common sense to apply them judiciously. Unfortunately, there is no one approach that will work unfailingly for everyone in every situation. Each of us has different goals, values, and attributes that influence our actions in a real life work situation, including our approach to those we manage. We need to develop a systematized approach to incorporating our values in our management practice.

THE ROLE OF THE NURSE MANAGER

In developing a style, managers at any level have a valuable resource in theories that have been formulated to explain important phenomena that occur within organizations. For example, there are theories of organizational design, decision making, leadership, motivation, and change. The best theory in any situation is the one that provides the most complete, useful, and accurate explanation of the organizational practice at issue. As described by Filley, House, and Kerr (1976), "Theory is the basis for practice and application—the real world, with all its complexities must be ordered in a systematic fashion before we can hope to act on it or upon it. Theoretical formulation is the ordering process" (p. 21).

Making decisions, especially in the midst of crisis, based on some proven theoretical concept applicable to the particular set of circumstances can enhance the decision-making process. Theory can provide a guide for action. However, in any given situation, one should not ignore that critical intuitive gut feeling one gets when faced with a difficult situation. Most managers can remember having made a significant mistake when they did not heed their own warning bell!

According to Filley et al. (1976), in addition to providing managers with a description of their environment, theory "also serves to broaden their range of knowledge, for by deriving predictions from theory in the form of hypotheses, they are able to relate specific facts to broader explanations. They use theory to guide their search for variables relating to practical problems and in their efforts to *produce* optimal solutions" (p. 29). Thus, nurse managers can review management theories that help them analyze or solve problems they encounter in their everyday life. Remember, those who want to apply theory to their practice must evaluate each theory individually and determine if it is applicable and pragmatic for their purposes.

MANAGEMENT THEORIES

The essential functions of management consist of planning, organizing, leading, and controlling. As mentioned earlier, management is a process of getting work done through people. The effective manager is aware of the role and power of human behavior in achieving organizational goals and objectives. Behavior is caused and goal directed. Observed behavior can be measured and motivated.

Within a health care organizational setting, the nurse manager seldom works in isolation, more often working in dyads (with a subordinate or colleague) or in small groups (peer groups, task forces, or committees). The nurse manager works with individuals or collectives of individuals. People are a composite of cognitive abilities (i.e., verbal aptitudes), noncognitive proclivities (i.e., individuals' different characteristics or personalities), and skills (i.e., task-related competencies). To most effectively manage, that is, to effectively get work done through people, one should be aware of the variety of motivators that operate to direct the behaviors of others.

Before drawing on any given theory of management, the nurse manager should first determine his or her managerial assumptions of people. For example, do you hold to the belief that the worker does not basically dislike work and can actually grow and develop under proper conditions? Or do you assume that the worker basically dislikes work and will avoid it if possible, forcing you as the manager to cajole, control, or coerce in order to get work done? The former view is consistent with McGregor's Theory Y (1960); the latter with Theory X. Or do you espouse the philosophy of Likert's System IV organization (1967), with its assumptions of the wisdom of decentralization, delegation, and participative decision making? Reflecting on one's basic assumptions about the human resource is the first step to more effective management.

It was production engineers Frederick W. Taylor and associates who conducted the first systematic U.S. study of management—in a machine shop. This study shifted an interest in production bonuses to a focus on management, and it launched the concept of scientific management (Newman and Warren, 1977). The principle behind scientific management was that one needs to separate planning and performance. It stressed developing the best method for doing a job, selecting the right person to do the job, and training the worker in the proper method of accomplishing the tasks involved. Scientific management focused on combining these factors and introducing an incentive system to pay each worker on the basis of individual productivity. It required close cooperation of managers and workers, with the managers planning the work and the workers accomplishing it (Filley et al., 1976).

Newman and Warren (1977) are cited as providing the most important contribution of the founders of scientific management in that they fundamentally altered the way we think about management problems. "Instead of relying on tradition and intuition, we now believe any management problem should be subjected to the same kind of critical analysis, inventive experiment, and objective evaluation that Taylor applied in his machine shop" (pp. 6,7).

Subsequently, the concept of the bureaucracy model was introduced. Although it is somewhat outdated, most of us still follow this and are uncomfortable when we deviate from it. Principles of a bureaucracy include the following:

- Scalar principle: There should be a clear line of authority and responsibility from the top to the bottom of the organization. Lines of authority (legitimate power) and relationships should be clear, codified, out in the open.
- Ultimate responsibility: Responsibility of higher authority for the acts of a subordinate is absolute in work-related areas. A manager cannot abdicate responsibility for work-related acts of subordinates. There are disadvantages to this, mainly that of a great tendency to centralization. Tight supervision tends to permeate the organization, with detailed involvement and too little or minimal delegation. The tendency is to restrict the flow upward throughout the organization.
- Hierarchy: The foremost proponent of bureaucracy was Max Weber (1864–1920), whose theory, according to Newman and Warren (1977), was based on a concept of "a 'bureaucratic or rational legal' authority that is accepted by subordinates because the exerciser of that authority occupies a certain position within the hierarchy" (p. 7). The principle of hierarchy rests in the premise that each office is under the supervision and control of a higher one. This principle can be evidenced in an organizational chart that, in effect, displays the chain of command within an organization.

Administrative organizational theory, which looked at the entire organization and developed principles for designing organization structure, was the next model to be explored. It classified management activities in a manner still used in management literature—planning, organizing, and controlling. This approach observed the entire organization and developed principles for designing organization structure.

MOTIVATION

The theories of motivation fall into two camps, those that deal with content (i.e., factors or elements) and those that deal with process (i.e., the hows and whys behavior is enacted and directed).

Content Theories of Motivation

Let us begin with an overview of and commentary on selected content theories of motivation. The major players for the content theories of motivation include Maslow (1943), Aldefer (1969), and Herzberg, Mausner, and Synderman (1959).

Maslow (1943) stated that a hierarchy of five needs exists for the individual, who must first satisfy basic physiologic needs before aspiring to the satisfaction of higher needs, toward self-actualization. Although nursing has almost universally accepted Maslow's theory and maintains a posture of reverential deference to Maslow, managers should know that Maslow's research consisted of chatting with friends and others (often anonymous) and reviewing written accounts of deceased public figures. From this biased and rather elite cadre of men, Maslow made the claim for his hierarchy of needs. The assumptions and limitations of his perspective of human motivations should be clear. As well, there is a dearth of cold, hard evidence to support the need hierarchy theory.

Aldefer (1969) proposed a somewhat different hierarchy of needs, existence (E), relatedness (R), and growth (G)—ERG. Similar to Maslow's theory in terms of the elements involved, Aldefer's theory differed in its belief that a frustrated attempt to satisfy one's "growth need" redirects behavior to satisfy the lower order relatedness need. As with Maslow, empirical verification of Aldefer's proposal is scant.

Herzberg et al. (1959) proposed a two-factor theory of motivation. They concluded that there were extrinsic conditions (job context) and intrinsic conditions (job content) to be considered. The extrinsic conditions were the dissatisfiers or "hygiene" factors. These factors must be present and adequate for the individual to be, at minimum, not "dissatisfied." The satisfiers or motivators, on the other hand, if present in the job should lead to good job performance. If they are not present, one is not necessarily dissatisfied. Of concern with Herzberg's work is the original sample, which consisted of about 200 accountants and engineers. Such a group is hardly an acceptable proxy for nurses. Additionally, the theory really concerns itself with job satisfaction, not performance motivators.

It would be reasonable to assume that, at this moment, the reader is a bit disheartened. The intuitive appeal of Maslow or Herzberg is understandable.

Each model is simple and so clearly human, if unsubstantiated. The one piece of insight the nurse manager gains from the content theorists is this—individuals are unique, and what motivates one person may have little, no, or (worse yet) negative effects on another.

One last class of content theory was derived from Murray's taxonomy of needs (1938). Atkinson (1964) and McClelland, Atkinson, Clark, and Lowell (1953) laid the theoretical background for the work in the area of need for achievement. When the need for achievement is high, it motivates behavior, which satisfies the need. Traditionally, research in achievement motivation was, for lack of a better term, simplistic. The Atkinson model was predictive of choice of task, persistence at a task following failure, and task approach/avoidance. The tasks generally consisted of puzzles and games. The subject pools were male-only or male-dominated.

More recent research into achievement motivation (Helmreich & Spence, 1978; Helmreich, Spence, & Pred, 1988) has demonstrated the multidimensionality of achievement motivation. These authors postulate a model of achievement motivation consisting of work, the desire to work hard, mastery, the desire to work well, and competitiveness—the enjoyment of engaging in interpersonal competition. The validity of achievement motivation for women and its capabilities to predict real world outcomes have been demonstrated (McCombs, 1991).

The reader who is familiar with the achievement motivation literature has no doubt heard of Horner's "fear of success" hypothesis (1972). Rest assured, women demonstrate no more fear of success than do men, and the motive is not particularly an important personality attribute of either sex.

Process Theories of Motivation

Now we turn our attentions to the process theories of motivation. The four most popular process theories are reinforcement, expectancy, equity, and goal-setting.

The skinnerian behaviorists are proponents of operant conditioning. Essentially, a person learns the desired behavior through a process of reinforcements. In reinforcement theory, generally speaking, desired behavior is rewarded and undesirable behavior is punished or ignored. Behavior modification concerns itself with behaviors, not personality, attitudes, or beliefs, and so the specification of desired behaviors is crucial. Behaviors are observable, and they are measurable. The selection of reinforcers and reinforcement schedules are important considerations in successful behavior modification. For the nurse manager, identification of a desired, critical behavior and application of the appropriate reinforcer may prove effective in selected situations. A caveat is in order: Remember that the change of behavior does not mean a change in values or attitudes. Behavior modification as a nursing management tool might be considered a stop-gap measure at best if more than just a change of behavior is needed.

Expectancy theory owes much to the work of Vroom (1964). The key components of the expectancy model are (1) instrumentality, the strength of the individual's belief that an action leads to an outcome, (2) valence, the strength of one's preference for an outcome (positive when the outcome is preferred, negative when the outcome is not preferred, and neutral or zero when the person is indifferent regarding the outcome), and (3) expectancy, a subjective probability that a specified behavior will result in a specific outcome. Effort is expended when there exists a probability of successful performance, successful performance will likely result in a defined outcome, and the outcome is valued. An additional consideration in expectancy theory is the specification of behavior as a function of motivation and ability. If one cannot, it makes little difference whether or not one would like to. Expectancy theory continues to be tested, and reviews on its success and applicability are varied. Some of the issues for concern center, first, on the operationalization of the elements and, second, on if and how an individual consciously calculates probabilities and valences.

Equity theory says in essence that individuals gauge their efforts and rewards according to those in similar situations. The key elements are inputs, the skills and abilities of the individual; outputs, rewards from the job, i.e., pay or recognition; and referents, the person(s) to whom one compares oneself. When the individual perceives that the ratio of inputs to outputs is unfavorable when compared to the referent, then inequity exists. To restore a sense of equity, the individual may reduce inputs, change outputs (under certain conditions), change referent, change his or her attitude, or change the situation. The limitations regarding research on equity theory are twofold. First, most investigations have focused on pay equity. Second, the identification of the referent is not always clear, consistent, or appropriate.

Locke (1968) is the father of goal-setting theory. The premise of this theory is that individuals' conscious goals are the determinants of behavior. Given specific, clear, and reasonably difficult goals and goal paths and provided unambiguous performance feedback, one can improve performance. The difficulties with goal setting are that it may be rather difficult to specify some goals adequately. Once a clear and sufficiently difficult (yet attainable) goal is identified, the importance of appropriate and timely feedback must not be overlooked for goal setting to effect the desired level of performance.

GROUPS

Having provided some conceptual foundations for considering individual motivation, we briefly review the concept of groups. Much of the work of the organization is done by groups.

A very simple definition of *group* would note that a group is any collection of more than two people interacting face-to-face. Within the organization context, one finds two types of groups, formal and informal. Formal groups are produced by the nature, structure, and goals of the organization. Informal groups are socially conceived. People join and leave groups for a variety of reasons. Some groups are specifically time and task limited; some endure for long periods of time. Groups have a life cycle, and most every group goes through a series of developmental and evolutionary stages, even groups of a relatively short-lived nature. Groups have a structure, and group members have roles. Depending on the nature of the group, some roles or positions may be assigned or may be attributed to an individual by other members of the group. Groups follow a specified or implied set of standards. These standards are norms. Nonconformity to a norm may result in punishment of the nonconformer by the rest of the group.

A sense of closeness among group members is usually referred to as cohesiveness or cohesion. Cohesion within the group may or may not be "good" from the nurse manager's perspective. In the ideal, one would find the organizationally defined work group (i.e., a service delivery unit) composed of persons who simultaneously view themselves as a social unit and whose goals are congruent with those of the organization. On the other hand, a highly cohesive group sometimes runs the risk of "groupthink." Named by Janis (1973), such a group is so cohesive as to perceive itself as invulnerable, morally validated, and unanimous in its decision making, which is usually markedly flawed. The pressure on individuals to conform is intense. The effective nurse manager needs to be able to recognize and address dysfunctional groups and group members. Dysfunctional groups consist of those who engage in groupthink or dysfunctional intergroup conflict. Conflict, in and of itself, is not necessarily a negative concept. Functional conflict, wherein groups confront and redress a problem to the benefit of the organization, is healthy. Dysfunctional conflict is disruptive, nonproductive at best, destructive at worst. Intergroup conflict may stem from differences in goals, differences in perspectives, competition for scarce resources, or reward structures (i.e., rewarding groups rather than the individuals' performances).

Following are a few of the techniques at the manager's disposal to deal with dysfunctional conflict:

- Problem-solving
- Negotiation
- Compromise
- A superordinate goal orientation
- Authoritarianism

CONCLUSION

At this point, the reader may feel that we are ambling about in a maze of theory and have lost sight of the purpose of this chapter, which is to give an overview of some management theories applicable to the nurse manager. As indirect as the approach may appear, we have done what we set out to do. It is important that the reader understand that every theory has its limitations and that, depending on a manager's unique perspective, some may be impossible to adopt in a particular situation. For example, adopting the human relations model faces the manager with some hard choices, such as whether the individual is willing to relinquish some of the decision-making process to buy employee motivation. Since much of people's self-respect in a job hinges on being a part of the process, they are more apt to accept a decision in a mature manner if they have participated in it. From the manager's perspective, it may be far more important that the decision be right than that people feel good about it, especially when it affects the overall goals of the organization. This is particularly true at the executive level, where spreading decisions around tends to politicize them. At that level, you probably have a good idea of the shortcomings of the major players in the decision loop and you should not tie your decisions to the political agenda of the cast of characters involved.

As another example, some managers prefer to look at situations from a change theory model perspective, which the human relations orientation was not particularly good at addressing. There continues to be a rapid rate of change in the workplace involving, among other factors, an increasingly complex technology and accelerating pressure on financial matters. In such an environment, individuals and organizations tend to downplay human relations, especially when they come under financial pressure. This is readily apparent in today's health care organizations, and managers must deal with the resultant dilemmas as effectively as possible. It may help to remember that there is no single best way to manage in all circumstances. In effect, what a manager does in any given situation is contingent on the needs of that situation. As Newman and Warren (1977) suggest, "only a quack doctor prescribes the same medicine to all his patients. The professional first makes a diagnosis then, drawing upon his knowledge of alternative actions and their likely effect, he prescribes for the individual case" (p. 10).

In closing, we urge you to adapt theory to your own needs and management style. Look at the issues involved in any situation; identify alternatives that have worked well in other circumstances; identify pros and cons of each, and select the most appropriate one for the particular situation. Deal with the issue within the context of the present event. Above all, remember that the apparently ideal solution is not always the best one in the particular set of circumstances. Trust your experience, judgment, and intuition in arriving at the one that is the best!

References

Aldefer, C.P. (1969, April). An empirical test of a need theory of human needs. *Organizational Behavior and Human Performance*, pp. 142–175.

Atkinson, J.W. (1964). *An introduction to motivation*. Princeton, NJ: Van Nostrand.

Filley, A.C., House, R.J., & Kerr, S.F. (1976). *Managerial process and organizational behavior* (2nd ed). Glenview, IL: Scott, Foresman and Company.

Helmreich, R.L., & Spence, J.T. (1978). Work and family orientation questionnaire. An objective instrument to assess components of achievement motivation and attitudes toward family and career. JSAS. *Catalogue of Selected Documents in Psychology, 8*(2), 35.

Helmreich, R.T., Spence, J.T., & Pred, R.S. (1988). Making it without losing it: Type A, achievement motivation and scientific attainment revisited. *Personality and Social Psychology Bulletin, 14*(3), 495–504.

Herzberg, F., Mausner, B., & Synderman. (1959). *The motivation to work*. New York: Wiley.

Horner, M.S. (1972). Toward an understanding of achievement-related conflicts in women. *Journal of Social Issues, 28,* 157–175.

Janis, I. (1973). *Victims of groupthink: A psychological study of foreign policy decisions and fiascoes*. Boston: Houghton Mifflin.

Koontz, H. (1961). The management theory jungle. *Academy of Management Journal, 4*(3), 174–188.

Koontz, H. (1980). The management theory jungle revisited. *Academy of Management Review, 5*(2), 175–187.

Likert, R. (1967). *The human organization.* New York: McGraw-Hill.

Locke, E.A. (1968, May). Toward a theory of task motivation and incentives. *Organization and Performance,* pp. 157–189.

Malsow, A.H. (1943, July). A theory of human motivation. *Psychological Review,* pp. 370–396.

McClelland, D.C., Atkinson, J.W., Clark, R.W., & Lowell, E.L. (1953). *The achievement motive.* New York: Appleton-Century-Crofts.

McCombs, L.L. (1991). *Achievement motivation predicting academic and career performance among hospital and health administration graduates.* Doctoral dissertation, University of Iowa.

McGregor, D. (1960). *The human side of enterprise.* New York: McGraw-Hill.

Murray, H.A. (1938). *Explorations in personality.* New York: Oxford University Press.

Newman, W.H., & Warren, S.K. (1977). *The process of management: Concepts, behavior and practice* (4th ed.) Englewood Cliffs, NJ: Prentice-Hall.

Shortell, S.M., Kaluzny, A.D., et al. (1988). *Health care management. A text in organizational theory* (2nd ed). Albany: DelMar Publishers.

Vroom, V.H. (1964). *Work and motivation.* New York: Wiley.

CHAPTER 2

LEADERS: YESTERDAY, TODAY, AND TOMORROW

KARLENE M. KERFOOT

EXECUTIVE SUMMARY

Today's nursing leaders will find themselves in many challenging situations. The successful nurse leader will have a clear vision of what nursing is and is not and of how excellence in patient care can be created regardless of the situation.

This chapter is about leadership. The differences between leadership and management are discussed. Places for both managers and leaders exist in nursing. The history of leadership in nursing is reviewed. The study of leadership and the consequent development of theories of leadership is discussed in detail.

New forms of leadership are now being discussed and used. The kind of leadership that is needed now is leadership that can innovate, enable large organizations to respond quickly to challenges, and develop semi-autonomous knowledgeable workers at the front line. The leaders of the future must think in terms of integrative, cross-functional teams and must restructure to promote innovation by empowering the front line. They must create a value-driven organization by developing a strong moral and ethical culture on which to base visions and strategy.

Effective leaders can envision a new reality and communicate it in a way that will make people become excited about the vision and believe in it. The leader can develop high levels of productivity if hierarchical arrangements are replaced with new collegial models and if synergistic teams can be formed.

The times are changing. As hospitals redesign, as we stretch for innovations in quality, and as we search for ways to deliver health care at lower costs, we find that the old models will not work any more. The leader today must be able to see beyond the traditional structures and paradigms and envision a new reality for the patient, for nursing, and for health care.

Dr. Olga Maranjian Church summarized the study of nursing leadership as follows: "However one cannot hope to understand the reality as experienced by the individual by only looking to the rhetoric of the leadership. One must also look at the milieu, the context, the social-political-economic times out of which such leaders and their followers emerged" (1990, p. 5). Church's point is that leadership is influenced by many factors. However, her analysis concluded that the mission as articulated by Nightingale for nursing was consistent over time. "The mission was perceived and presented by the leadership as 'serving humanity'" (Church, 1990, p. 5). The leader in nursing will find himself or herself in many challenging situations. The situations may change, but the clear vision for what nursing is and is not and how excellence in patient care can be created must not waver. This is what successful nursing leadership is all about.

LEADER VERSUS MANAGER

It is easy to confuse leadership with management. This chapter is about leadership. It is worthwhile to distinguish clearly between these two concepts. Zaleznik (1977) noted that managers and leaders differ fundamentally. According to this author, managers work on goals and projects as they are assigned, whereas leaders fervently develop and champion goals with a very personal approach. Managers accomplish the work through policies, predetermined outlines, and directions. Leaders, by contrast, are the pathfinders who develop innovative approaches to problems. Leaders are the ones who create new models and paradigms. Managers work to get the job done, and leaders concentrate on the meaning of the events and the impact on participants. Zaleznik noted that leaders have visions and dreams that managers are not capable of and that leaders get their positive rewards from new innovations and ideas, whereas managers feel fulfilled to maintain the status quo.

Obviously, there is a place for both managers and leaders in nursing. However, the person in the top level position needs to possess leadership qualities and the style of a leader. If positions are reversed and the person with managerial skills is at the top and the person with leadership skills is at the bottom, a sense of incongruence in the organization will develop.

In a classic article on the quality of leadership, Diers (1979) noted that leadership goes beyond setting and obtaining goals. She points out that a leader is a visionary who can dream and envision the future. She also notes that excellent visions live beyond the life of the leader and stand the test of time. Just as the Nightingale vision of serving humanity has provided an energy source for the profession of nursing over many years, a vision developed by a leader and the organizing framework to support it will outlive that person's tenure (Church, 1990).

THE HISTORY OF LEADERSHIP IN NURSING

Leadership in nursing has been influenced by the many situations in which nursing has found itself. The origin of nursing in religious orders and the military influenced many nursing leaders to take on an autocratic leadership style. The inspections made before nursing students went on the units and insignias on the student uniforms indicating rank by class were clear indications of a hierarchical autocratic culture. However, as more leadership theories were developed and as nurses obtained baccalaureate and higher degrees in schools where management and leadership were taught, a wide variety of leadership styles became viable options for nursing leaders.

THE STUDY OF LEADERSHIP

The study of leadership and the consequent development of theories of leadership have taken many routes. Initially, leadership was studied by examining the lives and leadership traits of highly influential leaders. This kind of study is common in biographies and has developed into a branch of the discipline history in which the person's life is studied in depth and documented by the historical researcher. In nursing, Christy developed this type of historical study of leadership in nursing as she studied famous nursing leaders (1969a,b).

After World War I and World War II, the study of leadership branched out in many new ways. Researchers began to study not only the personality of the leader but also the environment and situation in which the leader was placed. In addition to the leader, the quality and characteristics of the follower were studied. It became apparent that the success or failure of leaders was dependent on many factors both within the leader and in the situation.

Likert (1967) further developed the belief and support for the democratic/participative style of leadership. Likert's work described four styles of leadership that were ways of categorizing the leadership styles he observed. His four types of leadership were (1) the exploited authoritative style, (2) the benevolent authoritative style, (3) the consultative style, and (4) the participative leadership style. He concurred with previous writers that the participative style was much more effective and that productivity and job satisfaction were much better under this system of leadership.

Hershey and Blanchard's life cycle theory (1977) looked at the characteristics of the follower as they related to leadership and proposed that the maturity level of the follower should influence leaders to choose different leadership styles. They believed that the relationships between the leader and the followers were important to analyze and to work with in order to develop the most successful situation. These authors categorized leader behaviors on a scale of continuum of tasks from high to low and on a relationship scale from high to low. The best results were obtained when the leader could match the needs of the follower and do the kinds of tasks necessary at that point.

Fiedler's contingency theory (1967) noted that the effective leader had to consider both the leader's style and the situation in which he or she was working. Successful leaders could find difficult challenges in situations where their style did not fit the situation and they did not correct or modify their style. Fiedler's point was that leadership must be flexible and the success of the leader depends on the interaction and situational context of the leader and the group considered in total.

Blake et al. (1981) used a grid to analyze a leadership style based on two axes: concern for people and concern for getting the job done. Throughout this research, it became apparent that, in general, the highly participative style of leadership in which the follower could actively interact and develop a sense of pride and ownership in the work and in the organization was the style that produced the highest levels of productivity. It was noted through this research, however, that flexibility in leadership style also was necessary to meet the varied challenges in emergencies and other situations.

MacGregor (1960) proposed a categorization of leaders in terms of Theory X and Theory Y. Based on the leader's view of the workers, these theories supported a belief model about people in one of two areas. Theory X leaders considered people to be unmotivated and believed they needed to be closely supervised and monitored and were not to be trusted. Theory Y leaders, by contrast, believed that people enjoyed their work, wanted to do a better job, and could do well without major supervision.

From Theory X and Theory Y, Ouchi (1981) developed Theory Z. Ouchi combined Japanese management with MacGregor's Theory Y to develop the Theory Z. He believed that humanistic management would result in higher productivity and added the concept that the culture of the organization was very important. He studied companies he called "Z" companies and noted that they were very much like a family/clan in that the people's individuality was less important that their identity with their clan. By contrast, he noted that people in other work settings often have individualistic needs and do not think about the needs of the whole group or the corporation. He noted that people in the successful groups learn to synthesize their personal beliefs with those of the group. Therefore, he noted that Theory Z organizations were groups of people who were tightly bonded around a shared common purpose and were single-minded in their achievement of results.

LEADERSHIP FOR THE FUTURE

Much of the leadership literature has come under criticism because the kind of leadership that is needed now is leadership that can innovate, enable large organizations to respond quickly to challenges, and develop semi-autonomous knowledgeable workers at the front line. Knowledge is no longer acceptable only in the corporate office. Consequently, new forms of leadership are being discussed and used.

A landmark publication was that of Burns (1978), in which he studied famous people and drew conclusions about their leadership style. He believed that the traits of these famous people were applicable to people in all kinds of leadership situations. From his work, the concept of the *transformational* leader has risen. Burns believed that leadership is *transactional* when two people make contact and exchange information/projects for the purpose of exchanging a valued thing. Transactional leadership occurs when there is an exchange of a valued thing. By contrast, Burns discussed transformational leadership as the kind of leadership that allows people to reach higher states of motivation, morality, and productivity than is possible in transactional leadership. His point was that transformational leadership fuses values and creates a sense of wholeness and a unity of purpose among the employee, the leader, the organization, and the collective purpose of the organization. He believed that transformational leaders initiate and innovate social change and have a positive impact on themselves, their followers, their organization, and their society. Burns believed that transformational leaders actually transform organizations, themselves, and their workers.

Transformational leadership is very important for our future. At a time when the way health care is delivered has been virtually unchanged for the last 20 years, we need transformational leaders who can rethink and restructure the way we do things. Transformational leaders are able to look beyond the present and can see new possibilities in models of traditional settings. Transformational leadership is the kind of leadership that will restructure nursing for the future and will develop a new model that will be more applicable with the time.

Most organizations are coming to realize that the essence of a quality organization is not necessarily the firm's top management but rather the quality and synergistic relationships of the people who work within. "Human capital" is a term commonly used to develop the value to the organization of a highly competent work force. The emphasis is turning to the "knowledge worker" and the tremendous investment this person represents to the company. The truly successful companies of the future will be managed from within through structures that recognize that top-down management is not effective. Managing from above will be replaced by managing from within. Fully developing the potential of the staff will mean success for the leader of the future.

Our shared governance structures have just begun to scratch the surface of the potential for an exciting future for health care. Nursing has led the way with shared governance structures that have set a climate of participation and of empowering the front-line knowledge worker, the nurse, to develop innovative models to provide excellence in patient care. It is the job of the leader of the future to think in terms of integrative, cross-functional teams and to work with new and exciting organizational structures in which the boxes of organizational charts are replaced by concentric three-dimensional overlapping circles of energized and synergistic teams. The team will be excited and committed to make needed changes in the health care system. Leaders who can tap into this tremendous potential will certainly have the most effective, high-quality programs in the country today.

The more recent literature on developing innovation and self-managed teams demands a different kind of leader. Kanter's book, *When Giants Learn To Dance* (1983), and Manz and Sims' book, *Super Leadership* (1990), are examples of the literature indicating that the role of a leader is to empower the front line to think creatively and autonomously. As bureaucratic organizations reinvent themselves to more quickly meet the challenges of the day and as more literature becomes available on developing excellence (Peters and Waterman, 1982), nurse leaders must take a fresh look at what nursing leadership is all about. The work of Plunkett and Fournier (1991) and of Tracy (1990) are further examples of the move to empower people on the front line to achieve higher levels of productivity. As Naisbitt and Aburdene chronicle in their work *Reinventing the Corporation* (1986), successful companies are reorganizing differently to produce better results. Reinventing the corporation also means reinventing leadership.

QUALITIES OF LEADERS

One cannot discuss the quality of leadership without first discussing the values of the leader as a person and his or her ability to develop a value-driven organization. Without a strong sense of integrity and principle-centered leadership, such as Covey (1991) describes, the nursing leader is guided to develop a strong moral and ethical culture on which to base visions and strategy. Covey describes effectiveness of the leader as the degree to which "people recognize and live in harmony with such basic principles as fairness, equity, justice, integrity, honesty and trust" (p. 18). He notes that people instinctively trust those who base their lives on these principles. Blanchard and Peale (1988) further elaborate the five Ps of ethical behavior that help consistently to clarify and direct purposes and goals: purpose, pride, patience, persistence, and perspective. Autry (1991) believes that "Management is, in fact, a sacred trust in which the well-being of other people is put in your care during most of their waking hours. It is a trust placed upon you first by those who put you on the job, but more important than that, it is a trust placed upon you after you get the job by those whom you are to manage." With a firm set of values, a leader can develop a program of worth that will benefit not only the company but the people who work in that company and also the customer.

Leaders set a direction for the organization. The ability to be future-oriented and to have a clear sense of direction is the ability to envision the future and envision a new reality. Vision also happens when there is passion associated with that drive and an extraordinarily strong intensity to achieve that end. Leaders have distinctive visions that are often idealistic and intertwined with such concepts as excellence, uniqueness, and a drive to create the future, not to react to it. Leaders are forward-looking, proactive people who convey a sense that the impossible is possible. Successful leaders provide uplifting and inspiring visions for the organization. Their visions captivate one and create a sense of commitment and loyalty.

Leaders can envision a new reality but are not successful unless they can attract other people to that vision and can communicate it in a way that people will become excited about the vision and believe in it. People will bond to a vision if they can see a common link between their own hopes and dreams and how the vision will enable them to reach them. Vision cannot be delegated to others to implement. Instead, successful leaders must communicate well to develop a shared sense of direction by discovering the shared purpose in which everyone can participate. In this period of our history, the ability to achieve stated outcomes is of extraordinary importance. As the complexity of care rises and financial reimbursement does not, we are often left with a stated objective that cannot be met.

To enable and empower, systems and support must be in place so that the people in the front line can achieve their true potential. The leader must believe that nurses are bright, exciting people who can lead us into higher levels of clinical excellence if we provide them with the resources for support. We must lead nurses as professionals want to be led, not the way blue-collar technical people traditionally are led. Raelin (1985) makes the point that the overspecification of the means and the underspecification of the ends is the wrong way to manage professionals. This author believes that one cannot manage professionals. Professionals are schooled and socialized to think and work semi-autonomously. They are most productive if this is recognized. Nurses are also most productive when their professionalism is recognized. Therefore, the leader can develop high levels of productivity if hierarchical arrangements are replaced with new collegial models and if synergistic teams can be formed.

To truly achieve synergy, the concept of collegiality and the absence of hierarchical structure must be in place. Collaboration will not suffice in the health care models of the future. Interactive planning and collegial evaluations of our continuous improvement programs will lead us to higher levels of quality. There are relatively few areas where a health care professional can assume sole ownership of an outcome. Patient care has been so sophisticated that it takes many types of professionals to manage the outcomes adequately. These professionals must have a *we* orientation that will lead to highly synergistic teams. Hierarchical, rigid relationships are not effective. Blaming the doctor, the social worker, or the hospital administrator gets nowhere fast.

Diers and Kraus (1983) define collegiality as "an association of individuals bound together by a shared set of values and goals, bent on fostering mutual support and common effort. Essential to the notion of community and collegiality is the rule that a hierarchy of position has no place in the exchange of ideas" (p. 197). Collegiality is based on the flow of knowledge that is readily exchanged between professionals and is not impeded by hierarchical arrangements. In this synergistic, barrier-free flow of knowledge, patient care is safe, of excellent quality, and cost effective.

If we want people to act as professionals, we must treat them as professionals. Cultures that position professionals as infantile, underdeveloped people who are not to be trusted will produce people that live up to that concept.

ENABLING THE FRONT LINE

To get things done at the highest level of quality possible, leaders must form partnerships with people in the organization. Successful leaders build cohesive teams in which people work together, play together, and feel like a family. They find ways to make others strong and find joy in watching the development of colleagues as they grow to be even greater than they were. By enabling others to act, people develop a sense of ownership, of commitment, and of loyalty to the organization that is not possible in other models. When the leader gives people the tools, resources, and freedom within which to learn and grow, they achieve heights of success that were never dreamed possible. Health care moves too fast to wait for top-down decisions. The front line must be able to make decisions quickly to ensure the survival of the organization (Kanter, 1983).

There is more to liberating the front-line people to think and act than just concern for the bottom line. Helping people to reach their full potential is the right thing to do. No longer should nurses feel that the quality of their work life suffers because they choose to work in a bureaucratic hospital rather than a law office. When people are offered possibilities that provide them with new growth, their spirit is free and they can achieve higher levels of human dignity, creativity, and meaning in their lives.

Tracy (1990) makes the point that the ultimate way to achieve power is for the manager to give power to the people who work for him or her. Tracy delineates 10 principles (p. 163) for empowering people, for example:

1. Tell people what their responsibilities are.
3. Set standards of excellence.
7. Recognize them for their achievements.
9. Give them permission to fail.

Tracy incorporates these 10 principles into a power pyramid, which enables the person to act more independently within the framework of these tools.

Kouzes and Posner (1987) note that when people enable others to act, they foster collaboration and strengthen others. According to these authors, real leaders develop cooperative goals, seek solutions which are integrative, and build trust relationships.

The times are changing. As hospitals redesign, as we stretch for innovations in quality, and as we search for ways to deliver health care at lower costs, we find that the old models will not work any more. We have learned that we must empower people on the front line to think, innovate, and respond quicker because we know these are the people who really have the best and most practical ideas about reinventing the way we deliver health care. How do these new demands for redesign fit in the traditional models of management and leadership that involved planning, controlling, managing by objectives, and all those other truths we learned? We must rethink the paradigms we have traditionally used because they do not fit any more. We must question, rethink, and redesign everything we ever learned about leadership in order to meet the leadership challenges of our future.

Handy (1989) developed the thesis that we are in a period of time that he characterizes as "upside-down thinking," discontinuity, and fast, rapid changes that are propelling us into a world so much different from what we have known that we have no guidelines. He provides several organizational models for our future to cope with this new reality that consist of smaller subsidiaries of the larger organization that are attached in new and different ways to the parent organization. These models free people to create and innovate in new ways.

We have evidence of this kind of upside-down world everywhere we go in health care today. The old traditions that we learned are now sacred cows. The principles of management that we were taught to believe in, such as controlling and directing others by giving orders and dictating through policies and procedures, are no longer viable. We have also learned that managing people creates robots who are angry, unthinking creatures with no commitment to the organization. We have learned that we must treat knowledge workers (nurses) as professionals, not technicians, to achieve the highest levels of quality (Raelin, 1985).

LEADERSHIP CHALLENGES OF THE FUTURE

It is safe to say that the health care industry had its origins in an industrial, technical model. Hospitals were designed to send the patients through the facility in a conveyor beltlike process, which meant that the patient moved from the physician's office to the emergency room to the acute care unit to the operating room to the recovery room to an intensive care unit as the condition changed and on to a stepdown unit, an acute care unit, a rehabilitation unit, and a home health care unit. The nurse and other health care professionals were seen as highly specialized people who worked on only certain parts or conditions of the patient as he or she moved through the health care system. Hospitals, for all intents and purposes, were designed and still appear to be a giant assembly line in which the patient moves from one independent department to another and where highly specialized people do highly specialized things. In this same context, nurses have been seen as technicians who work with their hands and repair parts of the patient in highly specialized settings. Our patient classification systems even measure the time to do tasks and rarely account for the intellectual activity necessary to develop excellence in nursing care. Even though we have talked about interdisciplinary, integrated care, rarely has this been realized. We also have talked about organizing what we did around the patient, but in reality we built our health care system around the convenience of the health care professionals in the hospital. Various independent autonomous practitioners traditionally have worked independently on patients, and rarely have they worked in collegial teams that were patient focused. Consequently, the health care industry has been built on layers of people who duplicate each other's work and are so highly specialized that they cannot cross boundaries.

A leader must be able to see beyond these traditional structures and paradigms and envision a new reality for the patient, for nursing, and for health care. The leader of today must be able to bring diverse groups of people together to rethink and redesign. Most importantly, this leader must be able to tap into the creative potential of the people who are working on the front lines to redesign effectively. The leader of the future must believe sincerely that the best results will come from a work force that feels a sense of ownership of their unit, feels pride in the output of their group, and truly feels they are an integral, important piece of the success of the organization.

The only way these major changes can occur is to change the traditional managerial culture of health care. A culture where hierarchical thinking and superior/subordinate differentiations do not occur will transform organizations. A sense of collegiality and synergy will develop when people are intimately connected with each other by a shared vision and shared values. People who are committed to the principles and the values of the organization can carry out their day-to-day activities without direction.

References

Autry, J. (1991). *Profit and the art of caring leadership*. New York: William Morrow.

Blake, R., Mouton, J., & Tapper, M. (1981). *Great approaches for managerial leadership in nursing*. St. Louis: Mosby.

Blanchard, K., & Peale, N. (1988). *The power of ethical management*. New York: William Morrow.

Burns, J. (1978). *Leadership*. New York: Harper & Row.

Christy, T. (1969a). Portrait of a leader: Isabel Hampton Robb. *Nursing Outlook 17*, 26.

Christy, T. Portrait of a leader: Isabel Maitland Stewart. *Nursing Outlook, 17*, 44.

Church, O. (1990). Nursing's history. What it is and what it is not. In N. Chaska (Ed.), *The nursing profession* (pp. 3–8). St. Louis: Mosby.

Covey, S. (1991). *Principle-centered leadership*. New York: Summitt Books.

Diers, D. (1979). Lessons on leadership. *Image, 11*(3), 3–7.

Diers, D., & Kraus, J. (1983). Dean as administrator, scholar, and colleague. In M. Conway & O. Andreskiw (Eds.), *Administrative theory and practice* (pp. 167–205). Norwalk, CT: Appleton-Century Crofts.

Fiedler, F. (1967). *A theory of leadership effectiveness*. New York: McGraw-Hill.

Handy, C. (1989). *The age of unreason*. Boston: Harvard Business School Press.

Kanter, R. (1983). *When giants learn to dance*. New York: Simon & Schuster.

Kouzes, J., & Posner, B. (1987). *Leadership challenge: How to get extraordinary things done in organizations*. San Francisco: Jossey-Bass.

Hershey, P., & Blanchard, K. (1977). *Management of organizational behavior: Utilizing human resources*. Englewood Cliffs, NJ: Prentice-Hall.

Likert, R. (1967). *Human organization: Its managements and values*. New York: McGraw-Hill.

MacGregor, D. (1960). *The human side of enterprise*. New York: McGraw-Hill.

Manz, C., & Sims, H. (1990). *Super leadership: Leading others to lead themselves*. New York: Berkley Books.

Naisbitt, J., & Aburdene, P. (1986). *Reinventing the corporation*. New York: Warner Books.

Ouchi, W. (1981). *Theory Z: How American business can meet the Japanese challenge*. Reading, MA: Addison-Wesley.

Peters, T., & Waterman, R. (1982). *In search of excellence*. New York: Harper & Row.

Plunkett, L., & Fournier, R. (1991). *Participative management: Implementing empowerment*. New York: John Wiley & Sons.

Raelin, J. (1985). *The clash of cultures, managers and professionals*. Boston: Harvard Business School Press.

Tracy, D. (1990). *Ten steps to empowerment: Common sense guide to managing people*. New York: William Morrow.

Zaleznik, A. (1977). Managers and leaders: Are they different? *Harvard Business Review, 55*(3), 67–78.

CHAPTER 3 • • • • • •

ORGANIZATIONAL STRUCTURES FOR EFFECTIVE PATIENT CARE DELIVERY

ROXANE SPITZER-LEHMANN

EXECUTIVE SUMMARY

In a decentralized structure, whether product line management, matrix management, or creative composite, the role of the chief executive or chief nursing officer (CNO) is extremely important and strategic. The CNO must first participate in hospitalwide decision-making and policy-making activities, thus assuring nursing its central role. Visibility and dynamic leadership will help enhance nursing's role in the institution and at the same time promote nursing's image throughout the community by supporting the nurse managers in achieving high-quality services.

The chief patient care executive also serves as community representative and role model for nursing. Participation in community organizations, teaching in colleges, and participating in national conferences and professional organizations provide an important public relations and marketing function for both the institution and nursing as a profession.

V olatile forces operating on and within today's health care system require major changes in organizational structures and patient care delivery systems, structures, and processes. Flexibility, consumer and regulatory demands for high-quality service, cost constraints, and positive patient outcomes are central to hospital viability. Efficiency and efficacy, also known as productivity, have become the hallmarks of success for the nursing profession throughout the country as more and more people find it increasingly difficult to access and afford modern, high-tech health care services. New organizational strategies will be the critical success factors for health care institutions if they are to survive the 1990s.

In response to these concerns, hospital executives are drawing on the experience of modern industry and adapting to a decade of rapid change. Peters and

Waterman (1982), in their pursuit of the excellent companies, indicate that a successful firm in the 1990s will be:

- Flatter [in structure]
- Populated by more autonomous units
- Oriented toward differentiation
- Service conscious
- More responsive—much faster at innovation
- A user of highly trained, flexible people

Changes in workplace as well as the economic environment mandate innovation in managerial vision and organizational design. These changes require the skills most often stifled by traditional hierarchical bureaucracies and related rules and processes.

Jacobs and Macfarlane (1990, p. 152) describe the greatest invention of all time as the "something" without which all other inventions would be useless—organization. They call it the least appreciated, least admired of all the components of growth and prosperity, yet it remains the single greatest underused secret of real growth and productivity. It is the "lever and the fulcrum" by which any company can rise to the top.

That being the case, what are the components that describe those organizations that generate greater creativity, energy, and productivity? These may be defined as follows.

1. Authority must match responsibility.
2. Delegate as much responsibility as possible to the first-line level in the organization.
3. Harmonize (integrate) the units so they work together toward a common goal.
4. Put the right person in the right job—then train her.
5. Monitor results.

TRADITIONAL STRUCTURES

Traditional theory identified hierarchical, chain-of-command structures as the most effective means to accomplish both quality and efficiency. Although they do create a certain amount of security and accountability with clearly delineated lines of communication, well-regulated work relations, clearly defined responsibilities, and established policies and procedures to govern behavior, they are often too cumbersome to accommodate rapid change. Though they are assumed to produce fast, efficient, obedient responses in crises situations, this is often not the case. To better understand the problems inherent in traditional, hierarchical structures once taken for granted throughout the health care industry, it is helpful to examine its characteristics in greater depth (Fig. 3–1).

In this structure, the familiar pyramid, the labor force is on the bottom supporting the whole structure, with various layers of supervisors spread over the top, one above the other, to the highest executive levels. Information flows

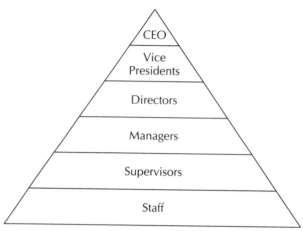

Figure 3–1 Hierarchy or pyramid structure.

up the chain, and orders flow down. Presumably, everyone has clearly defined responsibilities and knows her or his place, and logic and order prevail. One of the major problems here is the slow reaction time. It may take weeks for information to travel to the top and often months for a decision to be made. In the meantime, the entire situation may have changed or the problem may become seriously out of control.

True, as Drucker (1954) says, "Organizing is a process by which the manager brings order out of chaos, removes conflicts between personnel over responsibilities, and establishes an environment suitable for teamwork." However, when people overidentify with their place in the organization and begin to say, "That's his job, not mine," or "I don't know anything about that; this is my job," rigidity and territoriality issues arise.

Another problem in this model is that information gets distorted as it progresses up the chain of command, becoming cleansed and summarized as it goes until the person at the top actually has very little idea what is happening below. Flexibility and innovation are stifled. The person closest to the problem, with the most information, often has the least power to act. Thus, although these organization are assumed to produce fast, efficient, obedient responses in crises situations, this often turns out not to be the case. In addition, leadership development and managerial competence are retarded as lower-level personnel are constrained and confused by rules, processes, and controls often unrelated to the organization's desired outcome.

One of the primary concerns of management, and often the reason for pyramidal structures as opposed to flat structures, is control. Span of control, according to Drucker (1954), implies a limit in each management position to the number of persons an individual can manage effectively, although this varies with the situation of appropriate timely information and although the span can be stretched by the availability of the knowledge-based worker.

In service industries, the limiting factor is that managers are not present to oversee every act and cannot intervene to improve quality or prevent serious problems until after the event. The success of patient care delivery determines the manager's productivity yet often rests on the discretion and judgment of the caregiver. Thus, much of management's effort is devoted to developing judgment, discretion, and pride in quality of care given by their professional staff. The legacy of the industrial hierarchical structure has been an alienated, robotized, bored work force—totally counterproductive in the health care setting. Such a work force cannot deliver compassion, reassurance, or inspiration and hope for the patient. These qualities cannot be bought or coerced and often are stifled by the very structure designed to facilitate their development.

If professionals in health care are to be given the autonomy and discretion to exercise judgment, initiative, and innovation, innovative organizational structures and systems must emerge.

DECENTRALIZATION

Decentralization becomes the first step in the new direction. Decentralized management best serves the hospital working environment where the various departments and functions may be widely scattered throughout the facilities and work patterns, materials, and activities are as diverse as OR and maternity.

The power of an organization resides in the coordination of people and activities, that is, teamwork and communication. The power of decentralization is the job satisfaction found in people who now have control over their work environment and the autonomy to exercise both judgment and discretion. Decentralization of clinical units and decision-making delegation is advantageous because it

1. Establishes accountability closer to the point of service delivery
2. Places discretionary decision making nearer to sources of information and resources
3. Stimulates initiative and innovation
4. Provides a means to create profit centers within units and a related contribution margin for goal achievement

Decentralization, however, is as antithetical to the concept of laissez-faire as it is to the traditional bureaucracy. A successful decentralized organization maximizes management control systems. This does not imply controlling people but rather providing directions and defining outcomes while allowing autonomous units to use methodologies and processes to achieve these outcomes within defined parameters. Information that allows for timely decision making and communication is central to the success of a decentralized organization.

PRODUCT LINE MANAGEMENT (PLM)

Over the last few years, institutions across the country have been decentralizing their structures and establishing a product line form of organizational structure in place of the traditional pyramidal chain-of-command. In this struc-

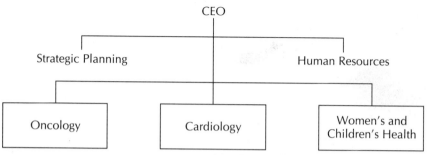

Figure 3–2 Service line management structure. Patient management functions for all departments (e.g., oncology, cardiology, women's and children's health) are included under one head. Management functions include finance, marketing, patient care delivery (e.g., nursing, pharmacy, social work, i.e., case management) and support services (admissions, laboratory, radiology).

ture, developed at Proctor and Gamble in 1928, the product manager becomes the focus of all information related to the product line, source and repository of all relevant data, planner, profit controller, and motivator. His or her responsibility is to develop, market, and sell profitable products by producing high-quality products or services at the least cost (Fig. 3–2). Some of the advantages of this organizational form are that it

1. Provides strong, clear communication channels
2. Places line authority over the product and its outcome with a single manager
3. Provides rapid response time
4. Develops a focal point for customer relations
5. Frees upper management time for strategic planning and prioritizing while developing future executives
6. Allows unprofitable product lines to be identified and eliminated
7. Creates flexibility in time, cost, and effort tradeoffs

There are, however, a number of disadvantages to PLM that may be discovered years later. There can be duplication of effort, facilities, and personnel that could make operating costs prohibitive to smaller institutions. Career opportunities and continuity can be jeopardized for personnel who become overidentified or specialized within the product line. Conflict may arise when two projects require the use of the same facilities or equipment at the same time. Most importantly, a mechanism must be in place to ensure that one product line does not overuse resources at the expense of another. The focus requires that a strong integrating function occur at the upper management levels to avoid power plays that may destroy the overall mission and direction of the organization. An example in health care constitutes assuring that the cardiovascular product line (also known as service lines) competes fairly and equitably for service resources (capital, personnel, and technology) with, for example, an oncology service line.

Coordination must occur based on the mission of the hospital, community

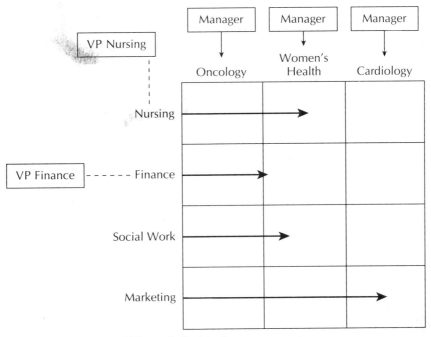

Figure 3–3   Matrix management.

demographics, and ethical decision making and not just on contribution margin or power czaristic behavior.

MATRIX STRUCTURES

Matrix management has become one of the industry's answers to the drawbacks inherent in the previous organizational schemes. In it, the advantages of a functional (traditional) structure and the PLM structure are combined (Fig. 3–3). Each project manager oversees a profit center and reports directly to the general manager or vice president. This manager has total responsibility and accountability, just as in PLM. However, the functional departments retain responsibility to maintain technical excellence, headed by a department manager whose primary concern is to provide a strong technical base and quality controls and to share information and expertise among projects. The ground rules are

1. Horizontal as well as vertical communication is essential.
2. A fast, effective conflict resolution procedure is needed.
3. The horizontal line must be allowed to operate independently in all but administrative arenas.
4. All managers need to be involved in planning, decision making, and prioritizing.
5. There must be an integrating process at the executive level.

In this model, *communication* is the key to problem prevention. The matrix structure can respond rapidly to changes, conflicts, and project needs because the manager's authority allows commitment of resources if scheduling conflicts are resolved quickly. She or he can establish needed policies and procedures to alleviate red tape so long as they do not violate institutional policy. Matrix management is an attempt to assure maximum technologic expertise delivered cost-effectively within time schedule constraints.

Some disadvantages may include the following.

1. More people may be required than for traditional structures.
2. Care must be exercised to avoid duplication.
3. Prioritizing must be handled jointly to avoid territoriality and personal priority issues.
4. Balance must be maintained between functional and project organization power.
5. Individuals must place the good of the organization over the success of the individual product line.

HORIZONTAL ORGANIZATIONS

Today, newer structures are even more exciting. The horizontal organization paves the way for collaboration and teamwork as never before. Focusing on the client, in our case primarily the patient/family, this new structure builds on the concept of value added; that is, what can we bring of value to our clients over and above what is required? The goal is to improve services and efficiency, providing an organized continuum of care through concepts of case management as well as through a system of implementation that improves the delivery of care and outcomes in a time-sensitive manner.

The horizontal organization in health care is the wave of the future. The December 20, 1993, issue of *Business Week* summarized the commandments of the horizontal organization as follows: Organize around process, not task; flatten hierarchy; use teams to manage everything; let customers drive performance; reward team performance; maximize supplier and customer contact; and inform and train all employees.

Each of these concepts is inherent in the mission of health care organizations. Focusing on process and outcomes rather than tasks is the role of the knowledge-based worker, the professional nurse. Hierarchy has frequently interfered with empowerment and the best time/place for decision making, that is, at the point of service. Teamwork has always been essential in the delivery of patient care. Recognizing and rewarding it is only common sense and provides the mechanism for changing the culture of separate professional isolationism to a "we" approach that focuses on cost-effective, quality outcomes for our clients and employers. Maximizing supplier and client contact allows for mutual interchange of what we expect and what is expected from us; this can only enhance our responsiveness and productivity as well as satisfaction for a job well done. Last but not least, we have always been committed to clinical education. Recently, education has been a victim of the cost-constrained environment. This is inopportune, since improved and continuous education in all areas inclusive of process and management enhances productivity and provides a better quality of employee with the self-confidence necessary to meet both client and organizational needs.

Horizontal organizations demand the dissolution of territoriality and historical fragmentation and require a massive cultural change in our organizations. As of 1994 only extreme pressures from business, the government, and our clients will promote this radical yet necessary change.

NURSING'S ROLE IN THE DECENTRALIZED MODELS

How do these patterns fit into the hospital environment? Which are most effective in the clinical setting, and how does the nursing unit function within these structures? These topics are addressed in this section.

The principal product in nursing is high-quality patient care delivered in a timely, cost-effective manner. A decentralized model allows nurse managers appropriate flexibility to provide quality and productivity while carefully monitoring costs and responding appropriately to economic constraints, regulatory standards, and consumer demands. A modification of the PLM model or the horizontal organization can suit this need well. Under either the nurse manager becomes the overseer of the development and implementation of specialty services, programs, or units. In this role, she or he

- Becomes the source and repository of all information of various types whether from automated, computerized statistical reports, management policies, standards manuals, unit-based policies and procedures, educational references, accounting data, or technical handbooks
- Becomes the planner, profit controller, and motivator
- Must develop her or his staff technically and allocate materials and equipment efficaciously as well as monitor and control both costs and profits

The goal, once again, is to produce a quality product—quality patient care with positive outcomes—at the least cost. As can be seen, this is no small task. The demands are many, and the skills required are extensive, not only in the knowledge requirements of clinical nursing practice but also in business management and, to some degree, entrepreneuring.

Timely decision making by those closest to the customer—the patient, doctor, family, and all others using health care services—is enhanced. Nurses are the production coordinators, being closest to the consumer, having clinical data on the patient's accessing ancillary department services and data, and being able to constantly assess patient changes. The nurse manager can most ideally manage resources efficiently, determine intervention efficacy, expedite patient education, oversee discharge planning, and allocate staffing resources in response to changes in customer demands.

To support the nurse manager, the organization needs to provide and promote development and maintenance of adequate clinical, interpersonal, and managerial skills of all caregivers. Top management must view all caregivers as bedside managers, developers, and revenue producers, often a difficult perspective to imbue. The Japanese, for example, have long emphasized the importance of recognizing that the people doing the job require the expertise to innovate and make needed improvements. In view of the increased job satisfaction, reduced turnover and absenteeism, and the personal investment in both quality and productivity, management would be well advised to keep this perspective in mind. In fact, it has been demonstrated that organizational systems combined with strong management support are major determinants of job satisfaction and a productive organization.

In major institutions, when this approach has been implemented, it has been seen clearly that unit-based decision making is an effective and efficient way to induce first-line managers as well as staff caregivers to exercise initiative in increasing productivity by redesigning unit work, restructuring staffing systems, or rearranging the work environment.

Peters and Waterman (1982) found in their search for excellent companies that those companies with the most productive performers on staff used rewards abundantly, "showering pins, buttons, badges, and medals on people" (p. 269) at every possible opportunity, strongly confirming the role of recognition in producing excellence. People need it and will respond enthusiastically to it. These companies found that productivity and profits increase when the organizational philosophy promotes respect and reward for individual contribution. Naisbitt (1984) stated that enthusiasm stems from the feeling of ownership in the process. The PLM, a modified product (service) line, or the future horizontal organization will provide the opportunity to enable this process.

NEW RELATIONSHIPS AND MATRIX STRUCTURE

According to Toffler (1985), the corporate leader must be willing to tolerate a diversity of assignments and organizational settings and must be able to adapt to continuously changing work relationships and personnel. In health care institutions, a vast array of project teams, ad hoc task forces, and various interdisciplinary committees, such as joint practice or joint operations committees, parade across the scene. As Peters and Waterman (1982) point out, the excellent companies employ fluid ad hoc task forces as the primary method of solving and managing difficult problems in a practical, timely manner.

Teamwork, task forces, and interdepartmental collaborations have become hallmarks of the innovative management trend. Hrebiniak (1984) points out that matrix management best suits environments with interdependent relationships and relatively unpredictable phenomena, typical of the health care environment today. In comparison with traditional bureaucracies, the organismic matrix structure establishes a weblike structure that is both resilient and strong enough to support professional functioning, individual initiative, and collaboration. It provides adequate psychosocial stimulus to energize team efforts among professional workers. Matrix managers use ad hoc committees to develop and implement new answers to changing issues and environments. Toffler (1985) suggests organizing "ad hocratically," not bureaucratically, for anticipating long-term trends and capitalizing on current opportunities. The matrix manager becomes a mediator/

facilitator who can integrate diverging roles and interdepartmental personnel. This implies a modular structure where each unit interacts with many others laterally. Teamwork and intradepartmental as well as interdepartmental relationships are enhanced for the benefit of the patient and the organization.

In effect, teamwork and networking are the hallmarks of the matrix structure. Cross-channel communication and collaboration are intrinsic to its success. Delegation of authority and accountability must be dovetailed with an interwoven communication web supporting the patient–nurse relationship along with the interacting flexible reporting system. The informal organization not apparent on the organizational chart becomes exceedingly important in matrix management relationships.

As can be seen in Figure 3–4, the weblike structure is comprised more of informal interactions than of the more formal reporting relationships. Extensive horizontal interaction is involved and probably exceeds, at least in quantity, that of the formal or vertical relationships. In Figure 3–4, the direct relationships between the vice president and the various directors are apparent for long-range planning and policy formulation, whereas day-to-day activities are coordinated by the nursing operations director, providing a basis for problem solving and decision making. To assure quality care in terms of technical excellence, standards of practice, and clinical policy making, the clinical specialists report directly to the clinical director. The nurse managers carry responsibility for day-to-day unit management, with support and counsel of the clinical directors and specialists, enhancing their technical expertise and assuring quality of care. This structure can be flattened even more depending on the size of the organization and the number of programs.

COMMUNICATION

Supporting nurses in this structure requires empowering the caregiver at the bedside and a strong reliable communication network assuring that information is shared, goals and objectives are maintained, and collaborative efforts are encouraged as essential to nurses' productivity and efficiency. High technology, unpredictable demands, and frequent crises require that nurse managers encourage staff participation in making innovations. In turn, the staff nurses need communication channels to

- Resolve frustrations and conflict
- Organize their ideas into plans
- Coordinate and support their professional practice

Open communication channels are essential to efficiency and success.

In a major west coast institution, a staff nurse advisory board consisting of 12 volunteers from various units met regularly to present this view on decisions and plans relating to patient care directly to the vice president. This assured that senior management was tuned into staff concerns without the filtering up and cleansing effect found in traditional hierarchies. In fact, the board was very forthright and served management well in its advisory capacity. The members

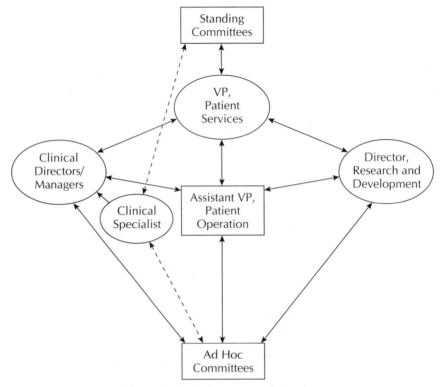

Figure 3–4   Patient care organization.

were responsible for relaying information back to their units and apprising staff of current developments. A much more direct communication link could hardly be found.

Policies and procedures were developed by the nursing executive council with staff nurse advisory board review and feedback. Thus, the communication link was complete. Some of the problem resolutions were the following.

1. Established verbal walking rounds, deleting the tape recording
2. Established primary nursing assignments
3. Established a patient liaison nurse
4. Improved physician–nurse communication through unit-based problem-solving groups
5. Minimized floating within shifts
6. Oriented new patients to the unit with a hostess-type approach
7. Floated the same nurse to the same unit consistently

There were many more similar procedural improvements. This increased job satisfaction and helped staff feel more involved in work environment.

Involvement, in reality, is key to this process. Participation in committees and task forces must be encouraged for the structure to be effective. A wide range of opportunities must be presented for involvement, such as

1. A nursing newsletter, which provides a forum for recognition of individual and unit effort as well as discussion of ideas and concerns
2. Recruitment and retention committee, which provides open discussion of job dissatisfiers with an eye to preventing problems and crises as well as developing reward and recognition programs to encourage excellence in practice
3. Quality improvement groups inter- and intradepartmentally (or product line), as well as central coordinating committee that oversees all quality activities
4. Open forums and "lunch with the VP" to encourage information flow and a sense of real concern from management for the day-to-day problems and frustrations of a caregiver's life
5. Regular department meetings and open door policies
6. Recognition banquets, nursing day symposia, and other professional recognition and educational events on a regular basis, not just once a year

All of these provided opportunities for staff to participate, realize professional fulfillment in their work, and effect real and meaningful changes in their working conditions. Additionally, joint education and joint practice protocols were developed to promote continuity of nursing and medical care, as well as collectively. Joining practice conferences, committees, and rounds facilitated nurse–physician communication and joint problem solving. In turn, iatrogenic complications were reduced, saving on the length of hospital stay and reducing costs. Of 120 cesarean sections, 80 patients were discharged a day earlier, representing $40,000 savings in a month.

Fundamental to the participative, matrix structure is ongoing education. Education of clinical care givers and experience represent a major resource investment in a hospital's enterprise, in terms of both cost and revenue. Assuring a common, solid body of skill and technical knowledge for all staff is essential to success and quality care. Though these programs can be costly, ways have been devised to reduce cost and time lost while assuming that competency and appropriate skill levels are maintained.

One solution has been competency-based education, coordinated and implemented on the unit. The first units of self-instruction introduced were 16 institutional competencies to be completed within appropriate time frames. Following this, self-education courses were presented in specialty-specific and unit-specific competencies, which are updated and expanded regularly to keep abreast of the changing technologies and environment. This is a genuinely economical and effective way to provide appropriate skills and knowledge in such a way as to minimize staffing impact and scheduling problems for nurse managers. All competency records are maintained on the unit for convenience and appropriate managerial monitoring. Supporting this scheme were clinical specialists and clinical instructors acting as resource persons, encouraging staff participation, and constantly reevaluating program effectiveness. Managers also acted as resource persons and were able to use the competency record in annual employee evaluations.

Some questions nurse managers need to ask themselves, if they are to adapt successfully in decentralized, consumer/patient-centered systems, are listed:

1. What strategies should I use to establish an appropriate, supportive environment for highly skilled staff to be most productive and efficient?
2. What services or products should I be developing to meet new consumer demands? (This includes patients, families, and physicians as well as third party payers.)
3. Does our nursing service provide positive, supportive, and dynamic leadership with vision and enthusiasm?
4. Are services delivered as efficiently and efficaciously as they could be? If not, what needs to be changed?
5. What programs can I initiate that will encourage staff participation and cross-channel communication?
6. Am I providing resources and leadership that stimulate innovation and program development by staff?
7. How can I involve the executive level leadership in improving education and resources at the unit level?

Many other such questions should be asked regularly in a self-inventory review if nursing management is to retain its central position in the health care enterprise of planning and marketing.

Nursing must be responsive to marketplace demands if its services are to meet consumer needs and adapt to changing socioeconomic environments. Reactive management will not suffice. Organizational structures need to promote and enhance these efforts. Customizing, specializing, or tailoring services to reimbursement and cost also must be part of the nurse manager planning process. Matrix management can go a long way in aiding this focus for managers, clearly delineating role responsibilities, goals, and outcome expectations for staff.

References

Drucker (1984)

Geneen, H., & Mascow, A. (1984). *Managing*. Garden City, NY: Doubleday.

Hrebiniak (1984)

Jacobs, G., & Macfarlane, (1990). *The vital corporation*. Englewood Cliffs, NJ: Prentice-Hall.

Naisbitt, J. (1984). *Megatrends*. New York: Warner Books.

Naisbitt, J., & Aburdene, P. (1990). *Megatrends 2000*. New York: Avon Books.

Pascale, R., & Othos, A. (1982). *The art of Japanese management*. New York: Simon and Schuster.

Peters, T., & Austin, N. (1985). *A passion for excellence*. New York: Random House.

Peters, T. (1987). *Thriving on chaos*. New York: Alfred Knopf.

Peters, T., & Waterman, R. (1982). *In search of excellence*. New York: Warner Books.

Spitzer, R. (1986). *Nursing productivity: The hospitals key to survival and profit*. Chicago: S-N Publications.

Spitzer, R., & Kralovic, J. (1989). *The new nursing organization*.

Toffler, A. (1985). *The adaptive corporation*. New York: McGraw-Hill.

Walton, M. (1990). *Deming management at work*. New York: Putnam Publishers.

CHAPTER 4

MISSION STATEMENT, GOALS, AND VALUES

KAREN S. EHRAT

EXECUTIVE SUMMARY

Vision, mission, and values statements in descending order of abstraction embody the philosophy of the organization. They provide a conceptual description of the organization as well as a framework for that organization's planning and operation. They provide information about the organization's desired future, its intent, and its beliefs. To drive the organization's operations, however, a strategic plan built on these statements must have sufficient flexibility and specificity to allow adaptation to changing dynamics. The statements of action in a strategic plan are those required to achieve the goals derived from the vision, mission, and value statements. The strategic plan, usually written for a three- to five-year period, is in turn the basis for developing annual operating plans and budgets. The provision of quality health care services has long been a theme of the mission statements of acute care health organizations, but the concepts of quality service and customer satisfaction have only more recently been integrated into strategic and operational goals as fundamental components. These more recent components entail thinking of health care service as a product—a perspective difficult for many health professionals to accept—and applying continuous quality improvement concepts to improve customer satisfaction with the health care "product." A number of support and structural changes are required to achieve continuous quality improvement, including work redesign to achieve barrier-free health care environments. The nurse manager is in a key position to influence these redesign efforts in ways that ensure improved patient care.

ORGANIZATIONAL PHILOSOPHY AND PLANNING

A shared set of beliefs and understandings assists organizations in channeling diverse discipline energies and interests toward desired outcomes. In a continuing era of diminishing resources and heightened interdisciplinary competition for those resources, common understanding of priorities and expected accomplishments is a prerequisite to organizational success or solvency.

From this author's perspective, precise definitions of mission statements, vision statements, values statements, guiding principles, strategic plans, goals, and operational objectives are less important than their intent. Each of those components serves as a necessary unit of an organization's planning process. In essence, the planning process seeks to achieve stakeholder consensus and support at various levels of planning abstraction, moving from strategic desires to concrete tactical actions that demand annual accountability.

Hierarchy of Planning Abstraction
Vision Statement

The hierarchy of planning abstraction typically begins with the development of a vision statement (Fig. 4–1) that captures in writing how the organization views, or desires to view, its future. Creating a vision statement is more akin to crystal ball gazing than a scientific process of inquiry. As one CEO noted, "There is a fine line between vision and hallucination" (Charan, 1991, p. 12). Creating a vision requires both imagination and imagery. The intent is to envision alternative scenarios or futures and then select accordingly. Despite the absence of a definitive process, creating a vision statement involves articulating and reaching consensus about an organization's desired future and direction. Typically, governance representatives, senior management, and medical staff leadership converge to create the vision statement (Table 4–1). In early American history, the vision of colonists was to build a free enterprise where self-government and religious freedom prevailed. Vision statements are typically sufficiently

vision statement   abstract articulation of an organizations's preferred future based on desire and imagination. Vision guides planning.

↓

mission statement   articulation of an organization's purpose and the public it services. Planning should be congruent with the purpose of the organization. It should reflect the organizational philosophy.

↓

values   articulation of concrete beliefs that guide organizational practices.

↓

guiding principles   statements of principle derived from values or foundation beliefs.

↓

strategic goals   broad statement of action necessary to achieve vision (3–5 years).

↓

strategies   more specific actions required to meet any given strategic goal. May be multiple strategies for each strategic goal (3–5 years).

↓

tactics or initiatives   concrete, well-defined actions that satisfy any given strategy. May be multiple tactics or initiatives for each strategy. Tactics may become annual operating goals.

↓

operational goals   statements of outcomes to be accomplished during the year at hand.

↓

objectives   specific actions necessary to meet annual goals.

Figure 4–1   Hierarchy of planning abstraction.

broad to engender a wide base of acceptance and support. Vision statements promote organizational focus.

Mission Statement

Mission statements, the second level of planning abstraction, tend to describe what an organization stands for or the purpose and philosophy of the organization. Most health care organizations have incorporated into their mission statements some language relating to both the rendering of services to the ill and disease prevention. Often, mission statements describe the populations served by the organization, special functions such as education and research, antidiscrimination statements relating to those populations served, contribution(s) to the community at large, and other broad statements.

Mission statements (Table 4–2) attempt to describe the essence of an organization. In a teaching hospital, education is the primary mission of the orga-

TABLE 4–1 Examples of Vision Statements

A. American Organization of Nurse Executives: shaping the future of health care through innovative leadership*

B. The collaboration of Mercy Health Services and Henry Ford Health System provides an opportunity for both systems to achieve financially viable delivery mechanisms that will better serve the health care needs of the population of Macomb County. Through this collaboration, the Henry Ford Mercy Health Services network strives to achieve in the Macomb region a system that provides

1. The best health care value in the community; value that combines continuous quality improvement, compassion, current technology, and cost advantage within a mechanism that continually assesses and improves clinical effectiveness through a philosophy of patient-centered care.

2. A comprehensive, vertically integrated range of services, drawing on the resources of St. Joseph's Mercy Hospitals and Health Services, Henry Ford Health System, and Mercy Health Services using innovative models of financing and delivery—urban, rural, suburban. The delivery system responds to the market imperative for managed care and has as its principal objective improved health status of those it serves.

3. Leadership in shaping a community health care system: fostering collaboration among community health care resources, attaining recognition as the preferred employer of the community, and determining ways to meet the community's health care needs as well as exceeding the community's health care expectations.

4. A governance and management structure that optimizes collaboration, integration, and continuity of care and minimizes duplication and competition.

5. A pluralistic medical staff that supports both group and private practices, seeking collaborative synergy in terms of joint use of resources, educational programs, quality improvement initiatives, and physician recruitment.†

---

*Courtesy of the American Organization of Nurse Executives, a subsidiary of the American Hospital Association, Chicago, Illinois.
†Courtesy of Henry Ford Health System/Mercy Health Network, Farmington Hills, Michigan.

nization, with the provision of health care services as a by-product. Similarly, in a research university environment, a university hospital may have the discovery of new knowledge, new treatments, and new technology as a primary mission, with education and the delivery of health care services as secondary activities. As consumer and regulator expectations change, payment bases further erode, and provider competition intensifies, many organizations are redrafting mission statements to acknowledge commitment to quality improvement and further define the populations served.

The mission statement serves to ground the organization and, in a gross sense, places parameters around organizational activity. Any development plan or budgetary request incongruent with the mission of the organization is unlikely to meet with success. Therefore, the manager should always consider plans and actions in relation to the mission. Any plan or action that furthers or supports the organizational mission is likely to meet with more support than one to the contrary. The organization's governance is the principal sponsor and protector of an organization's mission.

Though the intent of this chapter is not to belabor the discussion of mission, several key points are relevant. Like vision statements, mission statements tend to be broad and general in nature. The breadth of the organizational purpose statements allows agreement and support even in dynamic and politically charged environments. Halpern (1971) illustrated this point in his discussion of foreign policy bureaucracy. He concluded that consensus can be reached through the articulation of ambiguous policy (or mission) that avoids the major points of conflict. In his example, he stated that although various government and military representatives could conclusively support the production of weaponry to protect

---

TABLE 4–2   Examples of Mission Statements

A. The American Organization of Nurse Executives (AONE) is the voice of nursing administrative practice. AONE members are leaders in collaboration and catalysts for innovation. The organization provides leadership, professional development, advocacy, and research in order to advance nursing practice and patient care, promote nursing leadership excellence, and shape health care public policy.*

B. Mercy Health Services is a unified system of institutions, programs, and services established to carry out the health ministry sponsored by the Religious Sisters of Mercy–Providence of Detroit in collaboration with others committed to this ministry. Mercy Health Services addresses human needs and promotes an environment in which access to health care, especially for the economically disadvantaged, is achieved. To accomplish this mission, Mercy Health Services provides a comprehensive range of services either through direct delivery of high-quality, compassionate health care or through linkages with others in order to assure continuity of care in the communities we serve.†

---

*Courtesy of the American Organization of Nurse Executives, a subsidiary of the American Hospital Association, Chicago, Illinois.
†Courtesy of Mercy Health Services, Farmington Hills, Michigan.

the United States and foreign allies (mission), there was disagreement over issues relating to budget, timing, and impact on allied relationships. The budget for Skybolt (Halpern, 1971), the air-to-surface missile in question, was overrun, and production was delayed. Government officials responsible for the military budget favored scrapping the project. Air Force officials favored project continuation to avoid threat to the future of strategic manned bombers (Air Force mission). Had Navy officials been part of the Skybolt debate, they likely would have argued to abandon the costly project in favor of seafaring weaponry. Budget people support balanced budgets. Air Force personnel support air technology. Naval representatives give allegiance to seagoing concerns.

Similar to Halpern's example, the multiple disciplines and technical specialists found in hospitals tend to support broad missions aimed at stamping out disease and restoring health, without regard for sex, race, or socioeconomic status. However, in the day-to-day living out of the organizational mission, conflicts arise from competing professional and technical priorities or specialty missions. For example, the mission of environmental service workers is to provide a clean environment. At times, this mission conflicts with nursing's priorities. Similarly, pharmacists value accurately dispensing drugs, although their processes may inhibit nursing's delivery of timely medications. Part of nursing's mission deals with the coordination and sequencing of care components that are suited to patients' changing needs. At times, nursing's priorities for patient care disrupt physical therapy, surgery, and other schedules. An organization must actively subscribe to its written overarching mission if internal conflicts are to be minimized. In customer-driven organizations, the needs of users, rather than the needs of service providers, should establish operational priorities.

Values and Guiding Principles

A lower level of planning abstraction deals with an organization's shared values or guiding principles. Values (Fig. 4–2) represent the concrete beliefs that undergird the practices of an organization. Guiding principles (Fig. 4–3) are principles of practice derived from values or foundation beliefs. Commonly, values are articulated through an interdisciplinary effort and frequently have their roots in ethics or similar committees. Religiously affiliated hospitals often model their values after the sponsoring church or congregation. All components of a strategic and operating plan should support, or be congruent with, an organization's stated values. For example, Americans value life, liberty, and the pursuit of happiness. In theory, individual and collective actions should reflect those values. Clearly, in a diverse organization, written values or beliefs attempt to unify intent and actions.

Vision, mission, and values, to one degree or another, reflect the philosophy of the organization. They provide an introduction to the organization as well as a framework for planning and operation. In overview, written vision, mission, and value statements provide information about the organization's desired future, the intent or essence for organizational being, and beliefs guiding organizational activity. Although reviewed and modified from time to time, an organization's

↓ **Our Values** ↓

We, the employees, volunteers, professional staff and trustees of TMCare, are in partnership to provide caring, healing and hope to all we serve.

We believe health care is much more than a business.

Quality

We are a team dedicated to the highest possible performance, fulfilling with special care and compassion emotional, physical and spiritual needs.

Dignity

We will demonstrate integrity in all we do, with respect for the special gifts, needs and responsibilities of every individual.

Leadership

We will foster our position of excellence and preeminence in health care through the enhancement, development and evaluation of innovative systems, programs and services with commitment to implement those that maximize the clinical and financial benefits to our patients.

Stewardship

We are committed to maintaining the financial strength and performance efficiency that will ensure the future of our mission to serve our patients, physicians and community.

Partnership

We conduct our operations in effective collaboration with our physicians and all members of the health care team, sharing common values and in pursuit of common clinical and financial goals.

Development

We are dedicated to the personal as well as the professional growth and education of all members of our health care team.

Community

We are an integral part of the civic and social fabric around us and will be responsive and sensitive to the needs and concerns we all share as neighbors and fellow citizens.

Figure 4–2 Sample statement of values. (Courtesy of Tucson Medical Center, Tucson, Arizona.)

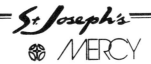

Guiding Principles

To create an organizational environment that enables us to achieve and maintain the vision of St. Joseph's, we must demonstrate a shared set of principles. These principles must be understood and practiced by all who work here and be consistently expressed to the communities we serve. The following principles, combined with our commitment to the values of our Catholic sponsors, will guide us as we anticipate and respond to challenges in the health care and social environment.

We value the individual; therefore, we will:

- respect and recognize the uniqueness of each person

- assist each individual in reaching his or her maximum potential

- be open, honest and trusting in our relationships

- treat each other with dignity

- provide clear and realistic expectations with constructive and honest feedback

- enhance communication by listening, relaying information and responding in a timely manner

- promote wellness to all employees and community members

We value our organization; therefore, in structure and practice, we will:

- be flexible, responsive and harmonious

- empower people, release authority and promote participation

- minimize bureaucracy

- promote shared use of resources

- encourage and support creativity and risk-taking in developing innovative solutions to new and traditional challenges

- value passion and persistence

- establish, prioritize and achieve goals, within our value system

- respect patients and their families as equal partners in treatment

We value the community in which we serve; therefore, we will:

- foster collaborative relationships with other organizations to identify and develop services which are responsive to the needs and expectations of the community

- advocate for the underserved and disadvantaged

- encourage participation by the community in defining our role

- demonstrate a unified commitment to providing accessible, quality health care to persons of Macomb County and surrounding areas, within the framework of our Catholic sponsors

- actively participate in shaping economic and social growth and changes within the community

Each of us hopes to build "energy" into this organization by modeling commitment to the above principles.

Figure 4–3 Sample statement of guiding principles. (Courtesy of St. Joseph's Mercy Hospital and Health Services, Mount Clemens, Michigan.)

mission and values tend to remain fairly constant. In contrast, the vision statement will be adapted as the desired future changes or as political, social, or economic forces negate the realization of a given, preferred future. In healthy organizations, plans and actions are congruent with those published statements, and employees are conversant with the content. It is the nurse manager's responsibility to ensure that his or her direct reports have an understanding of the organization's philosophy and to manage assigned areas within that framework.

Strategic Goals

Philosophy, although important, does not drive the operation in either a strategic or operational sense. To achieve its desired future, an organization must develop plans with sufficient specificity to guide the organization and of sufficient flexibility to allow adaptation to changing forces. The strategic plan is a document that attempts to lay out a series of broad actions necessary to achieve a desired future. Strategic plans are typically developed by teams of governance, senior management, and medical staff leadership and are built on commonly agreed upon assumptions. Although various labels may be used, the written strategic plan generally includes the vision and mission statements, a demographic and environmental assessment, broad goals, key strategic issues, strategies, and tactics or initiatives. Strategic issues may be discussed from the vantage points of strengths, weaknesses, opportunities, and threats (SWOT). Strategies tend to be general statements of action necessary over time to achieve the stated goals. Tactics or initiatives represent specific actions or activities to be accomplished. Beginning with the strategic goals, the plan becomes more concrete with each descending order plan component, strategic issues, strategies, and tactics (Table 4–3). Strategic plans generally are written for a 3 to 5 year period and should be reviewed and adapted annually. The rate of industry change suggests a need for frequent modification of an organization's strategic plan.

The formal strategic plan serves as the major guide for organizational activity over time. However, the written document must be accompanied by strategic thinking and action. "Strategic thinking describes a state of mind, an attitude that looks at a given situation and applies a disciplined perspective, an orientation that consistently seeks out opportunities for improvement and advantage" (Beckham, 1991, p. 38). This animation in thinking propels an organization toward its desired future. Strategies should be proactive in effecting desired change or organizational progress.

Operational Goals

The strategic plan becomes the guidepost for developing annual operating plans and annual resource/supply and capital budgets. Typically, senior management staff will develop broad annual operating goals consistent with the strategic plan, from which department managers can develop division- or unit-specific annual goals and objectives. Annual operating goals and objectives are specific in nature and generally represent actions or activities to be accomplished in a specific fiscal year.

TABLE 4–3 Example of Strategic Goal with Increasingly Specific Planning Subunits

Professional goal: Provide member services that support and enhance the management, leadership, educational and professional development of nurse executives and nurse managers to advance nursing practice and patient care.
  Strategic Objective: Provide and influence formal and continuing educational preparation for nurse executives and nurse managers.
    Operational Objective: Develop and deliver educational programs that are meaningful for nurse executives to members.
      Strategy: Strengthen current educational offerings.
        Tactic: Continue a fall national conference that focuses on executive development in 1992 and evaluate the impact at annual meeting.
        Tactic: Initiate joint venture with chapters to conserve resources and minimize competition.
      Strategy: Continue to implement alternative delivery formats for education.
        Tactic: Continue audiotape products of AONE educational programs in 1992.
        Tactic: Continue video and computer-assisted products in 1992.
      Strategy: Collaborate with American Association of Colleges of Nursing (AACN), National League for Nursing (NLN), Association of Hospital Schools of Nursing (AHSN), and schools of nursing to influence the development of academic curricula.

Courtesy of the American Organization of Nurse Executives, a subsidiary of the American Hospital Association, Chicago, Illinois.

The purpose for developing unit-based operating goals and objectives is to guide the manager during the year. Organization-wide operating goals and objectives serve to move the organization in total toward desired outcomes. Organizations vary in the degree of rigor applied to the formal development of goals and objectives. However, preplanning to achieve desired department, division, and organizational outcomes cannot be overemphasized. Unit-based or division-based goals and objectives should reflect the input of managers, staff, and customers.

Objectives.   Although in concept managers support the value of planning and subscribe to the identification of desired annual outcomes, individual managers often struggle with the actual writing of goals and objectives. Goals are written to express a general intended outcome, such as "improved patient satisfaction" or "reduction of medication errors." Objectives are specific statements written to indicate how a given goal will be met. Objectives describe the specific actions to be done, the parties responsible for the actions, the important conditions surrounding actions, and the criteria by which achievement will be judged (Mager, 1975). For example, to meet the goal of "improved patient satisfaction," the following two objectives might be written.

- Objective 1: Case managers will meet jointly with assigned patients, families, and attending physicians on a daily basis to plan continued care, review patient progress, and answer patient questions. Success will be measured by (1) quarterly improvements in patient satisfaction survey scores and (2) patient expression of satisfaction on open-ended, nonpartisan patient interviews.

- Objective 2: All staff members assigned to direct patient care will, before report, introduce themselves to assigned patients using patients' preferred names. Staff will communicate to patients their approximate time of return, following shift report. Success will be measured by (1) reduced call lights during report, (2) patients' recollection of staff names, and (3) quarterly improvements in patient satisfaction survey scores.

Although seemingly labor intensive, the development of precise operational objectives provides staff with explicit directions and convey management's expectations. To be effective, outcome or success indicators must be pre-established and openly communicated. Where possible, outcomes should be quantified rather than subjective. In all instances, outcome expectations are achieved more readily when staff are involved in goal setting, the crafting of operational objectives, and the development of evaluation or success indicators.

As acknowledged previously, for organizations to meet with success, the philosophy and planning components must be congruent and understood, in both the short term (tactical) and the strategic sense. Figure 4–4 attempts to draw together philosophy and planning components and their interrelationships. Throughout all planning aspects, organizations need to be focused externally, attentive to customers, competitors, the market, payors, and environmental changes. It is the role of management to convey to staff the intent and interrelatedness of organizational and unit goals. Figure 4–5 demonstrates organizational accountability for the various philosophy and planning components.

THE CONTINUOUS QUALITY IMPROVEMENT MOVEMENT

Provision of quality health care services has long been embedded in the mission statements of acute health care organizations. In recent times and in accord with reimbursement shifts, the themes of quality service and customer satisfaction have been integrated into both strategic and operational goals. Historically, customer satisfaction was viewed as a strategic tool to enhance market share. Today, customer satisfaction is a fundamental component of operations necessary to maintain market share. More and more, product differentiation or institutional choice is based on user perceptions of quality rather than on available technology, physical presentation, or cost factors. Prospective reimbursement, capitated plans, and purchaser discounts have all but leveled the price playing field. Hospitals are struggling to improve services while controlling costs per case in order to contend with declining reimbursement and accelerated health care product inflation.

The relatively recent quality and customer satisfaction movements have their roots in manufacturing, where free market forces have prevailed historically.

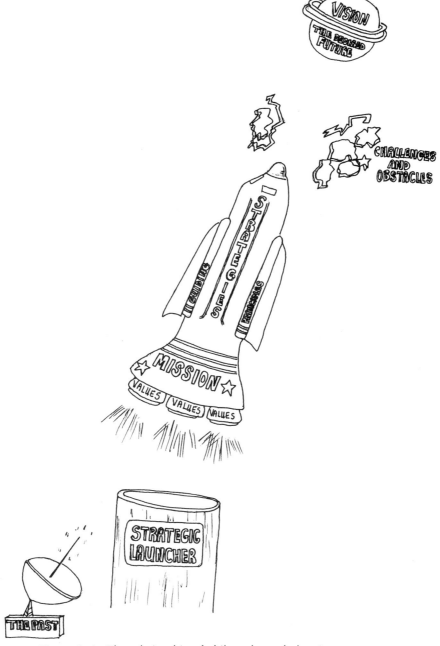

Figure 4–4 The relationship of philosophy and planning components.

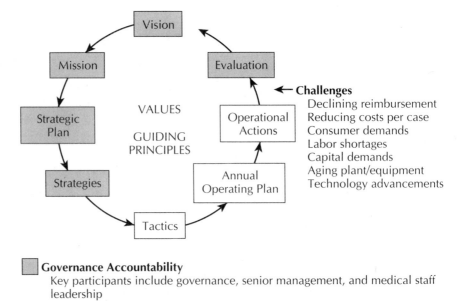

Governance Accountability
  Key participants include governance, senior management, and medical staff
  leadership

Management Accountability
  Key participants include senior management, department managers, and staff

Figure 4–5 Organizational accountabilities for philosophy and planning.

Given uncompromised access to similar products, purchasers select goods offering the highest quality or value at the lowest price. When the quality of like products is assumed to be equal, cost, convenience, or service will guide purchaser decisions.

Health Care as a Service Product

Often, health care professionals have difficulty thinking of health care services as a product. Albrecht and Zemke (1985) have attempted to assist that understanding by discussing service products. They distinguish a service product from a commodity by the following service characteristics (pp. 36, 37):

- A service is produced at the instant of delivery; it cannot be created in advance or held in readiness.
- A service cannot be centrally produced, inspected, stockpiled, or warehoused. It is usually delivered wherever the customer is by people who are beyond the immediate influence of management.
- The product cannot be demonstrated, nor can a sample be sent for customer approval in advance of the service. The provider can show various examples, but the customer's own haircut, for example, does not yet exist and cannot be shown.
- The person receiving the service has nothing tangible; the value of the service depends on his or her personal experience.

- The experience cannot be sold or passed on to a third party.
- If improperly performed, a service cannot be recalled.
- If it cannot be repeated, reparations or apologies are the only means of recourse for customer satisfaction.
- Quality assurance must happen before production rather than after production, as would be the case in a manufacturing situation.
- Delivery of the service usually requires human interaction to some degree. Buyer and seller come into contact in some relatively personal way to create the service.
- The receiver's expectations of the service are integral to his or her satisfaction with the outcome. Quality of service is largely a subjective matter.
- The more people the customer must encounter during the delivery of the service, the less likely it is that he or she will be satisfied with the service.

There is a growing intolerance among health care purchasers—government, industry, and individuals—to shoulder the increasing financial burden for health care service products. The health care industry is being pressured, economically and politically, to reduce price escalation and improve service. These external pressures have triggered competing forces within health care organizations: tradition vs change, margin vs mission, and short-term expediency vs long-term (strategic) viability.

The notion of providing quality health services has long been a goal shared by health care professionals and provider institutions. Given the nature of health care services and the rather poorly defined measures of outcomes, past judgments about quality were based on compliance with the various professional and accreditation standards. In general, the prevailing attitude of the 1960s, 1970s, and early 1980s was "the more services, the better the care." Rising costs, the shift to Medicare prospective payment (mid-1980s), the growth of managed care programs, and the shift to outpatient services called into question past definitions of quality and placed greater emphasis on organizational productivity. The U.S. Office of Personnel Management (1980) defined productivity as

> The measure of individual or organizational performance. It is not only efficiency (the ratio of inputs to outputs), but also effectiveness (to what extent the output satisfies program objectives). . . . It involves not just how much of a product is produced— or a service delivered—and at what cost, but also quality, timeliness, and responsiveness. (p. 3)

The late 1980s found health care organizations fixated on improving efficiency, with minimal attention devoted to effectiveness. Following industry trends and supported by the Joint Commission on Accrediting Healthcare Organizations (JCAHO), the 1990s ushered in a commitment by provider institutions to quality improvement. It is generally believed that poor quality is largely responsible for sluggish productivity, inhibiting competitiveness. It should be noted that the term "quality improvement" is an umbrella term that encompasses meeting customer expectations, reducing costs and service defects, improving efficiency, reducing redundancy, and using statistical methods for monitoring performance. This continuing shift in emphasis and thinking has found the health care industry in a reactive mode, scrambling to discover quick-fix programs. It is noteworthy that this transition in health care thinking lagged sufficiently behind the manufacturing industry. A plethora of vendor-developed and home-grown quality improvement programs have been unveiled in an attempt to fasttrack provider institutions to efficient, user-friendly enterprises that demonstrate commitment to their respective missions.

Band (1991) has put forth the argument that "quality and service are the means, but value for the customer is the end" (p. 19). Customers or purchasers of a given institution's health services products must perceive value superior to that offered by other providers if the organization is to prevail in the market. Albrecht and Zemke (1985) acknowledge that performance standards, sensitive and efficient feedback systems, a clearly defined service package, a good delivery system, proper training, and good management are all important to service improvement. However, they caution that "unless the shared values, norms, beliefs, and ideologies of the organization—the organization's culture—are clearly and consciously focused on serving the customer, there is virtually no chance that the organization will deliver a consistent quality of service and develop a sustained reputation for service" (p. 102). Organizational leadership must *walk the talk* and reward customer-sensitive service. In a special report, *Business Week* (1987) noted that "managing for quality means nothing less than a sweeping overhaul in corporate culture, a radical shift in management philosophy, and a permanent commitment of all the levels of the organization to seek continuous improvements" (p. 131).

Health care organizations exist to serve the customers or users of the various health services products. Customers are both external and internal. Many health care service delivery units or departments are sensitive only to external customers—third party purchasers, patients, and physicians. True quality improvement demands that service units support one another to improve the overall system.

Theories of Continuous Quality Improvement

The continuous quality improvement movement had its genesis in 1900 in manufacturing. Scientific management (Frederick Taylor) and Theory X style of management have been blamed by various experts for the inefficiency creep in the major manufacturing industries. These inefficiencies have their roots in the industrial revolution, when specialization of labor and economy of scale theories were put into place to correct inefficiencies of small cottage industries. Through that specialization, "business disaggregated work into narrowly defined tasks, reaggregated the people performing those tasks into departments, and installed managers to administer them" (Hammer, 1990, p. 107). Modern era U.S. industry losses to Japan made apparent the overall inefficiency of conventional production systems.

W. Edwards Deming is thought of by some as the U.S. apostle of quality management. Born and educated in America, he assisted post–World War II

Japan in census work and later in quality control statistical techniques. He first came to the attention of Detroit auto moguls in the late 1970s and began work for the Ford Motor Company in the early 1980s. Deming places responsibility for quality improvement on management. His approach involves identifying and correcting *special cause* variation in work production and then focusing on correcting common cause or predictable variation. Statistical methods are used to identify and monitor variation. Deming developed the following fourteen-point plan for improving processes and products and enlisting employee support (Walton, 1986, pp. 34–36):

1. Create constancy of purpose for improvement of product and service.
2. Adopt the new philosophy.
3. Cease dependence on mass inspection.
4. End the practice of awarding business on the price tag alone.
5. Improve constantly and forever the system of production and service.
6. Institute training.
7. Institute leadership.
8. Drive out fear.
9. Break down barriers between staff areas.
10. Eliminate slogans, exhortations, and targets for the work force.
11. Eliminate numerical quotas.
12. Remove barriers to pride of workmanship.
13. Institute a vigorous program of education and retraining.
14. Take action to accomplish the transformation.

Deming advocates a long-term management focus, with clearly defined vision and mission statements guiding day-to-day actions.

W.E. Deming is one of three quality improvement gurus (Walton, 1986). J.M. Juran, a Romanian immigrant to the United States, was another pioneer in quality improvement methodologies. Like Deming, Juran worked with Japanese industry, teaching management techniques to yield quality. Juran has been one of the leading total quality management (TQM) advocates in this country. He developed the quality trilogy as a way of thinking about quality and its organizational fit. The trilogy includes three interrelated processes—quality planning, quality control, and quality improvement (Juran, 1988). The planning activity relates to identifying customers and determining their needs and developing and implementing production processes to produce product features to meet those needs. The quality control function involves evaluating actual operating performance, comparing the actual performance to goals, and acting on the difference. The final component of the trilogy, quality improvement, represents a phased approach for achieving unprecedented levels of performance. Juran's universal steps for breakthrough (1988) include establishing proof of need, project identification, organization to guide the projects, organization for diagnosis—for analysis of projects, diagnosis, proof of the remedies under operating conditions, dealing with cultural resistance to change, and control at the new level.

Philip Crosby is the third leading American expert in quality improvement.

He served as the corporate vice president of ITT before forming his own consulting company. Crosby's quality improvement methods focus on prevention rather than appraisal, with zero defects as a goal. Quality measurement is based on the cost of quality and on nonconformance and conformance costs. Crosby's quality improvement process (1979, 1984) highlights commitment of senior management, error-cause removal, employee training, and worker awareness of quality problems.

There is more similarity than variation in the methodologies advocated by these key quality leaders. It is important to note that key disciples of quality advocate that 85% of organization problems relate to systems rather than to people. Quality improvement programs are thus geared toward improving the production process, using statistical techniques to identify and monitor variation.

Various U.S. manufacturers should be acknowledged for their ongoing commitments to quality improvement. Westinghouse, DuPont, AT&T, Kodak, IBM, Hewlett-Packard, and Corning Glass are often recognized as industry leaders. The basis for industry overhaul has been to achieve customer satisfaction and, through that effort, to gain or maintain market share and net gains.

Customer Satisfaction

Attaining a quality product and efficient production will not guarantee market success. The customer must also perceive a value addedness. Absent from the previous discussion is the notion of innovation. Old products, though superior in design and service, will not motivate customers. Witness the market entry of compact disc players, notebook computers, and the Mazda Miata. Technology advances or artistic innovation causes market paradigms to shift accordingly. In all cases, however, customer satisfaction remains paramount to market success. Given that premise, organizational missions should recognize the necessity of research and development activities geared toward satisfying the changing needs of customers.

Translating manufacturing models for quality improvement into service product industries is sometimes perplexing. The health care industry continues to struggle with the development of a perfect model for continuous quality improvement. The JCAHO is attempting to spearhead a transformation in thinking by demanding more focus on care delivery processes and patient care outcomes. Further, the JCAHO is requiring evidence of multidisciplinary attempts to improve overall quality. Third party payors, through their respective methods for ratcheting down reimbursement, are attempting to force efficiency and improve services. Although the health care industry traditionally has assumed a defensive posture toward external interference, it is apparent that many inefficiencies and quality variations exist. Witness the wide geographic variations in hysterectomy and cesarean section rates, the wide pricing gaps in local health care service areas, the functional redundancy in various caregiver roles, insufficient clinical information systems to assist in medical practice reform, and the overuse of diagnostic technologies, to cite but a few examples.

When functioning under a cost-based reimbursement system, there was little incentive for health care providers to promote efficiency. Similarly, when most Americans had the benefit of full health care insurance coverage and employer profits were escalating, there was no external pressure for health care reform. However, in a national climate of retrenchment, consumers are unwilling to tolerate the prevailing rate of health care cost escalation. The logical conclusion is that, whether voluntarily or secondary to intense public pressure, health care delivery systems will reform.

To illustrate the inefficiency and customer dissatisfaction in any given acute care institution, the manager may wish to count the aggregate number of steps, the person-dependent points of process breakdown, and the total lapsed time of transforming a discharge bed to a patient-ready bed or of completing a routine radiologic procedure, from the point of patient order to final report on the patient record. Suffice it to say that there is latitude for marked improvement. Retooling health care delivery systems will necessitate a focus on system efficiency, operational effectiveness, value to the customer, and innovation in work design and delivery.

REDEFINING ORGANIZATIONAL RELATIONSHIPS AND ACTIVITIES

Progressive health care organizations have abandoned bureaucratic organizational models in favor of task- or team-driven organizations. In these new models, the task(s) to be accomplished governs who works with whom and who provides leadership (Beer et al., 1990). Hospital leadership will continue to be a series of multilateral transactions focused on outcomes rather than on processes or specific functions (Flannery and Williams, 1990). Those operational transactions defy chain-of-command relationships and require leaders to be both creative and theoretical (Ehrat, 1990). Continuous quality improvement is an operating mindset rather than a prescriptive set of actions. Traditional quality assurance activities are but a small component of quality improvement efforts. To better meet the needs of users, organizations must define both their internal and external customers. In the final analysis, most internal departments are customers of other internal divisions. In the same fashion, most internal departments are service providers to other internal divisions. A service improvement attitude must prevail internally as well as externally.

The quality improvement cultural revolution demands that divisions and departments posture themselves differently and that organizations establish mechanisms to recognize and reward desired behavior. The modus operandi becomes one of incremental organizational successes and wins based on

- The satisfaction of customers and users
- Efficiency gains in the parts and the whole
- Overall system improvements that assist the service production process

Clearly, this type of thinking runs counter to discipline rivalry, division or unit competition, the collection of tin soldiers, and other political and power games commonly observed in organizations. Historically and now, disciplines and divisions within health care systems suffer from a lack of interconnectedness.

This lack of interconnectedness contributes to competition, inefficiency, and redundancy and drives up costs.

Continuous improvement has to do with empowering knowledgeable workers to make timely decisions in the service provision process. It further has to do with reducing inefficiency and duplication and, therefore, costs. Management consolidation has assisted these desired outcomes. The intent of these radical changes in health care delivery systems is to avoid self-liquidation (Bolster, 1989), an organization's "inability to earn a level of operating profit enough to sustain replacement of plant and equipment" (p. 1). Bolster notes that "business winners will be those organizations that learn to deliver improved care and reduce costs such that operating margins can sustain plant and technical advances" (p. 7).

Retooling Management Education and Support

To achieve continuous quality improvement, a number of support and structural changes are necessary. First is the retooling of management education and support. In speaking of education, Simpson (1962) suggested that the mark of an educated person is a versatile, flexible mind that can deal effectively with changing conditions. Clearly, discipline curriculums require modification to yield players oriented toward team accomplishments and customer satisfaction. Common languages are required across organizations to foster understanding and collaboration. What may be good for any given discipline, including nursing, may not add value to the whole.

Creating Barrier-Free Health Care Environments

The challenge for the various health care professions and technical specialties is to create new methods for achieving distinction and fame beyond those that further segment organizations. Organizations must overcome discipline and department barriers to become seamless from the perspective of the customer. In many instances, architectural constraints promote unnecessary service segmentation and contribute to both inefficiency and work redundancy. Solutions to these structural barriers require innovative thinking within cost constraints. Similarly, the redesign of both work and work flow is fundamental to speeding production and eliminating work redundancy. Although no blueprint for work redesign exists, it seems clear that many roles and jobs will, of necessity, become more general and flexible. The motivation for change is customer satisfaction, user convenience, and organization efficiency gains. At present, most patients move through acute care centers in a misguided and poorly coordinated, assembly line fashion. Perhaps the industry's greatest redesign success to date is implementation of the LDRP concept, where the customer remains stationary, and services are brought to the bedside as necessary. Work redesign is a function of barrier-free thinking among key disciplines and management. Given nursing's dominant role in coordinating all aspects of patient care, the nurse manager is in a key position to influence patient care redesign efforts.

In further attempts to streamline operations and reduce the costs of doing business, organizations have focused on decreasing the aggregate number of position titles and have sought coherence among the multiple job categories. Nursing has been a leader in that arena through its efforts in practice differentiation. Stimulated by demand-driven labor shortages, differentiated practice calls for licensed practicing nurses to be used in accord with their respective experience, ability, and formal and continuing education (Ehrat, 1991). Often, differentiated practice, as a human resource deployment model, has accompanied patient care redesign efforts, though it is intended to enhance any model of nursing care delivery. Frequently, differentiated practice accompanies the implementation of managed care or case management or other hybrid patient care models that are geared toward care continuity. Although there is, at times, frustration on nursing's part regarding the slowness of other organizational units to develop and implement service innovations, this situation supports the view that meaningful change begins at the periphery of organizations and works inward. Beer et al. (1990) cautioned that organizations cannot be transformed by leader-imposed programs but rather through transformations occurring at the periphery and supported by the leadership. Nursing has been the initiator of many shared service programs intended to improve both patient outcomes and organizational efficiency. For example, decentralized pharmacies and laboratory substations have contributed to care improvements in larger hospitals.

The Role of the Nurse Manager

Nursing's positive relationship with other organizational divisions is a prerequisite to establishing a barrier-free environment focused on meeting customer needs. To expand its professional scope of influence in work redesign, nursing has focused attention on the system as a whole. Whenever possible, key disciplines are part of nursing's planning and innovation efforts. The nurse manager can both spearhead and coordinate these activities. Resistance to nursing's leadership in these efforts will be diminished if improved patient care outcomes, rather than improved nursing care, is the focus.

Nurse leaders must continue to extend themselves and expand the thinking of their respective staffs to identify effective methods for diminishing departmental barriers. Multidiscipline quality improvement groups and collaborative practice forums have been effective strategies for engineering system and care delivery enhancements that improve the care delivery process. In all instances, nursing should hold on to the view that patient care enhancement is a multidisciplinary task and an organizational, rather than a disciplinary, success.

Hospital operations must continue to evolve in ways that place patients' needs rather than departments' needs in the forefront. Both the customer satisfaction movement and quality improvement philosophy have placed nursing at the helm of many organizational work redesign efforts. This positioning has served as a vehicle for recognizing nursing's expertise. In this new role, nursing must seek innovation rather than retooling outmoded delivery mechanisms and systems. To stimulate innovative thinking, the nurse manager can promote a "blow it up and start over" mindset. Processes must be reviewed from a system and organizational perspective. The objectives should be improved patient care outcomes and system efficiency. Efforts must be directed toward identifying and solving system problems rather than system symptoms. At the heart of system redesign is the notion of discontinuous thinking, where there is recognition of and breaking away from the history and assumptions that underlie operations and practice (Hammer, 1990). Hammer (1990) points out that work structures and processes need to be updated to match new technologies, demographics, and business objectives (vision and strategies). Hammer (1990) identified seven principles for redesign (pp. 108–112).

1. Organize around outcomes, or tasks.
2. Have those who use the output of the process perform the process.
3. Subsume information processing work into the real work that produces the information.
4. Treat geographically dispensed resources as though they were centralized.
5. Link parallel activities instead of integrating their results.
6. Put the decision point where the work is performed, and build control into the process.
7. Capture information once and at the source.

Nurse managers can facilitate and assist organizations in achieving work redesign. All processes should be reviewed with the customer and quality improvements in mind. Gavin (1987) proposed eight dimensions of quality adapted by the author to guide service improvement efforts (pp. 104–108).

1. Performance: how the service or product is delivered (promptness, consistency, wait times, etc.)
2. Features: characteristics that enhance the basic service (patient education, activities to occupy wait time, valet parking, etc.)
3. Reliability: the probability of performance breakdown over a prescribed period (influenced by equipment failure, staffing shortages, etc.)
4. Conformance: the degree to which provided services meet organizational, professional, and accreditation standards
5. Durability: the amount of long-term good one can derive from the services rendered
6. Serviceability: the speed, courtesy, reliability, and competence of follow-up
7. Perceived quality: the overall reputation of services provided by the facility

Whether service improvement attempts are unit based or organizationwide, Gavin's dimensions provide a framework for evaluating quality initiatives. The nurse manager can use this framework to evaluate planned changes in care methodology, teaching programs, multidisciplinary endeavors, and so forth. Clearly, new methods for evaluating and measuring quality must accompany service redesign efforts.

Although the continuous quality improvement philosophy has only begun to penetrate acute health care, its adoption will grow as external pressures increase.

The dissonance created between present-day realities and an organization's desired future becomes the driving force for innovation. A clearly articulated vision statement is fundamental to that effort. Quality improvement is a philosophy rather than a program, requiring intensive organizational commitment over time. In the manufacturing industry, significant outcomes from quality renaissance programs have required 5 to 10 years of committed effort. It is assumed that the same or greater amount of time will be required in health care institutions, owing to discipline diversity. Berwick et al. (1990) state, "the notion that quality is made not by people but by processes, flies in the face of a central myth of health care—that quality is made by doctors" (p. 15). Changing this historic physician perspective will require the intensive involvement of physicians in continuous improvement efforts. It will also require time.

The business of health care redesign and customer satisfaction is the responsibility of all levels of health care leadership. A manger's role in that effort is to design, to teach, and to serve others—to promote ongoing organizational learning (Senge, 1990). From their research on leadership, Kouzes and Posner (1990) identified 5 practices and 10 commitments common to leaders who achieve extraordinary goals in organizations (p. 14).

1. Leaders challenge the process by
   • Searching for opportunities
   • Experimenting and taking risks
2. Leaders inspire a shared vision through
   • Envisioning the future
   • Enlisting others
3. Enabling others to act by
   • Fostering collaboration
   • Strengthening others
4. Modeling the way by
   • Setting the example
   • Planning small wins
5. Encouraging the heart by
   • Recognizing individual contributions
   • Celebrating accomplishments

These practices and commitments can serve as guides for the nurse manager and can assist in promoting and supporting unit-based quality enhancements. For organizations in total to achieve quality improvement success, the collective leadership must subscribe to these or similar philosophies and behaviors. "Long term successful companies stand for more than just profit or market share. They also stand for people—people who contribute net value to society" (Belasco, 1990, p. 102). Sahney and Warden (1991, p. 14) note that

> Success will be achieved when senior management spends more time addressing the improvement of quality in the organization than solving its financial problems; when quality items appear for discussion on all management, medical staff, and board

meeting agendas, and when all employees, including managers, apply the concepts of TQM in their daily work

The nurse manager role and individual nurse manager's performance are vital to institutional quality improvement efforts. By guiding or participating in multidiscipline quality initiatives, the nurse manager can assist in improving patient care support operations. The breadth of nursing's understanding regarding patient care needs is additive in all patient care improvement initiatives. Working collaboratively with other operations managers, the nurse manager can gain a heightened awareness of internal and outpatient customer needs and can assist in redesigning processes to meet those needs. Nursing's expertise in problem identification and resolution is helpful in all redesign activities.

The scope of the nurse manager role provides a natural bridge for community interface. Through community involvement, the nurse manager can gather perceptions about institutional services provided and share information about ongoing quality improvement successes. The confidence displayed by nurse managers in external interactions assist in building customer support and institutional loyalty. As a further bridge to the community, the nurse manager can implement patient follow-up activities and programs to link past users with community resources.

The nurse manager can develop multiple methods for involving staff in identifying and resolving system problems that inhibit performance and efficiency. To be successful in those endeavors, however, the nurse manager must view himself or herself as a teacher and a mentor. Staff will perform according to the expectations established by the manager. If the nurse manager's attitude and behavior convey support for multidisciplinary collaboration, proactive thinking, a willingness to challenge past norms, and nondefensive support for change, staff will follow suit. In today's health care arena, there is little room for traditional management thinking or behavior. The evolving manager's role encompasses employee support and empowerment, the modeling of organization philosophy, and an orientation toward total system improvement. Owing to both the breadth of responsibility and organizational visibility, nurse managers are expected to be in the leading wave of transformed managers.

References

Albrecht, K., & Zemke, R. (1985). *Service America!* Homewood, IL: Dow-Jones-Irwin.

Band, W. A. (1991). *Creating value for customers*. New York: John Wiley & Sons.

Beckham, J.D. (1991, Nov.-Dec.). Strategic thinking and the road to relevance. *Healthcare Forum Journal*.

Beer, M., Eisenstat, R., & Spector, V. (1990, Nov.-Dec.). Why change programs don't produce change. *Harvard Business Review*.

Belasco, J.A. (1990). *Teaching the elephant to dance: Empowering change in your organization*. New York: Crown Publishers.

Berwick, D.M., Godfrey, A.B., & Roessner, J. (1990). *Curing health care*. San Francisco: Jossey-Bass Publishers.

Bolster, C.J. (1989). Current economic realities: Implications for the nurse executive. *Aspen's Advisor, 5*(3).

Charan, R. (1990, Sept.-Oct.). How networks reshape organizations—for results. *Harvard Business Review*.

Crosby, P. (1979). *Quality is free: The art of*

making quality certain. New York: NAL Penguin.

Crosby, P. (1984). *Quality without tears: The art of hassle-free management.* New York: New American Library.

Ehrat, K.S. (1990). Leadership in transition. *Journal of Nursing Administration, 20*(10).

Ehrat, K.S. (1991). The value of differentiated practice. *Journal of Nursing Administration, 21*(4), 9–10.

Flannery, T.P., & Williams, J.B. (1990). The shape of things to come. *Healthcare Forum Journal, 30,* 15–31.

Gavin, D.A. (1987, Nov.-Dec.). Competing on the eight dimensions of quality. *Harvard Business Review,* pp. 101–109.

Halpern, M.H. (1971, Spring). Why bureaucrats play games. *Foreign Policy.*

Hammer, M. (1990, July-Aug.). Reengineering work: Don't automate, obliterate. *Harvard Business Review,* pp. 104–112.

Juran, J.M. (Ed.). (1988). *Juran's quality control handbook* (4th ed.). New York: McGraw-Hill.

Kouzes, J.M., & Posner, B.J. (1987). *The leadership challenge: How to get extraordinary things done in organizations.* San Francisco: Jossey-Bass Publishers.

Mager, R.F. (1975). *Preparing instructional objectives* (2nd ed.). Belmont, CA: Fearon Publishers.

Quality special report. *Business Week,* June 8, 1987.

Sahney, V., & Warden, G. (1991). The quest for quality and productivity in health services. *Frontiers of Health Services Management, 7*(4), 2–40.

Senge, P. (1990, Fall). The leader's new work: Building learning organizations. *Sloan Management Review.*

Simpson, A. (1962). The marks of an educated man. In L. Locke, W. Gibson, & G. Arms (Eds.), *Toward liberal education* (4th ed.). New York: Holt, Rinehart & Winston.

U.S. Office of Personnel Management. (1980, Jan.). *Manager's guide for improving productivity.* Washington, DC: Office of Personnel Management.

Walton, M. (1986). *The Deming management method.* New York: The Putnam Publishing Group.

CHAPTER 5

BECOMING A MANAGER

SALLY EVERSON-BATES
LINDA JENKINS

EXECUTIVE SUMMARY

The essence of management is learning how to deal effectively with the needs of a diverse population. To the new nurse manager, this population includes clients, supervisors, peers, non-nursing managers, physicians, nursing staff, and support staff. In short, the new manager will be faced with trying to meet the needs of many others. These needs come in varying levels of importance and urgency, and they usually contain at least one surprise or twist just to test one's flexibility.

There are some basic skills that can help to make the transition to manager successfully. This chapter provides some guidelines for developing the skills required. There is a brief review of traditional management structures, followed by the hard part—how to do it. Examples are given of such management basics as clarifying values, prioritizing, delegating, dealing with procrastination, and effective decision making.

There is an insightful section on time management based on the core belief that time is used most efficiently when goals are set and prioritized. Information on how to chair a meeting and avoid wasting time is provided. The chapter concludes with a review of stressors and how we can control them to reduce our stress level.

This chapter contains valuable information for the new nurse manager, and it also serves as an excellent checklist for experienced managers.

T he decision to become a nursing manager is a significant step in professional development. It requires a shift in work patterns from direct clinical intervention to meet the needs of individual patients and families to indirect and less visible activities of enabling the work of caregiving staff. This chapter provides you as a new manager with a basic understanding of how nurses manage and guidelines for using several management tools. Because hospitals are in a period of significant transition, we begin with a description of traditional management structures and then analyze more recent trends in the management processes.

TRADITIONAL MANAGEMENT FUNCTIONS AND PROCESS

Traditionally, hospitals were structured hierarchically with multiple layers of managers, each typically having one job to perform. Managers' primary functions were identified as planning, organizing, controlling, and decision making.

How these functions were accomplished was described as management process, a series of interrelated events influenced by the environment and consisting of five elements: input, processor, output, controls, and feedback mechanisms (Table 5–1).

These concepts and language originated in industry, where outputs, or industrial products, were costed and measured. Emphasis on outcomes and the bottom line were a natural outgrowth of such an orientation. Hospitals adopted management practices from the industrial community as hospitals moved from a small service orientation to big business after World War II. These traditional management concepts were developed in a patriarchal structure, resulting in styles of hierarchical or military-like structure, presenting an autocratic approach to decision making and relying on positional power for authority.

Over the past 15 years, increasing costs of health care have forced hospitals to rethink their structures and style (see Chapter 3). As a result, many acute care

TABLE 5–1 Nursing Management Process

COMPONENT	DEFINITION
Processor	Nurse management group that has operations authority for Planning Directing Controlling
Outputs	Products or outcomes, such as Patient care Staff development Research
Controls	Monitoring of operations through tools, such as Nursing budget Performance evaluations Disciplinary procedures Union contracts Accreditation and licensure surveys
Feedback mechanisms	Information/data for evaluating Financial reports Nursing care audits Quality assurance surveys Peer review of employee performance
Output	Products of all operations targeted toward effective patient care

institutions have chosen to change from hierarchical to decentralized organizational structures, streamlining organizations by reducing the number of management layers and increasing the job responsibilities for those who remained. As a result of this transition, the role of the nurse manager shifted from primarily a clinical focus to one requiring clinical skills and business acumen.

Today, most first-line nurse manager responsibilities typically include

- 24 hour responsibility
- Hiring and firing
- Evaluation, coaching, and counselling
- Staffing, scheduling
- Fiscal management
- Patient care management; standards of care and practice
- Staff development, education
- Interdepartmental collaboration, coordination
- Public relations, representing organizations

These complex responsibilities often require simultaneous attention and, unlike clinical practice, must be accomplished primarily by working through others. How this occurs requires a brief discussion of several key concepts, the most critical of which is participatory management.

Decentralization of decision making in hospitals and the concept that staff should participate in those decisions are often linked. The linking of participation and decentralization is predicated on the notion that people who are closest to an activity, such as the care provider to the patient, have the most accurate knowledge and perspective, both of which are essential to making timely, effective decisions. Participatory management does not mean abdication of responsibility for decision making or decision outcomes but recognizes that staff who understand and are committed to a decision will be more motivated to accomplish the outcome.

Such management concepts are particularly familiar and comfortable for nurses because they are closely related to patient care management strategies. This style of management recently has been identified as a typically female management strategy.

WOMEN'S MANAGEMENT STYLE

Women's management style has been compared with many of the highly successful Japanese management strategies. Nurse manager roles, filled primarily by women, have been identified as having many similar traits. Such approaches are now widely recognized as both effective and productive but formerly had been criticized in traditional management environments as being more involved with process than outcome.

Typically, women

- Are more likely to build consensus among a group to obtain a wide base of support for an issue.

- Work with all levels of staff to maximize cooperation in accomplishing tasks or objectives.
- Encourage those involved in a project to discuss, debate, and examine potential approaches to that project's accomplishment.
- Gather information from multiple sources to apply in designing an approach that can be supported by all participants.

This approach increases motivation and the probability of a high-quality outcome. At the same time, overemphasis on process without a ratio that produces concomitant results must be avoided.

NURSING MANAGEMENT PROCESS: THE ROLE OF THE NURSE MANAGER

The most useful description of the nursing management process for new nurse managers is one derived from others experienced in the role. In a study by Everson-Bates (1990), experienced nurse managers were asked to characterize their role. Their descriptions suggested that most of their efforts required interacting with individuals or groups to influence behavior.

Establishing, Monitoring, and Maintaining Standards

The most common activity described was establishing, monitoring, and maintaining standards. These standards included such areas as clinical, fiscal, and personnel policies or social behavior, as in compliance with guest relations. Developing and maintaining standards requires definition of acceptable performance or behavior for staff and applying such sanctions as coaching and counseling or evaluations to ensure staff compliance.

Providing Resources

The second process nurse managers described was provision of resources, such as emotional support and goods and services for staff. Typically, this process is most highly valued by staff, and nurse managers who are skilled at this are labeled visible and available to staff. This activity includes helping staff with professional and personal development, for example, how to cope with death, drug addiction, or conflict. Providing goods and services includes equipment and supplies and visible hands-on clinical assistance when needed.

Translating, Interpreting, and Negotiating

A third management process was described as translating, interpreting, and negotiating. Nurse managers must interact with multiple disciplines, each with its own values, perspectives, priorities, and language. Negotiating working relationships and solving problems that arise with physicians, finance, personnel, dietary, laboratory, or other staff is a role expectation for most nurse managers.

Supporting and Providing for Change

The final management process described was supporting and providing for change. As the health care environment continuously changes, facilitating change is becoming a larger part of the manager's role. Small changes happen daily: new order forms are issued from purchasing, or documentation procedures for granting vacation time are revised. Large changes happen almost as frequently: managers resign, reporting lines are altered, or new programs come online. To create an environment that will facilitate change, managers need to build a common social bond of trust among staff. Trust occurs when staff know and accept the manager's values and are certain that decisions will be made consistently and fairly.

Trusting relationships with staff develop through both work and social interactions. The work-focused relationships evolve through repeated interactions where staff needs for resources are consistently met. Social relationships also are important and essential to bridging status barriers. Whether intended or not, a manager has a different status and possesses power that staff do not have. Collaborative professional working relationships require that staff view the manager as accessible and supportive. There are many ways to bridge this status gap, such as simply having lunch with staff.

As bonds of trust and working relationships evolve, staff will begin to reflect the beliefs and values of the nurse manager. It is important for a new nurse manager to develop and articulate clear, consistent values for staff to emulate. To clarify personal values, the nurse manager may ask himself or herself the following questions:

1. Where do I spend most of my time?
2. How do I structure my day?
3. Are there any activities I engage in no matter what else is happening?
4. What makes me angry enough to visibly display it?
5. What staff behaviors please me enough to say "good job" publicly?

Although health care management is increasingly oriented as a business requiring business strategies and using business language and concepts, such as *strategic planning, cost containment, market analysis,* and *cost–benefit,* first-line nurse managers are primarily women managing women who are providing a caring interactive service. Practicing, effective nurse managers state that the essence of the management process is

- Creating standards
- Providing necessary resources
- Facilitating interactions with multiple groups
- Assisting staff to incorporate change

The nursing management process facilitates these activities by creating an environment of trust and clear explicit values.

PRACTICAL APPLICATIONS

The components of the nursing management process are

- Achievement of productivity
- Decision making

- Prioritizing
- Delegation
- Avoiding procrastination
- Time management
- Stress management

Productivity

Nursing management is a process with measurable outcomes. The achievement of these outcomes is measured as productivity, which is an economic concept that compares the output of an industry to the resources or input required to produce products or provide services. Productivity also refers to the quality and quantity of that product or service.

$$\text{Output} - \text{Input} = \text{Productivity}$$

Input may include the costs of labor, technology, supplies, and services. Labor productivity is the ratio of the dollar value of the product to the labor hours used to produce it.

$$\text{Labor productivity} = \$ \text{ Product value} : \$ \text{ labor costs}$$

In most industries this will provide a simple estimate of production efficiency.

It is far more complex to define productivity in health care, since there are many variables in the measurement of input and output. Fewer problems exist in measuring labor, supplies, and equipment than exist in measuring the output of patient care quality. Measurement of labor costs for nursing personnel is complicated by the fact that nurses have varying levels of pay. Even those nurses with similar pay may vary considerably in efficiency and competence.

Difficulty in measuring productivity in health care, particularly in nursing, is due to the uniqueness of services provided and the lack of consensus about how to measure the results of those services. Productivity is directly affected by the nurse's ability to prioritize, delegate, and manage time. Productivity is also related to organizational goals, departmental objectives, and personal values. The more synchronized these expectations become, the easier it is to accomplish established objectives and improve productivity.

Prioritizing

Prioritizing is the ranking of the importance of tasks required to accomplish objectives. Prioritizing requires an understanding of the management role and an identification of objectives required to reach management goals. Every nurse manager faces the situation of having too little time allocated to perform all the planned activities. This is when the skills of prioritization need to be developed. These skills undoubtedly will be influenced by what the nurse manager values most in meeting his or her objectives.

Prioritizing is not something that can be accomplished in isolation. A new manager must be attuned to the values of the organization, the supervisor, staff, and colleagues, all of whom have a legitimate stake in influencing how the manager chooses to allocate his or her time and efforts. The nurse manager with strong values in the area of staff development may place a higher priority on daily interactions with staff than on daily preparation of operational reports. In this case, the task of completing reports can be delegated to qualified staff, allowing the manager to perform the higher valued function.

Judgments in prioritizing should be made carefully and negotiated with the immediate supervisor to determine whether the manager's priorities conflict with the expected job performance. Learning to prioritize effectively is a complex process that requires thoughtful attention. The following exercise is focused on short-term prioritizing of just 1 day, but the same procedure may be used on longer periods of time or larger projects.

The following is a prioritizing exercise:

1. Gather data
   - Compile a list of tasks that you are planning to accomplish in a day.
   - Place each activity on a small piece of paper, such as a 3 by 5 inch card.
2. Evaluate the list
   - Is it realistic? If yes, proceed to step 3.
   - If it is not realistic, place any cards that do not require accomplishing today in a separate *delay* pile.
3. Place cards in order
   - Rank order your cards from the highest value to the lowest.
   - Place the stack to one side.
4. Review the *delay* cards
   - When you have verified that those activities can be delayed, set them to one side.
5. Review prioritized activities
   - Request a colleague with more nurse management experience to review and prioritize the activities.
   - Request your immediate supervisor also to prioritize the activities.
6. Compare the results of each prioritization
   - Did each of you prioritize the same?
   - Did you learn that values varied?
   - Did you recognize any need to change your prioritization or to negotiate acceptance of your priorities by your supervisor?

There are no correct or incorrect answers to this exercise. It is simply a tool to assist in the development of prioritization skills and values.

A nurse manager has flexibility in developing his or her role and in prioritizing to meet the agreed on goals of the position. The objectives must be communicated clearly to the nursing staff in particular. In this manner, the nurse manager empowers staff to prioritize their activities and to take action that facilitates achievement of expected outcomes.

Delegation

One of the early lessons of every nurse manager is that there is never enough time, and learning what to delegate, why, how, and to whom does not come easily to many nurses. Delegation is an important aspect of time management and staff development. It is the process of getting results through people while facilitating their growth and controlling results, not people. The nurse manager needs to delegate in order to free time to manage and lead.

Benefits of Delegation

- It increases the results the nurse manager is able to produce.
- It frees time for the nurse manager to manage.
- It is motivational.
- It teaches people new things and allows them to grow both personally and professionally.
- It introduces new ways of doing things into the patient care unit.

The two most common reasons nurse managers give for not delegating are a lack of trust in the person's abilities and the belief that she or he can do it better. Whether the nurse manager can do it better is the wrong standard of assessment. A better question is: Can the staff nurse do it well enough? Delegation is also a process of staff development.

Delegating must be equitable, which means assigning both pleasant and unpleasant tasks as well as making sure the workload is shared. A common problem for managers is overusing high performers.

How to Delegate

1. Decide who can do the task by evaluating staff skills/abilities and workload.
2. Identify the kind of resources needed and the amount of coaching from the nurse manager.
3. Understand the assignment and be able to express it in measurable terms.
4. Clarify the desired outcome and responsibility, avoiding the three common causes of failure
   - Instructions/desired outcomes not communicated
   - Inadequate knowledge to complete assignment
   - Know how and what to do but need to know why to increase motivation and a sense of trust
5. Give the authority and its parameters, such as budget limits, along with the responsibility for the project.
6. Discuss the assignment in detail, including potential problems they may encounter.
7. Clarify the due date and arrange for feedback at specific time intervals where assistance can be provided if needed.
8. Help prioritize activities of the project.
9. Let the person know you are a team and will share the success or failure.
10. Praise the activity lavishly and immediately at accomplishment.

What Not to Delegate

1. Do not delegate disciplinary actions.
2. Do not delegate anything the nurse manager is legally responsible for.
3. Do not delegate morale issues.

Avoiding Procrastination

Procrastination is the action of not acting. It is making the choice not to choose. There are so many demands for the nurse manager's attention, it is all too easy to put off starting or finishing a difficult task. Reasons for procrastination include

- Lack of information
- Lack of discipline
- Lack of health, or physical debilitation
- Environmental or organizational chaotic scheduling of meetings, etc.

Following are some ways to avoid procrastination:

- Schedule activities when you are in your prime time for mental alertness and energy.
- Schedule the most difficult tasks during prime time.
- Break difficult or unpleasant tasks into small manageable pieces. Take a 2-hour project and divide it into 15-minute segments each day.
- Remind yourself through notes and other methods.
- Tie a tangible reward for yourself to the completion of the project.
- Use do-or-die dates. If projects are not done or initiated by the completion date, take the task off your list.
- Focus your attention.
- Fight perfectionism. Perfectionists procrastinate far more often than realists and may continually refine a project until time runs out.

Decision Making

A new nurse manager will be asked to make many decisions ranging from small to large, usually on a daily basis. The following guidelines may assist the nurse manager in making sound decisions in a timely fashion.

1. Take risks in making decisions; try to have enough information but do not go into information overload; determine the worst possible result of the decision and whether you could accept that.
2. Do not try to make a lot of small decisions, but focus on the larger ones.
3. Know the desired outcome of the decision and have alternatives available to help you reach that outcome.
4. Do not make decisions when you are tired, upset, or overstressed.
5. Make your own decisions. Intuition does count.

Time Management

Time cannot be managed, but it can be used efficiently. The nurse manager does not have total control over the 8 and sometimes 10 hours of work per day. Superiors, other managers, subordinates, other health team members, as well as patients and their families, control much of the time. The higher the manager's position in the organization, the more his or her time is controlled by others.

Effective use of time requires an organized approach to realistic planning despite the unpredictability of the day's events. Activities need to be scheduled in the appropriate sequence with sufficient time allocations. There should be enough time allowed to respond to new priorities that may arise on a daily basis. The manager must adhere to the plan/time schedule to produce desired results.

Time is used most effectively when goals have been set and prioritized. Organizational goals typically have time frames established. Personal and professional goals become more manageable when they are grouped into time frames, such as 2 years, 6 months, and daily. Identification of the desired results may be accomplished by prioritizing the long-term, short-term, and daily goals. It is rarely possible to accomplish all goals in each area. Unexpected events that reach crisis proportions are familiar to the health care industry and nursing management in particular.

Planned activities for the day may be interrupted by such occurrences as an equipment breakdown, a large number of admissions in a short time frame, or a personnel crisis. If priorities have been set for the day's activities, the nurse manager can then quickly decide which of that day's goals can be abandoned. Another advantage to prioritizing daily goals is the insight it gives into the manageability of staff's workload, morale among caregivers, and other dynamics of the patient care unit.

Scheduled time to work on longer-range goals needs to be integrated consistently into the daily or weekly plan for accomplishments. If the nurse manager is responsible for a project, such as developing a proposal for a new skilled nursing unit, blocks of time must be set aside during the week to do the necessary research. Selecting the days and times with the least chance of disruption requires evaluation of the daily activity trends. If meetings are typically scheduled for Wednesday and Thursday, and Monday often requires schedule adjustments to address incidents that occur over the weekend, Tuesday and Friday would be more appropriate for scheduling blocks of time.

There are several time wasters to avoid. Even though the goal may be clearly identified in the initial action plan, tasks may expand to the point that the goal is lost sight of. To avoid this trap of poor time use, the nurse manager must review frequently the relationships of tasks, time, and effort and their appropriateness in accomplishing the goal.

Other time wasters are unproductive meetings, drop-in visitors, and frequent or long telephone calls. Visitor and phone call problems can be reduced greatly by minimizing time spent in the office. The concept of management by walking around provides the opportunity to contact a large number of people on a frequent and consistent basis. Scheduling of rounds/availability provides timely information and recognition of potential problems for early resolution.

Meetings

A nurse manager functions as a central point for coordinating organizational activities that affect patient care and frequently is asked to participate in committees. The increase in participatory management concepts and decentralization in health care organizations has resulted in nurse managers attending an ever increasing number of meetings. With larger amounts of time being spent in meetings, it is necessary to maximize efficiency to avoid the frustration of wasting time. As a committee member, the nurse manager must evaluate the group dynamics and determine how best to facilitate group process. The committee chair should

1. Schedule the meeting time and place to facilitate prompt attendance
2. Prepare and distribute a written agenda in advance
3. Begin on time
4. Facilitate active participation by each member

Within a short period after the meeting, minutes should be distributed recording the discussion, action, and accountability for each agenda item.

Beepers have become important communication tools for the nurse manager. They have reduced overhead paging in most health care organizations, helping to lower noise levels. Beepers also have become one of the greatest causes of distraction and interruption of meetings where several managers are in attendance. If the nurse manager cannot delegate beeper response to an available associate, the beeper service should be instructed on how to screen calls. They should interrupt only if there is a crisis or emergency, as determined by the caller. When callers are given the power to make the decision of interrupting the meeting, waiting until the meeting is over, or dealing with the issue at hand, most will make the appropriate decision. Dealing with staff in this participatory manner will help reduce the number of meeting interruptions and will improve staff decision making. If the caller makes an inappropriate decision about interrupting the meeting, the situation should be discussed in a nondisciplinary fashion to help improve the caller's decision-making ability.

To use time effectively to accomplish goals, it may be necessary to say no to a co-worker's request for assistance with an interesting project that does not contribute to the nurse manager job responsibilities or goals. Saying no is difficult for most nurse managers, but it is an essential skill to learn to maintain efficient use of time and good interpersonal relationships.

Stress Management

Occupational stress has been studied by at least four disciplines, and each has developed unique definitions and conceptualizations of stress. As explored here in relation to the role of the nurse manager, a stressor is an environmental stimulus that an individual perceives as stressful and responds to with a physiologic or psychologic strain. For example, early research examining head nurse stress found the primary stressor to be incongruence between supervisor and head nurse expectations for the role, resulting in burnout (strain) and turnover (coping strategy) (Anderson, 1964).

Identifying Stressors

Identifying stressors and, perhaps more importantly, developing strategies for coping with stress are essential tasks for becoming an effective manager.

Stressors inherent in accepting a management position for the first time are well documented in the literature and can be most easily understood as environmental or job related. There are also sociologically based stressors that are derived from the fact that managers are all nurses and, commonly, women managing women.

Job-related stressors include both the need to learn new role responsibilities and behaviors and the simultaneous loss of traditional social support systems and identity. Concomitant is the need to acquire a new, role-appropriate support network and identity.

Learning the tasks and role behaviors of management are difficult but only minor stressors for most new managers. The greater source of stress will likely be the need to acquire a new identity that integrates and reconciles personal/professional values with those of the corporation/hospital. The burning need to contain costs and be more productive to maintain present-day corporate or hospital health is often at odds with the professional value of meeting all the health care needs of an individual patient and the patient's family. The nurse manager not only must find a personal resolution for these and numerous other conflicting values but also must give leadership to staff in such areas.

Equally stressful is the fact that as this identity is evolving, the nurse manager may be losing what have traditionally been supportive relationships with other nurses and physicians who give care at the bedside. These losses typically occur for two reasons. Most clinicians perceive the role of the ideal manager as one of enabling their work by providing resources. They also perceive most management as doing little more than going to useless meetings and thwarting the "real work" of hospitals by restricting resources. It is not uncommon for the manager to be confronted by clinical colleagues who ask such questions as, "You used to be such a good nurse. Why did you give that up?"

In addition, most effective managers are concerned with both appearing and behaving in a manner that is perceived as fair by staff. Developing or maintaining personal relationships with individuals one manages often is perceived as giving special privileges, whether or not that is factual. Thus, if the nurse manager has moved up the ladder in the hospital where he or she practiced as a staff nurse, the manager may be forced to give up previously supportive relationships and be savvy in the development of new, institutionally based supportive relationships.

Stressors are not only environmentally created but also are the result of the nurse manager's sociologic status as a woman. Several recent studies found that the typical nurse manager is a woman between 35 and 45 years of age, is currently (or has been) married, and has children or other familiar caretaking responsibilities (SEB/AONE/Hingley and Cooper). One study also found that at some point in this time frame, the study participants were currently or had attended school for an advanced degree. Whether carrying such complex and demanding roles simultaneously is realistic or why nurses make such choices is beyond the scope of this chapter. However, multiple, complex, and often conflicting roles are clearly a source of strain.

Stress Response

Strain, the response to these stressors, has been described by nurse managers as both somatic and psychologic. Typical somatic responses have been reported as high blood pressure, weight fluctuations, migraine headaches, and epigastric pain. The psychologic responses are those most frequently associated with burnout, chronic anxiety, fatigue and sleep disturbances, irritability, and generalized depression.

The turnover rate among nurse managers is problematically high, a strong indicator that one coping strategy is simply to leave the role. Although this approach will likely be successful in reducing stressors, there are experienced managers who have developed less drastic approaches to stress reduction that allow them to continue in the role.

The most common of these strategies are physical and typically include some form of exercise or hobby that is absorbing or physically demanding, such as jogging or gardening. Meditating has been used and is once again gaining popularity as a stress-reducing strategy.

Managers often try to develop barriers or boundaries that separate their roles, which is particularly difficult for women. Common techniques include working extra days if necessary but never bringing work home or choosing a particular point in the commute to and from work where thoughts are deliberately changed from one role to the other.

Stress is essential to growth and change and is likely to continue as an issue for health care managers. The challenge is to establish approaches to work that keep stressors under control and mitigate strains as they occur.

The nurse manager role is one of the most challenging, yet rewarding positions in acute care settings in the 1990s. This chapter describes several techniques to help to accomplish the goals identified as important to improve care when accepting the role. Maintaining a positive attitude and approach, keeping focused on objectives, and sincerely caring about the development of subordinates will lead to significant accomplishments.

References

Anderson. (1964).

Beehr T., & Franz, T. (1986, Fall/Winter). The current debate about the meaning of job stress. *Journal of Organizational Behavior*, 1986, *8*(2), 5–18.

DePree, M. *Leadership is an art*. East Lansing:

Michigan State University Press, pp. 23–29.

Everson-Bates, S. (1990). *The nurse manager: An ethnography of hospital-based first-line nurse managers practicing in an expanded role*. (Dissertation, University of San Diego).

Gillies, D.A. (1989). *Nursing management: A systems approach*. Philadelphia: W.B. Saunders.

Sanborn, M. (Speaker). (1989). *Managing your time, energy, and relationships*. Englewood, CO: ManagersEdge Corporation.

Sullivan, E.J., & Decker, P.J. (1988). *Effective management in nursing*. Menlo Park, CA: Addison-Wesley Publishing Co., Chap. 1, 2, 3, 4, 11.

CHAPTER 6

MANAGEMENT PROBLEM SOLVING AND DECISION MAKING

MARJORIE BEYERS

EXECUTIVE SUMMARY

Decision-making styles and methods reflect the organizational architecture and culture. In today's social and political environment, people are empowered because they have information. Decisions increasingly involve others in participative processes. Because decision making is integral to the managerial role, decision-making styles reflect personal management style. Using technology to support decision making and being clear about what information one needs for assessment, planning, and evaluation facilitate rational and objective decisions. Most decisions have a context, situation, and outcome that cannot be totally rationalized. The human factor in decision making is thus important. It can be expected that decision making will continue to change along with influencing changes in the organization. Effective managers can retain their edge if they acknowledge and master these changes.

A manager's life is spent making decisions. Management literature over time reflects not only the importance of decision making in the management process but also the way decision making is changing in today's highly technologic society. In this chapter, the reader has the opportunity to consider how decision making affects performance outcomes. The emerging concepts and methodologies for making decisions are presented. Problem solving and decision making are presented as key management attributes. Concepts of effective decision-making behaviors are integral to management behaviors in today's organizations.

It should be noted that problem solving and decision making may or may not be synonymous terms. One makes decisions when solving problems and may solve problems when making decisions. For the purpose of discussion, the term *problem solving* is used to relate to an immediate, more circumscribed element, activity, or issue. *Decision making* is the term used to relate to thinking things through—whether it be a work plan, a strategic approach to an action, a new policy, or a new project.

Managers at every level in the organization engage in complex decision making. All managers use problem-solving, decision-making processes to accomplish their respective assignments and responsibilities in the organization. Managers make decisions about who, what, when, where, and why of activities or tasks that should be performed in the organization. Making decisions is the manager's work and is thus the crux of management. The quality of one's management performance is closely related to one's effectiveness in decision making. The human factor in decision making is expressed in one's management style. To some extent, the effectiveness of decision making in the management situation is a matter of how one's personal style fits that of the work group and of the organization.

Management science is concerned with effective use of resources to accomplish goals and objectives. Performance measurement is essential to evaluate the effectiveness and efficacy of outcomes. Therefore, the manager is well served by thinking through a framework and conceptual approach to his or her problem solving/decision making. All types of managerial decisions relate the conceptualization of process, structure, and outcome to the application in work processes at every level in the organization. Decisions are tested through application within the organization in pragmatic operations, in executive management, and governance. A defining characteristic of a manager is the willingness to make decisions and the competence to make effective decisions.

THE NATURE OF DECISION MAKING

Decision making is rational behavior. It involves thinking. In today's environment, decisions are made by knowledge workers of all types. Decision making and problem solving are commodities that knowledge workers offer for compensation. The challenge today's managers face is how to manage people who are paid to make decisions. Managers are accountable for decisions made by those they manage. Managers at all levels in the organization are accountable to enable individual decision making and to create the environment in which individuals and teams make effective decisions. The manager must foster the relationships that support effective individual and team performance.

Decision Making in Traditional and Evolving Organizations

Managerial decision making is changing as organizations change. Organizations are thought to be evolving into new types. Transformation of organizations from the traditional bureaucratic type to a new dynamic, variously shaped organization is expected to be completed by the turn of the century (Drucker, 1992). In the meantime, the evolving organization will continue to change. Already, many organizations are quite different, and expectations for managers reflect the differences. Some of the differences are pertinent to this discussion. In the traditional organization, decision-making authority is conferred on a few persons, empowered by their positions in the architecture of the organization. Top level managers prescribe functions and who should implement them. Decisions are transmitted to others through policies, procedures, and rules that employees are expected to follow in their work. The well-managed traditional organization maintains order and control through uniformity and consistency (Rockart and Hofman, 1992).

In contrast, the evolving organization is well managed if people are empowered to make decisions about their work. In the new type of organization, individuals and teams are empowered to decide and to act. Policies are held to the minimum necessary for the common good, and procedures and rules support decision making. Managers thus foster plurality in behaviors.

Decision Making in Nursing Service Organizations

Nursing service organizations reflect the changes taking place in all types of business and social organizations. For example, in traditional approaches to nursing service, decisions are made about the tasks of nurses and assisting staff. Procedures are then formally written and promulgated in the nursing policy and procedure book. Procedures contain information about what should be done, by whom, in what sequence, and using what materials. Managers are responsible for writing procedures, for teaching employees to use the procedures correctly, and for ensuring competent performance. They supervise implementation, conduct routine evaluations, and update procedures as appropriate.

Compare the traditional expectations with the evolving ones. Nurse managers in evolving organizations are expected to empower nurses to make decisions about patient care. The manager's task has changed. Instead of deciding what others should do, managers now empower others to decide. Learning new behaviors may be difficult for the managers. It is difficult to dismantle good work, such as is found in policy and procedure books. To make the situation more complex, managers must support change in others while they work out their own change responses. The staff nurses and other employees may be having just as difficult a time accepting their responsibility for decision making.

It should be noted that empowerment does not magically create decision makers. Empowerment must be managed. People need to be clear about what they are empowered to do, may need preparation to enact the new functions, and require support during the time they are learning to become comfortable and effective in their empowered state (Bowen and Lawler, 1992).

APPROACHES TO DECISION MAKING

Historically, management texts have emphasized the importance of decision making. Current approaches to decision making have been evolving during the past 50 or more years (Beyers, 1991).

Scientific Problem Solving

The groundwork for scientific management was laid in the early part of the century. Much of what we know today about decision making has been influenced by development of the scientific approach to decision making and problem solving. In both, the manager defines the problem, collects and analyzes data, reaches conclusions, develops an action plan, and implements the plan.

Managers who make decisions in the organizational environment use the systematic problem-solving approach to reach rational, objective decisions.

The goal to achieve rational, objective decisions is critical when one considers all of the noncontrollable and potential emotional factors that influence decision making and the response to decisions once made. Because organizations are often complex, organizational decision making is complicated by relationships. The manager must consider responses to decisions because people's perceptions color their trust and relationships with not only the manager but also the organization. Part of the manager's job is to engender willingness to contribute to accomplishing work, to use talents of employees effectively. It has been shown that involving the parties who will implement the decisions in the decision-making process promotes participation in the implementation phase (Peter and Morton, 1978).

Participatory Decision Making

Managers may use participatory decision making as a powerful management approach. People may participate in any part of the decision process: defining the problem, collecting the data, analyzing data, identifying probable courses of action or remedies to the situation. The manager should strategize participation in decision making to achieve the greatest benefit from the process. The outcome is often rewarding. For example, a group often reaches the best solution to a problem. Usually, group members select the option that works best in the situation to resolve the problem. Participation in decision making is important when the solution or implementation requires buy-in from others. The process of selecting options for solution promotes understanding, a sense of ownership, and a feeling of acceptance.

INFORMATION TECHNOLOGY AND DECISION MAKING

The new science of informatics, of decision support systems, and other high technologic approaches to help people with decision making are designed to facilitate thinking. Technology is now available to format problem solving/ decision processes for orderly progression, for positing potential outcomes of various approaches to a problem or decision, and for developing cost-benefit analysis to evaluate a decision. Systematic decision making can be supported by software programs and computer databases that make information accessible. Decisions at every level of the organization are facilitated by information. Technology now supports a broad range of organizational decision making from simple decisions to complex strategic and futures planning. There are programs for developing operational business plans, project work plans, and the budget.

Information systems are changing the way people make decisions in organizations (Peter and Morton, 1978). There is some indication that data availability and processing are also changing the knowledge that nurses and others use for decision making. One of the questions raised in the current literature is whether managers will be needed in the future, given the technologic support for decision making. For example, will the technology replace decision makers (Drucker,

1992; Horton, 1992)? In service industries, such as health care, technology may replace people for routine, programmable tasks and will support decision making for caregivers, patients, and families. The availability of technology for systematic decision making does not replace or displace the need for clinical and managerial decision making.

THE HUMAN FACTOR IN DECISION MAKING

In the emerging organizations it seems likely that systematic approaches to decision making will continue to be used for routine matters as well as for support of complex decisions. It can be expected that technologic, social, and political forces will continue to require the human decision maker, willing to take risks and to be accountable for implementation.

Consider, for example, decisions achieved through negotiation; that is, give me what I want, and I will give you what you want. Face-to-face discussion and confrontation will continue to be normal behavior in complex organizations. The individual's beliefs, desires, goals, and competencies will continue to influence effectiveness. External events, such as policy decisions, backed by authority will continue to influence individual and organizational decisions. People will continue to use political processes to accomplish what they need to have done but cannot do in their separate and individual capacities.

THE SELF-CONFIDENT MANAGER

Problem solving and decision making are managerial tasks. For the manager, the personal and critical human factor in effective decision making styles is self-confidence. Confidence in one's own decision making is an essential behavior of effective managers. To be confident, the managers must accept their decision-making authority. The confident manager knows how to make decisions, who to involve in decision making, and how to recognize occasions for decision making.

ASSESSMENT IN THE DECISION-MAKING PROCESS

Nurse managers are fortunate because the decision-making process used in providing nursing care is very similar to the process that managers use. For every decision, there should be an assessment of the events, facts, or other contributing causes to the problem or to creation of the opportunity for decision. All sides of the topic or issue are examined. The manager observes the situation: the behaviors and the facility and resource aspects. Systematic assessment of these factors is supported by data collection: seeking input from involved individuals and groups, completing a literature review, examining the issues from different perspectives, and seeking input from experts. These typical assessment methods enable the manager to discern what is important in a given situation.

ORGANIZATIONAL RELATIONSHIPS

The assessment must also take into account the potential impact the decision may have on the organization. Decisions have an added dimension of complexity when organizational relationships, perceptions, and power issues affect the decision. Many decisions are more complex because the manager agonizes over who should make the decision, how the decision will be received, and other such factors. The situation of the decision affects the manager's response to and handling of the decision-making process.

For example, a manager may experience stress while making the difficult management decision, "Who should make the decision?" In some instances, the manager should decide to make the decision independently. Such factors as timing, confidentiality, or maintaining a strategic edge may indicate the need for an independent decision. In other instances, participation is critical to achieving a successful outcome. Managers, cognizant of their decision-making effectiveness, carefully consider who should be involved in deciding either the approach or the method for decision making or both.

Decision-making methodology is not much different from problem-solving approaches. Both are applied by people. Some problems must be solved independently; others should be solved by the group. The effective manager learns when it is appropriate to involve others in the decision-making process. The manager makes decisions about how to involve others in decision making. One of the keys to effective participative decision making is setting realistic expectations.

Different people may be involved in one or more steps in problem solving/decision making to define the problem/point for decision, collect data, analyze data, define options or various action plans, and discuss or make the final decision about action. Each step may involve different persons. Participation may be achieved by assigning each of these steps to someone or a group, by assigning different groups a different step or combination of steps, or by full participation in all of the steps. Another way to gain participation is to share the decision with another person or group and ask for assistance in developing an implementation plan. Depending on the type of decision, the situation, and the desired outcome, a manager decides what process to use for the decision making. The decision(s) may be reflected in a plan, policy, or other written materials that must be reviewed and approved. In this case, up-front participation by potential reviewers is helpful.

RECOGNIZING THE OCCASION FOR DECISION MAKING

Recognizing the occasion for decision making is a talent to be developed. The manager applies decision theory to practical situations and adapts decision-making styles to fit varying situations. Knowing what style to use for the desired outcome may be intuitive, gained through practice and developed through experience. The ability to make the right decisions at appropriate times and situations is the mark of an effective manager.

The situation/occasion for decision making may be analyzed to some degree by seeking some insights about the following points:

1. Identify the strategy or tactics that work best in this situation to achieve the goal. An example is deciding on a project to engage physicians and

nurses in improving the quality of care through data analysis and action planning.

2. Analyze and select the critical points of contact that must be considered in the decision-making process, the implementation, and potential consequences.

3. Evaluate the short-range and long-range impact potential to influence or affect behavior. Decisions with short-range potential to affect the organization may be structured for the short term, whereas those with long-term effects need to be designed to maintain a steady, focused course of action with built-in evaluation and revision of the decision at key points.

4. Project the probability that the decision/implementation may be changed in midstream because of factors, such as changes in staffing, personnel, resources, external regulations, or other pressures. The decision-making process must include evaluation of the potential factors with a backup plan for how to deal with any one of the possible events that might occur. A schedule for evaluating progress and for revising the decisions is critical.

The importance of decision relative to events surrounding the decision must be assessed. Factors include

- Impact of the decision
- Availability of decision support systems, including people/computers/software/experience data
- What is prudent
- What is valued
- Decisions about what to do/how to do it/when to do it/where to do it/why it is being done
- How to decide if you need help and when and where to go for help mentor/preceptor/experienced individual/analysis expert

DEVELOPING A PERSONAL DECISION-MAKING STYLE

Developing a personal managerial decision-making style is assisted by establishing a classification of the types of decisions one makes. An example of a useful classification a nurse manager might apply in practice is shown in Table 6-1. Readers are encouraged to use the classification to assess decision making in their own settings. For example, should individuals at the caregiver level be empowered to make decisions about care processes at the level of care delivery? Managers should match their decision-making objectives to those of the organization.

Newly appointed managers should also review the types and levels of decisions expected of them to ensure that their scope of decision making is appropriate for the position. One of the most difficult adaptations to a new position is matching one's own confidence and experience to the new position. Developing new relationships and keeping former relationships in perspective require thoughtful consideration and maturity. The tendency is to revert to the comfortable rather than risk the unknown.

TABLE 6–1 Classification of Health Provider Decisions

Care level decisions Assessment/plan/implement/evaluate.

Service level decisions Population of patients; grouping by some common characteristics to make sense of/garner and aggregate resources; what services needed; what resources required; how to provide the care level decisions.

Organization level decisions Architecture of the whole, that is the structure; how defined by purpose/expectation of outcome, that is, the mission, strategic plan, operating plan.

Community level decision How the organization relates to community; community services decision making. Within the classification of community level decisions, different approaches to decision making may be selected as appropriate to fit the demands. For example:

Individual, personal level decisions about patient care usually affect individuals on a more personal level. Both individual caregivers and members of care provider teams relate very directly to patient care decisions.

Management group decisions relate to service level decisions. Allocation of resources, cooperative interaction to complete an ongoing process, provide a service, or develop efficiencies or improved quality in one or more aspects of patient care are the types of topics managers make decisions about at the management group level. The management group may develop business and work plans for activities.

Manager to manager decisions may be related to policies, procedures, selection, employment, and discipline of employees; acquisition of capital; interdepartmental interactions; or sharing of resources.

Organizational level decisions often relate to employment practices and policies; facility use such as parking, locker rooms, and such employee supports; organizational mission, strategic planning, and goal setting. Infrastructure decisions relate to financing, facility planning and management, and external relationships.

Policy level decisions often reach beyond the organization to encompass the community/public policy/professional levels of interaction. These types of decisions require the manager to consider representation. If the manager is representing self, the decision may reflect personal perspective or bias. If the manager is representing the organization, the decision should reflect the organization's preferences.

An individual has choices about how to relate to decision making at a very personal level. Some considerations to use in thinking about one's own style include the following:

• Does decision making competence match desired performance?

- Does capability in making decisions influence behavior, quality, cost, or outputs?
- Does relationship to the group affect/influence outcomes?

Every individual and culture is guided by personal values and beliefs, and decision-making styles are grounded in the personal talents of the individual. As a manager, reflection on one's own background and experience is as important as reflection on the organizational structures and preferences for action. The organizational architecture is influenced by tradition and ideology. Today, as organizations are being transformed, much work is being put into deciding how to design the organization of the future. It can be expected that the organizational structure will reflect change for some time (Bowen and Lawler, 1992).

GUIDELINES FOR DECISION MAKING

Decision making in the transforming organizations differs somewhat from that in traditional organizations. Formerly, decisions were good or bad, right or wrong. In today's organization, the environment is dynamic. Few aspects of the organization remain the same for long, and the challenge is to make decisions that work in a turbulent environment. Decisions are not the end behavior but rather one aspect of a sequence of deciding, implementing, and evaluating in a learning mode (Weaver and Bryant, 1990). What can be learned from implementation of the decision may be as important as the decision itself. Decisions are viewed as choices. The first choice of the manager is deciding how to decide.

Decision-making methodologies have to be adapted to the new organization. Managerial decisions embody a set of activities that extend beyond problem solving. Managers must decide how to decide; they must decide who makes the decision and how to inform others of the decision. Managers are concerned about implementing the decision. They are also involved in evaluating performance related to the decision, particularly about learning how to do things better. Guidelines for these aspects of decision making follow.

1. What is the scope of this decision?
   - Who will be affected by the decision?
     Who needs to know?
     Who sets the criteria for the decision/outcome?
   - What are the consequences of the decision?
2. Who should make the decision?
   - Who is most qualified to make the decision?
   - Who has to implement it? understand and carry it out?
3. What are the interfaces for implementation?
   - What resources are affected by this decision?
   - Who provides, controls the resources for implementation?
   - How is evaluation of process and outcome accomplished?
   - In uncertain times, how do you weigh the cost–benefit of the decision?
   - Who or what is the targeted outcome for the activity involved?

- Which people will perform the tasks/activities implicit and explicit in the decision?
- Who has the ultimate accountability?

4. What are the implementation effects?
   - Who will follow through to ensure the desired outcomes?
   - How will the decision be evaluated?
   - Who will need to know whether the decision worked?

The type of decision being made is influenced by some critical factors in decision making. Consider the following about decision making.

1. What assumptions can you make about the decision?
2. What are the emotional factors in the decisions?
   - What individual beliefs color the way persons will make or receive the decisions?
   - How will people enacting the decision respond?
3. What are the risks?
4. What is pertinent?
5. What decisions will be effective?

Implications of each decision entail more decisions, such as how the decision will be communicated to others, how it will be promulgated, that is, presented and understood by the implementers. Implementing decisions means that they must be transmitted to others, taught, and marketed and that resources are deployed for implementation.

IMPLEMENTATION AND EVALUATION OF DECISIONS

In health care services, such as nursing, individuals are responsible for implementing the majority of the decisions. Thus the human factor in decision making also applies to the decision implementation (Young, 1992). The manager's leadership effectiveness, whether it be charisma or management authority driven, is important to obtain effective implementation buy-in. The manager thus should make decisions with conviction. The manager should also acknowledge when decisions do not work. Most managers recognize that decisions are made through a balancing of facts, beliefs, and motivation. The manager's self-confidence is thus important, and it takes maturity to be objective about one's own decisions.

Most managers consider the effects of their decision in relation to their position and ability to influence. Some guidelines for the manager in this aspect of decision making follow.

- Are you confident in your decision?
- Can the decision be carried out with others?
- Is there a logical basis for the decision?
- Are you able to appropriately justify the decision?
- Is the decision likely to be well received?
- How costly is the decision?
- Will it be popular? unpopular?

- Who/what will be affected by the outcome? If favorable? If not favorable?
- Will others respect you?

CREATING THE CYCLE FOR DECISION MAKING

Managers must think through all aspects of the managerial decision. One considers antecedent and future events related to the decision. One way to accomplish this perspective on the decision is to create a cycle of activities in which the need is identified for problem solving or decision making: the appropriate information is obtained, appropriate participants are informed and convened to make the decision, and the supports for decision making are in place. When decisions require process for buy-in, understanding, expertise, and other reasons, the manager makes sure that the decision cycle is communicated to others. Some guidelines follow.

- Keep individuals/teams/groups informed.
- Obtain input from others whenever possible about the decision substance, content, process, implementation, evaluation.
- Touch base with others about progress and results: learn reactions and responses.

DECISION-MAKING AUTHORITY

Because organizations are being transformed, decision-making authority is being questioned. Managers at all levels have to work through appropriate behaviors in decision making. It can be expected that managerial behaviors related to decision making will continue to be influenced by sources of decision authority. Traditionally, authority is derived from factors, such as position power in the organization: expert power based on knowledge or informal power based on leadership talents. In traditional organizations, knowledge and information are sources of power. Managers keep knowledge and information from employees to retain the edge in position authority.

Information as Empowerment

One of the major changes related to transformation of organizations is that managers can no longer constrain information. Consequently, information is now a source of empowerment for all who have access to it. Information is now available to individuals on a wide array of subjects. Many persons now have access to information that was restricted to managers. Information and thus power have been redistributed. It can be posited that knowledge is now more important than information to managers as a source of power. For the manager, this knowledge refers to knowing how to work with people whose place in the organization depends on having specialized knowledge.

Middle Managers and Their Supervisors

All managers, particularly first-line managers, can be stressed in decision making when attempting to discover the best way to relate to others in making decisions. First-line managers have to acknowledge and respect the authority and options for decisions of the person they report to in the organization. They must also satisfy the employees who report to them. Being in the middle requires managers to clarify what kinds of decisions they are expected to make autonomously, what decisions have to be communicated and to whom, and what decision-making authority is outside their domain. A framework for working with one's supervisor is useful to establish the relationships. Decision grids, such as pert charts, a pro forma budget, or others, help managers communicate the decision process and implementation. Knowing what is expected fosters positive interaction and trust in cooperative experience with one another. Developing the grids enables cooperative planning. Personal preferences of key individuals, the situational factors that should be figured into the decision-making process, and resource allocation aspects can be planned for in developing the grids.

DECISION MAKING AND RISK TAKING

Decisions often are associated with risk. Taking the risk to make a decision may be one of the first challenges for first-time managers or those in new positions. Routine decisions in traditional organizations are made thoughtfully, set forth in policies, and thereafter become the law. Transforming organizations require comprehensive thinking at every level of decision because the former consistency in management promoted by policies and procedures is being dismantled. There are advantages to having stable policy and procedure. People know what is expected of them. Without the stability, the organization has become more dynamic, and the focus is on the purpose and flow of the work.

MAKING DECISIONS IN TRANSFORMING ORGANIZATIONS

There are few guidelines to help managers with decision making in the transforming organizations. A beginning draft of guidelines is presented in this section. The manager has to ascertain what factors to consider when deciding how to decide and with whom. Helpful information is gleaned from observation and talking to others through formal focus groups, informal discussions, and other interactive techniques.

In all types of organizations there are some constants that probably will not change but that are critical in decision making. These are issues of trust, relationships, and, as mentioned previously, organizational culture. Trust can be assessed but not contrived. Relationships can be developed but not exploited more than once. Culture can change, but usually only with great effort, some pain, and considerable growth that most often occurs at an uneven rate in an organization (Horton, 1992). Consequently, it is not easy to decide how to develop one's management style to influence or to decide the appropriateness of a decision in a given situation.

Decision inputs for all types of organizations probably will remain constant over time. These factors are related to internal and external data sources for assessment of problems/occasions for decision. The manager needs to be observant and alert to identify and respond appropriately to occasions for making decisions. Systematic input from individuals who benefit from or who contribute to the activities about which decisions are being made is an imperative in informed decision making. This input is particularly relevant to making decisions about services that people need, want, or plan to use. Market trends continue to be a source of data important in all business and industry decisions that meet a service need, want, or desire. Managerial decisions relate to resource allocation and use with the expectation of a beneficial outcome, usually economic. Consequently, market share is a proxy indicator of whether the service/decision has potential to have an impact.

Technology analysis is critical in decisions that involve capital and facility aspects of activities. The cost of technology includes capital expenditures for acquisition, costs of maintaining and housing the item, and training staff to use it. The expected life span of technology, the potential for a new generation of the same technology, and a myriad of other technology-related factors must be included in the assessment for many decisions related to health care. Some of the current product acquisition cost–benefit analysis formats can be adapted to technology assessment analysis.

Managers, when making decisions, are shaping their own future. Selecting the key influential factors related in any decision is a practice that managers must develop. Some of the knowledge about influential factors is best learned through experience, by seeking advice from others, and from scanning the field and the literature to ascertain what is important and what is peripheral. Because managers have limited time, one must select what key factors to pursue in assessment and planning. Not all interesting factors can be pursued. Consequently, the manager selects those that potentially can make a positive difference.

FUTURE TRENDS IN DECISION MAKING

A new dimension of decision making in today's organization is getting ready for and maintaining optimal performance in an environment of turbulent change. Organizations employ many different types of decision making to prepare for and deal with constant change. Tapping databases to evaluate cost of care, to analyze variances in critical pathways or in patient care service budgets, to manage flexible staffing and scheduling, and to project future trends are a few of the decision supports available today.

Software programs are available to help organizations understand the uncertain environment and possible future events. Programs that allow modeling and scenario development or simulations can be used for problem solving and decision making about the future. Optimization models now provide an approach to determine the wider organizational system: a series or sequence of events to accomplish goals through algorithms. Heuristic problem solving, based on observations of human experience, enables managers to build descriptions of events that can be analyzed to improve the decision process.

References

Beyers M. (1991). Guest editorial. *Nursing Administration Quarterly, 15*(4), viii.

Bowen D.E., & Lawler, E.E. (1992). The empowerment of service workers: What, why, how and when. *Sloan Management Review, 33*(3), 31–44.

Drucker, P.F. (1992). The new society of organizations. *Harvard Business Review, 70*(5), 95–104.

Horton, T.R. (1992). Decision making: Does Rambo have it right? In *The CEO paradox, the privilege and accountability of leadership* (pp. 10–19). New York: American Management Association.

Peter, G.W.K., & Morton, M.S. (1978). *Decision support systems: An organizational perspective* (pp. 21–49). Reading MA: Addison Wesley.

Rockart, J.F., & Hofman, J.D. (1992). Systems delivery: Evolving new strategies. *Sloan Management Review, 33*(4), 21–31.

Weaver, F.M., & Bryant, F.B. (1990). An analysis of decision making in discharge planning. *Evaluation and the Health Professions, 13*(1), 121–142.

Young, S.T. (1992). Multiple productivity measurement approaches for management. *Health Care Management Review, 17*(2), 51–58.

PART TWO · · · ·

SKILLS OF NURSING MANAGEMENT

"**W**e have watched the golden era of the health care industry disappear. Resources have become more limited at the same time that the demand for services has grown. Health care institutions are recognizing that the public cares about the quality of services provided and the continuity of these services to the patient. To respond to these monumental changes, institutions need creative approaches to develop responsible, efficient delivery systems. No one administrator, nurse executive, physician, department head, or nurse can do this alone."

JANE FAIRBANKS NEUBAUER

CHAPTER 7

INFORMATION MANAGEMENT AND COMPUTER TECHNOLOGY

ROY L. SIMPSON

EXECUTIVE SUMMARY

As health care technology and staffing shortages increase, we find ourselves in the curious position of having to do more documentation and communication in less time. To make matters worse, there is also the issue of finding enough time to properly evaluate what we have documented. Although it is not the sole answer to these pressing issues, a well-designed computerized information system can free up valuable time by providing readily accessible data. This chapter offers a straightforward look at what is on the market and how it might apply to various needs.

The chapter begins with a few concise definitions that explain computer technology to the novice and provide an updated review for those in the know. This is followed by a look at the various types of information systems in use in today's hospital environment: nursing information systems, hospital information systems, decision support systems, and executive information systems. Clinical applications and research capabilities of computer systems are covered. The usual components of each type of system are described in user friendly language.

A fundamental decision in the area of hospital information systems is whether to use a single vendor or to assemble a niche-based solution from a variety of vendors. A word of caution here: Single vendors offer completely integrated systems, which may not provide full functionality. Niche-based systems offer more functions, but it may be less likely that the system components can talk and work with each other.

Practical guidelines are provided for selecting an information system and encouraging the staff and individual users to fully adopt the system. The chapter ends with a brief look at future technologies in health care information systems.

T echnology can alleviate many of the challenges and pressures nurses face in today's dynamically changing environment. Patient acuity and patient demands for quality service are increasing. At the same time, staffing shortages may leave many nursing departments chronically understaffed. Nursing information systems and hospitalwide information systems are particularly important in this environment because they can reduce the burden of documentation, communication, and planning.

In addition, information systems assist and provide definition, standardization, and uniformity to nursing practice, as well as to nursing phenomena. They also provide an important source of raw data for nursing research. As a result, technology can make a big difference in nursing's overall efficiency and professional standing. More importantly, technology supplies the means and potential to improve the quality of patient care.

UNDERSTANDING TECHNOLOGY

Before one can fully understand the scope of nursing informatics and hospital information systems, it is important to understand the technologic components involved. It is also important to remember that the pace of technology continues to accelerate. Solutions that are standard today may be made archaic in a matter of months by the introduction of new, better, and faster technology. Nevertheless, it is useful to get acquainted with the basics of today's technology in the nursing and hospital environment.

Hardware

The hardware is the actual box the system runs on—including all electronic components and peripherals. Hardware can be anything from a small, inexpensive, single-user personal computer (PC) to a giant, multimillion dollar mainframe system. The primary difference between the two ends of the spectrum (besides price) is processing power—how much information each box can process efficiently. Familiar hardware vendors in health care include IBM, Digital Equipment Corporation, Data General, and Hewlett Packard. In most cases, hardware vendors do not produce hospital application software, the actual program that runs on the hardware or tells the hardware components what to do.

Software

To help understand the distinction between hardware and software, it is useful to consider hardware as a stereo and software as a tape or compact disc (CD). There is usually only one hardware platform (stereo), but it can run many, many programs (cassettes or CDs). Software is called the *application* or *system*. In this chapter, software programs are referred to as *systems* when discussing nursing information systems and hospital information systems.

Operating System

The operating system is often called the brains of the computer or the master program. Without an operating system, the hardware could not operate, nor could it run the software programs. The operating system instructs the computer how to run. For single-user programs on a PC, an MS-DOS operating system is the most common. For larger systems involving multiple users, a multitasking, multiuser system is more appropriate. Multitasking means the ability to run more than one program at a time on a single computer (Cushing, 1991). For example, a user may want to use the system's word processing function at the same time that another program is compiling, running, and printing a scheduling and staffing breakdown report in the background. Common multitasking operating systems include OS/2 and UNIX/AIX.

A multiuser system allows more than one operator, on separate terminals, to retrieve and operate the same program at the same time (Cushing, 1991). Multiuser systems commonly are created with local area networks (LANs) and wide area networks (WANs) by linking or connecting several computers to one master computer, called the *file server* (Simpson, 1992). Operating systems that are both multiuser and multitasking include UNIX/AIX or other systems referred to as *open*.

THE NURSING INFORMATION SYSTEM

A nursing information system (NIS) is typically a software system through which nursing and health data are collected, stored, processed, retrieved, displayed, and communicated in order to administer nursing services, standardize the delivery of patient care, and link research and education to the practice of nursing (Saba & McCormick, 1986).

In a hospital environment, NISs typically are subsystems that are linked to the larger hospital information system (see next section). They include the following functions or subsystems: patient acuity or patient classifications for allocation and distribution of nurse resources, care planning and documentation, quality assurance, inventory, order entry and results reporting, discharge planning, and evaluation.

Patient Acuity or Patient Classification

A staffing and scheduling system is a by-product of a method by which patients are categorized and staff is distributed and allocated based on patient care needs. Acuity is determined by predetermined indicators. Staffing needs may be determined by some or all of the following criteria: the patient's routine self-care needs, the time required to carry out various nursing activities, specific or unique patient care requirements, and nursing diagnosis for patient dependency. The advantages of using a patient needs/acuity-based staffing and scheduling system include a more effective, efficient distribution of the workload, resulting in greater optimization of staff and more efficient use of personnel resources.

Care Planning and Documentation

Nurses spend an estimated 40% of their time managing, communicating, and documenting patient information. Hundreds of pieces of information must be entered into patient records on a daily basis—usually manually. A care planning and documentation system often can reduce this burden.

Many care planning and documentation systems focus on medical and nursing diagnoses using the nursing process. These systems often provide concise, organized, shift-specific medical and nursing care orders for the patient's stay-to-date care. These systems also may automatically issue individualized care plans (based on hospital-defined standards of care or critical paths) as well as station worksheets and DRG tracking tools.

Major productivity benefits can be accrued from these systems, including improved quality of information, improved documentation, greater efficiency, reduced errors, streamlined communications among clinicians, and increased communication between departments.

Quality Assurance

Quality assurance (QA) systems evaluate the quality of nursing services based on patient records, nursing care plans, patient observation and instruction, nursing personnel observations, and patient care criteria based on predetermined standards. QA systems not only help nursing track performance and plan care improvement goals but also provide performance comparisons among multiple hospitals.

Inventory

These subsystems streamline communications between the nursing department and materials management for supplies of pharmaceuticals, linens, and medical equipment. Nurses may create, change, or print purchase orders on-line (right on the computer) and send them electronically (the nursing computer speaks directly to the materials management computer to place the order). Patient charges for supplies often are entered via bar coding equipment. The system monitors and audits patient charges and ensures that they are reflected correctly on the patient's hospital bill.

Order Management/Results Reporting

Order management systems significantly enhance communications between nursing and other departments, including radiology, clinical laboratory, nutrition, and pharmacy. Nursing initiates orders on the system, and they are automatically generated in appropriate departments. Charges are logged as the orders are processed. Many systems also allow for *panel ordering and charging* or *order explosion,* where one transaction can set off an explosion of multiple orders and charges—streamlining work efforts and improving productivity. It is important to note that order explosions can be difficult to program in a system, not only because of its complexity but also because it represents the core of a results reporting clinical system.

With these systems, comprehensive results are reported for major departments as well as for smaller, specialized service areas. The results are communicated back to the point of origin for inclusion in the patient's medical record.

Discharge Planning

These systems allow nursing to standardize discharge plans and improve the effectiveness of communications regarding nursing patient orders and options for aftercare community support. The system effectively reviews the patient's to-date stay and progress and charts the patient's learning needs and requirements for exercise, nutrition, and physical therapy.

Evaluation

Many systems support the final step in the nursing process—evaluation—through a report writer capability that can help nursing managers analyze variances to treatment protocols. The report writer typically reaches into many areas of the hospital's network to extract the data nurses need to evaluate the quality of delivered care and the productivity and cost-effectiveness of staffing levels. Based on these reports and findings, nursing can modify both care plans and orders for intervention.

Point of Care Systems

One of the newer tools available to nursing departments is point of care technology. Point of care systems require special bedside terminals. These terminals collect data through integrated optical bar code readers that scan bar codes on patients, employees, and medications. Information entered once at the bedside flows directly to ancillary testing and clinical departments (sometimes even the physician's home or office) and to medical records and accounting/billing departments. Some systems allow data to be presented in clinically significant ways through the use of graphing, charting, and color coding. Thus, clinicians can graphically display and correlate vital signs, medications, and test outcomes in a variety of ways, significantly improving the quality of delivered care.

Because patient data are recorded accurately at the point of care, the system ensures improved charting and documentation, increased access to vital information, better risk management, and improved productivity and cost control. These systems allow nurses to work smarter and allow them to "get back to the bedside where he or she wants to be" (Childs, 1988). In other words, they support clinical practice at the bedside. However, bedside technology may represent a paradigm shift in the practice environment.

HOSPITAL INFORMATION SYSTEMS

Hospital information systems (HIS) are understood to encompass the information-processing needs of the entire hospital—from administrative to clinical functions, including radiology, pharmacy, and laboratory. However, it is always useful when dealing with HIS vendors/suppliers to have each supplier define its specific definition of an HIS. Some suppliers may call their accounting and administrative system a complete HIS, whereas others may call their ancillary department system (such as laboratory or radiology) an HIS. Nurses must clarify the vendor's operating definition and establish minimum requirements of a system to meet nursing's needs as well as the needs of the entire hospital or health care organization.

In general, hospital information systems process information for patient accounting and financial management, patient care (which includes nursing information systems), laboratory, radiology, and pharmacy. Not all HISs have functions for all these areas, although some of the leading suppliers offer unified and completely integrated systems that include all of them. These are commonly referred to as *single-vendor solutions* and offer distinct benefits, which include single-source accountability and system uniformity. On the down side, single-vendor systems do not always feature the kind of rich functionality that niche suppliers can provide for individual hospital departments.

Niche-based solutions means different parts of the information systems are supplied by different vendors. These niche systems then have to be patchworked together to create a full HIS. For example, one supplier may provide patient accounting and patient care, another may provide radiology and laboratory, and still another may supply pharmacy. The advantage of buying separate pieces of the total HIS from different vendors is that, often, these small subsystems offer greater functionality. Nevertheless, this approach means that it is harder for disparate systems to talk to each other and work as a unified whole. Therefore, the sum of the parts may not be equal to the whole of a unified system when interfaced.

For single systems to work together as a unit, interfaces must be created. An interface is a program that allows one system to talk to another and share information. It functions as a type of translator between systems, just as a translator is necessary for speakers of two different languages to communicate effectively.

Patient Accounting and Financial Management

Because financial accounting is easier to automate than the often subjective and ever changing area of clinical monitoring, many of the first HISs began as accounting and billing systems. Today's financial management systems often include admissions, registration, and discharge assistance. Basic patient ID data required for billing and medical records can be entered once at the point of entry and made available to all major hospital departments throughout the patient's stay, discharge, and beyond. These systems reduce data entry and potential for errors.

Financial management systems often include *patient accounting* for timely and accurate billing and faster collections, *medical records* for tracking of all diagnostic and procedural data, *accounts payable* for maximizing the hospital's cash flow, *general ledger* for monitoring the hospital's financial position, *materials management* for controlling the activities of purchasing, receiving, inventory maintenance, and accounts payable, and *payroll and human resources* for managing multiple types of payroll and personnel data.

Patient Care

To most clinicians, the most important aspect of an HIS is its ability to manage and monitor patient care information. A significant portion of a patient care system is also a part of the nursing information system, which includes order management and results reporting. However, a hospitalwide information system also benefits other clinical constituencies in the hospital.

Most patient care systems assist clinicians (including physicians and technicians) through scheduling capabilities that control workflows throughout the entire hospitals. For physicians, many system suppliers ofter physician registry and accessing systems, which allow doctors to access the HIS and use their own system for logging and receiving messages and consultations. Physicians may preadmit patients and access patient demographic and clinical data from their own systems. Terminal links can be placed at the physician's office or home for remote hookups to the system.

Laboratory

Laboratory information systems not only improve the quality of operational controls but also enhance the effectiveness of communications with external constituencies. These systems typically automate order management, clinical chemistry, microbiology, hematology, urinalysis and immunology, surgical and anatomic pathology, blood bank results reporting, quality control, workload recording, and contract billing.

Radiology

Radiology information management systems control and manage the flow of patients and information within the radiology department. They also provide a means for consistent, accurate, and clear results reporting. These systems typically automate patient scheduling, order management, examination reporting/resulting, film/file room management, management reporting, activity tracking, and QA measures.

Pharmacy

Pharmacy management systems are designed to help the pharmacy department support high-quality patient care through increased clinical screening and monitoring capabilities. They also assist pharmacy departments with business management and ambulatory care services for outpatient care.

DECISION SUPPORT AND EXECUTIVE INFORMATION SYSTEMS

Decision support systems (DSS) usually are considered management information systems. These systems allow managers to make informed operating and management decisions based on "what if" analyses and forecasts (Brown, 1991). Executive information systems (EIS) consolidate and summarize those analyses and forecasts, interpret them in light of the goals of the entire organization, then represent them in easy to understand visual formats (Simpson, 1991).

DECISION SUPPORT SYSTEMS

Hospital and nursing information systems are transaction-based systems that produce immense amounts of raw data. However, millions of bits of data do not provide managers with the information they need to make the proper decisions. DSSs are the vehicle though which raw data are turned into information on which managers can base their decisions. These systems typically cover the following areas of management concern.

Cost Accounting

Cost accounting is basically a process by which costs for every expense in the health care organization are accounted for, analyzed, and reviewed to determine how resources should be allocated and how much revenue is needed to continue operating. In a hospital environment, cost accounting can be broken down into *clinical cost accounting* and *management cost accounting*.

Clinical cost accounting can be considered a type of product costing, which helps health care organizations know whether they are making or losing money from each patient, groups of patients, doctor, nursing department, DRG, and third party contract. Management costing is the process of discovering whether the services provided to patients justify the cost of service. It brings the benefits of cost accounting to the world of operational control.

Some systems also assign *resource utilization* analyses to cost accounting functions, which allow highly detailed looks at resource consumption. Resource utilization reviews also provide an in-depth look at the quality and performance of individuals and groups of clinical providers.

Case Mix

These systems organize information on clinical performance, resource consumption, demographic patterns, and financial results to predict how changes in patient volume will affect costs, quality, and profits. Nursing managers can use case mix capabilities to predict staffing, recruitment, training and use needs (Simpson, 1991).

Departmental and Whole Organization Budgeting and Forecasting

DSSs actually began as budgeting systems. Because of today's industry pressures—including complex reimbursement schemes—sophisticated budgeting and forecasting capabilities are required for many midsized and large organizations. Many systems provide comprehensive financial modeling and budget applications for simplifying the budget process, improving performance monitoring, and providing detailed and accurate forecast models.

Marketing Planning

Many systems now combine external marketplace data with internal data from other DSSs. This allows hospitals to establish and review strategic plans and marketing activities. These systems often merge clinical and financial data with powerful industry databases. These databases may include patient demographics, service location analyses, market segmentation and targeting, and surveys of physician and consumer preferences.

EXECUTIVE INFORMATION SYSTEMS

In many health care and business circles, the last bastion of computer illiteracy is in the executive suite. Most users of computers are workers, and the typical executive involvement with computers involves reviewing the computer-generated output (reports). The advent of EIS threatens to change this pattern. EISs are the first systems designed for the executive user and not the staff user.

EISs typically depend on the information generated by DSSs, but instead of analyzing the raw data, executive systems consolidate it, interpret it, and visually represent it. Satisfying top management's need for better information is the most commonly expressed business objective for an EIS (DeLong & Rockart, 1988).

According to Brown (1991), "Executive Information Systems let corporate heads view and sometimes manipulate data from various corporate and external information sources. The systems are tailored to executives' needs in key ways: They display information in simple, often graphic, formats. They present timely information that the executive has determined is vital to his company. And they can be easily used by the rapidly decreasing population of computer illiterates" (p. 28).

EISs have been compared to the advent of television because they represent the news in visual, encapsulated stories—much like television news—using color, graphing, charting, and icons (Keegan, 1991). EISs inform executives on the status and performance of the hospital based on key indicators of hospital performance, including net income, census, cash balances, patient acuity, capital expenditures, staffing levels, and the level of patient or physician complaints (Simpson, 1991).

The purpose of an EIS is to provide executives with information, not just data. These systems are unique in that they allow executives to drill down to deeper levels of information. For example, one highlight report may tell the nursing administrator that the nursing department is over budget in staffing. The system allows the user to investigate which service area is the problem, then go further down to look at which shift, then which unit is responsible. At the same time, the system can be correlating those data with patient acuity. The major benefit of EISs is that they empower executive users to make better decisions and give them greater insight into the overall health of the organization.

CLINICAL APPLICATIONS OF COMPUTER SYSTEMS

The advancement of clinical computing has been hampered by clinician concern over quality of care and patient control. Much technology in the area of clinical applications, particularly in regard to medical DSSs, is either fairly new or concentrated in teaching centers where the technology is being continually researched, tested, and experimented on.

Historically, clinical computing has centered around these basic areas: ICU monitoring, medical records systems, patient monitoring in the operating room, and medical DSSs.

ICU Monitoring

The care of critically ill patients requires considerable skill and prompt, accurate treatment decisions. ICU monitoring systems can assist physicians and nurses in improving the quality of care through ongoing physiologic monitoring (Gardner, 1986).

Most basic ICU systems display the ECG and heart rate with sound alarms. They also typically analyze ECG arrhythmias, monitor intravascular pressures and respiratory status, and measure oxygen saturation (Gardner, 1986). Arterial and pulmonary catheters to measure blood gases are common. In addition, these systems typically automate infusion pumps, ventilators, urine output systems, chest tube drainage measuring systems, and ear oximeters.

The problem with physiologic monitoring systems is that each monitor is made by a different vendor. As a result, they often do not operate similarly or as a unit. For these systems to work together in a unified clinical information system or operate connected to the larger HIS, they must be able to communicate with each other. However, this is nearly impossible without the creation of interfaces (Simpson, 1992). An interface is a program that functions as a type of translator between systems, just as a translator is necessary between speakers of two different languages to communicate effectively. Although translated dialogues work fine, they can be at risk for misunderstandings and communication breakdowns. In addition, it can be very expensive and time-consuming for a hospital to undertake the creation and testing of numerous (sometimes up to a dozen) interfaces for the continuum of physiologic monitoring systems.

One common solution in the industry is to have each monitoring device share a common interface that can convert the unique system data communications needs (*protocol,* or the way each system talks) into a standardized hardware and software system (Hawley, Tariq, & Gardner, 1988). This is accomplished by creating a local area network (LAN) around each patient.

One LAN can have as much as 300 devices plugged into its network, each with its own identification code. Some systems can support thousands of device ID codes, each classified by type of machine—fluid delivery devices such as IV pumps, fluid collection devices such as urine output measurement devices, respiratory life-support instruments such as mechanical ventilators, and noninvasive measurement devices such as automatic cuff blood pressure (Gardner, 1986). Some advanced systems include audible sound production capability, pushbutton switches, and greater memory space for increased capacity.

Automating the ICU is made difficult by vagueness as to regulatory responsibility. Medical devices (which include physiologic monitors) are regulated by the Food and Drug Administration (FDA), whereas LANs and HISs are not (Simpson, 1992). Interfaces serve as the bridge between the monitoring systems and the rest of the information system. It is not clear whether the FDA considers interfaces within its realm of regulatory control, and if so, how that would affect the development of these systems.

Medical Records Systems

Medical records systems are computerized, time-oriented summaries of patient charts (Whiting-O'Keefe, Simborg, & Epstein, 1980). They are automated tools by which clinicians record progress notes and interventions during the patient's stay, replacing current paper-based, narrative documents. Medical records systems are still primarily in the research and testing phase, although prototypes have been used and developed by large teaching hospitals for more than 10 years. These systems, by virtue of the size of data requirements and complexity of automating clinical diagnoses, are typically immense in size and cost, making them virtually inaccessible to all but the largest teaching hospitals and best-funded medical centers.

Pioneers of medical record prototype systems include the Summary Time-Oriented Record (STOR) model from the University of California, San Francisco, the HELP model from Latter-Day Saints Hospital in Utah, the Regenstrief Medical Record from Wishard Memorial Hospital in Indianapolis, the THERESA system from Grady Memorial Hospital in Atlanta, and The Medical Record (TMR) from Duke University in North Carolina.

Electronic charting, though still in its infancy, can have a tremendous impact on the quality and productivity of a health care institution (Sisk & Rappoport, 1989). Because of their size and complexity, these systems commonly require large data storage dictionaries for storing and retrieving huge amounts of detailed clinical data, chronologic flowsheets that mirror the way nurses and physicians deliver care, computerized problem lists and standard forms that will still allow for individual notes, and coded data searches for easy data retrieval (Sisk & Rappoport, 1989).

Patient Monitoring in the Operating Room

Operating room (OR) systems typically include scheduling, intraoperative monitoring of patients, report generation, and permanent storage of perioperative information and research (Garfinkle et al., 1987). OR systems help clinicians improve care by linking OR data—mode of anesthesia, monitoring of heart rate and oxygen saturation, and recovery time for each patient—with patient demographic and health history data.

Medical Decision Support Systems

Medical DSSs are computer programs designed to help health professionals make clinical decisions (Shortlife, 1987). They deal with patients' medical data or medical knowledge necessary to interpret such data. Many HISs can be considered medical DSSs in that they focus the attention of the clinical provider on significant clinical issues. Other systems operate within either consulting or critiquing modes. With a consulting system, the program accepts patient data, asks questions, and generates advice regarding diagnosis or treatment. Critiquing systems serve as a sounding board for clinician suppositions and ideas and either express agreement or offer alternative options (Shortlife, 1987). The latter systems are highly complex and advanced and remain primarily within the domain of research and development. Medical records systems, such as HELP and TMR, are examples of critiquing systems combined with patient monitoring. Both these and other medical record systems are still in prototype form.

NURSING RESEARCH AND EDUCATION TECHNOLOGY

Systems for assisting nursing research include document retrieval systems containing bibliographic references to the nursing literature, statistical packages used for editing and analyzing data, and models used to depict the nursing process

(Saba, Johnson, Halloran, & Simpson, 1992). Nursing researchers and educators can use data line/modem technology to access computerized libraries, such as those at the National Library of Medicine (Simpson, 1991). The Library's major clinical and research family of databases includes Medical Literature Analysis and Retrieval System (MEDLARS), which contains the MEDLINE and GRATE-FUL MED databases. MEDLINE, according to the Library, is accessed 10,000 times a day by clinical researchers and practitioners. The National Library of Medicine also sponsors NUCARE (NUrsing CAre REsearch Conference), an electronic, interactive bulletin board and conferencing system that gives researchers the means to share and exchange nursing practice information relating to nursing research.

BARRIERS TO NURSING TECHNOLOGY: THE NURSING MINIMUM DATA SET (NMDS)

One of the most significant barriers to the advancement of nursing-related technology is the lack of a nationally agreed on taxonomy or nomenclature. Although nurses provide the primary care for a patient in a health care setting, nursing data typically are absent from the systems. Although systems have the capability to document, sort, track, and report on national data, the lack of a uniform coding format for nursing diagnoses renders these capabilities virtually useless (Simpson & Waite, 1989).

The purpose of a minimum data set is to establish a comparability of nursing data across clinical populations, geographic areas, and time through the identification of data categories, variables, or elements and through the uniform definition of these for use in nursing's clinical practice and administrative, research, and educational endeavors (Werley, 1988).

Without common language documentation, nursing's data will continue to be missing from health data used for health policy making. The American Nurses Association is sanctioning adoption of the data elements approved for classification by the North American Nursing Diagnosis Association (NANDA).

CONSIDERATIONS IN SELECTING A SYSTEM

In its 1991 nursing care standards, the Joint Commission on Accreditation of Healthcare Organizations (JCAHO) specified that nurses be involved in evaluating, selecting, and integrating all systems that affect patient care (Simpson, 1991). According to the Commission report, "The nurse executive, or a designee(s), participates in evaluating, selecting, and integrating healthcare technology and information management systems that support patient care needs and the efficient utilization of nursing resources (NC.5.5)." JCAHO plans to verify nursing involvement through evidence that shows a nursing representative was on the selection committee, primarily meeting minutes and nursing requisition orders.

To select an appropriate system for the nursing and health care environment, nursing leaders must be prepared to (1) appoint a clinical nurse specialist to the selection committee, (2) understand the importance and role of the request for proposal (RFP), (3) create an atmosphere that encourages education about technologic issues, (4) create an advisory committee of clinical nurses, (5) demand veto power for nursing representatives, and (6) participate in contract negotiations.

Appoint a Clinical Nurse Specialist

Although a nursing executive typically serves on the selection committee, it is also important to appoint a clinical nurse specialist. As an expert in clinical practice, the clinical nurse specialist offers a unique perspective that can guide the selection process: an unwavering commitment to and focus on the patient (Simpson, 1990). This focus on the nursing care and process perspective is requisite for quality nursing systems.

Understand the RFP

The RFP is a standard document used to solicit information about system standards from vendors, suppliers, and consultants. In the RFP, a health care institution announces the acquisition plan and states guidelines for responses. The RFP should (1) introduce the vendor to the environment for which the system is intended, (2) state general requirements for information to be supplied, (3) describe any performance bond or equivalent requirement, (4) state conditions of an equipment demonstration, (5) outline the method of financing, (6) specify training and orientation expected, (7) cite evaluation criteria to be used in evaluating proposals, (8) state the standards of performance that will be used in deciding whether the system is acceptable, and (9) state specifications for particular hardware and software components (Austin, 1988).

Many nurses make the mistake of not using weighted values or proper term definitions in identifying general requirements (Simpson, June 1991). For example, to ask a vendor whether it handles acuity or patient classification is much too vague a question. The question could be referring to nurse staffing, DRGs, or a nurse patient classification. Nursing must be rigorous in defining specifically what it requires and in using the proper terminology.

In addition, without assigning weighted values, it would appear that every requirement nursing makes is of the same value or importance, when, clearly, that is not possible.

Encourage Education About Technologic Issues

To make educated business decisions, the clinical nurse specialist and nursing executive on the selection committee will need to spend the necessary time educating himself or herself on technical and operational issues related to the acquisition, implementation, and use of an information system. This will involve a significant investment of time on the part of the nurses involved in the selection, particularly since a selection process can take as long as 2 to 5 years. Nursing managers and the nursing department must support selection committee members in their time-consuming, educational endeavor.

Create an Advisory Committee of Clinical Nurses

It is useful to have nursing selection committee representatives work with an advisory committee of clinical nurse specialists. This ensures that patient care issues will predominate and that staff clinical nurses will be more open to the system when it is finally selected and implemented. In addition, a committee of clinical nurses can provide useful feedback, ideas, and solutions to issues that may emerge during the process.

Demand Veto Power for Nursing Representatives

The clinical nurse specialist should have not only an affirmative vote on the system development/selection committee but also a veto vote (Simpson & Somers, 1991). Financial and administrative executives typically enjoy veto power, whereas veto power for clinicians is fairly new. Nevertheless, nursing representatives should demand this confidence to ensure that the proper system is selected for clinical as well as financial operations.

Participate in Contract Negotiations

Once a system is selected, it is important for nursing leaders to protect the interests of both the nursing department and the health care institution as a whole. In negotiating contracts, nursing leaders must be prepared to define and determine warranties, intellectual property, maintenance agreements, maintenance fees and obligations, and upgrade management. Insight from an outside systems consultant can be of great assistance in this phase of systems selection.

OVERCOMING STAFF RESISTANCE

Nursing and other hospital leaders may spend years planning and evaluating for the right system but often overlook the most important part of any technologic change—the effect it has on people. However, there is a proven methodology to change management, and it involves understanding why individuals resist change, soliciting buy-ins at the initial stage of the systems selection process, auditing current work processes, and assigning change sponsors and change agents.

Understanding Why Individuals Resist Change

The most important part of change management is determining not only why people might want to change but why they resist it as well (DeMark & Sisk, 1990). Often, system sabotage is related to the individual or group of individuals' perception of job viability and present working conditions. According to Dowling, overt sabotage can include such interferences as oral defamation, alleged inability to operate the system, data sabotage, and refusal to use the system.

Soliciting Buy-Ins at Initial Stage of Systems Selection Process

One of the most effective ways to overcome resistance is to include key individuals and constituencies in the planning process, preferably before a system is selected. In fact, soliciting buy-ins from all involved constituencies should be part of the initial system study—well before the selection and implementation process begins (DeMark & Sisk, 1990).

Auditing Current Work Processes

An operational audit of current work processes is critical to understanding what works, what needs to change, and why. Having key individuals and representatives involved in the audit process, particularly clinicians, helps prevent the automation of inefficient workflows. According to DeMark and Sisk (1990), it also helps each individual and each department identify present skills and needed future skills for training and development.

Assigning Change Sponsors and Change Agents

A change sponsor is often a high-level executive who understands the hospital's overarching objectives, goals, and missions and can effectively articulate them to managers and staff personnel. In a nursing environment, this change sponsor should be the nursing administrator or vice president of nursing. Sponsors must be responsible for generating enthusiasm for the change and maintaining the momentum and commitment.

Change agents serve just as important a role. Change agents are typically system managers or representative for the information systems (IS) department. These individuals are uniquely picked to move the project forward and manage the human factors or processes (DeMark & Sisk, 1990). They must be able to speak both clinical and technical languages and serve as the liaison between the two areas. As a result, good change agents are individuals who have an excellent understanding of the technical issues involved with implementing a new system and can also act as negotiator, motivator, and confidante to clinical users who may have concerns about the system.

EMERGING TECHNOLOGIES

To select the appropriate system for a health care organization, nursing leaders must be aware of the advancing technology in order to ensure the viability of the nursing information system for years to come. New technologies being tested in the marketplace include the following.

Video and Voice Processing

McDonald (1989) predicts that within 5 years, medical information systems will record more than text and will include such images as x-rays, snapshots of patient's faces, closeups of skin lesions, electrocardiographs, and perhaps even cines of a Parkinson patient's gait. In addition, human voices will be directly understood by computers without human transcription. Today, these systems are available, but prices remain out of reach for most health care institutions.

Cooperative Processing

Cooperative processing is a procedure by which powerful personal computers access clinical data on the host (mainframe or minicomputer), then manipulate that data on the workstation for sorting, displaying, reviewing, and printing. This is a form of distributed processing. However, data are not stored on the PC, despite the fact that it can be manipulated there.

Data Storage

The ever increasing amount of data that must be stored, retrieved, and analyzed on computers will be made available through inexpensive optical devices (such as CD-ROMs) that will permit indefinite retention of any text data. Data storage will probably include image storage. Organizing and searching for the data will be made easier through parallel processing, associative memory, and hardware-based text searching (McDonald, 1989).

References

Austin, C.J. (1988). Evaluating and selecting a computer system. In *Information systems for health services administration* (3rd ed., pp. 113–127). Ann Arbor, MI: Health Administration Press.

Brown, R. (1991, March). The evolution of executive information systems. *Systems 3X/400,* pp. 26–34.

Childs, B.W. (1988, November). Point of care: Being a pilot site. *U.S. Healthcare,* pp. 23–24.

Clayton, K., & Simpson, R. (1991, Winter). Automation: The key to successful product line management. *Nursing Administration Quarterly,* pp. 33–38.

Cushing, M. (1991). Getting to know your operating system. *M.D. Computing, 8*(5), 322–325.

DeLong, D., & Rockart, J. (1990). *Executive support systems.* Dow Jones Irwin.

DeMark, J., & Sisk, F. (1990). Clinical information systems management: The crucial difference. *HIMS* annual publication in the 1990 Annual Healthcare Systems Conference.

Gardner, R.M. (1986). Computerized management of intensive care patients. *M.D. Computing, 3*(1), pp. 36–51.

Garfinkle, D., et al. (1987). HORNET: Hospital Operating Room Network, a first description. *SCAMC,* pp. 817–821.

Hammond, W., & Stead, W. (1988). Computer-based medical records. *SCAMC,* pp. 625–629.

Hawley, W., Tariq, H., & Gardner, R. (1988). Clinical implementation of an automated medical information bus in an intensive care unit. *SCAMC,* pp. 621–624.

Keegan, A. (1991). Executive information systems: A new look at financial information. Submitted to *Healthcare Financial Management.*

McDonald, C.J. (1989). Medical information systems of the future. *M.D. Computing, 6*(2), pp. 82–87.

Saba, V.K., Johnson, J., Halloran, E., & Simpson, R. (1992). *Computers in nursing management.* Pamphlet submitted to the ANA.

Saba, V.K., & McCormick, K.A. (1986). *Essential of computers for nursing.* Philadelphia: J.B. Lippincott.

Shortlife, E. (1987). Computer programs to support clinical decision making. *JAMA, 258*(1).

Simpson R.L. (1990–1992). Technology: Nursing the system. *Nursing Management,* Columns dating July 1990 through March 1992.

Simpson, R., & Somers, A.B.D. (1991). The role of the clinical nurse specialist in information systems selection. *Clinical Nurse Specialist, 5*(3), pp. 159–163.

Simpson, R., & Waite, R. (1989). NCNIP's system of the future: A call for accountability, revenue control and national data sets. *Nursing Administration Quarterly,* pp. 72–77.

Sisk, F.A., & Rappoport, A.E. (1989). Moving the electronic chart to the community hospital. Prepared for *M.D. Computing*.

Werley, H. (1988). Introduction to the nursing minimum data set and its development. In H.

Werley & N. Lan (Eds.), *Identification of the nursing minimum data set*. New York: Springer-Verlag.

Whiting-O'Keefe, Q., Simborg, D., & Epstein, W. (1980). A controlled experiment to evaluate the use of a time-oriented summary medical record. *Medical Care, 18*(8).

CHAPTER 8 • • • • • •

BUILDING YOUR TEAM

JANE FAIRBANKS NEUBAUER

EXECUTIVE SUMMARY

This chapter reviews the various aspects of building an organizational team. Included are topics regarding organizational development concepts, review of basic group process theories, how to use the role negotiation structure to decrease conflict, and some suggestions on collaboration and committee workings. The purpose of this text is to assist the nurse manager to incorporate team building processes into her or his everyday work activities to enhance goal achievement and employee satisfaction.

As in no other time in the past, the health care team must work together to prosper in these turbulent times. There is no choice! We have watched the golden era of the health care industry disappear. Resources have become more limited at the same time that the demand for services has grown. Health care institutions are recognizing that the public cares about the quality of services provided and the continuity of these services to the patient. To respond to these monumental changes, institutions need creative approaches to develop responsible, efficient delivery systems. No one administrator, nurse executive, physician, department head, or nurse can do this alone.

Modern America was developed by men who believed and lived Horatio Alger's traditional notion of success. We all know the familiar tale of triumphant individuals and enterprising heroes who win riches and rewards through a combination of Dale Carnegie-esque self-improvement, Norman Vincent Peale-esque faith, Sylvester Stallone-esque assertiveness, and plain, old-fashioned good luck. Reich (1987) reminds us that these stories are more than entertainment and are like ancient myths that have captured and contained essential truth about our culture. He says that we must change our mythic celebrations to those of collective entrepreneurship if we are to adapt to today's complex world. "The Team as Hero" could be the title of this chapter. The concept of a few entrepreneurial heroes and multiple industrial drones—the inspired and the perspired—is no longer relevant.

We have known for years that there were problems with the delivery of comprehensive health care because of compartmentalization of services resulting from emphasis on and isolation of individual disciplinary services (George, Ide, & Vambery, 1971). Now the demand is for higher quality, better service, and increased efficiency (less cost), which cannot be accomplished unless we focus on the growth of the team as well as the individual. A commitment to team building and skills for developing teams are essential to every leader and every professional in the health care system. The nursing manager can be the leader of this movement. Cooperation and group accomplishment are not new concepts to nursing.

A successful team demonstrates a high degree of trust and works cooperatively rather than competitively. Communication is at a high level among all members, and the group is flexible and adaptable. A team is characterized by the following descriptors.

- A common goal
- Interdependence
- Cooperation
- Coordination of activities
- Task socialization
- Division of effort
- Mutual respect

Mutual respect within teams does not require agreement on every issue, but it does require a willingness to trust other's skills and expertise (Zenger & Miller, 1974).

If there are problems with goal achievement, there undoubtably are problems with process. Too many groups are not teams at all but collections of individual relationships with the boss in which each individual is vying with the other for greater power, prestige, recognition, and personal autonomy. Under these conditions, unity of purpose is a myth, and the team is inept at accomplishing objectives through group effort. Managers often feel that no one can do it as well as they can. High-level groups with strong personalities often are described as a team of wild horses rather than a group of people working together to achieve common goals. Other symptoms of poor team work include department heads telling other department heads how to manage their operations, several team members ganging up on one of their peers, people withholding information, failing to follow up, or meet commitments to the group effort, and team members not listening to each other and being unwilling to compromise.

ORGANIZATIONAL DEVELOPMENT

Focusing on the team rather than the individual in accomplishing work means changing the way in which people think, feel, and work. Some organizations might say: "What we need here is to improve our key people." In contrast, organizational development (OD) focuses on groups or teams of people and their relationships. It is the system, be it a unit or an entire hospital, that is the object of an OD effort (Sherwood, 1972).

OD is an evolving collection of philosophies, concepts, and techniques aimed at improving an organization's performance. It is neither a scientific management nor a human relations approach to organizational analysis but a combination of these techniques. It is a long-range effort to improve an organization's problem-solving and renewal processes. The actual interventions assist formal work teams in identifying their own creative resources, diagnosing problems, and developing alternative solutions while providing a mechanism for continual self-renewal (French & Bell, 1990).

Senge (1990) suggests that organizations will prosper only if they create continuous learning environments. New roles for leaders as designers, teachers, and stewards are described. Emphasis is placed on new tools to foster communication and collaboration and new skills to build a shared vision, challenge mental models, and engage in systems thinking. These are not new ideas to us in nursing, but it is refreshing to see them presented as one answer for the 1990s.

Necessary Conditions for Success

For an OD approach to be successful, certain conditions must exist in an organization. Key people must feel disturbed and pressured to initiate change. There must be a willingness by those key people to risk innovations involving new ideas and changes in relationships. The entire team must realize that the strategy will involve a long-term commitment. The organization must be willing to provide rewards, not punishment, for efforts to offer creative and innovative solutions to present problems. Once committed, managers can no longer view problems as situations someone else created. It is then no longer acceptable to operate under the premise that "they" did it to me. The manager must realize that he or she helped create the situation and must be involved in working out the solution. In other words, everyone must commit to being a part of the solution, not a part of the problem (Fisher, 1980).

OD focuses on groups or teams of people and their relationships related to getting their job done. Sherwood (1972) suggests a general set of objectives for an organization or a team embarking on an OD process.

1. To build trust among individuals and groups throughout the work environment
2. To create an open problem-solving climate in the work teams where people can confront problems and clarify differences
3. To locate decision-making and problem-solving responsibilities as close to the information and resources as possible
4. To increase ownership of goals and objectives
5. To move toward greater collaboration between interdependent persons and groups
6. To increase awareness of process and its effect on performance, helping the people involved become aware of what is happening between and to members of the group while the group is working on tasks

GROUP PROCESSES

The processes that take place in groups are an essential part of every group's working relationship. Nurses have studied the basics of group processes in relation to family theory or mental health and illness. A review of the concepts and assistance in applying them to the work group is appropriate, since these theories apply everyday. Work teams are work families.

Task Behaviors and Maintenance Behaviors

Two types of group behaviors have been identified: task behaviors, which relate to goal achievement, and maintenance behaviors, which relate to group process, norms, and feelings. Both are essential for group achievement. One must remember the premise, "If there are problems with outcome, there are problems with process!" It is critical for groups to review the various roles in groups from time to time and do a self-assessment to be sure that essential roles are being implemented and group members are being flexible. Individuals in groups must understand the importance of their participation in various roles to assist the group in achieving goals. A method to accomplish this is for a group to use a self-assessment form periodically and discuss group success and failure together after the assessment.

Each person begins in a group with self-oriented behavior that is seeking answers to the questions: What is my identity in the group? Am I included? How much power or control do I want or have? How much affection will I get and give? Will my personal needs be met? Each individual will demonstrate various behaviors in coping with his or her needs, such as aggressive, tender, supportive, and withdrawn. The group will not move forward if these issues are not resolved by each member (Schein, 1988).

Stages of Group Growth

There are several approaches to understanding the stages of group growth. It is critical to recognize that no group moves from one stage to another in perfect sequence. Issues may arise at any time and demand attention. Schein (1985) describes four stages in relation to confrontation with certain issues.

1. Dependency/authority
2. Peer relationships/intimacy/role differentiation
3. Creativity/stability
4. Survival/growth

Dependency/Authority Stage

In the first stage, the group must resolve the issue of authority—who will lead, and how much power and influence he or she will have. This is often illustrated by a power struggle with the leader and can be based on personal issues with authority. The group must resolve the dependency/authority stage in order to move ahead and focus on group issues as well as external problem solving.

Peer and Role Relationships

Peer and role relationships fall into stage two. How people relate to each other will be a part of the group's issues for the rest of its life and must be dealt with directly. Roles must be clarified, and group process issues must be discussed on a regular basis.

Creativity / Stability

A group cannot succeed without continued ability to create and innovate, but neither can it feel comfortable with abandoning all policies and norms. This is the challenge of the third stage. Constant creativity is disruptive and anxiety producing but necessary at times to maintain adaptiveness. The group's challenge is to balance stability and creativity.

Survival vs Growth

The survival vs growth question is the final stage of group development. It is essentially the evaluation of effectiveness. The question is whether the group continues to serve important functions and should survive or whether it should dissolve and allow a more adaptive set of solutions to be created by a new group. There are many groups in organizations that are no longer functional and need to be put to death, possibly with an appropriate mourning celebration.

Understanding group development is critical to leading and participating in groups. This brief summary is intended to assist in assessing and understanding groups in order to make them more effective.

THE ROLE OF THE NURSE MANAGER
Practical Applications
Assessment of Process

Multiple methods for assessing processes are available. There are many group process assessment tools developed specifically for work groups. They all generally cover such areas as goal clarity, purpose of meeting to reach goals, priorities, trust and commitment in the group, roles and participation of members, willingness of participants to talk straight and listen to others, ability to deal openly with conflict, leadership quality, closure on topics and schedules, post-meeting follow-up, and support of meeting issues. McGregor (1967) and Schein (1988) present suggestions on these topics.

After deciding on the issues or obtaining an evaluation sheet that meets the needs of the group, a class on group process should be held to familiarize members with group process theory applied to their work group. The most important follow-up is to regularly assign someone in the group to observe group success and give feedback to the group. A discussion about how to improve should follow. This process can be done in 5 or 10 minutes at the end of the meeting. Great progress can be made in group outcomes by improving the process. Initially, it may take more time to complete topic discussions when trying to include everyone in the group and come to consensus, but long-term commitment and goal achievement will increase tremendously.

Awareness of process is one of the original objectives of organizational development techniques and is essential to improving team effectiveness. The only way to improve a team's success in group process is to practice, assess progress, and discuss it regularly.

Building Trust

One of the most influential power bases is the extent to which people can trust the manager. This does not mean that they necessarily like the manager or approve of the schedule. It means they trust that the nursing manager will be consistent and fair and will incorporate his or her values in decision making. Getting to a high level of trust with others is a complex process. It is helpful to understand the four components of trust (Zand, 1972).

1. Intention
2. Actual behavior
3. Expectation of others
4. Perception of others

Intention to trust is entering a situation assuming mutual trust with co-workers. It is the preconceived ideas brought into the group: "I like working with these managers" vs "Here we go—another meeting with dietary—these guys are never honest."

Demonstrating trusting behavior includes eye contact, other body language, smiles, sincere greetings, and introductions. These seem simple but are very important. Beginning discussions with honesty about the situation is the next step. We have all met people for the first time and initially trusted them. In initial contacts with a new peer, intentions and behavior regarding trust are critical to the new person's trust in the new situation.

Lack of intention to trust and lack of demonstration of trusting behavior can affect a new person's perceptions and expectations. If, for example, a new nurse manager enters the room and group members continue their conversation and ignore her, they have not demonstrated trusting behavior. They appear to be withholding information, which indicates lack of intention to trust or trusting behavior.

Group members' expectation and perception of others' trustworthiness are just as critical. Hearing positive things about a new nurse manager inspires expectations and perceptions of his or her trustworthiness. An opposite reaction occurs when it is known that the nurse manager has just finished graduate school and a member thinks all people with graduate degrees are arrogant. Therefore, expectations and perceptions are set negatively before there is any experience with the nurse manager.

There is a role-playing situation in which two groups role play the same meeting in an organization with a specific problem. The only difference is that group one is told they can trust their co-workers and group two is told they cannot trust their co-workers. When observers rate the goal achievement and working relationship of the two groups, group one (trusting) consistently rates twice as high as group two (nontrusting). Trust is one of the most important aspects of group achievement (Zand, 1972).

Trust on the part of one person in a group encourages others to risk trusting. Trust must become a norm in a group for the group to be successful. The amount of trust necessary in a group depends on the significance of the group's goals, the time frame of the working relationship, and the degree of collaboration necessary to achieve goals. Each group in which a person participates will demand a different degree of trust. It is possible to increase the trust level in a group if the group understands how to do this and commits itself to the process. To increase trust, one must get and give feedback.

Getting and Giving Feedback

Feedback (or self-disclosure) is given by verbal and nonverbal messages to a person or group providing information on how their behavior is affecting one's feelings and perceptions. The objective of feedback is to be aware of how a group member's behavior affects other members. In other words, to change one's behavior, everyone in the group must be aware of how others see them as well as how they see themselves. Each person must get feedback from others and be receptive to that feedback as well as to give feedback to others. Awareness is the first step in changing behavior.

If a veteran group member realizes that his or her initial behavior was inappropriate when greeting the new nurse manager, the group member might say, "Welcome. I'm afraid we didn't start off very well, and I am sorry [disclosure of feelings]. You came in with a warm smile [giving feedback]. What would be most helpful for us to tell you in our introductions today [getting feedback and being receptive]?" This type of interaction will increase everyone's trust within the group. This shows that the process does not need to be formal but each group member does need to be aware of and implement the principles of increasing trust.

There are some ground rules to follow in the feedback process.

- Each person must report on her or his own perceptions—no one else can do that.
- Feedback should be related to a specific observed behavior.
- If the feedback is to be beneficial, the motive should be to help, not punish.
- Feedback must be confirmed with others for consistency.
- Feedback is not analysis—each person must decide what to do with the information received.
- Here and now feelings are most important.

A person must be open to feedback and willing to hear it. There is a great deal of information available to help a person be more effective in the job, but he or she must trust enough to get the information. One way to feel more in control is to ask for feedback rather than wait for it. Supervisors should review performance with the people who report to them every few months, or they can request this or do a self-evaluation and ask for comments from the supervisor. Most of the feedback available is positive (we tend to think that it will be negative), and much positive feedback is never shared if there are no mechanisms designed for sharing.

Feedback is given in many ways. It must be given clearly so that it is most helpful to the receiver. Chances of growing by seeing ourselves as others see us are improved considerably if we tend to be open, understanding, and interested in feedback [see JOHARI window, a model designed by Luft & Ingram (1966), which illustrates the interaction of sources of information about oneself].

To build trust in any situation, it is necessary to be honest, be open, be constructive, be adult to adult, and be accepting and respectful.

Role Negotiation

Organizational conflict often is rooted in role issues. The causes for conflict are many: changing institutional priorities, scarce resources and reallocation, and the militancy of various professional groups. One common reason for conflict is change in employees' roles. Any change that is perceived as diminishing the role's importance is likely to generate conflict. Therefore, to learn to prevent some disruptive organizational conflict, managers must understand the concepts of role behavior and facilitate role negotiation (Veniga, 1981).

Although conflict is not always negative, it must be dissipated to some extent so that the organization and the manager do not spend excessive energy on it. Too much energy is spent in organizations sidetracked on role issues rather than on goal achievement. If one is to enhance productivity, one must assist with resolution of these conflicts. Conflicts generally arouse feelings of inadequacy and such questions as

- How much power do I have?
- Is someone taking my authority?
- Who values me?
- Am I necessary?

With the rapid changes in organizations today come constant role alteration and, therefore, the necessity for constant role negotiation. Each person in the organization has expectations from superiors, peers, health team members, subordinates, other departments, and self. These discrepancies lead to role ambiguity (expectations not clearly defined), role conflict (incompatible expectations), and role overload (inability to meet multiple expectations). Each team member is faced with pressure to reduce these conflicts but still maintain an equilibrium between his or her internal values and beliefs and the external expectations. Many believe the success of organizations is determined largely by the organization's ability to clarify roles among employees.

Most people's role concerns are related to ambiguity rather than actual conflict. Clarification is needed. Much energy is spent while people try to second guess what others want rather than clarifying and discussing and agreeing on expectations. There are some administrative activities that must be implemented to assist this process. Programs should be held that describe the major roles in the organization for all employees, including administrators and physicians and nurses and housekeepers. Job functions must be outlined clearly in writing so staff members know each other's expectations and responsibilities.

This is only the beginning, however. Even with these processes in place, the organizational goals are constantly changing, and priorities and activities for the day or the year are evolving. Individual needs and concerns are critical. Therefore, there must be regular dialogue concerning role expectations and role negotiation. Questions to be answered in this process include

- What do I want from you?
- What do you want from me?
- What am I willing to do to help you be successful?
- What are you willing to do to help me be successful?

The answers are essentially a role message (Rubin et al., 1976). From this message, negotiation takes place about what each person agrees to do. These questions can be answered in many settings—from a formal discussion of each person's role on a project to a quick discussion with a supervisor or a physician.

In a formal setting, to obtain some general information about roles to be shared, there is another subset of questions that may be helpful. These include (Harrison, 1973)

- What would the person or group like the same of? (activities to be continued that are functional)
- What would the person or group like more of?
- What would the person or group like less of? (activities to increase or decrease that would help others do their jobs)

In the supervisor/supervisee negotiation, a formal discussion using a facilitator is best. For instance, the director of nursing should have a session with her nurse managers, preferably in a retreat setting. These questions are answered between the director and the group. The outcome would be a role agreement between the nurse managers and the director. This should be followed by individual sessions with each nurse manager and the director on a regular basis. The nurse manager should use a facilitator to have this type of discussion with her staff. The director might also be there to describe the organization's expectations of the role of the nurse manager. This probably sounds threatening, but there are so many nurse managers who never hear all the things their staff appreciates and the one or two things they could do that would help the staff tremendously. Most staff ask for things like rounds on other shifts or more information about the budget.

The process can be used very effectively with physicians. The discussion can take place without ever saying, "Now we are going to do a role negotiation." Many physicians are frustrated because we have never asked them what they want and then tried to achieve it. The nurse manager could go to the physician and say, "What is the most critical issue for you in the next month on my unit?" The manager might ask for assistance with the budget or a problem physician or some other concern. Discussion with the physician should take place yearly about what must be accomplished next year and what each person should do to reach those goals.

Role negotiation does not make the conflict go away, but it brings it out in the open so that it can be discussed. Nothing can be resolved if it is not acknowledged. If it is necessary to tell the director that the QA project will not be done on time, it is better to say it upfront and explain that time is being spent on other projects.

These discussions can be helpful also with staff and line issues, for instance, negotiation of staff development programs for the unit between the nurse manager and the staff development instructor. Both their supervisors should be present for the discussion so that their expectations are clear. This process should be done at least yearly. Often, formal agreement is written concerning programs for the year, with informal follow-up and renegotiation several times during the year as necessary.

Most people are anxious about these kinds of discussions initially but often much of the information is positive. People go back to work aware of the many things they do that are helpful to others in doing their jobs, the few things they need to change, and areas for growth.

Jourard (1964) says that "roles are inescapable. They must be played or else the social system will not work" (p. 22). One of our major roles as managers is to facilitate role clarification.

Committees and Work Groups

Middle managers in industry may spend as much as 35% of their work week in meetings. That figure can be as high as 50% for top management (Seibold, 1979). There are many resources for learning how to chair a meeting. The chairperson's job is demanding—an amalgam of planning, promoting, leading, directing, informing, interpreting, encouraging, stimulating, refereeing, judging, moderating, and conciliating. It is critical for a chairperson to prepare for a meeting.

The success achieved by a head of a committee or formal group will depend largely on the person's ability to preside and guide the meetings of the group to a definite goal. Some suggestions for this include

- Start on time.
- Work from an agenda.
- Clarify purpose of meeting.
- Get materials to members ahead of time and expect them to have been reviewed.
- Keep things moving.
- Retain control but encourage disagreement so it can be dealt with.
- Remain neutral as chair.
- Summarize at the end.
- End on time unless there is an unusual situation.

Minutes are critical, since they are the record of accountability and the history of the group. Public minutes on newsprint keep everyone focused. Minutes should be distributed quickly with assignments and clear accountability (Seibold, 1979).

The real challenge, however, is to be a positive, active member of a work group. This role is in some ways more taxing because one has less control. Leadership is not the only issue in a group. Some organizations are experimenting with setting up work groups with no leader, and there have been some positive successes.

The Role of the Followers

Effective followers share a number of essential qualities.

1. They manage themselves well.
2. They are committed to the organization and to a purpose outside themselves.
3. They build their competence and focus their efforts for maximum impact.
4. They assist in managing process as well as task in groups.
5. They are courageous, honest, and credible.

These are people who see themselves as equal to the leader in responsibility and see colleagues as allies. They truly are focused on the goal and hold high standards of performance for themselves. A courageous follower can keep a leader honest and out of trouble (Kelley, 1988).

To cultivate effective followers, we must redefine followership and leadership. Good leaders know how to follow, and they set an example for others. One approach is to structure work groups so that followers can be developed. This can be done by rotating leadership or creating leaderless groups. Performance evaluation should include feedback on followership as well as leadership qualities and should come from peers and subordinates as well as supervisors.

There are so many more positions for followers than leaders. Organizations must find ways of rewarding followers and bringing them into full partnership. The power of an organization cultivating fully engaged, fully energized, fully appreciated followers can only be imagined.

Collaboration among Groups

In health care and nursing, we have discussed collaboration for years. It is suggested, however, that we have never achieved a working relationship with other individuals or groups if it interfered in any way with building our own department or professional power base. As managers and employee positions are decreased and rework and double work interfere with economic survival, the time has come to finally truly improve our collaboration.

We are all members of multiple teams. Making a list of them might help to comprehend the magnitude of this issue. Our role in each team is a little different.

Ways to Enhance Collaboration.   Collaboration can be enhanced through several mechanisms. Executives and high level managers must make a commitment to delegate decisions and conflict resolution to the appropriate level. This means refusing to make the decision alone. Getting several people together to assist them in making the decision may help. Assisting subordinates to think through issues and come to their own conclusions calls into play the role of the leader as teacher again. This means asking questions rather than giving advice. A leader must focus on this continually to avoid being trapped into making decisions that need to be made elsewhere. People must be taught how to accept delegated responsibility.

One organizational process that can be used to enhance collaboration is management development. Organizing in-house classes can accomplish several goals. It can educate and assist others to practice new skills with peers, which enhances collaboration. Executives can be encouraged in their role as teacher/facilitator. The content and structure could be designed by a task force based on a needs assessment. Topics might include leadership, conflict resolution, change theory, and team building. The focus must be interdisciplinary, including nurse managers, other professional managers, and ancillary managers.

Many outcomes can derive from this interdisciplinary, in-house design. In one large university hospital, managers met people who they had worked with over the phone or in formal situations. They practiced problem solving with others before they had to deal with real issues. They participated in classrooms where their executives were teachers and did not always have the answer. Executives had exposure to a different side of themselves and another opportunity to affect the culture. Some class groups met together after the formal classes to support each other and problem solve. Many reported positive new feelings about working in a large organization and increased optimism that problems could be solved and conflicts resolved. One nurse manager negotiated with the environmental services supervisor to clean the unit IV poles regularly. (Many of you realize what a feat this was.) Many participants believed that the processes in the classes were team building at its best.

The Use of Consultants

The literature is full of descriptions of consultants' activities and successes. The major focus of a consultant, whether an internal or an external consultant, is to help the consultees to help themselves. Consultants are sometimes referred to as trainers, change agents, or facilitators. They generally are people experienced in psychologic and sociologic research regarding human behavior. They are trained in personality theory and group dynamics and have studied organizational culture and social systems.

The consultant's work is to plan and implement an intervention into the client system, which may comprise the entire department or a part of it. There are different approaches to the consultative process. The consultant may function as a technical expert with skills to solve a particular problem, or a consultant can function in a very process-oriented way by assisting the organization in understanding itself and its members and how they can work together more effectively (Lippitt & Lippitt, 1978).

There are advantages and disadvantages to using an internal vs an external consultant. External consultants provide a new and fresh approach to problems.

They are objective. However, it takes time and effort to understand a complex organization. They must become familiar with the organization's structure and processes and acquire a knowledge of the culture, values, and norms.

The internal consultant has the advantage of being familiar with the way the organization functions. This person understands the structural processes, knows its values and norms, and can provide continuous attention to the process of change. However, the internal consultant may not be regarded as an expert by others in the organization. Also, the internal consultant depends on the organization's reward and penalty systems and consequently may not take the risks he or she otherwise might take if not so tied to the system. The internal consultant's objectivity may be limited.

People in other parts of an organization who can assist the nurse manager include clinical specialists, staff development specialists, faculty in the school of nursing, people in the human resources department, and peers. These people have the advantage of having some knowledge of the organization, yet they can be objective about specific areas. The functions of the consultant are to help the department understand its current behavior, determine areas of desirable behavior change, and facilitate change from old dysfunctional behaviors to new functional ones (Beckhard, 1969).

Each organization must choose the right options for itself. At times, it may be necessary and appropriate to have a full-time internal consultant or use someone in the organization as a consultant part time. Other times, an outside consultant can bring a new perspective, offer knowledge not available in the organization, or focus on the issue when only a short period of time is available. In any case, it is critical that the person hiring the consultant be very clear as to what the goals and expectations are and the processes that will be used to meet these goals. This upfront negotiation is critical to a positive, productive outcome of the process.

Organizations are using consultants more and more as dollars for full-time staff support are less available. Their expertise can be obtained for the time needed. To hire a consultant, it is necessary to identify the needs of the group or organization and then identify two or three consultants who could be helpful and have the right fit for the team. It is best to work with the consultant for a period of time to gain full advantage of the perspective he or she has gained about the organization and the advice he or she has to offer.

Building Effective Teams

These are some thoughts to review when trying to improve the effectiveness of a team.

1. Develop a better understanding of each team member's role in the work group.
2. Develop a better understanding of the team purpose.
3. Improve communication among team members about issues that affect efficiency of the group.

4. Develop more support for team members.
5. Develop a clearer understanding of group processes by working through problems inherent to the team at task and interpersonal levels.
6. Use conflict in a positive rather than destructive way.
7. Increase ability to work collaboratively with other groups.

References

Beckhard, R. (1969). *Organization development: Strategies and models.* Readington, MA: Addison-Wesley.

Fisher, W.F. (1980, October). A review of organizational development. *Journal of Nursing Administration.*

French, W.L., & Bell, C.H. (1990). *Organizational development* (4th ed.). Englewood Cliffs, NJ: Prentice-Hall.

George, M. (1971, March–April). Ide, K., & Vambery, C.E. The comprehensive health team: A conceptual model. *Journal of Nursing Administration,* pp. 9–13.

Harrison, R. (1973). Role negotiation: A tough-minded approach to team development. In W. Bennis, et al. (Eds.), *Interpersonal dynamics* (3rd ed.). Dorsey Press.

Jourard, S. (1964). *The transparent self.* Princeton, NJ: D Van Nostrand & Company, p. 22.

Kelley, R., (1988, November–December). In praise of followers. *Harvard Business Review,* p. 144.

Lippitt, G., & Lippitt, R. (1978). *The consulting process in action.* LaJolla, CA: University Associates.

Luft, J., & Ingram, R. (1966). *Group process: An introduction to group dynamics.* Palo Alto, CA: The National Press.

McGregor, D. (1967). *The professional manager.* New York: McGraw-Hill, p. 172.

Reich, R. (1987, May–June). Entrepreneurship reconsidered: The team as hero. *Harvard Business Review,* pp. 77–78.

Rubin, I.M., et al. (1976). *Improving coordination of care: A program for health team development.* Cambridge, MA.: Ballinger Publishing Company.

Schein, E.H. (1985). *Organizational culture and leadership.* San Francisco: Jossey Bass, pp. 164–165.

Schein, E.H. (1988). *Process consultation: Vol. I. Its role in organizational development.* Reading, MA.: Addison-Wesley.

Seibold, D. (1979, Summer). Making meetings more successful. *Journal of Business Communication,* p. 49.

Senge, P. (1990). *The fifth discipline: The art and practice of the learning organization.* New York: Doubleday Currency.

Sherwood, J. (1972). An introduction to organizational development. In W.J. Pfeiffer et al. (Eds.). *Annual handbook for group facilitators.* LaJolla, CA: University Associates, p. 153.

Veninga, R. (1981, December). Resolving role confusion: A source of employee conflict. *Hospital Progress,* pp. 41–45.

Zand, D. (1972). Trust and managerial effectiveness. *Administrative Science Quarterly, 17,* pp. 553–572.

Zenger, J., & Miller D. (1974, March–April). Building effective teams. *Personnel.*

CHAPTER 9 • • • • • •

EXECUTIVE SELF-DEVELOPMENT

JIM O'MALLEY

EXECUTIVE SUMMARY

Taking career management seriously and getting on with planning a career means living in the present and future simultaneously while preparing oneself for the reality of constant change. Managing a career means taking charge and accepting responsibility for developing a path to reach identified career goals. For the 1990s, the focus of career planning is to cultivate networks, respond to investigate recruiter's potential opportunities, and continually evaluate each assignment and position to determine if it enhances further growth and development as well as future employability (Hirsh, 1987). This list of activities identifies some of the mechanisms to operationalize achievement of career goals and outcomes. Executive success in the era of changing world economies, the emerging information-based society, and the systemization of entrepreneurship and innovation will require old as well as new skills. Drucker (1992) encourages executive development of a series of new skills, including (1) being outside where the results of a service or business occur, (2) identifying and meeting one's own information ends, and (3) continually focusing on building learning into the system.

Ultimately, managing careers in an era when opportunity hopping has replaced corporate ladder climbing is contingent on developing self-reliance, collaborative abilities, commitment to achievement of projects that show results, and willingness to learn (Kanter, 1989).

Evaluation of career developmental progress should be formalized and conducted every 2 to 3 years. The evaluation process should focus on progress made, incremental goal attainment, and the ability to stay on course in order to facilitate ultimate goal attainment (Cotham, 1989). In turbulent times, change is the only certainty, and periodic reviews help us to identify midcourse corrections and action plans to facilitate proactive executive development and, ultimately, personal and professional goal attainment.

CRISIS IN HEALTH CARE LEADERSHIP

Change has become the only constant in health care. The array of rapid and complex changes in the provision of health care services has resulted in a new definition of what health care is today, including how it should be priced– packaged–marketed and who can best provide it as well as what is the most effective design for delivery. These fundamental changes have significantly taxed even the most progressive health care executives. Nursing leaders, in an effort to manage the cost–quality agenda, are initiating changes to reposition their organizations for a successful future. They have launched a profusion of strategic initiatives to further develop clinical services based on defined needs, benefits, and product differentiation, as well as dramatically shifting the internal culture to improve quality and customer service, productivity, and overall management performance (Bader & O'Malley, 1992).

In the face of this turbulence, the crisis in health care leadership is creating a paradigm shift in the culture of management. As new definitions of what it will take to successfully manage health care emerge, the need and the pressure to develop effective executives have never been more critical. Understanding that executive leadership has always been more of an art than a science and that successful executives are self-made and ultimately accountable for their own development provides the underpinnings for the important work at hand. The opportunities encompass a diversified range of experience with a balance in lessons learned, as brilliantly articulated by Bronowski (1973, pp. 115–116): "We have to understand that the world can only be grasped by action, not by contemplation . . . . The most powerful drive in the ascent of man is his pleasure in his own skill. He loves to do what he does well and, having done it well, he loves to do it better."

NEW WORK FOR LEADERS: LEARNING

The transition of nursing leadership characterized by shifting roles and changing organizations has placed a compelling emphasis on learning. Senge (1990), in his acclaimed book *The Fifth Discipline: The Art and Practice of the Learning Organization,* underscored the critical need for understanding how individuals within organizations learn is greater today than ever before. His important work provides a framework for organizational learning and ascertains that changing the way we think is the basis of the discipline of mental modeling. The application of his work is based on surfacing, challenging, testing, and altering shared mental models as pivotal to personal as well as organizational learning. The challenge for us within the context of our own development as executives is to move from single loop learning to double loop learning. Most of us are good at single loop learning in changing the strategies that we use, but we are not good at changing the underlying assumptions and values we hold. We need to become good at double loop learning, which allows us to change the underlying mental models behind our strategies. As the turbulent health care world has become increasingly dynamic, complex, interdependent, and unpredictable, no longer is it possible for any of us to have it all figured out. On a daily basis, the pressures to be fast on our feet have become intense. Senge's work reminds us that "learning has very little to do with taking in information. Most fundamentally, learning is about enhancing capacity . . . building the capacity to create that which you previously couldn't create. It is intimately related to action, which taking in information is not" (Kim, 1990, p. 1).

PLANNING FOR GROWTH: GOAL SETTING

The first step in executive development is setting goals. Identifying goals provides direction and purpose for a developmental plan. As individuals, each of us is responsible for charting the course of our lives and careers. Cotham (1989) describes how the goal setting processes should be operationalized. "Too many people's careers are dictated by the actions of other's rather than by their own plans. It shouldn't work this way. The secret is to establish your own plan and take charge of your own future" (p. 65).

Critical to the success of executive development and career planning is charting short-term and long-term goals. This activity is difficult for most people because we tend to be focused on the here and now. The skills involved with goal setting are easy to learn and include three basic processes.

1. Identification of desired outcomes
2. Development of specific action plans
3. Establishment of measurement criteria

A formalized goal setting process can facilitate responsibility and accountability for growth and development for self and others who work for you. The goal setting process may open us up to fresh ideas as well as new directions.

CAREER DEVELOPMENT ACTION PLAN

Name:_____ Date Prepared:_____

Career Goal:_____

Developmental Needs	Developmental Actions	Timetable
What experiences, knowledge or skills are needed?	What actions are to be taken and by whom?	When will the actions be taken?

Figure 9–1 Examples of goal planning tools.

TRACKING YOUR PROGRESS

Name:

Career Goal:

Start Date: Target End Date:

Activities	Month	1	2	3	4	1	2	3	4	1	2	3	4	1	2	3	4	1	2	3	4
	Week																				
	planned																				
	actual																				
	planned																				
	actual																				
	planned																				
	actual																				
	planned																				
	actual																				
	planned																				
	actual																				
	planned																				
	actual																				

Figure 9–1   *Continued*

As you know, setting goals is the easy part—goal accomplishment is the hard part. It requires committing yourself intellectually and/or emotionally to a course of action.

A number of useful tools are available for committing your goals to writing. A goal planning form is valuable in clarifying goals, establishing action steps, identifying time frames, and measuring outcomes. Figure 9–1 illustrates examples of goal planning tools.

CREATING A DEVELOPMENTAL PLAN

The focus of this chapter is a presentation of activities to support individualized executive development. It is based on the belief that leadership as an art requires the consistent upgrading of skills as a way of life and that development is synonymous with taking time to educate oneself and enrich personal purpose. The fundamental processes include keeping abreast of issues, broadening horizons and contacts, developing new skills that work, and training and supporting the development of staff and colleagues. The summary discussion lists a menu of developmental activities from which an executive may select to facilitate self-development. This listing is by no means exhaustive or all inclusive but rather provides a beginning framework to stimulate thinking and moving to create an individualized self-development plan.

Individualized Skill Assessment

Assessment of leadership strengths and personal characteristics provides useful data to confirm areas of strength and identify shortcomings. Assessment of one's current skill level in a series of functional areas may be crucial to the initiation of a developmental plan. The skill assessment process uses a series of psychometric instruments, situational assessments, observer feedback, written feedback, and group processes to identify how one's current leadership style and managerial skills influences one's overall effectiveness.

One of the most expensive and elaborate techniques for assessing future potential and predicting success is the assessment center concept. These centers, which use standardized exercises, common criteria, and multiple raters, have demonstrated a strong record in predicting future success. Assessment centers provide sophisticated skill assessments in a variety of functional and content clusters to achieve the following outcomes.

1. Identification of leadership strengths and weaknesses
2. Identification of dominant learning and leadership styles
3. Identification of competency level for a series of specific skills
   - Problem solving
   - Group processing
   - Negotiation
   - Conflict resolution
   - Developing staff
   - Analytic assessment
   - Project management
   - Developing systems
   - Strategic planning

Literature Review

Critical to a nurse executive's success and career development is the nurse executive's ability to increase the speed of acquisition, comprehension, and integration of information. During this era of rapid growth and technologic innovation, the reality is that much of what we have learned previously is not useful in the ever changing health care environment. Most of us are inundated with a myriad of professional and technical journals, newsletters, business magazines, and fiction and nonfiction books that may have relevance as metaphors to the workplace.

Steps to enhance one's timely literature review and knowledge integration of written materials include

- Be selective.
- Subscribe to abstracts of articles and books.
- Ask the librarian or a secretary to photocopy the table of contents of key publications identified as providing potential sources of needed information.
- Scan the abstracts and table of contents, selecting only those directly affecting your work for photocopying and perusal.
- Newsletter and journal scans can provide one with industry and professional trends in abbreviated and summary form.
- Read for ideas, not words.

- Scan key headings and summary paragraphs before deciding whether to read articles in their entirety.
- Adjust your reading speed to the material being read with the goal of reading as quickly as possible with the greatest possible comprehension.
- Make a mental summary of what you have integrated and the source of the material.
- Keep and circulate copies to those in the organization who could also benefit from newly found information.

Audiotape Listening

Unlike reading, listening to audiotapes can be effective in enhancing learning during such activities as commuting or exercising. Listening to audiotapes, whether they be news summaries, technical summaries, book summaries, or skills development tapes, can assist a nurse executive in keeping current with a minimum expenditure of time, energy, and expense. As with written abstracts, audiotapes usually focus on the highlights of the written word. Regional and national seminars and workshops often are recorded in their entirety and provide an inexpensive alternative for knowledge acquisition for those who did not attend.

Variable speed audio recorders permit speed listening, which has been shown to enhance learning efficiency as well as retention (Calano & Salzman, 1988). Learning efficiencies and effectiveness can be enhanced also by identifying goals for listening. The following are helpful hints or guidelines for listening to audiotapes.

- Do not bother listening to tapes that initially sound as if they will not meet your developmental needs.
- Replay tapes to gain new insights or focus on specific concepts.
- Jot down concepts that might be useful at a later time.
- Once you have mastered speed reading and listening, discipline yourself to continue the habit.
- Listen and read to learn!

Workshop and Seminar Participation

Attendance and active participation in workshops and seminars are an investment in ongoing lifelong learning. These short-term courses, which vary in length from one-half day to a week, are extremely valuable in providing practical and up-to-date information on a specific issue or topic. Participants can match their individual learning needs and level of expertise with anticipated program outcomes before deciding whether to attend a seminar. Success seminars energize participants by immersing them in the knowledge and skills they need, and they often provide experiential exercises. In addition, participating in workshops and seminars broadens one's perspective by stimulating new thinking and providing opportunities to network. Active participation may confront participants to relook at their careers, examine their role in an organization, and evaluate their personal growth and progress toward their own developmental goals. Making contacts at seminars with peers as well as content experts in a given field validates one's approach to a particular organizational challenge as well as stimulating new thinking related to possible solutions to old problems.

Recommendations for getting value from a seminar include (Calano & Salzman, 1988)

- Make sure it is a quality offering.
- Ask the sponsor for feedback from past participants and if a refund is available if the offering does not fit your learning needs.
- It is important to focus on your goals—formulate questions you need answers to or issues you hope to resolve as a result of attending.
- Use the opportunity to network by renewing old contacts and establishing new ones. Interactions with other participants and the speakers are activities that facilitate learning.
- Use the time to focus not only on learning but application in your professional as well as your personal life.
- Do not call the office.
- Use the seminar time to focus on your own development.
- After the seminar, capitalize on its value for your own as well as your organization's development by creating action steps, sharing new insights with your staff as well as your boss.
- Remember seminars should pay back either in savings or profits at least five times their fee.

Journal Writing

Journal writing is a useful developmental tool that uses reflection on one's thought processes and interactional patterns. Seeing innermost thoughts and feelings on paper can literally change perceptions of workplace issues by assisting in separating the writer from his or her thoughts, feelings, and ideas. Journal recording of workplace experiences is not like the diary from childhood. The journal is a tool for self-discovery and, ultimately, self-development. It can be used as a receptacle for the mind chatter that plays mental ping-pong with workplace decisions that have to be made. It can be used as a tool to train oneself to listen to increase awareness of the underlying beliefs and assumptions governing attitudes, behavior, and decisions. Listening through the printed word can unlock patterns that prevent looking at things in a different way. The journal can be a valuable mirror to see oneself and one's thinking from a different perspective. The journal can be used as a validation tool by highlighting and recording achievements and successes. The following (Carter-Scott, 1989) are some guidelines to assist in maximizing the benefits of the journal writing experience.

- Record your feelings, reactions, and thoughts.
- Focus on your internal experience.
- Write about all of the things your mind is chattering about.

- Tell your truth to the best of your ability.
- Ask yourself such questions as
  "What is the truth about that?"
  "Is there something even deeper?"
- Listen and write whatever answers you receive.
- Use the journal to get to the bottom of issues that surface.
- See if you can experience a catharsis releasing the emotion on an issue or incident.
- Whenever possible, use your journal in the midst of conflict.
- When your emotions are most intense, you can use the journal as a tool to delve beneath the surface and assess what is really going on.
- When you feel out of sorts and do not know why, use the journal to outflow whatever is there.
- Do not worry about making sense or being responsible; write whatever you feel, think, sense, judge.
- Forget about punctuation, grammar, syntax, and spelling.
- No one but you is going to read your journal, so tell it like it is.
- Make sure that it is legible so that you can read it later, but do not edit, rehearse, censor, or withhold.
- Use your journal daily.
- Set aside a specific time everyday to write in your journal—it usually works best to have a specific place to do your writing.
- Even if you have nothing to say, write that you have nothing to say, but do not go a day without writing.

Professional Presentations

Professional presentations and formal speaking engagements are opportunities for growth in determining both what is important to communicate and how best to communicate it. The outcomes as a developmental opportunity include (1) the period of reflection and planning that precedes a presentation provides opportunities for clarification of current values and knowledge, assimilation of new learning, and evaluation of successes and contributions of organizational change, and (2) presentation skills, group interactive skills, and self-confidence may be enhanced as a result of delivering the presentation. As an activity that facilitates individual development, speaking in public forums enhances one's learning by developing new insights and provides opportunities to sharpen both formal presentation skills and informal questions-and-answers response skills. In addition, developing competency and high-level expertise in making formal presentations positions one as a recognized leader and opens the door to future opportunities.

Writing for Publication

Professional writing for publication provides many of the same developmental opportunities as professional speaking. Preparing manuscripts forces one to think about a topic or issue that not only is important but also forces commitment of those thoughts and ideas to paper, with the potential to be read widely through the profession. The high level thought processes associated with preparing a manuscript for publication can be a powerful self-development tool that is both reflective and creative. Personal growth resulting from internal dialogue can be a primary motivator for preparing manuscripts, or the growth associated with writing may be a serendipitous event. Publication, similar to professional speaking, is an activity that positions one in a leadership role.

Personal Discovery in the Wilderness

Using nature and outdoor adventures as a learning laboratory, professional development courses, such as those developed by Outward Bound, have become a creditable vehicle for executive self-development. The core focus of survival in the wilderness courses is enhancing confidence by building leadership skills in risk taking, cooperation, analytic problem solving, task assignment, communication, and team building. Understanding that leaders in today's world face multiple issues, including personal and life transitions, thwarted expectations, and the fear of change, the Outward Bound courses are structured to enable participants to

- Reflect their day-to-day views
- Develop fresh perspectives
- Gain new insights into career goals
- Develop new skills

Feedback from participants in this type of learning experience has impressively documented the value and direct application of these multienvironmental courses to the everyday executive workplace.

Planning/Teambuilding Retreats

All day or multiday sessions away from the workplace provide the opportunity for management and executive teams to plan strategically as well as grow and develop as a high-performing work team. In addition to providing the internal resources to develop strategic and business plans, retreats facilitate individual and team development. There is profound value in teams spending extended periods of time together away from the workplace. Using a professional group facilitator with expertise in organizational behavior enhances the developmental process for the nurse executive and all members of the team to build on their own leadership, communication, problem solving, and planning skills. If properly structured and facilitated, retreats provide the catalyst for individual and team learning by facilitating (1) exchange of honest feedback, (2) identification of insights and strategies for self and team growth, (3) reflection of perspectives and reality, and (4) recommitment to individual and organizational goals.

Mentoring

Participants in a successful mentoring relationship can be a powerful adjunct to nurse executive development. For the developing executive, a mentoring relationship enhances exposure and visibility within a professional organization and facilitates development of leadership skills. In addition, mentoring relationships are pivotal in supporting risk taking and orchestrating opportunities for challenging assignments. The experience of nurse leaders who have participated in mentoring relationships has demonstrated that learning from a mentor's experience, role modeling, and counseling is a valuable opportunity.

As a developmental activity, mentoring relationships usually span an 8- to 10-year period and are characterized by a high level of trust, open communication, and intense interpersonal interactions. Participants in successful relationships self-select each other. Powerful, secure, competent executives who are good teachers and role models and are perceived favorably within the organization are sought as mentors (Zey, 1984). They, in turn, seek people who have an enhanced capacity for "on-the-job" learning, are risk takers, are committed to their organization, and have the potential to be a star. Careful selection of a mentor and periodic evaluation of the mentoring relationship can validate the value of the mentoring process and facilitate its success as a developmental activity for nurse executives for both the student and the mentor.

Networking

Networking, one of the highest forms of collaboration, is a two-way executive developmental tool for the nurse executive. It uses one's abilities to assist others in goal achievement and provides a cadre of associates who can assist in support of one's outcome attainment (Calano & Salzman, 1988). Whether networking is pursued as an unstructured or a planned activity, it is critical to successful development of a nurse executive. Using the collaborative relationships of networking validates data and enhances access to inside information. In addition, networking provides valuable insights into problem solving and may assist the nurse executive in finding new employees, suppliers, or customers.

The process of establishing networking relationships (Calano & Salzman, 1988), although not a comfortable or well-developed skill for many of us, is really easy to cultivate and includes the following.

- Force yourself to broaden your perspectives.
- Explore various environments for networking and then focus on those that have the greatest potential payoff for your development.
- Most of us already have a network. It is in our telephone directory, business card files, and correspondence files.
- Attend conferences and professional organizations or service clubs.
- Publishing and speaking facilitates networking opportunities through establishing one's position of authority on a current topic.
- Be proactive and seek new contacts as well as affirming current ones when the opportunity arises at workshops or meetings.

- Sponsoring another person by sharing resources in your network with others not only increases your value as a networker but provides an opportunity to a colleague who can best provide the information.

Successful networking is contingent on keeping in touch with individuals in one's network as well as competitors. Contacts within one's network perpetuate its stability and usefulness, whereas the benefits of gaining fresh insights from competitors can have a positive impact on thinking without sharing trade secrets. Expressing gratitude to those who have provided information powerfully reinforces a network. Networking facilitates problem solving, validates information and decisions, and provides information that is readily accessible with the advent of information technology among a network of colleagues. This process can facilitate the development of the nurse executive not only from the perspective of establishing collegial relationships but from the perspective of creating a large information base to facilitate information gathering and decision making.

Therapy

The complexity of the external world coupled with the advent of sociotechnical models has challenged us to examine the assumptions we make about ourselves and our work environment (Mitroff & Mason, 1981). Old paradigms of the world and methods of handling organizational problems have not prepared us for the paradigm shifts in today's knowledge-based health care organizations.

Managers, who in the past have focused on learning finance and operational skills, have come to realize that learning theories of human behavior drives the development of productive relationships needed to cope with complex issues in the workplace environment. In modern organizations, the boundary "where the inside of the mind of the individual leaves off and where the outside of the forces of society supposedly starts or takes over is increasingly blurred" (Mitroff, 1983, p. 161).

Most nursing leaders spend most of their waking hours within an organization. It is my hypothesis that "work families," just like "home families," can be dysfunctional and require therapeutic interventions to develop effective interactional patterns. Leaders in organizations, just as parents, must learn to lead, teach, grow, and use change creatively within an ever changing environment to facilitate individual and team development.

Therapy is a logical developmental activity if one believes the hypothesis that neither the behavior nor institutions can be understood independently of one another and the premise that human interactions in the workplace can be facilitated by leaders. In its broadest sense, therapy facilitates our reframing issues and learning more effective coping skills. From this perspective, a therapeutic relationship may be facilitated by a mentor, organizational development specialist, or those with expertise in clinical counseling and therapy roles. As a credible tool for executive self-development, therapy can facilitate the understanding of human systems and the motivation of individual and group behavior, which translates to a higher functional level for individual leaders and their organizations.

Institute and Fellowship Programs

A number of specialized and fellowship programs are available in nurse executive development. Among the most roleworthy are the Western Institute for Nurse Executives, Johnson and Johnson/Wharton Fellows Programs in Management for Nurses and HealthCare Executives.

Active participation in these programs provides the nurse executive opportunities to explore leadership strategies, examine their roles, and evaluate challenges of the nurse executive role. Specific benefits of these programs include

- Exploration of management and leadership advanced concepts tailored for nurse leaders
- Interaction with multidisciplinary leaders
- In-depth analysis of complex health care and nursing issues
- Opportunities to challenge old assumptions by exploring new insights and possibilities

Selection of participants is highly competitive, and most programs require active participation of the nurse executive's boss. In addition to participant selection criteria, program structure and curriculum have resulted in strengthening nurse executive management skills and application of financial and planning techniques (Rovin & Ginsberg, 1988). Institute or fellowship programs use social events and networking as another mechanism to facilitate growth and development for nurse executives.

Sabbatical Leaves

Traditionally, the opportunity for sabbatical leaves has been limited to the academic teaching environment, where tenured college professors were granted leaves every 7 to 10 years for rest, travel, academic enrichment, or research. Recently, there has developed a trend across corporate America from the high tech industry to the fast food industry to send people off for self-development with full or partial pay and benefits as well as job guarantee for the same or comparable position on their return (Naisbitt & Auberdene, 1985). Although sabbatical leaves have not been commonplace in the service sector of the health care industry, they are more and more frequently finding their way into executive employment packages. They serve as an excellent vehicle for providing a break or change in the normal routine of employment for the purpose of personal and professional enrichment. It is important that they are carefully structured and planned in advance to effectively facilitate self-development for the health care executive. As a developmental activity for the nurse executive, they can provide once in a lifetime opportunities for individuals to achieve one or more of the following outcomes: (1) acquire new and diverse perspectives, (2) experience paradigm shifts in reality thinking and testing, (3) prepare for short-term role changes, (4) acquire experience in other disciplines or service industries, (5) learn new skills that may fill experiential gaps, and (6) continue or complete formal education.

On-the-Job Learning

Rising to the challenge of specific jobs and mastering difficult assignments perhaps are the best experiences for developing executives. In fact, health care organizations with the best reputations for being on the cutting edge in delivering cost–quality outcomes have made extensive use of on-the-job learning to develop their leadership talent.

Among the most effective job assignments that promote true on-the-job learning are those requiring leading by persuading others. These often include special project and task force assignments that are temporary and discreet and focus on major organizational problems. These assignments are short term in nature, requiring outcome attainment within weeks to months, and exist above and beyond one's regular full-time position. Frequently, these persuasion-centered assignments involve a line to staff switch where accountability and authority no longer go hand in hand. These assignments usually are a developmental stretch and require learning new skills, such as developing new product or service lines, starting new businesses, or opening new markets. Usually, these assignments involve an increase in responsibility in terms of being both broader and different from one's usual role. Some assignments actually require moving into new businesses or assuming responsibilities for significant increases in numbers of people, dollars, and functions (McCall, Lombardo, & Morrison, 1988). The manager or executive who is truly committed to self-development is one who early seeks out and chooses on-the-job assignments that stretch his or her perspective and skills. For the aspiring executive, these assignments are stimulating and highly rewarding.

References

Bader, G., & O'Malley, J. (1992). Transformational leadership in action. *Nursing Administration Quarterly, 17*(1), pp. 38-44.

Bronowski, J. (1973). *The ascent of man.* Boston: Little Brown.

Calano, J., & Salzman, J. (1988). *Career tracking: The 26 success shortcuts to the top.* New York: Simon and Schuster.

Carter-Scott, C. (1989). *Negaholics: How to overcome negativity and turn your life around.* New York: Ballantine.

Cotham, J. (1989). *Career shock.* New York: Donald Fine.

Drucker, P. (1992). *Managing for the future the 1990s and beyond.* New York: Truman Talley Books.

Hirsh, P. (1987). *Pack your own parachute.* Reading, MA: Addison Library.

Kanter, R.M. (1989). *When giants learn to dance.* New York: Simon and Schuster.

Kim, C.L., ed. (1990). *The fifth discipline: The art and practice of the learning organization; A conversation with Peter Senge.* Framingham, MA: Innovation Associates.

McCall, M., Lombardo, M., & Morrison, A. (1988). *The lessons of experience.* Lexington, MA: Lexington Books.

Mitroff, I. (1983). *Stakeholders of the organizational mind.* San Francisco: Jossey Bass.

Mitroff, I., & Mason, R. (1981). *Challenging strategic planning assumptions.* New York: Wiley.

Naisbitt, J., & Auberdene, P. (1985). *Re-inventing the corporation*. New York: Warner Books.

Rovin, S., & Ginsberg, L. (1988). Johnson and Johnson Wharton Fellows Program in Management for Nurses. *Nursing Economics, 6*(2), 78–82.

Senge, P. (1990). *The fifth discipline: The art and practice of the learning organization.* New York: Doubleday.

Zey, M., (1984). *The mentor connection*. Homeward, IL: Irwin.

CHAPTER 10

EFFECTIVE COMMUNICATION AND NURSE MANAGER SUCCESS

Dixie Cornell

EXECUTIVE SUMMARY

A manager is called on to do many things: motivate people, delegate work, evaluate performance, understand financial spreadsheets, prepare a budget, and much more. All of these varied tasks require that we work with other people, that we communicate with our peers, supervisors, clients, and public. To be effective in this role, we must listen so that we can understand and speak so that we are heard.

In this chapter, I have attempted to address the issue of how we communicate and the impact that communication has on the success of the nurse manager. The material provides an overview of communication pathways and outlines strategies for improving both personal and departmental communication. I have also included an overview of the very complex issues of managing agreement and conflict resolution. I have used situations that I have experienced and have referenced material or programs that I find helpful in understanding these concepts. You will find a short section on written communication that may be helpful when you must commit your thoughts to paper or computer screen.

As a nurse manager, you have important work to do. I hope that the issues presented in this chapter can, in some way, be useful.

THE ART OF COMMUNICATION

What is it that can rob us of valuable time, make us snap at the people we love, ignore issues until they ignite into full-blown problems, and even do things we know are wrong? Stress? Deadlines? Conflicts? People? All of these are viable answers, and they all have a common thread: thoughtless communication. By "thoughtless" I mean that we do not give much thought to what we say or how we say it.

Over the years, we have learned that people are more comfortable and more productive in a work environment where communication is open, honest, timely, and accurate. Although this simple concept is not difficult to grasp, it can be a challenge to cultivate and support.

We must cultivate and support it, however, if we wish to provide the highest quality care and, ultimately, to survive in the marketplace. Not only must we be able to communicate our own needs effectively, but we also must understand the needs of the staff, peer, and administrative culture within which we work. There is also a business side to all of this. Kanter's research (1983) shows that organizations with open communication systems have increased potential for innovation, which stimulates financial growth. In the health care business arena, where prospective payment systems demand the delivery of quality care at the lowest possible price, the link among open communication, nursing performance, and job satisfaction becomes very clear (Wolf, 1986). Yet we continue to hear things like this.

> So, Marque called me into his office and said, "I heard you let Miranda leave early last evening and both Jamie and Kim had to work overtime to finish up. Where was your head to do a thing like that?" When I started to say something, he pointed his finger at me and barked, "Just shut up and listen." I've been the assistant head nurse for 3 years, and he treated me like a child. I think I may have to ask for a transfer.

> I've talked to her before about coming in 5 or 10 minutes late. Today, when she did it again, I lost it and I yelled at her in front of everyone at report. It wasn't very professional of me, and I feel terrible about it now. Maybe it's time for me to consider another career.

These examples are symptoms—symptoms of thoughtless communication—and they can take a serious toll on our self-esteem and well-being. The results of such experiences are fairly predictable: high turnover, increased absenteeism, nonproductive work, and even leaving the profession. What we hear sounds something like this.

> There's too much stress in my job. I can't take the pressure.
> I don't feel like I get any recognition for what I do.
> I just don't like the work any more.

In reality, much of what is expressed in these statements—stress, lack of recognition, burnout—has at its roots an element of poor communication. In this chapter we review

- Communication pathways
- Communication strategies for saying the right thing at the right time
- What to do when everyone agrees
- How to manage differences
- Written communication
- The relationship between poor communication and stress
- How nurse managers can model and promote proper communication

THE ROAD TO COMMUNICATION—HOW WE TALK. DO WE LISTEN?

A helpful way to look at communication is to view it as a pathway between two people. In far too many conversations we see this path.

Person 1: → Person 2: →

Two people are, in fact, talking. However, they are each intent on making a particular point, getting their own way, or hurrying through the conversation in order to move on to other business. As one person speaks, the other appears to be listening. In reality, however, the listener is gathering her thoughts and thinking about what she will say next. She is planning how to score that really big point. There is little evidence of active listening in these situations. Here is a comment that might be heard after this type of conversation takes place.

I don't understand why Scott handled the staff meeting like that. I told him exactly how he should approach the issue of staff reductions. It's as if we never talked!

The truth is, Scott probably was told and, in fact, agreed to chair the meeting and inform the staff members of the upcoming cutbacks in a certain way. The trouble was that he did not really hear his instructions because he was intent on making his point clear. In fact, Scott could be on the next floor saying

I don't understand why Barb is so upset. We agreed to tell the staff about the cutbacks at the in-service meeting.

Another common communication pathway looks like this.

Person 1 (supervisor, physician): ↘

Person 2 (staff nurse, head nurse): ↗

What we see here is a lot of talk coming down and very little going back up. We can imagine who is listening. If immediate action is needed, for example, in an emergency situation, this type of communication works. However, if you are trying to build an ongoing relationship and achieve certain goals, this path leaves much to be desired. We see this pathway at work in the situation where Marque called the assistant head nurse into his office and did not offer her the opportunity to speak. What future do you think these two have based on this communication style?

There is another important implication to this communication pathway. Information that starts at the top has a way of losing its original message or intent as it works its way down. It is sort of like the grade school game of gossip, where one child tells the next child a short piece of gossip. The information is repeated down the line until what the last child hears bears little resemblance to the original thought.

Nurse managers should also be aware of a slight twist to this communication pathway. It looks like this.

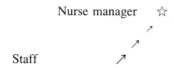

The boss—the star—is still on top and the staff people are still on the bottom. In this situation, however, information coming up the pathway is being filtered for the manager's ears. This pathway generally develops when staff members try to protect the manager from hearing disparaging news, not as a malicious attempt to keep news from the manager. The astute nurse manager should be aware that well-meaning staff members have been known to soften the blow so that by the time information reaches the manager it does not sound quite so bad as it once did. Unfortunately, it is also not as true as it once was. In fact, the higher you go in an organization, the more difficult it may be to get at the truth.

The most effective way to deal with this issue is to make sure that the information coming down the pipeline is timely and honest. This maximizes your chances of being treated in the same manner. In other words, what goes down might come up. However, if you have ever blurted out, "I didn't need to hear that just now," in response to a piece of nasty information, you may be protected in the future.

The ideal in communication pathways looks like this.

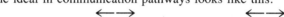

What we have is very simple: two people talking, two people listening. If solid working relationships and lasting results are the goal, this is the best path to take. When both people take their turns talking and listening to what the other is saying, we have a solid base for respectful working relationships.

A COMMUNICATION PRIMER FOR THE NURSE MANAGER

In the 1970s and 1980s, many of us attended a seminar or class on assertiveness training. In some of these sessions, the emphasis was on getting what you want—winning at any cost. Unfortunately, this often turned into a win-lose scenario. Now we are in the 1990s, the age of partnership. We finally have realized that we must work together to reach common goals and that we must do so without hurting each other in the process. The glue that holds many of these partnerships together is the ability to handle communications in a respectful yet assertive manner.

Paying attention to what we say and how we say it can bring a stressful, potentially explosive, or just plain bothersome situation to the point of negotiation. Use of the communication techniques discussed in this chapter in no way guarantees that we will get what we want. That is not the purpose. The goal is to bring the troublesome situation to the surface—lay it on the table—and discuss it like adults. If used properly, assertive communication can help us to

- Get the work done
- Reduce stress
- Be more productive
- Improve the quality of our lives

Some guidelines follow.

Always Think before You Open Your Mouth

Sometimes we open our mouths and unformed thoughts or opinions just tumble out. Insert a filter by thinking through what you want to say and the best manner in which to say it. Some people count to ten before they speak. My recommendation is to think, not count. It greatly improves the quality of what you say and reduces the chances that you will want to kick yourself later.

Believe That You Are Important and Deserve to Be Heard

This is extremely important. You must come to the belief that you have a human right to be heard—it is all in how you say it. In the example given earlier, we heard how an assistant head nurse was treated by Marque, her head nurse. His attempt at communication was certainly not professional or acceptable. What could the assistant head nurse have done? She could have asserted her rights to be treated with dignity and to be heard. For example, "Excuse me a minute Marque. You seem upset and I certainly want to discuss the situation. But I cannot sit here and allow you to yell at me."

What do you do if it was you who flew off the handle, as the person in the second example did. As soon as your behavior hits you, and it will hit you, go to the other person and start over. For instance, "Gail, I'm sorry that I yelled at you in front of the staff this morning. I realize I shouldn't have done that. That doesn't mean, however, that I can forget what happened. You are constantly 5 or 10 minutes late and we need to talk about how to correct this situation."

Structuring What You Want to Say

How many times have you said or heard, "What I'd really like to tell her is. . . ." It is odd that we usually know what we would like to say but develop some kind of block when it comes to actually saying it. The next time you say or hear, "What I'd like to tell him is . . . " pay attention to the message. Using the previous example of the manager who yelled at Gail, you might want to say, "You're always late, you hold things up and make people wait who were on time. It's not fair and it's got to stop." If that is the issue you want to bring to discussion, choose your words carefully and stick to the facts.

The Words You Choose
"I" Messages

The use of "I" messages conveys your concern and shows that you take responsibility for your feelings. On the other hand, statements that start with you can rapidly put the other person on the defensive.

- You should have had this report to me 2 days ago!
- You are always late.
- You make me so mad.

If your goal is to discuss the situation and take steps to improve it, "I" statements are required. For example, look how the examples given would sound if the person speaking took responsibility for her actions.

- **I** asked for this report to be on my desk by Wednesday.
- **I** see a pattern of tardiness developing.
- **I** am really angry.

Saying I asked, I see, I am does not change the message, but the blow is softer.

To use "I" statements effectively

1. State your feeling.
   - **I** am concerned.
   - **I** am frustrated.
2. State why you feel this way.
   - **I** am concerned because people who report to work (to the meeting, etc.) on time must wait for you.
   - **I** don't feel that this is fair.
   - **I** am upset because I feel that you don't respect my feelings.
3. State desired action.
   - **I**'d like to discuss this with you. Do you have some time this week?
     Asking to set a meeting time allows you both to think rationally about the situation and to calm down. However, if the person says, let us talk now, you should be ready to go.
4. Repeat steps if necessary.
   - As **I** said, **I** need to clear the air on this. When can we meet?
     Sometimes people just do not get it, and you must repeat your statement. Sometimes they never get it, but at least you have tried.

The use of "I" messages also helps to avoid another trap—assigning blame. No one wants to be held responsible for another's feelings. If you blame another, it lays the groundwork for getting even. Blaming an individual for something, especially in the presence of others, sets you up for a counterattack. Remember, your goal is to bring the problem to the point of discussion.

Personal Reflection Time

Think of a situation that has been bothering you recently. Would it help to bring the issue to discussion by using a few "I" messages? Give it a try.

1. State your feeling.

I _____

2. State why you feel this way.

I _____

3. State desired action.

I _____

Jargon

Every profession has its terminology and buzzwords. In nursing, this parlance can be as specialized as the unit on which you work. Jargon can be useful when people who understand it communicate with each other. However, more and more business situations call for the use of teams from a variety of professional groups (Pell, 1992). If specialized terms are used, make sure that everyone involved knows their meaning.

It is fairly common practice for a buzzword to be coined by a corporate officer or upper level manager, and suddenly everyone is using it. That does not mean that everyone understands its meaning. It just means that they are using it because it seems to be the thing to do. The chosen word starts appearing on reports and in strategic planning meetings. Soon the custodial staff gets wind of it, and someone asks, "What's 'downsizing' supposed to mean anyway?"

The use of jargon can cause people to feel intimidated when no such feeling is intended. Unless you are talking to individuals within your own specialized group, it is best to leave jargon out of the conversation.

Stick to the Facts

We are very aware of the distinction between objective and subjective. In human communications, the facts of a situation provide objective, useful data. On the other hand, an individual's behavior is a subjective reading and not really very useful. You must, of course, make sure your facts are correct.

If a head nurse repeatedly ignores your request for information, say so.

> *Fact:* "I asked you for this report 2 weeks ago, and I want it on my desk in 2 days."
> *Rather than:* "I can't wait all year," or "What do I have to do to get that report from you?"

If someone is consistently late for a regularly scheduled meeting, say so.

> *Fact:* "This meeting starts at 2 PM each Tuesday. The other group members count on you to be here on time."
> *Rather than:* "What's your excuse this time?"

Facts can then be used as a steppingstone to get to the real question—Why is this situation happening? For example

> *Fact:* "I notice you've been late three times this week and at least twice last week."
> *Ask the question:* "What seems to be the problem?"

Location

Another consideration is where you hold your discussion. Sometimes in the heat of disagreement, we tend to air our problems in front of anyone who happens to be in the vicinity. If this occurs, you can rest assured that the person you disagreed with will find an opportunity to get even. Whenever possible, conduct your discussion in private. It is well worth the trouble of moving to another area.

For example, years ago when I was a critical care head nurse, I entered the unit to find a surgeon yelling at a staff nurse for something I knew she had under control. Under his verbal attack, she broke down and cried. My first impulse was to yell at him and make him feel like the staff nurse. Common sense intervened, however, and I was able to say, "I'd like to talk with you in the hall please." He reeled on me and yelled, "the hall!" as if I had said the inquistion. Quietly I replied, "Yes, the hall." Then I turned and left the unit. He arrived in a moment, and we were able to discuss the situation calmly. Later, he apologized to the staff nurse, in private. The staff nurse felt supported, and, I believe, the physician learned something. Had I tried to discuss this situation with the physician in the unit, in front of the other nurses and physicians, I am quite certain the outcome would have been different.

How to Deal with Coded Messages

How many times have we said or heard, "Reading between the lines, I think . . . ." or "She didn't say it in so many words but I got the feeling that . . . ." What we are dealing with in these cases are people who, for whatever reason, are not being clear about what they need or want to know.

We all have made our contributions to muddy communication waters. We do this when we hint at what we really want to say. This is not fair to the person with whom we are talking and, in the long run, is not productive for us. What frequently happens is that we assume the other person knows what we are talking about. This assumption generally is not true, and what is obvious to us may not be so to others. We must say what we mean.

There are many situations where communication is unclear and results in mixed messages or total misunderstanding. For example, the supervisor who asks, "When do you expect to have the patient education project completed?" might be saying, "I have something more important for you to do." Or an innocent question, such as, "Do you have any travel money left in your budget?" could mean anything from, "You've been working so hard, you should take advantage of a conference," to "I need you out of my hair for awhile."

We hear these coded messages at home also. The wife who asks, "How long are you going to watch TV?" may really be saying, "When are you going to fix the back door as you promised?"

Some individuals use coded messages as veiled threats or innuendos that they know something you do not, for example, "The patient education program is running over budget isn't it?" Ask what they mean. Depending on the messenger, it could simply be a reflection of jealously. If the person will not elaborate, forget it. Do not dignify such behavior. If a problem exists, you will find out anyway.

It is difficult for relationships to prosper when communication is in code, but we can all get caught in this type of communication trap. You can help avoid coded comments by

- Being clear and direct
- Using "I" messages to convey feelings and needs
- Not accepting mixed messages; ask the person to say what he or she means

For example, "The patient education project will take another 2 weeks. Is there a problem?" Only when that question is answered can the conversation be meaningful to both of you.

Handling Feedback

If there is anything we have learned in the partnership age it is that people closest to the work have the best ideas—and we want to hear them. We want input, we need feedback. Suggestion boxes, unit idea books, and good idea contests come and go, and the staffs' reaction to them varies. One thing is certain—if a staff member offers an idea and if he or she never hears an acknowledgment or sees a tangible result, you will stop hearing ideas.

According to Tanouye (1990), you will be watched for how you react to the first suggestion. If you have asked for feedback and your staff feels that your request is a sincere one, how you react to that first offering is critical. Use positive comments, such as "That's helpful," or "That's important to know," over an overtly negative "I don't buy that," or the annoyingly neutral copout, "That's interesting." Tanouye recommends the use of a public thank you for feedback or simply a hand-written note: "Thanks for the support—I know it wasn't easy."

If we are sincere about wanting feedback, we must act responsibly when we get it. If feedback is not acknowledged, the people who provide it soon doubt its worth. Even if the idea is not workable, the courage to share it with a supervisor is worth a response.

THE HANDLING OF AGREEMENT

A former colleague recently talked at length about attending a monthly meeting, which I had attended many times in the past, that is now directed by a new upper level manager. My friend was appalled at what he saw. All comments were directed to the manager, with little if any exchange of ideas among those at the table. Meeting participants sat straight in their chairs with arms folded in front of them, and at the end of each subject, the manager looked around the table and asked, "Have we reached a consensus?" The answer in each case was, "Yes, we are all in agreement."

If you have not attended this type of meeting, I am sure that you have been involved in the following situation. A particularly hot item is brought up by the manager, vice-president, or director running the meeting, who asks for input.

Silence, followed by more silence. Finally, someone says something that absolutely no one can disagree with, such as, "This really is a problem. It's going to hurt us if we don't change our policy/stand/procedure. Our clients/patients/staff have been complaining about this for months." This statement is just the opening you have been waiting for, so you speak up. You give specific examples—dates, names, cost figures. And what are you greeted with? Silence, followed by more silence. At this point the manager/vice-president/director asks for more input and some trivial things are brought up and agreed on. In the end, it is decided to form a subcommittee.

Later, a friend confides, "Good for you for saying that. I feel the same way." Two or three other people approach you and pat you on the back for your bravery. It appears that everyone agreed with you, but while you went out on a limb, they sat back and listened. A few suggestions that may help this situation.

1. If you bring up a subject, encourage someone to join you. A comment such as, "We talk about this all the time. I know some of you have other examples or strong feelings about this issue," may bring out one more response, which could lead to another. In many cases, the only way a problem gets solved is by some brave person who is willing to take a stand.

2. When we see and hear a colleague attempting to get things done, we have a responsibility to contribute positively.

The Abilene Paradox

Another twist to the issue of agreement was discovered by Harvey (1988), a professor of management science at George Washington University. It is called the Abilene paradox, after the first situation in which Harvey saw the paradox at work.

Harvey and his wife were visiting his in-laws on a hot July afternoon in Coleman, Texas. The temperature was 104 degrees, dust was blowing everywhere, and he and the family were in about the most comfortable spot they could be, playing dominoes on the back porch surrounded by a fan and lemonade. Things were going fairly well, considering the heat, when Harvey's father-in-law suggested they all drive 53 miles to Abilene to have dinner at the cafeteria. While Harvey was thinking about the unair-conditioned car, his wife said she thought it was a good idea. His mother-in-law commented that she had not been to Abilene in a long time. Four hours and 106 miles later, the family returned home—hot, exhausted, and irritable. They all blamed each other for an event they had initially agreed was a good idea. In the end, the father-in-law admitted that he never wanted to go to Abilene but he thought the others might be bored. He just wanted to make sure they all had a pleasant visit!

This situation, followed by many more that Harvey witnessed in organizations, led him to develop his theory. He contends that organizations frequently take actions in contradiction to what they really want to do and, therefore, defeat the purpose they are trying to achieve. As a result, the inability to manage agreement is a major source of organization dysfunction.

Briefly stated, the Abilene paradox unfolds when group members agree on the nature of the situation and on the steps needed to cope with the problem but do not communicate their agreement. In other words, group members know what to do but are unable to do it. At this point, they tend to do just the opposite and lead each other into misperceiving reality.

What Harvey calls "action anxiety" then sets in as the members think about what could happen if they act in agreement with what they believe. Unfortunately, this anxiety gets them off the track of thinking about how to improve the situation. The anxiety seems to come from negative thoughts the participants have when they think about taking action based on their beliefs—Will they be separated from the group? Will they lose status? There are, in fact, real risks to speaking out in these situations, but members tend to exaggerate the risks rather than evaluating them realistically.

All of this results in frustration, anger, and dissatisfaction among members. In an attempt to deal with these feelings, subgroups of trusted co-workers are formed and the discussions center around who is to blame. Subgroups then start blaming other subgroups or certain authority figures for the problems they are facing.

I suspect many readers have been to Abilene and would like to avoid the trip in the future. There are a few things you can do.

1. During a meeting, listen to all the facts and to yourself.
2. Think about the real risk of not taking action.
3. Tell it the way you see it.
   • In a neutral tone
   • Avoid trying to influence others
   • Avoid blaming others
   • Avoid trying to control others
4. Ask if anyone shares your view.
5. Wait. If nothing happens, at least you have had the courage to state your views.
6. If someone else in the group breaks the agreement cycle and you feel the same, you owe it to yourself, the other person, and the group to speak up.

Harvey makes the point that if you do not speak up, you are colluding with the others in creating the dilemma. He sums it up by saying, "It takes a real team effort to go to Abilene."

For a more in-depth look at managing agreements, Harvey's book *The Abilene Paradox and Other Meditations on Management* (1988) is highly recommended.

MANAGING DIFFERENCES

In a 1992 survey conducted by Accountemps, a temporary personnel service firm, 200 executives in 1000 of the largest companies in the United States were polled about how they spend their time. These managers, all vice-presidents or directors, reported that they spend 6½ weeks each year, or 13.4% of their time, dealing with personality conflicts between employees. If people at this level spend this much time dealing with conflict issues, think of the time most managers must spend.

Conflict management, managing differences, or whatever you choose to call it is not only a time-consuming issue, but it is a complex one as well. The prevalence and outcome of conflict situations depend as much on varied work environments as it does on individual personalities. This section is intended to review the dynamics of conflict and to offer some suggestions and work practices that may help the nurse manager handle conflict with more confidence.

What's the Problem?

Bolton (1986) admits that he and most everyone else intensely dislikes conflict. He points out, however, that there are benefits to conflict. He believes, as others do, that confrontation is a necessary ingredient of organizational renewal. It prevents stagnation, stimulates interest, and fosters creativity. The answer is to learn to manage conflict in a way that minimizes the risks and maximizes the benefits.

There is, of course, a great deal of information on this topic. One only needs to look in any bookstore under the self-help and business sections. However, much of this material seems to come down to the same thing, which is communication skills. Knowing how to listen—and hear—and knowing how to speak clearly and nondefensively will serve you well in this arena.

Conflict or differing opinions are universal. They occur anytime there is a disagreement or perceived disagreement about what the situation or problem is and what should be done to correct it. These situations can crop up at performance review time, during negotiation meetings, and in needs assessments. Maselko (1992), a specialist in the area of managing differences, states, "In short, we can have a conflict situation whenever **'I'** meets **'YOU'** " (p. 1).

What to do?

In most models of conflict resolution, the first issue is to deal constructively with the emotional side of the conflict. I think we would all agree that it is much easier to talk after the yelling has subsided. According to Bolton (1986), we can only get at the substantive or real issues after the emotional decks have been cleared. Here is Bolton's model of conflict resolution.

1. Treat the other person with respect. This means that you listen until you feel that you understand the other person's feelings and views.
2. Restate what the other person said, to the other person's satisfaction. If you truly understand the meaning the issue has for the other person, this will be different than merely repeating the same words the person said.
3. Briefly state your views, needs, feelings. This is your turn to clearly state your position.
4. Always ask: what have I learned from this situation?

Maselko's view of managing differences includes the use of a set of skills he calls support and confront (1992). He defines support as accepting the reality of the other's perceptions, even when yours are different. Support, he says, is always for the other person. Confrontation, on the other hand, allows you to state your position. Maselko believes that support and confront should be used on the same issue as close in time as possible. As an example, *support* by saying: "You are convinced your method will reach the stated goals" *and confront* by saying: "I feel my method will reach them better."

In using this tact, avoid the word "but," as it only heightens emotions. "I know you really feel strongly about this, but I think it can't be done," is a sure lead-in to an argument. According to Maselko, "but" is not a supportive word. It takes away the reality of the other's position and does not really identify the difference. "And" is the better choice: "I know you really feel strongly about this and I feel differently. I think it cannot be done." This statement clearly indicates that you have heard the other's position and affirms your beliefs. It says that your position is valid for you and mine is valid for me. The next statement of course is, "What are we going to do?"

Maselko also believes there is a myth to conflict management. "Many people feel that if I'm interpersonally competent I can handle all conflicts," he says. "But the truth is that we must use diagnostic skills; we have to examine the symptoms. That's the only way to get at the root of the conflict" (1992, personal communication).

You can work toward the root issue by clearly establishing your individual positions and feelings. Then the task is to work toward resolving the differences. Throughout the resolution period, stick to facts and make every attempt to keep your emotions in check.

What's an Organization to Do?

As stated earlier, conflict is inevitable. However, there are a number of things that can be done to reduce it.

1. As policies and procedures are being developed, make sure they are
   - Clearly stated
   - Supported by those involved
2. Assess how your organization handles change. Bolton (1986) asserts that the amount of change and how we handle it influence the amount and severity of disputes within an organization. Rapid change coupled with ill-prepared people can and does create needless conflict.
3. Provide training on handling differences. This includes skill development in the areas of listening, asserting, and problem solving.

Whose Problem is it?

I think we would all agree that there are enough difficult situations to go around, and no one wants more. Sometimes, however, we get into situations where we unconsciously take on problems that we should not. This happens with some frequency to those in management positions.

For example, Amanda, one of the nurses in your department, comes to you with a problem. Every time she reports to work at 3 PM and Jeffry, another nurse, has been in charge, the medications room is, in her words, "a pigsty." Amanda contends that Jeffry never wipes up anything he spills or throws away anything he has unwrapped. She thinks that the medication area should always be clean, so she spends the first part of every shift cleaning. You listen to her and then ask, "Have you talked with Jeffry?" She has indeed talked to Jeffry, once, and he reportedly said that the shift had been busy and that he thought the next shift could help clean up. You suggest that since the situation occurs with regularity and that it apparently bothers her, perhaps Amanda should talk with Jeffry again.

A few days later, Jeffry comes into your office. Amanda did talk with him and accused him of being a sloppy male. He tried to laugh it off and assured her the medications room would be clean in the future. Amanda then started to list a number of other things that Jeffry was not doing. For example, she heard him on the telephone with a friend at the end of a shift, and she found a chart where a physician's order had been missed. She then accused Jeffry of being a poor supervisor. In exasperation, Jeffry yelled, "What's your problem?" loud enough for some visitors to hear. He now asks if you, the manager, will talk with Amanda and straighten this out.

The real question is whose problem is this? As the manager, you are responsible for the efficient operation of your department and the quality of care provided to patients. Although you cannot be responsible for the sniping between staff members, you are troubled by these comments. A solution that has worked for me on many occasions is to bring the two individuals together, on neutral time—between their shifts—with you acting as facilitator. Some key questions are

1. What are the facts? Who is doing or not doing what?
2. What are they willing to take responsibility for?
3. How can they work this out?

You will note that the emphasis is on the behavior of the two nurses. Your responsibility is to get Amanda and Jeffry to see the facts and to work toward a resolution. Although you want to discuss and resolve the problems, you are not required to act as a go-between.

I believe we must always remember when managing conflict that we are dealing with **people.** Most people are not intentionally cranky, perverse, or ornery. They are just people—people who have their own families, plus an odd assortment of quirks, values, hot buttons, and favorite athletic teams. In other words, do not take conflict personally.

WRITTEN COMMUNICATION

Face to face is generally the best way to handle both casual and complex communication needs. There are times, however, when a memo, letter, or note will do or when you must compile a report or dash off an item via electronic mail. This section is not intended to be a grammar guide, style manual, or specific tool for memos, letter, or reports, but it assumes that when you write any of these items, you would like it to be read. Hopefully, some positive action will follow.

I urge you to use oral communication in conjunction with written forms whenever possible. It is a lot more effective to call and say I am sending you a memo this afternoon, and I would like to know your thoughts on it by Monday. Even if you specify Monday in the memo, your voice message or voice mail carries more urgency. Of course, face to face contact is even better.

There are three core guides for written communication

- Keep it clear and clean.
- Keep it concise.
- If you want action, ask for it.

All the principles discussed in regard to clarity of spoken communication apply to written communication. People seem to have some kind of block, though, when it comes to writing. "Does this look right?" they ask. Generally, we answer, "Looks OK to me." The real question is: Will people read this? If your memo is four pages long and full of multisyllable, academic words, you are severely limiting your chances of readership. If you want a reply, ask for it. Do not assume that people know they should get back to you. More likely, your memo has been relegated to the things to do pile.

The best way to create your written communication is as follows.

1. Think about the situation and what you want to say. You can usually find what you want to say by completing this sentence: What I would like to say is. . . .
2. Write down what you would like to say.
3. Consider this your draft and craft your memo from these thoughts. Use words that come naturally.
4. After another draft, go through your work and remove any extra words, or "clutter," as Zinsser calls it (1980).

In his excellent book, *On Writing Well*, Zinsser (1980) gives an example of clutter that involves President Franklin D. Roosevelt. Roosevelt's office issued the following memo regarding a blackout order in 1942.

> Such preparations shall be made as will completely obscure all Federal buildings and non-Federal buildings occupied by the Federal government during an air raid for any period of time from visibility by reason of internal or external illumination. (p. 8)

Zinsser says he much preferred President Roosevelt's attempt.

> Tell them that in buildings where they have to keep the work going to put something across the windows. (p. 8)

I believe that when we write we sometimes feel that we must show the extent of our education and vocabulary. If you are writing for a scholarly journal, you should write this way, but if your intent is to transfer information quickly (why else would you use a memo, for instance) use short, to the point sentences. Humanize your writing. People relate to people much better than they do to institutions or institutional policies.

If you want to announce a new education reimbursement policy, for example, even if the policy itself could probably use some decluttering, the memo to announce it should be clear.

Rather than

Enclosed you will find the revised Educational Reimbursement Policy approved June 17, 1993, by the Board of Directors of Fairmount Municipal Hospital and Clinics. This policy is intended to provide a comprehensive and equitable educational reimbursement package to all participants. Please note that awards are limited to $500.00 per semester. All coursework must be approved by the Director of the Educational Reimbursement Program. A listing of eligible coursework is enclosed.

Completed applications must be accompanied by the signature of the individual's immediate supervisor. Refer all questions to your immediate supervisor or call the Educational Reimbursement Program secretary at extension 123.

Why not try

We are pleased to send to you the revised Educational Reimbursement Policy recently approved by our Board of Directors. The new policy offers up to $500.00 per semester on approved coursework (see list of courses inside). We feel this is a thorough and fair guideline for all participants.

If you are interested in applying for reimbursement, simply fill out the enclosed application and have your supervisor sign it.

If you have any questions, ask your supervisor or call extension 123 and ask for Wendy.

It takes practice to write naturally, but the reward is that more people will read it. Practice on a few of the forms or policies you must have somewhere in your desk.

EXAMINING THE RELATIONSHIP BETWEEN COMMUNICATION AND STRESS

Based on many years of people watching and problem solving, I believe that many of the situations we call stress are the result of thoughtless communication. Although learning to communicate positively can help immensely, there is one more thing that can help you stay ahead of these feelings. Become aware of how stress affects you—in other words, learn your stress pattern.

- Who or what causes you to feel stressed?
  Knowing the signs of stress will help you track down the stressors. Physically, the stress zone is the jaw, neck, and shoulder area. Tension builds

up here causing headaches, neck and shoulder pain, and backaches. Emotionally you feel on edge and are sharp when you talk to others.

List your stressors here

People _____

Situations _____

• How do you react to these situations or people? Do you vent by yelling or throwing things, or are you a quiet reactor?

My reaction to stress is _____

• When do you react—right away, or do you sit and stew and react later?

I react to stress _____

Understanding your stress pattern can make some situations predictable. For example, if you know that meeting with a particular person or department causes you to feel stressed, take some time and think through what you will say. It can help move the conversation or meeting in a positive direction and keep your blood pressure down as well.

It is beneficial to try to understand the stress patterns of the people with whom we live and work. Knowing that you are an instant reactor to a stress situation and that your spouse takes some time can help you get through stressful events.

The best way to use this information is to be aware of your stressors, then choose your words carefully. Speak clearly, concisely, and with conviction. And remember, anyone can bring a problem to the attention of another regardless of differences in role or perceived status. It is all in how you say it.

MODELING AND PROMOTING PROPER COMMUNICATION

Before we look at some ways of promoting proper communications within your department, take a moment and think about the best boss or mentor that you ever had. What was it that made this person so special? Chances are the person you have identified really listened to you, did or said things to make you feel important, and took time to recognize your contributions. All of these factors work to build trust, promote openness, and develop a more productive work setting.

It is helpful to think about those special individuals who played an important role in our early development. We have learned a lot from them. As nurse managers, we have an opportunity and a responsibility to pass on some of what we have learned to the people we work with. It does not take a lot to show our concern or respect for another, yet in our increasingly busy lives, we seldom do it. Some very simple things can improve communication within your department.

Make Time to Ask, "How Are Things Going?"

Once the question has been asked, listen to the answers you get—it is amazing what you will find out. Interestingly, some people will say that the manager should not become too friendly with the staff, that it puts everyone on an equal standing and makes supervision more difficult. I say that if you limit your staff interactions to the annual performance review you do not really know your people. If you do not know your people, how can you honestly evaluate their performance. In fact, casual questions throughout the year will make the performance review an even better tool.

Provide Regular Feedback

Feedback should be given throughout the year. An astute nurse manager is constantly looking for opportunities to catch people doing something right. She or he takes every opportunity to communicate when things are going well or when some development is needed. People who work for this type of nurse manager do not wonder how they are doing. They know (Wolf, 1986).

For some reason, we tend to use feedback sparingly and only for negative situations or at performance review time. People need to know, and have the right to know, how they are doing throughout the year. If you have questions about this, just think: When was the last time you received too much feedback?

In addition, if one of your staff is having performance problems, you owe it to that person to discuss the issue and provide opportunities for improvement. If you wait until performance review time, it could come as a shock. The most common factor in unsatisfactory performance is the employee's belief that he or she is doing all right (Bolton, 1986).

Offer an In-service Program on How to Communicate Effectively

Act proactively and discuss differing aspects of communication on a regular basis instead of waiting for problems to occur. If a yearly in-service schedule is determined, try to include the topic at least once a year.

Promote Team-building Activities

In his classic book on Japanese management theory, *Theory Z*, author Ouchi (1981) talks about a powerful yet simple concept: worker involvement. He sums it up by saying, "What people help create, they support" (p. 185).

Involving people in a team effort can range from simple duties, such as turning over the classroom bulletin board to a small committee, to more complex ones, such as compiling and prioritizing all suggestions received in a unit idea book. Another group could design the in-service programs for a year, and yet another could review the patient education programs. Do not overlook the person who complains about certain rules or procedures. Rather than view her as a troublemaker, channel her energy in a positive direction by assigning her to a committee, or even appoint her as committee chair. It could do wonders for her ego while allowing her to make a real contribution to the unit operation. After a while, she will develop ownership and could very well become your biggest supporter. Think about how you can do this within your area.

Review Job Descriptions and Orientation Programs

Many problems start at the beginning. A job description that is less than complete or an orientation period that is little more than a tag-along program are grounds for future problems. Look for the following.

1. Are job descriptions clear, and do they cover all aspects of the position?
2. Are expectations of the job clearly set and documented?
   For example, "As a member of this unit, you are expected to attend the regularly scheduled monthly meetings."
   Or, "Periodically our department must go through an accreditation process. It will be your responsibility to prepare for this event and to work with the evaluators when they are here and to assist with any reports that are needed for the process."
3. Does the orientation period give a true picture of the real workings of the unit or department? For instance, is it necessary for the new person to work a shift other than the one for which they were hired to gain an appreciation for departmental operation? This often is the case for midmanagers or administrative personnel who are hired on a straight daytime shift. Experiencing how the other shifts feel can go a long way toward helping these individuals understand what really goes on.
4. Are performance reviews discussed during orientation so that the person knows how the areas of performance, promotion, and salary increases will be handled? Is there an opportunity for a 6-month review for newly hired personnel?
5. Do you provide an opportunity for feedback on your orientation problem, say 2 or 3 months after a new person starts a position?

The ideas presented in this chapter can help to promote open, honest communication within a department. Treating staff and co-workers with respect and dignity will increase job satisfaction for the manager and the staff. The success of the nurse manager is dependent on inspiring the staff to provide the best quality service. Saying what must be said, in the proper manner, at the correct time, goes a long way toward this modest goal.

References

Accountemps (1992, Jan-Feb.). Bosses or babysitters. *Financial Executive*.

Bolton, R. (1986). *People skills: How to assert yourself, listen to others and resolve conflicts.* New York: Touchstone Books, Simon and Schuster.

Harvey, J.B. (1988). *The Abilene paradox and other meditations on management*. Lexington, MA: Lexington Books.

Kanter, R.M. (1983). *The change masters*. New York: Simon and Schuster.

Maselko, C.J. (1992). *Support/confront* (handbook from the program "Managing Differences and Agreement"). Plainfield, NJ: Designed Learning.

Ouchi, W. (1981). *Theory Z*. Reading, MA: Addison-Wesley.

Pell, A. (1992, April). Making things clear to them. *Managers Magazine*.

Tanouye, E.T. (1990, April). What is your staff afraid to tell you? *Working Woman*, 35–38.

Wolf, G. (1986, September). Communication: Key contributor to effectiveness. *Journal of Nursing Administration*, 26–28.

Young, L., & Hayne, A. (1988). *Nursing administration: From concepts to practice*. Philadelphia: W.B. Saunders Company.

Zinsser, W. (1980). *On writing well* (2nd ed.). New York: Harper & Row.

PART THREE • • • •

STRATEGIES OF NURSING MANAGEMENT

*"**I**ssues and trends affecting nursing and health care provide a context in which we will have to lead. In short, there will be more to do, less to do it with, and tremendous pressure to do it better than anyone else. Positioning ourselves for the challenge requires an incredible ability to look at who we really are and to bring about a fundamental shift in how we think about and do things. . . .The twenty-first century will not arrive as if some unknown intruder has come upon us and taken us by surprise. We know it is on the horizon and that it represents a future filled with many new possibilities. Essentially we have two choices. We can watch it happen or we can accept the challenge to create it."*

SUSAN CHAMBERLAIN WILLIAMS

Part A. Managing Human Resources

CHAPTER 11 • • • • • •

IN SEARCH OF THE PERFECT MATCH

JANET A. SECATORE
SUSAN SUMNER STENGREVICS

EXECUTIVE SUMMARY

Finding just the right person for a position is a labor-intensive process that generally involves a great deal of people, time, and money. Without adequate planning, the process and its consequences can consume even more of these increasingly scarce and valuable resources. Though the pressure to identify, attract, and select the very best staff they can is considerable, many nurse managers face the task unprepared. A well-orchestrated recruitment plan and nurse managers skilled in its implementation increase the likelihood that the matching of a candidate with a position will be successful.

The recruitment process involves many people in an organization. The effectiveness of the plan depends on how well these people work together, how well they function as a team. This in turn depends on their ability and willingness to reach consensus about key issues. First, there must be agreement on and commitment to the values, attitudes, and behaviors that are the foundation of the organization and that govern decision making. Second, there must be recognition of and respect for the expertise and contribution of each member of the team. Finally, it is imperative that all members of the team understand and abide by the rules and regulations governing hiring practices. Failure to comply in this arena can have grave consequences for an organization.

Before candidates can be screened and selected they must be attracted to the organization. Reputation, market competitiveness, and visibility are all important. Historically in nursing, energy and resources have been directed to recruitment rather than retention, even though it has been demonstrated that nurses are attracted to organizations that retain other nurses. An organization's reputation as "a good place to work" is its best and most powerful recruitment tool. Understanding the importance of market competitiveness, a measure of an organization's position in relation to others in its market, is the responsibility of everyone involved in the process. Continued monitoring of and adapting to changing market forces requires that everyone on the team gather, analyze, and share information so that decision making is as well informed as possible. Finally, strategies must be developed to communicate information about the organization and its needs. There are many means by which powerful images and messages can be conveyed, and there is much room for creativity and ingenuity.

The primary responsibility for matching a candidate with a specific position rests in the hands of an individual nurse manager who will work directly with the candidate. The most important aspect of the selection process and the one that creates the most stress and anxiety is the selection interview. There are several steps and phases of an interview, including (1) preparation, (2) the interview itself, which has six phases, (3) follow-up, and (4) making the decision. It is important to recognize that interviewing is a skill that improves with practice. Strategies, such as developing questions that uncover values, attitudes, and behaviors, and involving other staff in the selection process can assist managers in ensuring that they achieve the best match possible.

Being adequately prepared for conducting a process that has important implications for an organization is critical and is the responsibility of nursing leadership at all levels.

F inding just the right person for a position is a labor-intensive process that generally involves many people and much time and money. Without adequate planning, the process and its consequences can consume even more of these increasingly scarce and valuable resources. There is probably nothing more time consuming, disruptive, or upsetting to a unit than someone who just does not fit. The time spent up front in the selection of the right person is time very well spent.

The successful matching of a candidate's skills, abilities, and talents with the needs and requirements of a position is both an art and a science (Harvey, 1985). The science derives from the systems and methods available; the art from a manager's personal style and skills. As with most things, success comes with practice, education, and a willingness to learn from past mistakes and the experiences of others.

Although there is helpful information available—books and articles that outline the process—many nurse managers face the task unprepared. They disregard the science, saying that the methods and techniques offered are too time consuming or too structured or do not match their styles. In addition, they attribute the success of others to personality or other personal characteristics. We hope that the information in this chapter will help nurse managers in their search for "the perfect match."

IT BEGINS WITH VALUES

Through the selection process, a manager tries to match a candidate's skills, abilities, and talents with the needs and requirements of a particular position. A more important goal of the selection process, however, is to match a candidate's values with those of the organization and with the values of the people with whom the candidate will work. Managers, therefore, must know what their values are and how these values translate into personal characteristics and behaviors (Eubanks, 1991; Halamandaris, 1989; Paillard, 1990). It sounds simple enough, but often it is not. Most of us have a sense of or a feel for the things we value but have difficulty putting it into words and communicating it to others.

Before beginning the search for the perfect match, managers must spend some time thinking about their values. What are they? Are they palpable? What values guide their own actions? If managers have trouble answering these questions, they must do a little self-analysis, examine their own behaviors, and consciously try to link them to their values. For example, how much do they value decentralized decision making as a management approach? How is that value translated into practices and structures on a unit? In relation to staff, what characteristics and traits are most valued in a nurse? How important is technical competence? How is it rated compared to compassion, tact, maturity? How important is educational preparation? How would experience compensate for education? Is independence valued over team work? To determine the traits and characteristics most important in a clinical nurse, study the best performers. Most of us can recognize the things we value when we see them. Each of us can point to the nurse we would have care for us or a member of our family if we were ill. An understanding of the relationship between values and behaviors is critical. Walt Disney once said "If you know what your values are, all decisions become easy." This prescription is found in discussions of virtually all successful individuals and successful companies. It should be the basis for decision making in the selection process.

THINGS TO CONSIDER

Before continuing, two issues that can undermine an organization's ability to identify, attract, and select staff must be discussed: (1) the relationship between nursing and human resources departments and (2) laws governing hiring practices.

Relationship Between Nursing and Human Resources

There is often disagreement about who should do what in the complex process of attracting and selecting staff. In many settings, there is considerable friction between nursing and human resources and conflict about boundaries of responsibility. Debates about who does what and how the work is divided can be symptoms of power struggles within an organization and can be reflected in the simple question, "To whom does the nurse recruiter report in your organization?" In the presence of such conflict, focus on the goal of hiring the very best candidate for a position is jeopardized. The selection of personnel should be the work of a team of people who bring different skills and knowledge to the process. The team establishes a common goal, gets to know one another, and respects the skills, talents, and contributions of each member.

Human resource professionals have specialized knowledge nurses do not have, including (1) the latest information regarding Fair Labor Standard Act provisions and other rules and regulations governing hiring practices, (2) experience working with advertising agencies and media outlets, (3) an in-depth knowledge of an organization's benefit packages, personnel policies, and the relationship of nursing to other hospital departments, and (4) sophisticated computerized databases and tracking systems. On the other hand, they may not have a good understanding of (1) nursing practice and (2) the nature of the differences between graduates of various nursing education programs, and (3) they may not have spent much time with nurses or even on patient care units. This is the specialized knowledge of a nurse manager. In reality, recruitment is most effective when there is a partnership between nursing and human resources departments. The most important partnership is that between a nurse manager and a nurse recruiter.

To appropriately screen and steer candidates to a unit, nurse recruiters must know the nurse managers and the units with which they work. They must learn about the patient population, staff mix and pace, what the culture is like, what the predominate values are, and how the staff relate to one another, patients, and colleagues. Strategies to help recruiters gain this understanding and develop this partnership include shadow-a-nurse programs, rounds on patient care units, attendance at staff meetings, meetings with clinical nurses, and membership on recruitment and retention committees. It would be helpful if nurse managers simply invited recruiters to their units, giving them a chance to see and feel what it would be like to work there. When this kind of partnership exists, the question, "To whom does the nurse recruiter report?" becomes irrelevant.

Laws Governing Hiring Practices

Failure to abide, intentionally or unintentionally, by the rules and regulations governing the hiring process can have grave consequences for an organization. It is imperative that everyone involved in the process know what the rules are and what they can and cannot say and do. In addition, these rules and regulations are continually changing. For the most part, they originated in the 1960s and 1970s with passage of affirmative action legislation that prohibited hiring discrimination based on race, religion, national origin, sex, age, and the like. Later legislation extended these prohibitions to other circumstances—marital status, health and criminal records—and to other groups. Among other things this legislation restricts the kind of information that can be required from candidates. The recently passed Americans With Disabilities Act, the latest to have significant implications for employers, will not be the last. A knowledge of the rules and regulations governing hiring practices is essential. This is an area in which human resources personnel have considerable knowledge and expertise and can be of great assistance to nurse managers. Development of the partnership described earlier is one mechanism to ensure that an organization's hiring practices are in compliance with existing and ever changing rules and regulations.

RECRUITMENT PLAN

Once you know what your values are and have assembled a team, it is time to develop a plan to recruit nurses to your setting. As with most things, there is no one way to do this—no magic formula to follow. The plan for a rural hospital, which for all intents and purposes is the only place to work for 75 miles, will be quite different from that developed by an urban teaching hospital, surrounded by competing organizations and several schools of nursing. The plan for a specialty teaching hospital, a children's hospital, for example, even though it is part of a medical center complex, will be different from that of other hospitals in its neighborhood. There is, however, one constant—the existence of a plan. A fragmented, uncoordinated approach to hiring will result, most likely, in random achievement of the desired outcome, namely, the successful matching of an organization's or unit's needs with those of an applicant.

ATTRACTING CANDIDATES

A combination of variables contributes to an organization's overall attractiveness to candidates. Reputation, market competitiveness, and visibility are all important.

Reputation

An organization's reputation as a good place to work is its best and most powerful recruitment tool. Nurses are attracted to organizations that retain other nurses. Even in the midst of the nursing shortage of the early 1980s, there were organizations relatively unaffected by it. They were identified as magnet hospitals—those that attract and retain nurses—and were studied by McClure et al. (1982). These organizations focused on retaining nurses by creating environments that allowed, encouraged, and expected nurses to carry out their full professional role.

A focus on retention rather than recruitment requires a paradigm shift. Historically, more energy and resources were spent on recruiting rather than retaining nurses. Recruitment was an unquestioned budget item. The supply of nurses seemed endless. However, as supplies decreased and health care costs rose, questions regarding the cost of replacing a nurse were raised. The replacement cost of a nurse is considerable—varying from $2500 to $12,000/nurse (Cassidy, 1991; Curran, 1991; Jones, 1990). The supply of nurses is predicted to lag behind demand, and health care costs will continue to rise. A paradigm shift to an emphasis on retention may be the most important recruitment strategy an organization can devise (Spitzer-Lehmann, 1990).

Market Competitiveness

Unless an organization occupies a specialized niche, an enviable but uncommon circumstance, knowledge of where it stands in relation to its competition is essential. Although wages, benefits, and working conditions are not the only factors a candidate uses to make a decision, they are very important. An organization must make some decisions about where it wishes to position itself in relation to its competitors and take actions to get there. Where it finds itself should be the result of a carefully conceived strategy, not chance or serendipity. How each organization decides to use its financial resources will vary. An organization must know how it compares to its competitors in relation to wage and benefits packages, opportunities for advancement, and working conditions.

Visibility

Almost all organizations use a combination of strategies to attract candidates. These include print advertising, liaisons with schools of nursing, and appearances at professional meetings, job fairs, and career days.

Print Advertising

Print advertisements project an image, provide the candidate with information, and communicate an organization's needs. Good advertisements are clear and direct and convey powerful images and messages. They leave impressions, prompt responses, and attract candidates. An organization must spend some time thinking about what its image and message will be.

Most organizations contract with advertising agencies to develop advertising campaigns. In selecting an agency, it is important to remember who works for whom. These agencies are full of people with writing, graphic arts, and design skills. What they generally lack, however, is first-hand knowledge of the field, market, competition, and goals of the potential client. Good advertising agencies take time to learn these things. They learn what is special and unique about an organization so they can communicate it to others. An agency will help an organization convey its message in a more attractive and effective manner. Together, the agency and the organization can create a formidable team and a compelling campaign.

With the help of advertising agencies, organizations can develop quality recruitment materials for newspapers, professional journals, and other publications and materials for displays at national meetings, job fairs, and career days. Often this is as far as production of quality materials goes. All the money spent on expensive print advertising may be wasted if follow-up material sent to prospective candidates is of poor quality and does not convey respect for the individual or the process. To illustrate, the National Center for Recruitment and Retention Resources in Ann Arbor, Michigan, sent a mock letter from a baccalaureate graduate nurse inquiring about a position to 300 randomly selected hospitals. They used six questions to evaluate the materials sent by the 254 hospitals that responded.

1. Was the information well organized?
2. Did the layout and design enhance the written copy?
3. Was the letter written from the nurse's point of view?
4. Did the letter ask the reader to call or follow up in some way?
5. Was there too much/too little information in the packet?
6. Did the organization respond quickly?

The Center concluded that 79% of the responses they received were not persuasive recruitment tools and that 10% of the responses would actually repel candidates. In general, they found that the material sent was written from the organization's point of view, citing its accomplishments and range of services. Second, less than 10% of the organizations addressed issues of particular interest to nurses. There was little information in any of them to suggest why a nurse might like to work in their organization, what nursing practice might be like, or what other nurses said about working there. Third, the materials described the organization in terms of beds rather than patients. Fourth, photographs high-lighted places and architectural features rather than staff interacting with patients. Finally, the material was generally of very poor quality, consisting of photocopied letters and outdated and inaccurate information.

The researcher's message is clear, "If you want to help people make one of the most important decisions in their lives, you have to focus on them" (Perry, 1989, p. 41). Recruitment material should address issues of concern to nurses and be written from their perspective. That is good advice. When were your recruitment materials last reviewed? Are the image and message clear?

Liaisons with Schools of Nursing

Developing liaisons with schools of nursing is another means of recruiting candidates. This is easier to do, of course, when schools are nearby. In some places, developing links with schools of nursing requires creativity and ingenuity.

Having students in an organization has advantages for all involved (Table 11–1). The school of nursing gains clinical placements for its students, and faculty have access to the latest in practice innovations and technologic advances, ensuring that their knowledge is relevant and up to date.

The benefits to the organization are greater.

1. Students bring new ideas, energy, and enthusiasm to a clinical area.
2. They learn first-hand what it would be like to work in the organization and what a particular unit may have to offer them. They get a chance to observe the way nurses interact with patients, other colleagues, and most importantly for a new graduate, how they treat one another. They get a feel for the place. Obviously, if they like what they see and hear, they may choose to work there.
3. Faculty often influence their students' future employment choices. They can become an important referral source for the organization by encouraging students to work there after graduation. A faculty outreach program that acquaints faculty with the organization and offers them the opportunity to meet their own professional goals can pay handsome dividends.
4. The organization gets the opportunity to observe students as potential candidates for positions.

TABLE 11–1   Benefits of Partnerships

School of Nursing	Organization
1. Student placements	1. Stimulate environment
2. Faculty development	2. Student exposure to organization
	3. Faculty exposure to organization
	4. Preview potential employees

Before admitting students to an organization, a comparison between the values, philosophy, and goals of the school of nursing and the organization should be made. It is important to ensure that they are consistent. An organization may choose not to affiliate with a particular school of nursing if there are fundamental differences in philosophy, approach to patient care, professional commitment, and so on. On the other hand, it may be possible that through such a relationship an organization can influence change in a school of nursing. In addition, an organization should investigate a school of nursing's record in relation to state board passage rates, for example, and review the performance of graduates already on the staff. Contracts outlining terms, roles and responsibilities, liability, and professional conduct must be negotiated with each school of nursing. Attention to these issues at the start of a relationship reduces conflict and misunderstandings later. Contracts should cover broad issues but may include such specifics as parking, expenses, and dress.

Finally, there is another reason for an organization to consider developing liaisons with schools of nursing. One of the hallmarks of a profession is its commitment to prepare its future members. Through its liaisons with schools of nursing, an organization makes a statement about how it views that professional responsibility.

Appearances at Professional Meetings, Job Fairs, and Career Days

The partnering of nurse recruiters and clinical nurses at these events can be a very effective strategy to achieve organizational visibility. It provides potential candidates with information about the organization and gives them direct access to clinical nurses, those individuals who can address the day-to-day realities of working in the organization. In addition, clinical nurses are exposed to the greater nursing community and develop the skills needed to represent the organization and themselves in a professional arena. The investment in clinical nurses pays dividends in terms of their commitment and overall growth and development. Nurse recruiters, of course, can respond to questions covering broader organizational and human resource issues.

SCREENING INTERVIEW

The screening process is a preliminary review of a candidate's application, resume, work history, and education to determine if the candidate meets the basic requirements of the position. Screening can occur even before a candidate fills out an application. In a brief conversation over the telephone, it may be determined that a candidate is not qualified for a position and should not proceed in the process.

Who actually screens the candidates depends on an organization's structure. In most organizations, human resources personnel or the nurse recruiter or both screen candidates for qualifications and organizational fit. They also try to match a candidate with a unit or department. This is easier for recruiters to do, of course, when they have developed the kind of partnerships with nursing that were discussed earlier. In some organizations, clinical nurses have been used to screen applicants. Whatever the circumstances, the process should be fair, efficient, and respectful of candidates.

SELECTION INTERVIEW

The overall goal of the selection process is to find the best-qualified candidate for a position. The purpose of the selection interview is to learn as much as possible about the candidate to determine how well the candidate's skills, abilities, and talents meet the needs and requirements of the position. The selection process and interview often are used to weed out or narrow down a field. The emphasis should be on learning what strengths a candidate brings, how well these strengths match the needs of the position, and how likely it is that the candidate will be able to enhance those strengths with experience (McCluskey & Erickson, 1990). The interview should try to uncover a candidate's strengths rather than weaknesses.

Steps in the Interview Process

Steps in the interview process include (1) preparation, (2) interview, (3) follow-up, and (4) making the decision.

Step 1. Preparation

No matter how many interviews a manager has conducted, being prepared is always the first step. Before meeting a candidate, a review of the application, resume, and other available material is important. A manager thus can decide what points need to be validated or clarified or need more discussion. Questions targeted to elicit specific information can be planned at this time. A manager may choose to defer a review of a candidate's references, if they are available, to prevent prejudging a candidate.

Preparation in the form of time and space is important, too. The goal is to control as many variables as possible. Managers should try to determine their best times for conducting interviews. Are they better in the morning or afternoon? Tuesdays or Fridays? On which days of the week is their time most heavily scheduled? On which days do they tend to get backed up? When is payroll due? When are staff and budget meetings held? The selection of a quiet, comfortable setting without distractions and interruptions is important. Managers making critical decisions must be able to focus on the interview and not be preoccupied with other matters. The process and the candidate deserve a manager's complete attention.

Step 2. Interview

The selection interview is the central feature of the hiring process. Even when other methods, such as aptitude and psychologic testing and skill assessment techniques are used, the personal interview is still given the most weight in the decision-making process. Candidates can look pretty much the same on paper. In a face-to-face interview, distinctions are more apparent. Given the importance of the interview, it should be carefully done. Consider what is at stake. A decision to hire a particular candidate affects dozens, if not hundreds, of people—patients, co-workers, other colleagues, and most directly the manager and the candidate. A well-planned personal interview, although it will not guarantee a good hire, will contribute to that end. The phases of the interview process include (1) greeting, (2) information gathering, (3) information giving, (4) tour, (5) closure, and (6) interview write-up.

Phase 1. Greeting. An applicant should be greeted warmly. If the interview is viewed as an opportunity to uncover and examine the skills and talents of an applicant rather than a mission to uncover hidden faults and weaknesses, a friendly tone is easier to set. Small talk about traffic, parking, or weather can serve as an icebreaker and may help ease some of the tension at the start. The tone of the interview is established by the manager, whose comfort, ease, and confidence will be communicated to the candidate. The seriousness with which the manager conducts the interview conveys a message to the candidate of its importance to the manager.

A word about first impressions. The notion that managers make decisions about candidates within 2 to 6 minutes of meeting them has become part of management folklore. It is based on work done by Springbett and is widely reported and quoted. His findings resulted from a study in which interviewers were asked to make accept or reject decisions, for a very specific job with well-defined qualifications, after a 15-minute interview with a candidate. His study has never been replicated. Critics argue that given the study design, it is not surprising that Springbett found that interviewers made quick decisions about candidates. Perhaps, they suggest, no other conclusion was possible (Buckley & Eder, 1989). Despite the criticism, the myth persists. It is difficult to know just how quickly nurse managers make decisions about candidates. Many relate the agonies of decision making. Others say they make decisions quickly. Perhaps, in some cases, it is possible to do so. Managers should not think, however, that the ability to make quick decisions about a candidate is a mark of expertise. What they should strive to develop are the skills needed to conduct a thoughtful and fair assessment of a candidate.

It is important to note that during an interview, impressions are being formed by both parties. The candidate is developing impressions about the manager, the work setting or unit, and the organization. The manager represents the organization to a candidate and will probably be the person the candidate remembers most. Making a good impression is important to both parties.

After the greeting, as transition to the more substantive segment of the interview, the manager can outline the format of the interview. The purpose, agenda, and time frame can be reviewed. For example, the manager may say

> Ms. Thomas, this interview is scheduled for 1 hour. During that time, I will ask you some questions, give you some information about the position, the unit, and my expectations of staff, and will answer any questions you might have.

If a tour of the unit and involvement of staff are part of the interview process, this should be mentioned at this time so the candidate knows what to expect and how the interview will progress.

Phase 2. Information Gathering.   The goal of the longest and most important phase of the interview is to gather as much information as possible to determine how well a candidate's skills, abilities, and talents match the needs and requirements of the position and the environment. Thoughtful questioning can elicit information about a candidate's previous work experience or educational background, particular skills, abilities, talents, and interests, personality traits, characteristics, and personal style, integrity, values, and beliefs, sense of professional identity, potential for growth, ability to change, and ability to handle stress and challenging patient situations.

Methods to gather information from candidates vary from the use of structured interview guides with accompanying rating scales to a loose, go-with-the-flow approach. Those who recommend the use of guides and rating scales believe they reduce subjectivity in the process, provide structure for inexperienced managers or those with poor hiring histories, and ensure that comparisons between individuals are fair. No one really recommends the loose approach, although, in effect, it is used when managers are unprepared to conduct interviews.

During this phase, the candidate should do most of the talking. Recommendations range from 75% to 90%. The exact percentage is not critical. It is difficult enough to conduct the interview, especially when new at it, without having to worry about just how much the candidate is actually talking. The rule of thumb is to keep the candidate talking as much as possible. This can be a challenge if a candidate is particularly shy or anxious. It may be awkward and somewhat uncomfortable for managers to endure silences during interviews, but they should resist the temptation to fill those silences with talk themselves. Considering what may be riding on their responses, candidates need and certainly deserve time to think the questions through and formulate answers.

Open-ended questions and comments, those carefully phrased to avoid yes and no responses, will usually yield the most information during an interview. For example, a comment such as, "I see from your application that you once worked on an oncology unit. Tell me about the unit," will elicit more information than, "I see from your application that you once worked on an oncology unit. Is that correct?" The latter would only be all right if for some reason the manager thought that that piece of information required validation or clarification. Examples of other open-ended questions are found later in the chapter. Open-ended questions are useful for another reason. The candidate self-selects events and incidents to share with the manager. What the candidate chooses to share gives the manager an idea about what is important to the candidate. Even when a candidate answers a general question, such as, "Tell me a little about yourself," what is shared can give a manager insight into the candidate's values, goals, and personality.

Managers should have an idea about how much time they wish to devote to this phase of the interview. They must monitor the time so that they do not end up rushing through or eliminating other phases. Managers must be alert, keep the discussion relevant, and skillfully interrupt if the conversation wanders or if the candidate volunteers information that cannot be legally discussed during an interview. A comment, such as "We don't have to get into that now," followed by, "Why don't you tell me about what you have been doing since you gradu-ated?" may be needed to refocus the discussion.

The debate about notetaking continues (Meyer & Donaho, 1979; Smart, 1983). When a manager is well prepared, extensive notetaking during the interview usually is not necessary. Brief notes—words or phrases—that will recall an important point, a significant strength or concern, or information that requires follow-up are useful. Formal rating scales usually facilitate notetaking by allow-ing managers to check off or circle key points or impressions as the interview progresses. Managers can develop their own lists of characteristics, skills, and abilities to use during an interview.

Although notes can be helpful later, notetaking should not compromise the interview itself. When managers take extensive notes, they are less interactive and cannot maintain eye contact with the candidate or observe body language and nonverbal cues or be an active listener. Notetaking generally decreases as experience increases and as managers develop their own styles and tools.

Phase 3. Information Giving.   During this phase, managers do most of the talking. They outline specific information about the content, terms, and condi-tions of the position. Expectations should be stated clearly. For example, specific information might include details about the nursing care delivery system, rotation patterns, orientation, staff activities, the evaluation process, advancement op-portunities, and relationships between nursing and other colleagues. A manager may say

> My practice is to meet with new staff at the end of their orientation to review their progress and establish goals for continued growth. These in turn are reviewed at 6 months. At 1 year, a performance appraisal tool is completed by the new staff member and myself and goals for the next year are developed together.
>
> Primary nursing is the nursing care delivery system on this unit. I expect all staff to carry a full load of primary patients and to work collaboratively with their associate nurses and with other members of the health care team. That means participating in rounds with physicians, social service, and other clinical services.

It was stated earlier that what candidates choose to share is significant and meaningful. The same applies to managers. What they convey to a candidate generally represents those things that are most important to them. There is not enough time nor is it necessary in a 1-hour interview for managers to convey everything to a candidate. What is highlighted, therefore, is significant and usually represents those aspects of the position or the environment of greatest concern to the manager.

At this point, candidates are making their own assessments, trying to decide whether their skills, abilities, and talents match the requirements of the position and if this manager is a person with whom they can and would like to work. Although more emphasis is usually placed on the manager's impression of a candidate, it is often the case that the manager must sell a candidate on a position. What the manager chooses to share and the manner in which it is shared can be instrumental in the ultimate decision a candidate makes.

During this phase, the manager answers a candidate's questions. A simple,

"Now what questions do you have for me?" is usually all that is needed. Again, the questions asked by candidates usually reflect the things of greatest concern to them. Questions regarding time schedules, time off, workload, although important, convey different concerns than questions that seek an understanding of the relationships between colleagues, developmental opportunities, and the presence and type of nonclinical supports available on a unit or in an organization. Careful listening on the part of the manager is important.

Finally, managers must be prepared for discussions about salary. Practices vary from one organization to another. It may be that formal offers are not made at the time of interview or that a manager exercises discretion within a designated range. Managers must know what they can do in each situation, and they must be prepared to do it.

Phase 4. Tour (Optional).   Incorporating a tour of the unit is beneficial for both the manager and the candidate. The manager can observe candidates' responses to the environment and their interpersonal skills during casual introductions to members of the staff. The manager can evaluate a candidate's comfort, maturity, and self-confidence. Candidates form impressions, too—about the overall environment, tone, and climate. Candidates are asking questions too. "What is the environment like?" "Is there an air of tension, stress?" "How do the staff interact with or treat one another, the unit secretary, physicians?" "What's the pace?" "The noise level?" The most important question they are trying to answer is, "Could I work here?" Managers may delegate a tour of the unit to a staff member. Candidates usually appreciate the opportunity to speak directly to someone doing the job they are applying for, and staff develop their assessment skills. A discussion of staff involvement in the selection process is found later in the chapter.

It is important to leave time at the end of a tour to ask candidates about their impressions of the unit. Managers can evaluate a candidate's memory, powers of observation, and ability to express thoughts and feelings. Candidates may have questions or may need more information to fully understand or interpret something they observed. A tour can provide both parties with information that will aid them in the decision-making process.

Phase 5. Closure.   Exactly what the wrapup includes depends on the circumstances. At the end of the interview, the manager essentially has three options—to hire, to reject, or to defer the decision. The last is the usual and recommended course of action. For one thing, even if a manager is really interested in a candidate and wants to make an offer, references may still need to be checked, and the smallest area of question or concern must be investigated. This will not take long and is worth the time.

The manager may already have scheduled interviews with other candidates. Unless the current candidate is extraordinary and is being courted by others, an explanation of the projected timetable for decision making is usually acceptable to a candidate. If it is not, the manager will have to decide whether to hire the candidate on the spot or take the chance that the candidate will be available later.

If, on the other hand, it becomes clear that the candidate is unsuitable for the position, rejection of the candidate is an option. In general, however, the decision is best deferred. First, rejecting a candidate is a difficult thing to do. A measure of comfort comes with experience, but one generally needs time to prepare for the discussion. Second, out of respect and consideration for candidates, managers have an obligation to explain why they were not the best match for the position. Most candidates welcome feedback that will help them in future interviews. Third, a commitment to the professional development of colleagues and to the next generation of nurses, particularly in the case of the young inexperienced candidate, is the responsibility of the manager as well. Fourth, on a practical note, a candidate who is unsuitable for one particular position may be qualified for another at a later date. The manner in which candidates are treated influences their impression of the organization, what they tell others, and their future employment decisions. Managers who think only in terms of their own needs can jeopardize an organization's ability to attract suitable candidates in the future.

Regardless of the manager's decision about hiring the candidate, it is most important that a candidate knows what the next steps in the process will be. For example, a manager may say

> I plan to make my decision by the end of next week. I can call you on Friday. Will I be able to reach you at this number at about 11 AM?
>
> I would like you to meet some of the staff. Can we schedule an appointment to do that now?
>
> I will check your references, talk to human resources to discuss salary options, and call you the day after tomorrow.
>
> I have other candidates to interview. I hope to schedule their appointments soon. I will call you in 2 weeks to let you know if I have been able to do that and when I expect to make my decision.

Even if circumstances or timetables change or references are not forthcoming, managers need only call candidates to fill them in on how things are going and what to expect next. It is more than a courtesy. It is an important part of the process. If nurse managers have business cards, they can be given to candidates at this time. This ensures that they have the information they need to contact a nurse manager if that becomes necessary.

Phase 6. Interview Write-up. Virtually everyone agrees that the final phase of the interview is the writing of an interview summary. This is best done immediately after the interview when impressions are still fresh. Notes taken during the interview can be expanded to provide an in-depth description of a candidate's strengths, abilities, and talents. In addition, next steps and follow-up actions can be planned.

Just as it is important to set aside time to prepare for an interview, scheduling time after the interview is a good habit to get into. If an interview is scheduled for 1 to 2 PM, for example, the write-up can be scheduled from 2 to 2:30 PM. Running to a meeting scheduled immediately after an interview reflects poor planning at best and at worst the relatively little value placed on this phase of the process. Despite general agreement on its importance, managers frequently put off writing the summary. Taking a few minutes to complete this last phase can save considerable time later, especially if there are several candidates for a position.

Step 3. Follow-up

No matter what a manager's impressions of a candidate may be, it is important to do some follow-up and to check references before making a final decision. Most organizations require that requests for references be handled by the human resources department, which usually only verifies that an individual was or was not employed by the organization. When a candidate lists specific individuals as references, however, a manager may be able to learn more about the candidate. In some cases, it is possible to speak directly with a candidate's previous manager or co-workers. The ease with which a manager can get information about a candidate may be an indication in itself of a candidate's previous work experiences and relationships.

Step 4. Making the Decision

Once the manager has interviewed all the candidates, solicited feedback from others involved in the process, and followed up on references, it is time to make the decision. There is no magic formula to use. Some use graded rating scales. For those who do not, following are some guidelines.

1. Compare candidates as fairly as possible
2. Be honest with yourself
3. Weigh the recommendations of others
4. Follow your instincts
5. Resist hasty decisions
6. Beware of desperation hiring

Using the same questions in interviews makes it easier to compare candidates. How did each candidate answer the questions? Be honest. Does the candidate share the values of the unit and the organization? Does the candidate possess those characteristics most valued? Remember, newly hired staff will be able to learn the technical and procedural requirements of the position more easily than they can adopt different interpersonal skills. It is important to listen to the comments of others involved in the selection process. What are their impressions of the candidate? How well do they think the candidate will fit in on the unit? They have valuable information and a vested interest in the outcome.

Most managers can tell a hiring horror story, one where they knew as soon as they hired someone that they had made the wrong decision. In retrospect, they recognize that they may have suppressed some concerns or a gut feeling they had during the interview. This may happen more often in times of high turnover or expansion. From these experiences, most managers have learned to follow their instincts and to listen to that nagging little voice in the back of their minds. When they have ignored these warning signs, they have usually paid a price. Desperation hiring is always a mistake.

INVOLVING OTHERS

Involving staff in the selection of new staff has become commonplace (Ott et al., 1990). In fact, in many cases, a good idea has been carried to an extreme, with candidates being put through a series of often repetitive interviews. In general, however, involvement of others improves the outcome and benefits the staff and unit. First, although it is not a guarantee, it increases the likelihood that the best candidate will be selected for a position. Other clinical staff know the job, can speak more directly to the realities of the role, and can answer candidates' questions. Second, when staff are involved, they learn more about the philosophy and values that guide practice and decision making on the unit, and they learn how to convey that to others. That is an exciting and very worthwhile outcome. Third, involvement of the staff develops professional behavior among the staff, increases morale, and promotes team building. The staff become invested not only in finding the right match but also in that new person's integration into the unit. They can gauge a candidate's style and think ahead, perhaps, to orientation and the selection of an appropriate preceptor. Finally, when managers involve staff, it sends a strong message that their input is truly valued. Many managers say they believe in management concepts of decentralized decision making, participation, and team building, for example. Involving staff brings these concepts to life on a unit. The advantages far outweigh the concerns.

There are two very important caveats, however, regarding the involvement of staff. They must be adequately prepared to participate, and their role and responsibilities must be clearly outlined. This is an important process, and managers must take the time and effort to prepare staff so that the integrity of the process and the self-esteem of all involved are preserved.

QUESTIONS, QUESTIONS, QUESTIONS

There are no right or perfect questions. Knowing what kind of information a manager wants from a candidate will determine what questions are asked. That sound simple enough, and it really is. Asking good questions involves identifying the desired values, skills, abilities, and talents and developing and selecting questions that elicit them. What is important to one manager may not be as important to another. Units develop different cultures. A candidate rejected by one manager may be hired by another. This does not mean that one manager made a bad decision or that one missed a major weakness or deficit. The goal of the interview is to match the candidate with the setting. Most managers develop a set of questions they use in interviews. Over time, they learn that certain questions elicit useful information. They usually have questions they always ask and others they will ask based on the circumstances.

As with most other skills, developing and asking just the right questions is one that improves with practice. Some examples of questions that relate to specific values, skills, abilities, and talents may be seen in Table 11–2.

TABLE 11–2   Sample Interview Questions

Teamwork
- Tell me about a time—anytime, it doesn't have to be work related—when you were part of what you would describe as a "great team." What did the team accomplish? What role did you play?
- Tell me about a time when you were part of an ineffective team. Why do you think it was ineffective?
- What role do you think you generally play on a team?
- What sorts of people do you enjoy working with most? What is it about them that you like?

Flexibility
- How do you feel when you're involved in a project or situation where the goals are unclear or ambiguous? What do you try to do? Give me an example.
- What experiences have you had with being part of the start-up of anything? It doesn't have to be work related. What was it like?
- What kinds of things do you find most stressful in a work situation? What do you do about them?

Nursing identity
- How do you define nursing?
- Tell me about the person in nursing who has influenced you most.
- How do you distinguish the practice of nursing from the practice of medicine?

Patient care situations
- Tell me about a patient care situation you have had that is meaningful for you for any reason.
- Tell me about a patient care situation you have had that represents the essence of nursing to you.
- If a patient said to you, "Get out of my room," what would you say and do?
- Tell me about the most challenging situation you have faced as a clinical nurse/as a student.

Future goals
- What do you think your options for the future are? How do you feel about each one?
- What would you like to be doing in nursing in 5 years?

Reflection—insights into own character
- What three adjectives would your friends use to describe you? Why would they use them?
- How would a previous manager/teacher describe you? Why?
- What motivates you generally?
- List your strengths for me. (Then)
  I'd like to follow up. What did you mean when you said "creativity" or "hard working", etc.?
- In what areas do you think you need more experience?
- What criteria would you use to measure your own performance over the next year?

Table continued on following page

TABLE 11–2   Sample Interview Questions *Continued*

Additional questions

- Can you tell me why you are applying for this position?
- What were your favorite courses in school? Why did you enjoy them?
- Tell me about your most recent position. What was your role? What were your responsibilities?
- What aspects of your current (or last) position did you enjoy most?
- What do you think might be the challenges for you in this position?
- How do you handle stress? What relaxes you?
- We all make mistakes. What would you say were the most significant mistakes you made on a job?
- Give me some examples of the most important decisions you have made in the last year/few years.
- What sorts of college or community activities have you been involved in? What was your level of involvement?
- All jobs have plusses and minuses. What were the most enjoyable and rewarding aspects of your previous job? What were the least enjoyable aspects?
- Why are you leaving your present position?
- Did you ever make a decision that was unpopular with your peers? Tell me about the circumstances.
- What do you have to offer this unit? What do you think this unit has to offer you?

Hypothetical Questions

It is generally better to ask candidates to describe actual situations in which they have been involved. Although the specifics of the incident they relate is important, what they choose to relate may, at times, be more valuable. Their stories will generally reflect their concerns. A nurse manager once related that she notes how many times a candidate mentions the word "patient" in an interview. She began doing this after she had interviewed a candidate who had never once in the course of the interview uttered the word "patient." Needless to say, it made an impression on that manager and influenced her subsequent interviewing practice.

In general hypothetical questions—"What would you do if?"—might give insights into a candidate's notions of ideal behaviors or even their creativity, but they are not as predictive of future behaviors as questions that ask them to relate real past experiences.

CONCLUSION

There is a revolution taking place in American organizations today. The spread may be slow, but it is relentless. The radicals in this revolution (DePree, 1987; Peters, 1987; Senge, 1990) challenge us to change fundamentally the structures and relationships in our organizations. They argue that success results (1) when teams of people work together to achieve common goals and (2) when those on a team truly respect and value the role and contributions of each member. This kind of thinking represents a radical departure from traditional management practices.

Formerly, personnel were considered expendable and an easily renewable resource—a raw material, a production need, as it were. This was especially true in health care organizations. Nurses were seen as interchangeable cogs in a wheel. The refrain, "A nurse is a nurse is a nurse" was commonly heard. Today, things are entirely different. Leaders of today's successful organizations realize that people are an organization's most precious resource, that people are the organization's source of value and wealth, and that the success of the organization is dependent on its people. Organizations with this view are, in effect, leading this revolution and clearing the path to success for the rest of us.

Surely, the process which ensures that an organization has the very best people it can have is an important one. The pressure on nurse managers to identify, attract, and select the very best people they can will increase steadily. Being adequately prepared for this challenge is critical. It is the responsibility of nursing leadership at all levels.

References

Buckley, M.R. & Eder, R.W. (1989). The first impression: Interviews will measure job candidates' presentation and reasoning skills. *Personnel Administrator, 34*(5), 72–74.

Cassidy, J. (1991). Desperately seeking nurses: Recruitment and retention strategies. *Health Progress, 72*(4), 14–16.

Curran, C.R. (1991). Why can't they be like we were? . . . Scarce, expensive, and new nursing graduates. *Nursing Economics, 9*(4), 220, 231.

Depree, M. (1987). *Leadership is an art*. New York: Dell.

Eubanks, P. (1991). Hospitals probe job candidates' values for organizational "fit." *Hospitals, 65*(20), 36–38.

Halamandaris, V. (1989). Essentials of personnel management. *Caring 8*(9), 4–6.

Harvey, A. (1985). Hiring smart. *Nursing Success Today, 2*(8), 24–28.

Jones, C.B. (1990). Staff nurse turnover costs: A conceptual model. Part I. *Journal of Nursing Administration 20*(4), 18–23.

McClure, M., et al. (1982). *Magnet hospitals: Attraction and retention of professional nurses*. Kansas City, MO: American Nurses Association.

McCluskey, R.L., & Erickson, B. (1990). Se-

lection of talented employees is no accident. *Provider, 16*(4), 26–27.

Meyer, J.L., & Donaho, M.W. (1979). *Get the right person for the job*. Englewood Cliffs, NJ: Prentice-Hall.

Ott, M.J., et al. (1990). Peer interviews: Sharing the hiring process. *Nursing Management, 21*(11), 32–33.

Paillard, M. (1990). Selection and development of professional nurses in an in-patient setting. In J.C. Clifford & K.J. Horvath (Eds.), *Advancing professional nursing practice: Innovations at Boston's Beth Israel Hospital* (pp. 171–181). New York: Springer.

Perry, L. (1989). Recruitment materials can impede hiring of nurses. *Modern Healthcare, 19*(3), 41.

Peters, T. (1987). *Thriving on chaos: A handbook for a management revolution*. New York: Alfred A. Knopf.

Senge, P. (1990). *The fifth discipline: The art and practice of the learning organization*. New York: Doubleday/Currency.

Smart, B.D. (1983). *Selection interviewing: A management psychologist's recommended approach*. New York: Wiley and Sons.

Spitzer-Lehmann, R. (1990). Recruitment and retention of our greatest asset. *Nursing Administration Quarterly, 14*(4), 66–69.

CHAPTER 12 • • • • • •

STAFFING AND SCHEDULING: A SYSTEMS APPROACH

MARIE SMITH

EXECUTIVE SUMMARY

Current staffing and scheduling systems often do not fit patient care delivery models and fiscally constrained health care environments. This chapter uses a systems thinking framework to discuss strategies that will assist the nurse manager to identify and provide the number and type of personnel necessary to deliver care to a group of patients while meeting patient and organizational outcomes.

A HISTORICAL PERSPECTIVE
Challenges Past and Present

An NIH Division of Nursing report found the shortages of personnel, high cost of nursing service, and work overload of nursing staff to be the major issues facing nursing executives, with staffing problems taking a large proportion of their time. This report was published over 20 years ago, but it describes all too well today's reality (Aydelotte, 1973). Given its impact on the quality and cost of nursing care, the staffing and scheduling function may well be the number one critical management function confronting the nurse manager. Simply stated, staffing and scheduling practices translate abstract organizational goals into concrete plans and determine the achievement of clinical, service, and financial objectives (Stevens, 1980).

Staffing and Scheduling Goals

The primary goal of a staffing and scheduling system is to identify and provide the number and type of personnel necessary to deliver care to a group of patients. There are three major components that must be considered both individually and collectively when evaluating the system's ability to meet its primary goal.

- **Care delivery model:** The processes of care and associated work of the patient care unit and how it is divided and assigned to various caregiver roles. It ideally drives the other two components
- **Staffing plan:** The written plan that details how many staff and what classification are needed to implement the care delivery model for each unit on a shift-by-shift basis.
- **Schedule:** The assignment of individuals to work specific days and shifts for a specified period in order to meet the demand created by the staffing plan.

Each component interacts with and is influenced by the other components. An important concept to keep in mind is that each component functions primarily to achieve the overall goal of the staffing and scheduling system for that unit. The care delivery model is specific to the types of patients on a particular unit and their requirements for care. Hence, a critical care unit with a model of care calling for a higher ratio of registered nurses will have a very different staffing plan from that required by a unit with patients requiring less intensive nursing intervention.

Factors Influencing Staffing and Scheduling

In addition to influencing each other, the three components of a staffing and scheduling system are influenced by several other factors that should be taken into consideration when developing a new or evaluating an existing staffing and scheduling system (Table 12–1).

For decades, nurse managers have attempted to balance such factors to provide care to patients. Over the years, the factors have grown in numbers as well as

TABLE 12–1 Factors Influencing the Components of a Staffing and Scheduling System

Care delivery model	Staffing plan	Schedule
• Patient care requirements	• Variabilities in patient care requirements	• Existing labor contracts
• Patient expectations of care	• Job descriptions	• State and federal labor laws
• Staff competence	• Budget resources	• Budget resources
• Staff educational preparation	• Personnel policies	• Staff requests and expectations
• Medical practice	• Equipment, supplies, and technology	• Personnel policies
• Standards of nursing care	• State and federal regulatory requirements	• Current market conditions for selected staff categories
• Financial reimbursement	• Existing labor contracts	
• Physical design of the patient care unit	• State and federal labor laws	
• Organizational mission	• Budget resources	
• Administrative support	• Staff requests and expectations	
• State and federal regulatory requirements	• Personnel policies	
• Market availability of staff classifications	• Current market conditions for selected staff categories	

complexity. Additionally, most staffing and scheduling practices today arose in response to past problems. Senge (1990) postulates that today's problems are most often the result of yesterday's solutions. The growth of all RN staffing plans occurred in response to cost-based reimbursement before the advent of the DRG reimbursement system. After the DRG system was introduced, the focus was on reducing full-time equivalents (FTEs), and when faced with cuts, hospitals kept the position that could do more, the registered nurse. The resulting problem is registered nurses performing nonnursing tasks at a very high cost and often in lieu of professional nursing actions.

Breaking Away from Traditional Practices

Most nurse managers struggle with practices that no longer make sense in a rapidly changing and fiscally constrained environment. Yet questioning these practices often is akin to acknowledging that the emperor has no clothes. How can today's nurse manager break away from yesterday's solutions that no longer fit to develop better solutions all around? A good place to start is to recognize that a different way of thinking is required to create new ways of performing the complex function of staffing and scheduling. It is no longer possible to isolate and attempt to solve parts of the problem to make lasting, successful change.

SYSTEMS THINKING
A New Way of Thinking

An antidote to increased complexity is what Ackoff (1992) describes as "systems thinking," which can be used to provide a new way to organize and understand the factors involved in staffing and scheduling. According to Ackoff, we have moved from a machine age, where the world was viewed mechanistically, into a systems age, which views the world as a collection of elements interacting with each other. Systems thinking places emphasis on the interaction between the elements and the performance of the whole rather than the individual performance of the elements. A systems age dictates a new way of thinking, called "synthesis," meaning we can understand systems only by looking at their functions in the larger wholes of which they are parts.

Systems Defined

What exactly is a system? Systems are sets of components that work together to accomplish specific objectives (Arndt & Huckabay, 1980). An open system is one that interacts with its environment by taking inputs (information from its environment) and processing or transforming them into outputs, or products that return to the environment. System survival depends on a continuous cycle of input, processing information, and output. The environment continually evaluates the outputs and provides feedback to the system in the form of new inputs. As the environment is continually changing, its response to a system's output changes. Thus, what worked yesterday may no longer work today. An important concept to consider is that there may be nothing inherently wrong with the output. It is just a matter of it not fitting any longer. Inability to recognize this results in holding on to good ideas that have outlived their usefulness. For example, nursing departments in the 1980s responded to the input of decreased resources from the health care environment by transforming their model of care and providing staffing plans with less overall staff but higher RN ratios. This satisfied the demands of the environment for a short period, but the environment is dynamic, not static, and when changes in RN salaries (an input) occurred, the cost of care (an output) went up. The health care environment did not respond by increasing reimbursement but rather provided feedback that costs must go down. One of the major criticisms of health care institutions has been their inability to rapidly respond, as other businesses do, to changes in the environment. Feedback is an essential ingredient that is necessary to rapid response and successful system functioning. The system relies on feedback to tell it to either maintain or adapt based on changes in the environment. A system that cannot respond to feedback from its environment is doomed to extinction.

The traditional ways of managing are based on machine age problems and take the approach that if there is a systems problem, the way to resolve it is to rely on using analysis to break out and examine parts of the whole, then trying to reassemble them into an understanding of the whole (Ackoff, 1992). Solutions are invariably short-lived because systems and their environments are rapidly changing. Systems thinking requires the ability to see the forest and the trees (Senge, 1990). Emphasis is placed on keeping overarching goals, or a vision of the whole, constantly in mind. Planning becomes a high-priority, continuous process necessary to integrate the interacting elements in a system toward a vision of the whole.

Applying Systems Thinking

The application of systems thinking to staffing and scheduling is an opportunity to develop better solutions through

- Considering the environment in which staffing and scheduling exist
- Recognizing that there may be some good practices that no longer fit
- Establishing goals for the system rather than its individual components
- Realizing that planning and feedback processes are essential to linking the three components together to accomplish the goal of cost-efficient and effective patient care

Figure 12-1 describes a systems model for the staffing and scheduling functions. Each of the three components of the staffing and scheduling system is related to the other and part of a larger organizational system. The organization transforms inputs, such as the patient's disease state, available resources, and expectations, and transforms them into outputs, such as health outcomes and satisfaction with care. A change anywhere creates a ripple effect throughout. For example, recent pressures on hospitals have resulted in across the board reductions in the nursing care hour, with subsequent changes to the staffing plan. The unit's ability to deliver care according to an established model of care is severely hampered if the model of care has not been altered in a planned fashion in response to the change in staffing plan. Staff are left to figure out how to provide care in a model that does not match the staffing plan. A systems approach would recognize that the staffing plan is developed from the model of care, and if the cost of the staffing plan to be reduced, the model of care should be the starting point from which changes begin. Furthermore, planning is carried out throughout the process, linking one element to the next.

STAFFING AND SCHEDULING FROM A SYSTEMS PERSPECTIVE
Current Health Care Environment

Much has been said in this book about the state of the current health care environment. Technologic advances, the AIDS epidemic, increasing numbers of the medically indigent, and shortages of certain health care providers are all factors that have influenced the shape of health care institutions. Perhaps the single greatest challenge has been that provoked by the change in how hospitals are reimbursed for the care provided, with the radical shift from a cost-based, fee for service charge system to a prospectively determined, fixed-rate method of reimbursement. Hospitals responded in a rather disjointed fashion and, even 10 years after the advent of DRGs, are still struggling to adapt to ensure survival. Initially, only certain hospital functions changed in response to a major change in the environment. There was little if any view of the hospital as a system

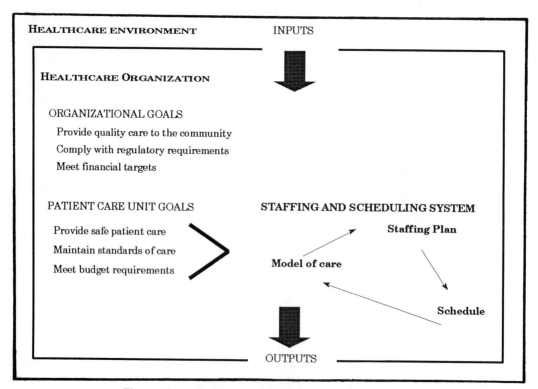

Figure 12–1 Systems model for staffing and scheduling.

composed of interacting elements, all of which were profoundly affected by the change in reimbursement.

A patient care model in a cost-based reimbursement environment could afford to be driven primarily by patient needs, which Stevens (1980) describes as the "do everything the patient needs" or goal model of care. Although there is no doubt that this approach may lead to excellence in practice, it does not take into account today's harsh economic realities. Donaho and Kohles (1992) cite cost control as the critical management issue and challenge management teams to rethink past decisions and, in essence, rethink the care delivery system. The most significant change for nurse managers is the acknowledgment of the need to shift from a goal-driven model of care to a resource-driven model in which goals for patient care are determined based on an assessment of available resources.

Most nurses, management and staff alike, have difficulty accepting the concept of resources determining care level, yet experts predict that rationing of health care is inevitable and that the denial of some potentially beneficial care to some patients will be required as part of any successful and sustained reduction in resources flowing to hospitals (Aaron & Schwartz, 1985). Health care systems that can control costs and maintain quality outcomes will be the systems that adapt and survive. The task for nursing management is to shake current models of care to the ground and rebuild them with an eye to preventing the restriction or rationing of essential elements of care.

Care Delivery Model

The goal of a staffing and scheduling system is to identify and provide the number and type of personnel necessary to deliver care to a group of patients. The necessary steps in developing a model of care on which staffing plans and schedules can be based include the following.

- Determining patient care requirements
- Assessing the roles necessary to provide the care
- Deciding how the roles will be assigned to meet the care requirements

Taking a systems approach, developing a care model in a resource-constrained environment dictates that assessment of available resources, as well as patient care requirements, be a major input to the process. Budgeted labor dollars set for nursing units are the available resource and become the target to meet when designing a care delivery model. Although it is recognized that the nurse executive is in the position to negotiate for the labor dollars necessary to provide for patient care, those dollars are rapidly evaporating as the budget becomes smaller each year. Patient care requirements and budget targets become the parameters that guide development of new models of care. This acknowledges the reality that both must be satisfied to achieve the goals of the unit.

Determining Patient Care Requirements

Methods to quantify patient care requirements arose in the 1960s, when it was recognized that fixed staff/patient ratios did not take into consideration the variability among patients in their need for nursing care. Pressure came from external sources, such as the Hospital Cost Containment Act of 1977, for nursing to justify their requirements for additional resources and from internal sources within the nursing profession to establish valid and reliable methods for developing nursing staffing patterns that reflected patient needs and cost containment (Giovannetti, 1978). A cost-based reimbursement system supported the approach that as long as patient care needs for increasing amounts of nursing care could be quantified, this would justify the increased consumption and costs of nursing service. As a result, patient classification systems (PCS) were developed as a means for assessing and quantifying patient requirements for nursing care and recommending staffing levels. Given the change from a cost-based reimbursement model to a fixed-rate payment, the use of patient classification systems to recommend staffing levels in isolation of the budgeted resources needs to be closely examined.

Patient classification systems are based on the concept of categorizing patients according to an assessment of their nursing care requirements over a specified period of time. Categorization is accomplished through the use of a patient classification instrument. Instruments commonly fall into one of two categories: a prototype evaluation tool, which uses broad descriptions and characteristics of the typical patient in each category, and a factor evaluation tool, which uses a listing of specific elements of care for which the patient is rated independently (Giovannetti, 1978). Descriptors used to classify patients are assigned nursing care time, which provides the quantification of patient care requirements. Although acknowledged as less than perfect in terms of maintaining instrument reliability and validity as well as deriving time standards, PCS met the needs to identify and justify the expenditure of more resources. When over 100 nurse executives at a recent leadership conference were asked how many were satisfied with their patient classification systems, they groaned and did not raise their hands. Judging by this response, the application of PCS developed for a cost-based era no longer fits in a fixed resource-based system of care. The focus should shift from precisely assigning time standards to nursing tasks for the purpose of recommending staffing levels to a broader approach of obtaining reliable data about the critical elements of care required by a group of patients. Trending variations in aggregate patient care requirements and unit workload is far more valuable for prospective planning.

The elements of care need not be limited to what nursing alone can provide. This is particularly true as nursing leaders heed the advice of Donoho and Kohles (1992) and create patient care models that centralize all patient care activities to a patient-centered unit and incorporate roles, such as pharmacy technicians and respiratory therapists, into the patient care model. Staffing projections based on the scientific methods employed by most patient classification systems are accurate only to the degree that the assumptions on which classification systems were based remain static (Barnum & Mallard, 1989). Given today's environment, it is unreasonable to expect that projected revenues, patient care requirements, technology affecting work methods, and other departments' work systems are not going to change. More practical, albeit less scientific, methods need to be employed that rely on the judgment and experience of the nurse manager and professional staff. Hoffman (1988) echoes this sentiment when she declares that much of management science relies on good common sense. Variability in patient care requirements should be acknowledged and used to plan a priori alternative models of care that respond to workload fluctuation and meet labor cost targets.

In many hospitals, one model of care is developed with a corresponding staffing plan that uses the maximum budgeted hours of care, with no written staffing plan for the times when variations in workload occur. Consequently, during periods of high workload, staffing clerks or managers scramble to call in staff. Last minute staffing augmentation is usually the most expensive, as a price is paid for ready availability. Unfortunately, increased workload does not necessarily result in increased revenue for the hospital. This is a good example of nonsystems thinking that fails to consider the relationship of the model of care to scheduling and staffing, approaching problems in each of these areas separately rather than as interrelated parts of a whole, and neglects to plan appropriately. This is not necessarily a result of poor design but rather a lack of connecting changes in the environment with system goals and modifying the parts accordingly. Ackoff (1992) believes that planning is the necessary effort required to deal with the problems, such as meeting increasing demands for complex care with decreasing resources, as part of a system of interdependent and interactive elements. This approach would call not only for flexible models of care that can adapt to changes in workload but also flexible staffing plans and schedules to meet the variable demands for staff.

Exploring New Methods

The ability to break out of old molds and into new possibilities needs to be valued, developed, and nurtured. Just as medical technology has enhanced our ability to diagnose and cure once fatal diseases, information technology should be used wherever possible to enhance the nurse manager's and staff's ability to create solutions to complex problems and plan accordingly. Computer simulation is one example of a useful tool that allows staff to explore different models of care within budgeted labor parameters (Flynn-Hollander, Smith, & Barron, 1992). Computer simulation can be used to explore new models of care within budgeted labor dollars (Fig. 12–2). Simulation acknowledges the interrelationships among the model of care, the staffing plan, and the budget labor resource. The nurse manager gets immediate feedback on the cost of a care delivery model.

Although patient care requirements and available labor resources are primarily what influence the type of care model chosen for a particular unit, the factors listed in Table 12–1 also should be considered when determining an appropriate model. Review of available data and identification of the key factors will increase the probability that the model designed makes sense and fits that particular organization. Conflict arising from opposing factors should be brought to the surface and negotiated. This is best accomplished by involving the stakeholders, which includes patients, nurses, physicians, and ancillary department staff, in

Total Patient Care Model

Mon/Tue/Wed/Thur/Fri Plan

Census	Budget Targets 134.60 $/PD	5.2 H/PD	MGR D-8	CHG D-8	RN D-8	LPN D-8	TECH D-8	CLK D-8	RN E-8	LPN E-8	CLK E-4	RN N-8	LPN N-8
30	133.93	5.2	1	1	4	2	1	1	4	2	1	3	1
31	129.61	5.0	1	1	4	2	1	1	4	2	1	3	1
32	132.56	5.1	1	1	5	2	1	1	4	2	1	3	1
33	128.55	5.0	1	1	5	2	1	1	4	2	1	3	1
34	133.36	5.3	1	1	5	3	1	1	4	2	1	3	2
35	129.55	5.1	1	1	5	3	1	1	4	2	1	3	2
36	132.80	5.2	1	1	5	3	1	1	5	2	1	3	2
37	136.17	5.3	1	1	5	3	1	1	5	2	1	4	2
38	132.59	5.2	1	1	5	3	1	1	5	2	1	4	2

Patient Centered/Case Management Model

Mon/Tue/Wed/Thur/Fri Plan

Census	Budget Targets 134.60 $/PD	5.2 H/PD	CCM D-8	RN D-8	LPN D-8	TECH D-8	NA D-8	CLK D-8	RN E-8	LPN E-8	TECH E-8	NA E-8	CLK E-8	RN N-8	LPN N-8	NA N-8
30	129.32	6.1	2	3	2	1	2	1	3	1	1	1	1	2	1	2
31	125.15	5.9	2	3	2	1	2	1	3	1	1	1	1	2	1	2
32	121.24	5.8	2	3	2	1	2	1	3	1	1	1	1	2	1	2
33	125.37	5.8	2	3	2	1	2	1	3	1	1	1	1	3	1	2
34	128.27	5.9	2	4	2	1	2	1	3	1	1	1	1	3	1	2
35	131.77	6.2	2	4	2	1	2	1	3	2	1	1	1	3	1	3
36	130.80	6.2	2	4	2	1	2	1	3	2	1	2	1	3	1	3
37	133.92	6.3	2	4	2	1	2	1	4	2	1	2	1	3	1	3
38	130.40	6.1	2	4	2	1	2	1	4	2	1	2	1	3	1	3

Figure 12–2 Alternative care models: computer-generated staffing simulations by PolyOptimum. (Courtesy of PolyOptimum, Inc., San Francisco.)

the patient care delivery model. Once a model of care has been determined that depicts the work to be done and the roles necessary to accomplish the work, the next step is to develop a staffing plan.

Staffing Plan

The staffing plan is the quantification of how many staff by category are required to implement the model of care. Historically, the standard for the number of staff needed has been captured by nursing care hours per patient day (HPPD), which were based on data gained from patient classification tools, community standards, and internally derived productivity standards, with the assumption that future staffing could be predicted on past experiences. The weakness in this approach is that it assumes that no changes in medical and nursing practice will occur, patient caregiver roles will remain constant, community standard is best practice, and revenues will keep up with inflationary expense growth. Using an hour-based approach does not account for differences between hours as new roles are introduced. Using a systems approach, the staffing plan of the future will most likely be derived from a consensus-building process as staff develop models of care that have to meet dollar not hour standards. Processes of care will be scrutinized closely and modified to decrease the resource demand. Staff will go back and forth between the model of care and the dollar standard, developing a staffing plan that takes both into consideration. Just as computer simulation assisted staff in the design of a care delivery model, it can be used in development of the staffing plan. Flexibility can be achieved in holding the plan to a dollar instead of an hour standard, with staff adding hours as long as the plan does not exceed the dollar target.

Alternative Staffing Plans

Understanding peaks and valleys in workload within a 24-hour day, as well as between days of the week, enables the manager to evaluate different shift lengths and starting times and the need for different plans based on the day of the week. Once a standard plan is developed, the next logical question is how much variability from the plan is expected based on changes in patient care requirements. A workload tracking system that provides reliable data can help the manager develop alternative plans that match the variations that occur. Workload tracking captures not only patient acuity but additional information that affects unit workload, such as admissions, transfers, discharges, and outpatients receiving ambulatory care on an inpatient unit. This information is most helpful if it is known relative to the time of day and day of the week that it occurs. It need not be collected on every shift, every day but can be obtained periodically as a snapshot of unit workload and used in conjunction with the model of care in developing a unit staffing plan. Thus, alternate staffing plans can be developed that take workload variability and patient acuity into consideration. A patient care unit may have several staffing plans, such as those in Figure 12-3. What this reflects is a systems approach that links staffing plans that provide the amount of staff necessary to a model of care that the unit staff have agreed previously will meet patient care needs and budget targets.

Target	$PPD 136.96	HPPD 6.3	D A Y S					
Title			MGR	RN	RN	LPN	LPN	NA
# Hours			4	8	4	8	4	8
Census								
18 A	124.93	6.0	1	3		1		1
B	116.34	5.8	1	2	1	1		1
C	129.98	6.4	1	3		2		
D	124.75	6.4	1	3				2
19 A	130.28	6.1	1	3		1		1
B	113.64	5.7	1	2	1	1		1
C	135.06	6.1	1	3		2		
D	132.26	6.9	1	3				2
20 A	123.76	5.8	1	3		1		1
B	109.16	5.2	1	3		1		
C	135.46	6.2	1	3		2		
D	132.22	7.0	1	3		1		3
21 A	119.67	5.9	1	3		1		2
B	115.23	5.9	1	3		1		1
C	130.25	6.3	1	3		2		1
D	129.81	6.7	1	3		1		3

A = Standard Plan
B = Low Acuity
C = High Acuity-Licensed
D = High Acuity-Unlicensed

Figure 12–3 Alternative staffing plans by PolyOptimum. (Courtesy of PolyOptimum, Inc., San Francisco.)

Creating Positions

Once the staffing plan or plans have been established, the next step is to determine the number and types of positions necessary to fulfill the staffing plan. The positions can be calculated directly from the staffing plan using the following method.

1. Take the number of staff required in each classification for a shift, at the budgeted or most frequently occurring census level
2. Multiply by the hours in the shift and number of days per week that the plan will be followed

		P M s				N I G H T S				
NA	US	RN	LPN	LPN	NA	RN	RN	LPN	LPN	CNA
4	8	8	8	4	8	8	4	8	4	8
	1	2	1		1	2		1		
	1	2		1	1	2			1	1
	1	2	2			2		2		
	1	2			2	2		1		1
	1	3	1		1	2		1		
	1	2	1		1	2			1	1
	1	3	2			2		1		
	1	3			3	2		1		1
	1	3	1		1	2		1		
	1	2	1		1	2			1	1
	1	3	2			2		2		
	1	3	1		2	2		1		
	1	3	1		1	2		1		
1	1	3	1		1	2			1	1
	1	3	2			2		2		
	1	3	1		2	2		1		

3. Divide the total by the full-time equivalent factor of 40 hours

This method takes into consideration different shift lengths and different plans by day of the week and is described in Table 12–2, using a very simple example of a day shift staffing plan for an inpatient unit with an expected daily census of 21 during the week and 18 on the weekend. The result, in FTEs, represents the amount of productive hours that are required to staff that unit according to the plan. This figure will match the budgeted hours and dollars to the degree that the staffing plan was developed to budgeted labor dollar targets. The FTEs are then distributed to full-time or part-time positions, taking into consideration

TABLE 12–2 Calculating Productive Full-time Equivalents (FTEs) from the Staffing Plan

Expected census 21 Mon–Fri	*Staffing plan Monday–Friday day shift*				
Staffing plan	MGR	RN	LPN	NA	US
	1	3	1	2	1
Multiplied by hours in shift	×8	×8	×8	×8	×8
	8	24	8	16	8
Multiplied by days in this plan	×5	×5	×5	×5	×5
	40	120	40	80	40
Divided by hours/FTE	40	40	40	40	40
FTEs for Mon–Fri plan	1.0	3.0	1.0	2.0	1.0
Expected census 18 Sat & Sun	*Staffing plan Saturday and Sunday day shift*				
Staffing plan	MGR	RN	LPN	NA	US
	0	3	1	1	1
Multiplied by hours in shift	×8	×8	×8	×8	×8
	0	24	8	8	8
Multiplied by days in this plan	×2	×2	×2	×2	×2
	0	48	16	16	16
Divided by hours/FTE	40	40	40	40	40
FTEs for Sat & Sun plan	0	1.2	0.4	0.4	0.4
Total productive FTEs (Mon–Sun)	**1.0**	**4.2**	**1.4**	**2.4**	**1.4**

- The need to cover 7 days a week
- Existing agreements or contractual requirements governing the frequency of weekend rotation
- The benefit costs of part time positions
- The need to create positions that facilitate the recruitment and retention of staff

Once the positions required to meet the productive hours have been determined, the next step is to calculate the amount of nonproductive time or time that staff in those positions will not be available to work due to paid time off (e.g., vacation, holiday, sick, education leave). Determining nonproductive time varies considerably from institution to institution, and the approach taken by the nurse manager should be internally consistent. Typically, a ratio of nonproductive/productive time is established, based either on the amount of nonproductive time that is accrued automatically or on the past actual usage relative to productive time. This ratio is applied to the productive FTE required in the staffing plan to determine the amount of additional productive hours (FTEs) that will be needed to cover nonproductive time (Table 12–3).

If alternate staffing plans for periods of workload fluctuation have been developed, a similar approach would be taken to determine the positions required to augment the unit staff and where they should be allocated. The frequency

TABLE 12–3   Relief FTE Calculations: Day Shift

	RN	LPN	NA	US
Total productive FTE × nonproductive rate 18%[a]	4.2	1.4	1.4	1.4
Additional FTE to cover nonproductive	0.76	0.25	0.25	0.25

[a]Rates may vary by category of staff.

with which the alternate plans are expected to be implemented should be factored into the calculations to avoid creating excess positions (Table 12–4). Combining the positions required for alternate staffing plans and for providing relief for nonproductive time in the same pool provides economies of scale and improves the chances of having staff available to meet workload peaks and valleys.

At this point, a choice can be made as to whether the additional FTEs should come from full- or part-time positions or from per diem staff who work only when needed and are not guaranteed a minimum number of hours. A decision as to where the hours are to be allocated is required as well. Environmental inputs influencing these decisions include

- The philosophy regarding floating staff between units
- Maintaining continuity of patient care and unit staff integrity
- The ability to recruit and fill relief positions
- The cost differential between full-time, part-time, and per diem positions
- Constraints placed by labor contracts on staff assignments

The goal is to strike the right balance of staff scheduled or available to match that required by variations in workload. Often, hospitals will offer additional work to its part-time staff, providing a differential for the additional hours worked. Caution should be exercised here to prevent creating disincentives to full-time work and costly short-term solutions that may be difficult to reverse as the economic environment changes. Reliable trend data on staff attendance patterns, unit workload costs, and the use of computer simulation can

TABLE 12–4   Alternate Plan FTE Calculations: Day Shift

	RN	LPN	NA
Additional productive FTE required by alternate Plan C		1.4	
Plan D			1.4
Frequency factor (% of time the alternate plan is projected to occur)		10%[a]	15%[a]
Additional productive FTE necessary to augment standard plan		0.14	0.21

help determine the right mix of full-time, part-time, and per diem staff for a given unit.

Relief positions can be allocated to the unit level or to a larger relief pool. The benefits of decentralizing the relief positions to the unit level are that the nurse manager is given control of scheduling relief coverage and can be held accountable for providing a balanced schedule. Continuity of care and team integrity can be maintained as long as the staff scheduled equal the staff required. The disadvantages to this approach are that economies of scale are lost and it may not be possible to match staff scheduled or available (in the case of per diems) to nonproductive usage and workload variations. In cases of excess, staff will either have to float out to another unit or take time off. Typically, since most staff dislike floating, this ends up being rotated among the entire staff, resulting in a lack of continuity of patient care. Not having enough staff will result in additional cost to the unit as costlier replacement staff, if available, are brought in to staff the unit.

Another approach to assigning relief positions would be to assume that the unit would be allocated the positions needed to meet the productive hours required by the staffing plan, with additional hours required to cover nonproductive time and alternative plans assigned to a relief pool that would be shared by several like units. For example, the typical grouping of units by specialty, such as medical, surgical, critical care, perioperative, psychiatric, and maternal–child, could be used to develop corresponding relief pools. The advantages to this would be that the unit positions would be augmented with staff who have been specifically hired and oriented to a relief position within a clinical specialty area. The floating in and out of unit staff would be minimized, with less negative impact on continuity of care. Since the staff would cover several units within a specialty, there is increased probability of covering the unplanned, last minute nonproductive times, such as sick time of unit-based staff. This approach dictates a systematic approach in determining how individual unit managers will be able to access the relief staff and to whom the relief staff would be reporting. Making the relief positions attractive can facilitate recruiting experienced staff who can very rapidly assume different assignments from unit to unit and day to day. Some hospitals have made the float positions an advanced position on a clinical ladder.

An approach used frequently in the past to allocate relief staff is to develop a large central relief pool, with staff hired specifically to relief positions but managed from a central pool rather than being unit or specialty specific. Although this theoretically increased the probability of having the right number of staff available to provide relief, it was impractical as well as undesirable to expect a nurse to maintain competence in all areas.

Thus, the approach to scheduling would begin with the standard staffing plan as well as any alternate or contingency plans to determine the productive positions or FTEs required to implement the plan, the assumptions about the amount of nonproductive time that will need to be covered, and where the relief staff positions will be allocated.

Scheduling

The scheduling component is the process by which individuals are assigned to work specific days and hours in order to meet the staff demand created by the staffing plan. Creating the schedule is the final planning step that pulls all the components together. The outcome of the scheduling process not only determines adequate staff to implement the staffing plan but profoundly affects staff personal life as well. Staff's primary concern is to have a work schedule that allows them the ability to plan and balance their personal life with their work commitments. Producing a schedule that satisfies staff and meets unit demands is a challenging and time-consuming management task. Providing 7-day-a-week coverage in a 5-day work world requires a thorough understanding of the cost implications of various choices, a sensitivity to reasonable work schedules, and knowledge of contractual agreements as well as state and federal labor laws governing work time.

Computer Technology

Advances in computer technology have provided managers with powerful decision support tools to assist them in considering the myriad of factors necessary to developing the right mix of positions and the most appropriate schedule. Linear programming is one such tool in that it employs sophisticated mathematical calculations to search for scheduling solutions that meet staffing plan demands, maximize the low-cost alternatives, comply with the various labor rules, and consider staff requests. This approach can be applied not only to determine the right mix of full-time to part-time positions but also to schedule the resulting positions optimally. Schedule patterns can be generated that allow staff to choose acceptable work schedules that also meet the staffing plan demand and budget target. Using computer technology not only relieves the manager from the tedious tasks that do not require professional judgment but also insures that all the factors necessary to relate the schedule to the staffing plan and model of care have been considered in the most cost-effective way. The result is a schedule that balances these factors in meeting the bottom line demand of the staffing plan. The understaffed days become the demand to which a relief pool is scheduled. The manager is freed to focus on the more important planning and evaluating activities necessary to insure that the staffing and scheduling system is meeting the patient care and financial goals of the unit.

IMPLEMENTING AND EVALUATING A STAFFING AND SCHEDULING SYSTEM
Centralized vs Decentralized

Once a staffing plan and schedule have been developed, the responsibility for implementing the plan has to be determined. The decision to centralize this function to a central staffing office or decentralize it to the unit level will depend on how much of the process has been computerized, the availability of clerical support on the patient care unit, whether economies of scale would be lost if each unit made staffing decisions in isolation from the rest of the patient care units, and staff responsibility and accountability for decision making. The advantages of decentralizing the function are that staff assume more responsibility for staffing decisions and the relationship among the staffing plan, schedule, and care delivery model is more visible. Decentralized staffing works best if the unit professional staff have responsibility and accountability for decision making and meeting the goals of all three staffing and scheduling components. The disadvantages include staff nurse time being used on nonpatient care activities and staffing inefficiencies when staffing decisions are made for one unit without knowledge of activity on other units. Centralizing the function to a central staffing office offers the advantages of looking at the whole staffing picture and gaining economies of scale, with a clerk performing the nonprofessional aspects of the function. The disadvantage historically has been that it sets up adversarial relationships among the nurse manager, unit staff, and the person making the decisions from the central office. This person, often a nursing supervisor, must balance the staff's request for additional resources with the pool of available relief staff and the manager's need to live within budget.

The conflict can be minimized through a systems approach that would identify that rather than an either–or choice of isolating the functions to a centralized or decentralized location, it is an integration of interacting functions. This can be accomplished by establishing a clearly articulated description of what the final results should be, clarifying roles of the respective staff, mutually agreeing on

Date:_____

Indicator: Established unit budgeted $PPD will be adhered to providing availability of qualified staff mix.

Unit	D-E-N	Census	Budgeted Established Skill Mix	Mix Scheduled	Variance Between Budgeted & Scheduled Skill Mix	Actual Staff Mix	Variance Between Actual Staff & Budgeted	Unit Floated To: a) sick b) absent c) vacation
CCU	D							
	E							
	N							
SICU	D							
	E							
	N							

Figure 12–4 St. Luke's Hospital staffing office QA audit tool. (Courtesy of St. Luke's Hospital, San Francisco.)

plans to achieve the desired results, and developing feedback loops so information passes back and forth to maintain and evaluate system functioning.

Chaney* has identified the ideal balance as "decentralizing the decision-making functions to the professional staff at the unit level while centralizing the technical functions necessary to implement the plan.

Feedback Loops

A continuous quality improvement approach facilitates integrating these important functions and provides feedback loops. Uskert† applied the JCAHO ten-step quality assurance model to monitor the important aspects of staffing and scheduling and provided managers with feedback on the ability of the central staffing office to implement the unit staffing plan (Fig. 12–4, Table 12–5). This information became a stimulus for mutual problem solving to remove obstacles to staffing according to the unit plan.

Evaluation

The three components of the staffing and scheduling system should be evaluated periodically to ensure that the primary goals are being attained. Information

*Gerald Chaney is Vice President of Nursing Services, Ukiah Valley Medical Center, Ukiah, California, a member of the Adventist Health System West.

†Ilse Uskert is Administrative Nursing Supervisor, St. Luke's Hospital, San Francisco, California.

** Indicate type of substitution and/or augmentation by # of people:_____

**SUBSTITUTION-AUGMENTATION **

RN			LPN			NA			Comments
House S/A	ST S/A	Reg S/A	House S/A	ST S/A	Reg S/A	House S/A	ST S/A	Reg S/A	

TABLE 12-5 Patient Care Services Quality Assurance Program: St. Luke's Hospital, San Francisco, California

GOALS AND OBJECTIVES

1. To develop a program of monitoring and evaluating staffing accuracies in an ongoing systemic manner
2. To assure that all entries affecting staffing are done on a timely and identifiable basis
3. To assist the nurse managers to stay as close as possible to their budgetary manpower allowances through
   3.1 Careful adherence of preset skill mix on a shift by shift basis
   3.2 Analysis of cost factor when substituting skill mix
4. To reduce need for registry usage
5. To maximize usage of available Spiriteam members
6. To identify staffing issues/problems and develop strategies to deal with them
7. To communicate relevant information on a regular basis to the nurse managers

Courtesy of St. Luke's Hospital, San Francisco, California.

gained can be used to plan any changes that may be required to align system functions to achievement of the overall goal. A systems approach would require that the outputs and inputs be measured to evaluate overall functioning. Outputs, such as clinical outcomes, length of stay, critical incidents, and cost, are good indicators of an adequately staffed model of care.

Patient, physician, and staff satisfaction are inputs or environment responses to the model that provide valuable evaluation data. These data would be looked at collectively to assess the functioning of the three components and the staffing and scheduling system as a whole.

SUMMARY

The demand to change the way in which health care is delivered dictates that new paths be taken in hospitals today. A systems perspective and the right tools can assist the nursing leader to develop new, cost-efficient, and care-effective staffing and scheduling systems.

References

Aaron, H.J., & Schwartz, W.B. (1985). Hospital cost control: A bitter pill to swallow. *Harvard Business Review, 63*(2), 167.

Ackoff, R.L. (1992). Address to participants in Strengthening Hospital Nursing: A Program to Improve Patient Care. *Gaining Momentum: A Progress Report*. FL: National Program Office of the Strengthening Hospital Nursing Program.

Arndt, C., & Huckabay, L.M. (1980). *Nursing administration theory for practice with a systems approach*. St. Louis: C.V. Mosby.

Aydelotte, M.K. (1973). *Nurse staffing methodology—A review and critique of selected literature*. DHEW Pub No. (NIH) 73-433, Washington, DC: U.S. Government Printing Office.

Barnum, B.S., & Mallard, C.O. (1989). *Essen-*

tials of nursing management. MD: Aspen.

Donoho, B.A., & Kohles, M.K. (1992). *Gaining momentum: A progress report*. FL: National Program Office of the Strengthening Nursing Program.

Flynn-Hollander, S., Smith, M., & Barron, J. (1992). Cost reductions Part 1: An operations improvement process. *Nursing Economics 10*(5), 325–330.

Giovannetti, P. (1978). *Patient classification systems in nursing: A description and analysis*.

DHEW Pub. No. (HRA) 78-22). Washington, DC: U.S. Government Printing Office.

Hoffman, F. (1988). *Nursing productivity assessment and costing out nursing services*. Philadelphia: J.B. Lippincott.

Senge, P.M. (1990). *The fifth discipline: The art and practice of the learning organization*. New York: Doubleday.

Stevens, B.J. (1980). *The nurse as executive* (2nd ed.) MA: Nursing Resources.

CHAPTER 13

JOB SATISFACTION AND RETENTION

GAIL A. WOLF
CAROL A. OREM

EXECUTIVE SUMMARY

It is no secret that a satisfied nursing staff can have a positive impact on overall morale, patient care, and productivity. The trick is to keep the nursing staff satisfied. This chapter takes an in-depth look at job satisfaction for nurses and offers some strategies for retention and recognition of staff.

The chapter opens with a review of the major factors of nursing job satisfaction and suggests that the issues of autonomy and inadequate staffing and scheduling of work hours have particular significance. Several strategies, such as case management to increase autonomy and a shift to flexible work hours, are reviewed as ways to increase satisfaction.

Since the impact of job satisfaction is clear, some measure of satisfaction must be undertaken. Several sources of ready-made job satisfaction assessments are provided. However, the use of an employee opinion survey that can be tailored to a particular nursing division also is recommended. If an employee survey is used, there are several things to remember. First, retention data indicate a trend for unhappy employees to leave within the first year and for those who stay at least 3 years to stay even longer. Effective employee surveys must include both groups. Second, employee surveys must be done in an atmosphere of trust. This includes sharing survey comments and informing the staff of any changes that will be made as a result.

We offer a guideline for a successful retention program spearheaded by a competent and well-informed nurse recruiter. The relationship between the nurse recruiter and the unit management is examined. Recognition systems, ranging from the clinical ladder to an exemplar program where nurses write about their experiences, and tips for creating a positive work environment round out the chapter.

In virtually all nursing organizations, the issue of maintaining employee job satisfaction is a major concern to managers because of its potential impact on morale, quality patient care, productivity, and cost. This is not an easy accomplishment, for although the rewards of nursing are great, the demands are equally so. In recent years, the nursing profession has made substantial progress in discovering ways of retaining a satisfied work force.

The purpose of this chapter is to review the major factors that influence job satisfaction, explore methodologies that can be used to measure satisfaction, discuss retention and recognition strategies, and examine the role of the manager in creating a positive work environment.

FACTORS INFLUENCING JOB SATISFACTION

Over the years, numerous research studies have been conducted to investigate factors that have an impact on nursing job satisfaction and its relationship to turnover (Hinshaw & Atwood, 1983; MacPhail, 1988; Parasuraman, 1989; Wolf, 1981). The data reveal that there are multiple factors contributing to job dissatisfaction, intention to leave an organization, and actual turnover. Although those factors are important to understand from an academic perspective, it is critical for the nurse manager and nurse executive to realize that each organization is different and has its own unique environment that will contribute to the satisfaction or dissatisfaction of its employees. It is essential for nurse managers to assess their unique environment accurately to determine effective intervention strategies.

For assessment purposes, the major factors influencing job satisfaction can be categorized as follows:

1. Nature of the work
2. Work environments
3. Salary and benefits
4. Career advancement opportunities
5. Supervision / management

Nature of the Work

In general, people enter a field because the nature of the work appeals to them. This includes role responsibilities, task requirements, personal satisfaction derived from work, perceived importance and challenge of the work, and the amount of control one has over work. In nursing, the appeal for entering the field typically is helping others in a time of need, providing comfort, and being influential in the healing process. Graduates of nursing schools enter the profession with enthusiasm about the contributions they can make in caring for patients. They become disillusioned and dissatisfied if this is not allowed to occur.

In a research study by Wolf (1982), nurses were found to be satisfied with their role as nurses but were more satisfied with the kind of work than with the amount of work. Satisfaction with work was found to be highly correlated with job satisfaction. The same study found that two aspects of nursing work predicted both work satisfaction and role satisfaction: providing for the psychologic needs and the educational needs of patients.

Autonomy, or control over work activities, has been identified repeatedly as a major factor in job satisfaction of nursing professionals (McCloskey, 1990).

In the past several years, more and more organizations have decentralized clinical decision making to the staff nurse and have developed systems, such as primary nursing, case management, and shared governance, that foster increased autonomy.

Work Environments

The conditions in which nurses perform their work have a significant impact on their satisfaction with the job. One of the most significant and common predictors of dissatisfaction is inadequate staffing to meet workload demand. Factors influencing this include the number of personnel, educational level, experience level, and mix of professional and nonprofessional staff.

Insuring adequate human resources is especially challenging for the nurse manager, since the workload often is unpredictable and the consequences of inappropriate decisions are significant. Overstaffing has major financial ramifications, especially in this time of cost controls. Understaffing can potentially result in decreased morale, increased turnover, and inadequate quality of patient care. Patient acuity systems have helped to a degree in determining the amount of nursing care a patient requires. However, most acuity systems are not capable of totally capturing nursing workload.

A second significant factor in the work environment is related to scheduling of work hours. This includes scheduling patterns, the time frame for posting of work schedules, scheduling fairness, difficulty of patient assignments, shift rotations, the amount of overtime required, and being required to work on other nursing units.

There is a direct correlation between scheduling and staff satisfaction, and as a result, most hospitals have moved away from rigid shifts to more flexible working hours. In addition, many organizations have allowed nurses to control their own scheduling to a large extent. Computerized scheduling, cyclical scheduling, and self-scheduling have become common methodologies to decrease dissatisfaction with this aspect of the work environment.

In addition to insuring adequate human resources through staffing and scheduling, it is important to have a clean work environment, with adequate equipment and supplies available. Although this is not typically cited as a major factor in job dissatisfaction, a poor working environment or failure to have the necessary tools to perform a job results in frustration that, coupled with other frustrations, can lead to increased dissatisfaction.

Relationships with co-workers often are cited as a factor in job satisfaction. This includes peer support, mutual respect, the amount of cooperation within the work group, and the relationship with physicians. A study by McCloskey (1990) demonstrated that social integration contributed to job satisfaction, commitment, motivation, and intent to stay on the job. This was found also to have a buffering effect on other factors shown to contribute to job dissatisfaction. Good work relationships have a positive impact on both morale and productivity and need to be fostered through effective communications and team-building activities.

Salaries and Benefits

In recent years, salaries and benefits have taken on an increased importance to nurses in terms of job satisfaction. A study of 416 nurses from five hospitals indicated that pay and benefits were the most important factor related to job satisfaction (Neathawk, Dubuque, & Kronk, 1988). This same study indicated that 51.5% of the staff was dissatisfied with their salary and benefits, which was the highest level of dissatisfaction of all the factors measured.

The increased perceived importance of salaries and benefits may be at least partially attributed to the declining economic stability throughout the country and the increased incidence of women as heads of households. In response to nursing shortages throughout the country, salaries for staff nurses have increased substantially over the past several years. Many hospitals have implemented clinical ladders that reimburse nurses based on performance and allow experienced staff to be promoted while still remaining at the bedside. Creative benefit packages that allow employees to choose from a menu of benefits, including child care, tuition reimbursement, health insurance, dental insurance, disability benefits, and retirement, have been implemented across the country.

Career Advancement Opportunities

Career advancement opportunities are important to nurses and are a contributing factor to job satisfaction. These include continuing education, professional growth opportunities, opportunities for promotion or for transfer to different clinical areas, and opportunities to try new ideas. Clinical ladders are a common strategy for meeting this need, but hospitals have numerous other mechanisms available, such as committee appointments, recruitment activities, and community projects.

Supervision and Management

There is a strong correlation between management style and staff nurse job satisfaction. Management style includes a number of factors, such as decision making, fairness, goal setting, communicating, establishing controls, leading and motivating staff, staff development, employee evaluation, ensuring adequate working environments, and staff relationships.

Research indicates that nurses prefer to work in a participative environment as opposed to one that is autocratic (Lucas, 1991; Taunton, Krampitz, & Woods, 1989), and there has been a definite trend in this direction throughout nursing organizations over the past several years. Visibility and access to senior administration are considered important, but the management style of the unit manager is paramount. Organizations are investing in management development strategies and are experiencing a shift to higher educational preparation for those in leadership positions.

APPLICATION OF RESEARCH FINDINGS

As mentioned previously, each organization is unique in regard to its work environment and work force. It is often difficult for nursing managers to determine where they should place their efforts in terms of the many variables relating to job satisfaction.

Two classic studies may help in this endeavor. The first is the well-known Magnet Hospitals study (ANA, 1983). This study examined 150 hospitals that were known for excellence and for their success in retaining staff nurses. The common characteristics of these hospitals included the following.

- A nurse/patient ratio that assures quality patient care
- Flexible staffing to support patient care needs
- Flexible scheduling and elimination of rotating shifts
- A strong supportive nursing administration and hospital administration at all levels
- Primary nursing
- Clinical advancement opportunities (so that RNs can remain at the bedside but still advance professionally)
- Participatory management
- Open communication in all directions
- In-service and continuing education opportunities on all shifts
- Good nurse–physician professional relationships
- Longevity benefits for staff RNs
- Tuition reimbursement

A similar but smaller study was conducted by the Secretarys' Commission on Nursing and was published by the Department of Health and Human Services in 1988. Hospitals that achieved substantial reduction in nurse turnover and vacancy rates were found to share certain common elements.

- Management commitment to nursing and nurses
- Strong nursing leadership
- Competitive salaries and benefits

Although there are numerous tools available for measuring job satisfaction, it is recommended that these concepts be incorporated as a baseline assessment for determining areas of focus for each organization.

MEASUREMENT OF JOB SATISFACTION

When discussing measurement of job satisfaction, we are attempting to ascertain what a nurse's attitude is toward her or his job. A person who is satisfied with the job has a positive attitude toward work. Conversely, a dissatisfied person usually feels negatively about the work situation. Nurses who do not like what they do look elsewhere or demonstate behaviors that are, at best, nonsupportive of their peers and the organization. How do we determine the level of job satisfaction of our nursing staff? Quite simply, we ask.

Assessment Tools

Assessment tools are one way to measure a staff attitude about their work situation. Individual interviews, group meetings, and surveys also are useful. A review of the standard tools can be found in organizational psychology texts. Some of the most common tools include the Minnesota Satisfaction Questionnaire

(MSQ) (Weiss, Davis, England, & Lofquist, 1967), which has both a short version of 20 questions and a long version of 100 questions. The MSQ uses the fixed-response question format based on the assumption that satisfaction and dissatisfaction are part of the same bipolar attitude continuum.

The Job Descriptive Index (JDI) (Smith, Kendall, & Hulin, 1969) also uses fixed-response questions. The JDI has separate scales for satisfaction with pay, promotion, supervision, work, and people.

A third assessment tool for job satisfaction is Porter's Need Satisfaction Questionnaire (1961), which is based on the discrepancy theory of satisfaction and uses fixed-response questions to scale what "should be" and "is now" (Wexley & Yukl, 1984).

An employee opinion survey, using the fixed-response format alone or in combination with open-ended questions, can be developed within a nursing division. Developing an individualized tool permits questions to be structured according to the particular organization. This can be updated to address current issues if administered on a yearly or repeated basis.

Administration of the assessment tool and collection of the data should be accomplished in an environment of trust. It is of paramount importance to communicate to the staff that their honest, sincere, and well-thought-out opinions and ideas are wanted, needed, and valued. One way to elicit these responses is to share the results and demonstrate attention to the information gained. Changes made as a result of the survey should be acknowledged. An in-house publication is an excellent way to disseminate the news, as is frequent mention at meetings within the nursing division committee structure.

Turnover Rate

Turnover, or the ratio of total number of positions to the number of times vacant positions are filled in a given period of time (usually a year), is frequently correlated with job satisfaction. The satisfied employee is less likely to leave her or his position than a dissatisfied one. Therefore, satisfaction data can be used as a predictor of turnover rate, although this should be tempered with other factors. For example, voluntary turnover is much lower in periods of economic hardship (Lawler, 1973). The strength of the relationship between jobs satisfaction and turnover varies from one time period to another and also from organization to organization. Even those individuals who feel positively about their job can be tempted by prospects of better pay, career advancement, or more opportunity (Organ & Hamner, 1982). However, if in general satisfied employees stay with an organization and those who are dissatisfied leave, the importance of retention efforts becomes clear.

Retaining quality staff is again emphasized when considering the cost of nurse turnover. In a 1987 report on Nurse Recruitment and Retention prepared by the Health Care Advisory Board, the cost of nurse turnover was estimated to be between $2600 and $17,500 per nurse—and thought to be rising. This figure included the cost of recruitment and orientation as well as productivity loss and agency replacement if applicable.

A recurrent theme in retention is the 3-year job tenure factor. This pattern suggests that if a nurse stays 3 years with an employer, longer retention usually occurs (Benedict, Glasser, & Lee, 1988). According to data gathered by the Health Care Advisory Board, nurses tend to repeat a pattern of dissatisfaction with employers but continue an interest in a nursing career by repeated stints of approximately 3 years with consecutive employers.

These data support a policy of surveying the nursing staff annually to identify factors that are satisfying and dissatisfying. Communication about results and intent to make change is of paramount importance, since the time period for impressing a nurse considering a job change is relatively short. The need to communicate change is intensified in times and areas of economic opportunity when a better job may appear to be an easy acquisition. Strategies to minimize turnover should be directed toward job satisfiers and dissatisfiers among a nursing staff, with particular attention to staff employed less than 1 year and those with the organization approximately 3 years.

Vacancy rate, the ratio of open or unfilled positions to the total positions available, is closely related to the turnover rate. Both are an indication of recruitment and retention strategies and successes. Both also have an impact on staff. A high rate of turnover is detrimental to morale. Nurses who are dissatisfied are rarely quiet about it. Negativism can sap the creative energy of a unit and pull younger, less hardy staff members into a web of hopelessness. Likewise, a high vacancy rate can exhaust a unit staff who are habitually understaffed or who are, at best, deprived of the joy of group cohesiveness when they consistently work with pool or agency personnel.

A prolonged high vacancy rate may affect a manager's hiring decisions and practices. A unit with a high turnover or vacancy rate may develop a reputation that impedes the recruitment process and diminishes the pool of candidates from which the manager can choose. The astute candidate will ask for the turnover and vacancy statistics and may consider these numbers in her or his decision about accepting a job offer. Finally, a manager in an effort to be sensitive to staff concerns for vacant positions may extend an offer to candidates more quickly than she or he might if many applicants were available for a single opening.

RETENTION PROGRAMS

Since a hospital's largest potential nurse market is the nurses it already has, the need to place equal or greater emphasis on retention as on recruitment is apparent (Neathawk et al., 1988). After assessing the level of job satisfaction, analyzing the turnover and vacancy data, and developing strategies for retention of staff, the next step is implementation of a retention program.

The initial tactic is to recruit for retention. The nurse recruiter must be knowledgeable about the conceptual framework of the nursing division and its future direction and be articulate when presenting them to prospective candidates. Indeed, the very presence of a nurse, a member of nursing administration, as a recruiter is evidence of empowerment of the nursing division. Many candidates perceive this as a demonstration of strong nursing leadership and as proof of organizational commitment to nursing. Additionally, the nurse recruiter must be knowledgeable about benefits and salary and the competitive standards of the surrounding community to provide a realistic description to the candidate. The recruiter's ability to present the nursing division truthfully and help the candidate compare values and expectations sets the tone for the applicant. Kersten and Johnson (1991) state that recruiters form the crucial frontline in the recruitment game. It might be more accurate to say they begin the retention process.

Employee retention is a challenge. One critical factor in a retention program is continuing to market your organization internally. Expending as much energy and effort as possible to keep nurses attracted to the concepts and values that first piqued their interest and contributed to their initial commitment to the organization should prove to be productive. In other words, you must deliver on the promises you made to expect them to remain with the organization. Considering the high cost of recruiting and orienting, retaining a nurse is protecting an investment.

After attracting and employing candidates whose values match those of the organization and monitoring the levels of job satisfaction of the staff, an additional critical factor in a retention program is to design, implement, and evaluate a strategic plan for retention. Recruitment activities take much time and energy, but retention functions are the challenge to address long-term issues (Wall, 1988). The organization should establish acceptable levels for vacancy and turnover rates and monitor them periodically. Corrective measures should be instituted if a trend surfaces before serious consequences are felt. For programs to be successful, they must be fluid enough to meet the changing needs of each hospital (Hoffman, 1989). Having the nurse recruiter as an integral part of the management team provides a source of constant feedback for trends and information about staff expectations and satisfaction. The nurse recruiter is a conduit for information about staff nurse feelings, perceptions, and concerns. She or he is a lightning rod for attracting and grounding anxiety and misunderstandings generated by changes in a progressive nursing division. By providing a safe place for staff to express these feelings and a viable source of information regarding change, the nurse recruiter can dissipate feelings and perceptions that may become job dissatisfaction factors.

Retention programs are successful if integrated into the nursing management structure of the organization. The impact of the middle manager has been recognized previously as an important factor in retention of professional staff in hospitals (Taunton et al., 1989). There must be a trust and comfort level between the nurse recruiter and unit directors that permits a free flow of ideas and exchange of information. When this occurs, the unit director perceives the nurse recruiter as a resource in the unit retention plan, and the recruiter uses the unit director as a key player in the nursing division retention program. An example of this beneficial interplay is the invitation from a unit director to the recruiter to conduct focus groups on the unit to assist the staff in problem-solving issues having an impact on unit turnover, such as old staff–new staff conflicts. Another intervention for the nurse recruiter might be an offer to teach interviewing skills to staff members when a new unit director wants to involve staff in the selection process for unit candidates. Furthermore, unit directors recognizing the more global perspective of the nursing recruiter may recommend that employees seek career counseling from the recruiter when needing or seeking a transfer or considering a career move. Finally, when it is necessary to downsize departments, the manager will find the recruiter a valuable ally in her or his efforts to assist the staff to cope with the change and seek new areas of practice.

It has been suggested that to retain staff, nurse managers need to be more attentive to the human aspect of their jobs (Landstrom, Biordi, & Gilles, 1989). To this end, the nurse recruiter can be a support to both the employee and the manager.

As stated by Lassiter (1989), retention opportunities are limited only by the creativity of nurse executives and managers. One such approach to retention of nursing division personnel is to bring students into entry level positions, such as nurse aide, and promote them to graduate positions at the completion of their academic programs. This allows an extended period for value comparison on the part of both employee and manager. A similar and more structured approach is the nurse extern program, which provides selected applicants a learning experience to augment their educational program and provides a bonding opportunity for the exemplary student and the sponsoring organization.

Recognition Systems

The essence of a retention program is recognition of those people you want to retain. Whether someone is adequately recognized can play a critical role in the building—or destroying—of trust in the workplace (Levering, 1988). Retention activities can be the setting and the stage for recognition opportunities. There can be formal, structured systems that recognize achievements of nursing division members as well as day-to-day integration of recognition into institutionalized activities. Staff should expect that their achievements will be acknowledged. They can and should be involved in the design and implementation of recognition systems. They should be encouraged to respect the accomplishments of their peers and should be afforded opportunities to participate in public celebration of those contributions.

Clinical Advancement System

A clinical advancement system, or clinical ladder program, provides the opportunity for advancement, professionally and financially. Ideally, the program is based on clinical knowledge, competence, and performance and should be developed with staff nurse input. It encourages and rewards commitment, expertise, and leadership ability for clinical practitioners. If peer review is a part of the advancement process, it can further demonstrate the respect nursing professionals extend to one another on a daily basis.

Shared Governance

Another formalized structure for the recognition process is shared governance. In 1987, Stanfill reported that by expanding the staff nurse role, morale and nurse retention rates increased, as did the effectiveness of the nursing department. Jenkins (1991) suggests that professional governance is the missing link to all the efforts made to retain nurses. She believes that when high-quality personal services are not rewarded beyond mediocre ones, people lose the motivation to seek better approaches to delivering services.

A participative management structure encourages staff members to contribute to change within the organization. In times such as these, when the health care delivery system is in constant flux, a dynamic management approach is necessary to keep pace with the challenging environment. A shared governance structure empowers staff and enables them to be recognized for the ability to cope with change. As evidenced in a mature professional practice model, the rewards of quality care are felt by the patient, by the staff, and ultimately by the hospital (McDonagh, Rhoades, Sharkey, & Goodroe, 1989).

Exemplar Program

A third example of a recognition system is an exemplar program. Such a program is relatively easily implemented, is cost efficient, and can be accomplished from inception to publication in approximately 1 year. Exemplars, or stories written by nurses about patients or other nurses, illustrate the delivery and impact of quality patient care.

Exemplars are stories about the art and science of nursing, about what happens between the nurse and the patient. By writing and telling these stories, nurses begin to realize and acknowledge the impact of their practice. Consequently, they can articulate for others the complex interactions that make up the nursing process.

Exemplars should be collected, published, and celebrated. A collection printed in magazine format is a useful recruitment tool when distributed at career days, open houses, and similar functions and is a very beneficial addition to a marketing packet. It provides applicants an intimate view of professional practice and care delivery and demonstrates the organization's valuing of clinical practitioners.

It is important to have public celebration of the writers and the stories. A high visibility recognition event for the nurse exemplars and their significant others might be an annual dinner, with hospital administration and board members in attendance.

Nurses' Week

Finally, no review of recognition systems would be complete without discussion of nurses' week. This celebration can become a pivotal event in a nursing division's recognition structure.

If the nurses' week events are planned and executed by a committed recruitment/retention committee or a similar group comprised of staff and management, this assures that the theme and tone will be meaningful to the nursing staff. If the planning group is invited to focus the celebration on professional practice and given the occasion to illuminate the depth and richness of the nursing resources of their peers, the week can become a celebration of the art and science of nursing.

When one or several staff members are afforded full accountability for the nurses' week program and budget and are recognized both before the week and after successful completion, it becomes an honor and an opportunity for visibility within the nursing division and the hospital structure.

The direction of the week's activities can be channeled by concerns or issues prevalent in the organization, and forums scheduled during the week can be opportunities to present solutions in a positive light. For example, programs can be offered that specifically address dissatisfaction factors identified in the staff satisfaction survey and can introduce a responsive action plan.

When the themes of celebration of professional practice and open communication are introduced and encouraged by staff committee members, nurses' week can become a recognition system for celebrating the accomplishments of individual practitioners, the nursing division, and the nursing profession.

CREATING POSITIVE WORK ENVIRONMENTS IN THE FUTURE

The primary role of the nurse executive is to create an environment where people can be excellent. Creating a workplace in which people are not just satisfied but are challenged and fulfilled requires vision, commitment, energy, and mutual trust. As difficult as that is to do, the future promises to be even more challenging. Future health care systems will contain greater demands and fewer resources than those of today. How will we be able to meet those demands and still maintain a positive work environment? The answer lies in developing an effective value system that supports those changes, providing vision and direction to accomplish the changes, empowering our staff, and developing effective communications and trust. Specifically, the following must occur.

We Must Change Our Paradigms and Value Systems

As nurses, we are socialized to believe that increased staffing will result in greater quality of care. In reality, it is not the quantity but the quality of time that is important. We will not have the resources to meet all the needs of every patient. We will need to use those resources wisely. Care must be highly individualized, rather than relying on routines as we do currently. Patients will need to be truly involved in planning their care along with the health practitioners in order to identify the most critical needs and most effective methodologies of meeting those needs.

We Must Develop Systems to Support These Changes

From a care delivery perspective, systems need to be developed that allow the authority, responsibility, and accountability for clinical decision making to be decentralized to one specific clinical practitioner. Without this, care will regress to common routines and will lack the necessary individualization.

We must develop systems that accurately measure the amount of nursing care needed to meet necessary patient requirements. With resource limitations, there will be a strong motivation to reduce nursing hours. A system must be developed that differentiates accurately between critical and noncritical nursing requirements of patients.

Operational systems within hospitals must be refined to maximize efficiency. We will not be able to afford the time or the frustration of nurses struggling through a bureaucratic maze or being engaged in rework. Systems that support innovative thinking and creative solutions will be our foundation.

As Administrators, We Do Not Need to Have the Right Answers, Only the Right Questions

The key to the challenges of tomorrow is developing partnerships with our staff. The clinicians are the experts on clinical practice and have the knowledge of how to make that practice more cost effective without compromising quality. They want to have a voice in their practice and in creating their future. Through open, honest communications, trust, and mutual respect, we can create an environment for the future that is both effective and satisfying.

References

American Nurses' Association. (1983). Task Force on Nursing Practice in Hospitals. *Magnet hospitals: Attraction and retention of professional nurses.* Kansas City, MO: American Academy of Nursing.

Benedict, M., Glasser, J., & Lee, E. (1988). Assessing hospital nursing staff retention and turnover. *Evaluation & The Health Professionals, 12*(1), 73–96.

Hinshaw, A. S., & Atwood, J. R. (1983). Nursing staff turnover, stress, and satisfaction: Models, measures, and management. *Research on Nursing Care Delivery, 6,* 133–153.

Hoffman, H. (1989). A nurse retention program. *Nursing Economics, 7*(2), 94–108.

Jenkins, J. (1991). Professional governance: The missing link. *Nursing Management 22*(8), 26–30.

Kersten, J., & Johnson, J. (1992). Recruitment: What are the new grads looking for? *Nursing Management, 23*(2), 44–48.

Landstrom, G., Biordi, D., & Gilles, D. (1989). The emotional and behavioral process of staff nurse turnover. *Journal of Nursing Administration, 19*(9), 23–28.

Lassiter, S. (1989). Staff nurse retention: Strategies for success. *Journal of Neuroscience Nursing, 21*(2), 104–107.

Lawler, E. (1973). Job satisfaction, absenteeism, and turnover. In B. Straw (Ed.), *Psychological foundations of organizational behavior* (2nd ed.) (p. 80–95). Glenview, IL: Scott, Foresman.

Levering, K. (1988). *A great place to work.* New York: Avon Books.

Lucas, M. D. (1991). Management style and staff nurse job satisfaction. *Journal of Professional Nursing, 8*(2), 119–125.

MacPhail, J. (1988). Job satisfaction in the nursing profession. *Recent Advances in Nursing, 19,* 98–119.

McCloskey, J. C. (1990). Two requirements for job contentment: Autonomy and social integration. *Journal of Nursing Scholarship, 22*(3), 140–143.

McDonagh, K., Rhoades, B., Sharkey, K., & Goodroe, J. (1989). Shared governance at St. Joseph's hospital of Atlanta: A mature professional practice model. *Nursing Administration Quarterly, 13*(4), 17–28.

Neathawk, R., Dubuque, S., & Kronk, C. (1988). Nurses' evaluation of recruitment and retention. *Nursing Management, 19*(12), 38–45.

Nurse Recruitment & Retention. (1987) (pp. 69–71). Washington, DC: Health Care Advisory Board.

Nursing News. (1992). *Nursing 92, 92,*11.

Organ, D., & Hamner, W. (1982). *Organizational behavior.* Plano, TX: Business Publications.

Parasuraman, S. (1989). Nursing turnover: An integrated model. *Research in Nursing & Health, 12,* 267–277.

Secretary's Commission on Nursing. (1988). Support studies & background information (Vol II). DHHS (pp. vi–vii). Washington, DC: U.S. Government Printing Office.

Smith, P., Kendall, L., & Hulin, C. (1969). *The measurement of satisfaction in work and retirement*. Chicago: Rand McNally.

Stanfill, P. (1987). Participative management becomes shared management. *Nursing Management, 18*, 26–30.

Tauton, R., Krampitz, S., & Woods, C. (1989). Manager impact on retention of hospital staff: Part 2. *Journal of Nursing Administration, 19*(4), 15–19.

Wall, L. (1988). Plan development for a nurse recruitment and retention program. *Journal of Nursing Administration, 18*(2), 20–26.

Wexley, K., & Yukl, G. (1984). *Organizational behavior and personnel psychology*. Homewood, IL: Richard D. Irwin.

Weiss, D., Davis, R., England, G., & Lofquist, L. (1967). *Manual for the Minnesota Satisfaction Questionnaire*. Minneapolis: University of Minnesota, Industrial Relations Center, Work Adjustment Project.

Wolf, G. A. (1981). Nursing turnover: Some causes and solutions. *Nursing Outlook, 29*, 233–236.

Wolf, G. A. (1982). *Causal attributions for job performance by registered nurses and the relationship to work satisfaction*. Unpublished dissertation. Indiana University, Indianapolis, IN.

CHAPTER 14 • • • • • •

WAGES AND SALARIES

SHIRLEY FREDERIKSEN
BARBARA MARION HILL
CHRISTEEN A. HOLDWICK
JUDITH E. JOHNSON

EXECUTIVE SUMMARY

The compensation plan and practices for any organization must be tied to the philosophy, mission, and values of the organization. The basic goals of any compensation program are to meet the goals of the organization, contribute to the achievement of operational objectives, maximize opportunities for growth in the business, and meet the reasonable expectations of employees and owners. Sound compensation plans contribute to the success of an organization. Given that wages and salaries comprise a large percentage of hospital operating costs, typically 60% or greater, the actual program policies are critical to the strategic success of an organization. The basis for the development of a sound and fair pay structure is the maintenance of accurate and up-to-date job descriptions. Adequate salary administration requires a consistent set of policies and procedures. Methods to insure that all employees understand the pay program should be developed and implemented. Current thinking challenges the historic belief that nursing salaries are poor and contribute to periodic nursing shortages. One study found that only 63.8% of nurses' total salary is accounted for by base wage. Special incentive programs, differentials, and bonuses contribute to total compensation.

As the work of delivering patient care is redesigned, so too compensation for the caregivers can be redesigned. New pay practices must be developed to change the hourly wage mindset of nurses. The future of wage and compensation packages is well-designed variable pay programs that increase commitment, involvement, and job satisfaction while decreasing job turnover. Gain-sharing, pay-for-performance, pay-for-knowledge, and differentiated pay and salary models are examples of future compensation structures. The nurse manager plays a vital role in shaping the development and implementation of the compensation program. Key responsibilities of the nurse manager are communication, confidentiality, consistency, and currency. Nurse managers are placed in a valued position in the organization, close to the staff, which allows them direct information on staff needs for compensation programs. With the national movement toward total quality management, the environment is right to test new, creative approaches to meeting the needs of a changing workforce.

IMPORTANCE OF A SOUND COMPENSATION PROGRAM

The compensation plan and practices for any organization, including hospitals and nursing services, must be tied to the philosophy, mission, and values of the organization. For many hospital organizations, mission statements include a commitment to the treatment of all individuals served, both patients and employees alike, with dignity, justice, respect, and concern for their total well-being. Part of that commitment to employees includes a fair and competitive compensation program.

The basic goals of many compensation programs are to meet the goals of the organization, contribute to the achievement of operational objectives, maximize opportunities for growth in the business, and meet the reasonable expectations of employees and owners. Policymaking around compensation programs is an essential responsibility of management. Sound compensation plans contribute, in a major way, to the success of an organization. Good compensation programs are a significant tool for the recruitment and retention of talented staff.

ISSUES IN NURSING COMPENSATION

Given that wages and salaries comprise a large percentage of hospital operating costs, typically 60% or greater, the actual compensation program policies are critical to the strategic success of an organization. Although wages and benefits generally are not the top priority in surveys of nurses' job satisfiers, it does rank among the top five.

The nursing shortage of the middle to late 1980s saw hospital nursing vacancy rates average 11%, with some hospitals developing severe shortages up to 20% (Marc, Minnick, Ginzberg, & Curran, 1989). Local competition for the same pool of nurses forced hospital advertising budgets to soar and an increase in the dollars spent to implement many new recruitment strategies and programs. Reports, such as the Magnet Hospital Study, the Health and Human Services Commission on Nursing Report, American Hospital Association 1989 Report of the Hospital Nursing Personnel Survey, and The Commonwealth Fund Paper, are among published works that indicate that recruitment incentives, including salary increases, are a short-term strategy to keep hospital beds open. The long-term strategy lies in retention of staff. Compensation is both a short-term and long-term strategy.

Significant gains were achieved in nursing salaries in certain geographic areas based on the law of supply and demand. The Commonwealth Fund Paper reports that starting salaries vary widely from $15.00 an hour in urban hospitals to $10.65 an hour in rural hospitals (Marc et al., 1989). The Hay-Modern Healthcare Nursing Compensation Survey, which collected data from 211,772 nurses at 897 hospitals across the country, showed that as of January 1, 1991, for-profit hospitals last year offered the greatest average salary increase of 11.2%. Secular, not-for-profit hospitals offered 7.9% pay increases, and religiously affiliated hospitals offered 8.7% increases (Perry, 1991, p. 27). It would appear that increases over the last 5 years have placed nursing in a more equitable position with other professions. What these reports fail to examine are national inflation trends during the same time periods or the percentage of nursing practitioners who are not part of the hospital data, which account for 32% of the total. When compensation for nurses who practice in all settings is computed and compared to the base salaries of other professionals, the data show that nursing salaries continue to lag behind those of other professions related to potential career earnings. During the course of a nurse's career, there is a mere 69% growth in earning potential. By comparison, accountants can expect to see a 209% growth in salary, attorneys a 226% growth, engineers a 183% growth, and medical machine technicians a 92% growth during the course of their career (Joel, 1992).

Nurses can enhance their base earnings through differentials, overtime, and weekend premiums. According to the Hay-Modern Health Care data, nationally hospitals paid an average of $1.47/hour for evening shift, $2.07/hour for night shift, and an additional $2.31/hour for weekend shifts. Therefore, nurses who worked the night shift for a full year could add as much as $4804 to their salary. A beginning nurse then could earn as much as $29,572/year, and a nurse earning the average maximum could earn $41,972/year (Joel, 1992, p. 15). However, off-shifts and weekends do not lead to riches, nor are they particularly satisfying to the majority of nurses. Traditionally, entering management and leaving the patient bedside have been viewed by many nurses as the road to higher salaries and better working conditions. To reverse this trend and thinking, nurse managers and nurse executives must look at the total salary dollars available and address the recruitment issue around entry level salaries, compensation for unpopular working conditions, and the long-term career earning potential.

To have highly paid registered nurses at both the entry level and the expert senior clinician level, nurse managers and nurse executives must acknowledge that the health care organization can afford to have only a limited number of registered nurses. The escalating national health care bill is forcing state and federal government reimbursement to shrink each year. Buyers of health care, such as employers, are questioning their costs for employees and are scrutinizing local hospitals' cost per case. This, in turn, is forcing hospitals and health care agencies to examine how to decrease their costs and continue to provide quality services.

Since nursing is the largest employee group within a hospital and registered nurses are the highest paid in the group, the number needed is being questioned. It is appropriate that nurse managers and nurse executives identify services that are required by licensure and patient setting to be provided only by registered nurses and services that can be performed by other staff.

COMPENSATION PROGRAM STRUCTURE

Every compensation program is a complex, integrated structure consisting basically of six components that support each other in meeting both organization and employee needs:

1. Compensation philosophy
2. Job descriptions

3. Job analysis process
4. Salary structure (pay grades and ranges)
5. Policies and procedures for administration
6. Communication policies and methodologies

These components provide a framework for developing, implementing, and evaluating the program. Because organizational needs, environmental conditions, and employee needs and desires are constantly changing, the elements must be continuously evolving and being modified to maintain a current, sound compensation program.

Philosophy

Underlying the compensation program is a philosophical base, usually written but sometimes unwritten. The philosophy will drive the other elements, providing direction for establishing a market position, determining how job analysis is conducted, establishing eligibility for benefits and premiums, determining elements of total compensation, and defining how pay policies are administered. By reviewing the philosophy of an institution's compensation program, a nurse manager should be able to understand the underlying values that will be operationalized.

Sibson (1990, pp. 13–14) identifies the following issues to be considered as part of a compensation philosophy for any organization:

- What should be the pay of jobs compared to comparable positions and roles in relevent markets?
- What is the policy with respect to pay for performance?
- Is there a commitment to pay with relation to inflation, and what is that commitment?
- There is the matter of providing health and retirement benefits and the reasons for providing such benefits. This also involves the issue of employee contributions to benefit coverage.
- Equivalency of compensation treatment is a policy issue—whether all persons or all jobs are treated the same way.
- Communication questions relative to the right-to-know and need-to-know are policy matters.
- What is the basic philosophy of pay—for example, do you buy people's time, use their knowledge, or pay for results?
- Should all employees or some employees share in the company's success?
- What are the at-risk and contingent compensation policies?
- How should compensation consider employee needs or corporate ability to pay?

Job Descriptions

The basis for the development of a sound and fair pay structure is the maintenance of accurate and up-to-date job descriptions. Since all pay structure decisons are based on job content, absent, inaccurate, or incomplete job descriptions can result in both internal and external equity problems. In addition to their use for pay determination, job descriptions are used to specify job requirements, set expectations at hire, and structure performance feedback.

Job descriptions may take many formats, but all should include at least

- The job title
- Department name
- Approval date and signatures
- General summary of the job's primary purpose
- A list of principal job duties

Other optional elements include

- Minimum requirements—education, skills, and abilities
- Degree of supervision received and given
- Working conditions
- Physical and mental effort required
- Scope of responsibility (size of budget, number of FTEs, size of unit)

Pay Structure

Using existing job descriptions and an objective job analysis process, jobs are evaluated and clustered into like groupings (levels, job families, grade). Job families are ranked from lowest to highest, and a pay range is established for each based on internal and external market comparisons.

Policies and Procedures

Adequate salary administration requires a consistent set of rules, determining, for example, how base pay is set, how promotions, demotions, and lateral transfers are handled, and how premiums and incentive programs are administered (Table 14–1). Policies cannot address every conceivable situation, however, and provisions must be made for an exception process. Frequent use of an exception process usually indicates that existing policies are perceived as inadequate and require formal revision to address the most frequent exceptions.

Communications Expectations

Methods to insure that all employees understand the institution's pay program, particularly as it affects their own pay changes, should be developed and im-

TABLE 14–1 Typical Pay Policies

Compensation program planning and design
Job descriptions
Job evaluation, pay grades, and rates
Market-sensitive positions (MSPs)
Determining pay rates when employees are hired, promoted, transferred,
    reassigned, or demoted to another job classification
In-range pay increases for nonmanagement employees
Shift differentials
Restricted on-call pay, nonrestricted on-call pay, and called-in pay

---

Courtesy of Catherine McAuley Health System, Ann Arbor, Michigan.

plemented. The role of the human resources department and the employee's supervisor/manager in pay program communications should be spelled out and differentiated (Table 14–2).

TOTAL COMPENSATION

Historically, the belief that nursing salaries are poor has been widespread, and this has been thought to contribute to periodic nursing shortages. More current thinking challenges this notion. When data from 1572 full-time RNs from 26 not-for-profit hospitals were analyzed, the average annual salary was $42,087, not including health and dental benefit costs, Worker's Compensation, and Social Security. Only 63.8% of the nurse's total salary was accounted for by the base wage (Strassen, 1992, p. 14). Special incentive programs, differentials, and bonuses contribute to total compensation but are seldom publicized or analyzed in formal salary surveys. Common supplementary pay practices include shift and weekend differentials, on-call and called-in pay, differentials for education and degree completion, and speciality unit premiums (Management Science Associates, 1992; William Mercer Co., 1991).

In addition, the cost or cash value of paid time off and other benefits contributes to higher total compensation packages (Fig. 14–1). Human resource experts within institutions struggle to develop total compensation programs that meet the needs of an increasingly diverse workforce. One strategy that is gaining in popularity is the use of cafeteria-style benefit programs where employees can select from the benefit choices offered those that best meet their personal needs. Paid time off, which incorporates sick time, vacation, and personal time, is

TABLE 14–2   Pay Program Communications Responsibilities

| | PRIMARY COMMUNICATION RESPONSIBILITY | |
INFORMATION NEED	DIRECT SUPERVISOR	HUMAN RESOURCES DEPARTMENT
1. Employee's pay grade, pay range, and pay rate	Yes	No
2. Change to employee's pay grade, pay range, or pay rate	Yes	No
3. Date eligible for next pay increase	Yes	No
4. General pay program design	Yes	Yes
5. Employee's job evaluation ratings	No	No
6. Job evaluation plan	No	No
7. Labor market data	No	No
8. Pay grade or pay range of another job	Yes, with human resources department input	Yes
9. Pay rate of another employee	No	No
10. Other information needs	Yes, with human resources department input	Yes

Courtesy of Catherine McAuley Health System, Ann Arbor, Michigan.

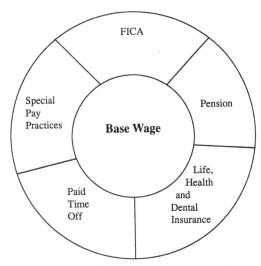

Figure 14–1 Total compensation program elements.

another flexible benefit option allowing employees to use their accrued time off in a variety of ways. Employer contributions to long-term income (FICA, pension, matching contributions to tax sheltered annuities/401K programs) also add to total compensation but may not be highly visible to the typical employee.

Base Pay

As the foundation of the total compensation package, base pay (usually expressed as rate of pay/hour or annual or monthly salary) continues to constitute the most important element of a salary program. Base pay can be either fixed or variable (at risk). Base pay structures are developed using several different basic methodologies. Two frequently used approaches are market data analysis and job content analysis. In market data analysis, key benchmark jobs are selected (usually jobs whose duties are well understood and fairly consistent across the industry), then priced by external market comparisons. Other jobs within the organization are then slotted around the benchmark jobs based on their content.

In contrast, job content analysis is a more objective process in which the primary focus is on understanding and grouping jobs based on the duties and responsibilities of the position. This can be accomplished through qualitative approaches, such as paired rankings, or by predetermining the number and nature of job families and pay grades and then assigning each job to a family based on a reading of the job description. Quantitative job content analysis involves evaluating each job on a factor-by-factor basis to produce a numerical score. The analysis can be done through review of the job description, interviews of employees and supervisors, or direct observation of the work as it is being performed.

Factors against which jobs are evaluated and how much weight is associated with each vary between management and nonmanagement jobs but typically include such elements as

- Required minimum level of knowledge, education, and training
- Experience-based knowledge needed to acquire skills to meet quality standards
- Analytic and problem-solving skills
- Degree of independent judgment exercised
- Impact on organization performance and probable consequence of errors
- Responsibility for resource deployment and use
- Responsibility for the welfare of others
- Necessary communication skills
- Interpersonal relationships
- Physical effort
- Mental/vision effort
- Working conditions and environmental hazards (American Hospital Association, 1984).

As each factor is analyzed by human resources staff, points are assigned. Total points for each job are summarized and plotted with totals for other jobs. Clusters are established around natural groupings or predetermined ranges of scores. These clusters then become the job families for which pay grades are established. Employees often question how their job can be worth the same as a very different type of position in another department. A general description of how base pay structures are established usually will allay fears and resolve potential conflicts.

External market analysis is the next step in the process of constructing base pay structures. Methods can be mail or phone surveys or review of a variety of industrywide or regionally published surveys. External market analysis should always be conducted by human resources staff to insure that accurate data are collected from legitimate sources, assure that salaries for equivalent benchmark jobs are considered, and determine the appropriate geographic and demographic parameters of the market. Word of mouth, information from casual sources, and recruitment advertising are never to be considered as valid market data. Market data usually are analyzed in comparison to several points within the pay range: at minimum (entry rate), midpoint (the median point of the salary range, usually meant to represent the pay rate of an individual who is fully competent and has demonstrated satisfactory performance), and maximum (the highest salary to be paid for that position). The point that is used for the primary comparison is based mainly on the individual organization's philosophy, needs, and strategy. Once appropriate range rates are established for job families containing benchmark jobs, other ranges can be constructed based on internally agreed on range widths (the percent difference from minimum to maximum) and differences between the midpoints of ranges within the hierarchy. Salary ranges may overlap, but a midpoint–midpoint difference of 8% to 10% will usually be sufficient to prevent compression and motivate staff to seek promotional opportunities (American Society for Personnel Administration, 1981).

Determining the base rate for an individual employee usually occurs at the time of hire, promotion, transfer, or demotion and when pay scales are adjusted. Although individuals seeking jobs are often encouraged to bargain for the best available base salary rates, most institutions develop and use a predetermined series of steps within the pay range, or breakpoints, for establishing starting salaries for all but high-level managerial and executive positions or positions with only a small number of incumbents. Breakpoints are usually determined by the years of experience of the applicant and possibly by educational credentials. The fairness achieved by using a consistent method to establish hiring salaries is important to prevent employee morale issues, compression, and frequently unnecessary internal equity salary adjustments.

Base salary determination in most other instances is done by a flat percent change (i.e., 5% promotion increase/pay grade), or range adjustments of a specified percentage. On occasion, these strategies can result in salary exceptions (American Hospital Association, 1984, pp. 134–135).

- Green circled—employee's rate is below the minimum for the range. The rate is usually brought up to minimum.
- Red circled—employee's rate is above the maximum for the range. Base rate is usually held constant until the range catches up.
- Orange circled—employee's rate is within the range but in the wrong relative position. The rate is usually adjusted upward or held constant based on a salary review of all incumbents with the pay range and job classification.

Once the employee's base rate is established, changes to that rate occur in one of three ways: the entire range changes due to market forces (range adjustment), the employee's rate moves within the range (in-range movement), or the employee is promoted or demoted to a job in a different pay range (out-of-range movement). Range movements occur either at predetermined periods of time, based on market pressures, or when job content has been reevaluated. Since the external marketplace often varies from job to job (even within the same job family and pay grade), it is possible for certain job ranges to be adjusted independently of others and to result in rates of pay exceeding predetermined ranges for the job family. These market-sensitive positions (e.g., RNs, CRNAs, physical therapists) are highly skilled and in-demand professionals, who are vital for operations and have experienced documented problems with recruitment and retention.

When ranges are adjusted, individual employees may receive an equivalent adjustment to maintain their relative position within the range or some percentage adjustment less than the range adjustment, or their salaries may be held constant. With either of the latter two options, the possibility of compression between the salaries of newly hired staff and existing staff must be closely monitored.

In-range adjustments or increases are a current debate and controversy. Traditional cost of living adjustments (COLA) tied to price indexes and across-the-board (ATB) increases, granted to all employees, have done little to promote the achievement of personal or organizational goals and rapidly come to be viewed as entitlements by staff. Step increases (annual or periodic increases) granted to employees, although easy to communicate and administer, reward longevity but are viewed by some employees and managers as pay for living another year. Merit or pay for performance systems for groups or individual employees is rapidly being implemented to motivate and reward high levels of performance and achievement of predetermined goals (AHA, 1984, pp. 109–110). To be successful, merit pay systems need to be based on differences in performance that are significant enough to measure and require skilled and committed managers, receptive employees, and skillful compensation professionals. Percentage increases for performance need to be great enough to motivate staff, ranges must be wide enough to accommodate increases over a number of years, and control and monitoring systems must be in place (American Society for Hospital Personnel Administration, 1981).

Movement out of range most often occurs as a result of promotion to a position in a higher pay grade. Depending on how it has been constructed, a nursing clinical ladder system can represent a way to recognize either superior performance within a job (merit based, in-range) or new additional duties and responsibilities (promotion to a different job).

Additions to Base Pay

Additions to base pay may be either mandated by law (overtime pay, FICA contributions), based on market pressures, or established to respond to a particular business need. The Fair Labor Standards Act of 1938 (amended, 1966 and 1974) requires that employers pay all employees not exempt from its provisions at a rate equal to 1½ times the regular rate for hours worked in excess of 8 hours/day or 40 hours/week. Because of the 7 day/week nature of their operations, hospitals may elect to pay for either 8 hours/day or more than 80 hours/2-week period. Employee groups exempted from these provisions include executives, administrative positions, professionals (including RNs), and staff employed in outside sales. A number of qualifying tests must be met. Where uncertainty exists or where precedent has been set, employees usually are classified as nonexempt and, therefore, eligible for overtime (AHA, 1984).

Additions to base pay not mandated by law are at the discretion of the institution. A clear understanding of how special pay practices, such as premiums, bonuses, and alternative scheduling/pay programs like the Baylor Plan, contribute to organizational and employee goals must be articulated, and evaluation measures must be established and reviewed regularly. Staff input to the development and evaluation of these programs is an important contributor to acceptance of and ultimate success of the program. Programs that do not achieve their stated objectives or whose objectives no longer contribute to current organizational goals should be modified, eliminated, or phased out through an open evaluation and decision-making process involving managers, and affected staff.

The fundamental wage and salary structure consists of objectively determined base rates, systematic processes for base salary adjustments, and supplements to base pay. Understanding the structure of the system and implementing it consistently are important contributions of the nurse manager to maintaining the integrity of the system. Nurse managers are in a strategic position to influence the development and testing of creative and new approaches to compensation.

FUTURE PERSPECTIVE

As the work of delivering patient care is redesigned, so too the compensation for the caregivers can be redesigned. Throughout the United States, there are many creative and exciting compensation approaches being studied and implemented. While nurses have strived for their professionalism, many of the features of the traditional salary and compensation structure for nurses have reinforced the hourly wage mentality. New pay practices must be developed to change that mindset.

As health care institutions adopt the principles of total quality management and continuous improvement, any compensation packages developed must be based on a system of employee involvement. The future of wage and compensation packages is well-designed, variable pay programs that increase involvement, commitment, and job satisfaction while helping to decrease unplanned turnover. The increased productivity and improved quality that can result may mean the difference between a hospital's merely surviving and its being highly successful (Jones & Hauser, 1991). Gainsharing, pay-for-performance, pay-for-knowledge, differentiated pay, and salary models are examples of future compensation structures.

Gainsharing

Gainsharing as a method for rewarding performance has been found to be successful in the manufacturing sector and now is receiving increased attention in health care. Gainsharing is a term that describes any system or program that shares with employees the financial gains accrued from improvements in some form of organizational performance. It is by definition a group incentive, and all employees in the defined group share in the gains in some equitable fashion (Berman, Markham, Scott, & Little, 1992, p. 59). Gainsharing provides clear and direct reinforcement for individuals and teams contributing to the improved organizational performance. Employees' personal goals for improving their financial status are met by working toward the achievement of the broader team and organizational goals. Gainsharing provides the opportunity for hospitals to share financial success with employees through its process of continuous improvement.

The IRS Tax Code states that an organization that has a not-for-profit tax status cannot pay employees gains based on profit or net earnings. If the compensation program focuses on reducing costs or improving productivity, it is possible to pay employees a percentage of the savings realized. Rewards are given for efficiencies and improvements—and employee performance is the key to success (Vestal, 1989).

A gainsharing system is effective only as an adjunct to an existing market competitive wage and salary system. To be successful, an organization's culture must support participative management and have a high priority for communicating organizational indicators of success and results. Success indicator measures that might be used in a hospital program include staffing ratios, expense improvements, customer satisfaction, employee satisfaction, and achievement of a designated volume target.

Incentives, such as gainsharing, can be the impetus needed to help nurses and other employees to shift their paradigms, to end the, "It's always been done this way" thinking, and encourage positive changes. Nurses, nursing staff, and other direct care staff have the ability to influence the cost of delivering care significantly. They are equally influential in improvement of the quality of care. Gainsharing increases the accountability of nurses and other caregivers for the predetermined outcomes, and the program is self-funded through actual savings.

In January 1991, a national study of gainsharing programs in health care was completed. Sites identified in this study included the laboratory staff at St. Joseph Mercy Hospital in Ann Arbor, Michigan, Cottonwood Hospital Medical Center in Utah, Center Ambulatory Care in Sacramento, California, South Central Mental Health in Bloomington, Indiana, and three other anonymous sites. The frequency of payouts from these programs ranged from quarterly to annually, and the amount was either a percentage of base pay (ranging from 2% to 6%) or a lump sum payout of between $2000 and $2500/year (Berman et al., 1992, p. 59).

Differentiated Compensation

Another future trend in nursing wages and salaries is to differentiate compensation. Nursing is a diverse career, a profession rather than a job, yet traditional salary and wage packages treat all nurses the same regardless of their clinical performance or their working conditions. Compensation can be differentiated based on education, clinical expertise, clinical area, and working conditions.

Saint Joseph Mercy Hospital (SJMH), a 720-bed community health care system in Ann Arbor, Michigan, allocates salary dollars for registered nurses using a differentiated compensation model based on clinical level of expertise and support of the business working conditions.

The Staff Registered Nurse Wage Grid is a new approach to the compensation of staff nurses and a transition away from an hourly wage model toward a professional salary model. The Staff Registered Nurse Wage Grid established separate job codes and pay scales to recognize differences based both on professional achievement (clinical ladder level) and working conditions that support business operations. As with gainsharing, employee involvement is essential in differentiated compensation programs.

In the case of the SJMH experience, staff input was gathered to validate data regarding what they believed was their major contribution to the business (i.e., which working conditions were considered the least favorable). Based on that feedback, three levels of working conditions were identified. Working conditions were placed on a vertical axis, and clinical ladder levels were placed on a horizontal axis to create a 12-cell grid. Each cell has its own job code and individual, seven-step pay scale (Fig. 14–2).

This system has been in place since 1988, has been through several revisions, and continues to be successful. Recruitment into areas with less desirable working conditions improved, a low and stable overall RN vacancy rate of 1.3% was achieved, and a dramatic decrease in attrition occurred. The Staff RN Wage Grid system provided a challenge to the payroll system and the yearly budget process. Keeping nurses accurately placed on the grid requires additional monitoring by the nurse managers (Johnson, Frederiksen, & Holdwick, 1989).

Differentiated compensation programs also exist that are based on educational preparation as another variable. The success of differentiated compensation lies in recognition of the diversity of the demands placed on nurses and recognizes nursing as a career with opportunities to grow professionally and be rewarded financially. It emphasizes the important role of nurses in the business operations of the hospital because the improved retention and recruitment and nurse satisfaction are essential to the efficient and effective operation of the hospital.

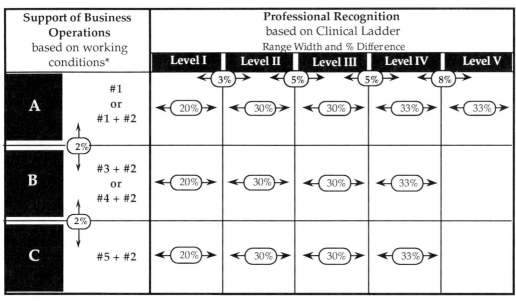

Copyright © 1989 Catherine McAuley Health Center

*Working Conditions
   #1 Monday through Friday, day shift
   #2 Weekend and holiday work
   #3 Straight evening or night shift
   #4 Shift rotation less than 33% of the time
   #5 Shift rotation equal to or greater than 33% of the time.

Figure 14–2   1989 Staff RN Wage Grid. (Copyright © 1989, Catherine McAuley Health Center.)

Salary Model

A frequent criticism of nurses is the tendency to cling to the mentality of an hourly wage earner. That mentality has a factual basis, since nurses are often paid based on an hourly rate. Many nursing leaders say that in order to eliminate the hourly worker mentality, the hourly pay structure must be eliminated. Salaries, annual or monthly, are common in educational institutions and in non-hospital-based health care organizations and are now beginning to be tried in acute care hospital settings.

In many peoples' minds, an annual or monthly salary as a measure of compensation is a distinguishing characteristic of a profession. Typically, the annual compensation is divided equally among pay periods. The amount paid to the employee does not vary from paycheck to paycheck. A system for the use of paid or unpaid time off must be developed as part of the system. The salary structure provides the ability for flexibility that is not possible in an hourly wage system. The nurse or the health care worker works until the job is done rather than working a predetermined number of hours and earning overtime for additional hours. Many nurses experience frustration with colleagues who watch the clock rather than concentrating on organizing their work, believing that the hourly method of pay penalizes the efficient, organized nurse and rewards the nurse primarily for the amount of time it takes to complete the work.

Several hospitals have experienced success with the use of salary models within the departments of nursing. Beth Israel Hospital, a 472-bed teaching hospital in Boston, implemented a professional nurse compensation program (PNCP). This was developed to support a professional nurse practice model. This approach identifies four salary categories that define and categorize variable hours that nurses are scheduled to work in the course of a year and the salary to be received for each category (Bauman & Powers, 1988).

Compatible with a salary structure is the concept of nurses forming professional group practices and entering into a contractual arrangement with the employer (the hospital) for the delivery of ageed on services. At St. Joseph Mercy Hospital in Ann Arbor, Michigan, the cardiothoracic and orthopedic perioperative nurses have formed group practices. The base compensation for each group is in accordance with the hourly rate within the hospital, and lump-sum bonus payments are distributed quarterly based on achievement of predetermined volume targets. The group members are responsible and accountable for the delivery of nursing services for all cardiothoracic and orthopedic cases, and among themselves they cover scheduled and unscheduled time off, on-call, and called-in situations. No members are eligible for overtime (Schmeckel, 1991). These group practice structures have resulted in strong, cohesive groups of professionals similar to professions such as physicians and attorneys. The members of the group practice experience autonomy and accountability.

Pay-for-Knowledge

In traditional systems, nurses' or nursing staff members' pay was determined by job classification and position. In a pay-for-knowledge approach, the pay is determined by the number of tasks the employee is capable of performing.

Many nursing organizations have formally implemented shared governance as a framework that empowers nursing staff, giving them many of the responsibilities that traditionally belonged to the manager. The greater the degree of autonomy that is accorded a team, the more important it becomes to implement cross-training and job flexibility, and the more critical it becomes to reward employees' multiple skills and broader contributions.

Pay-for-knowledge or skill-based pay supports the concept of team that is essential to the total quality management process by rewarding nursing staff for gaining new skills and enhancing their ability to work as a maximally flexible team.

Some managers may be fearful that increasing employees' skills and flexibility will involve increased compensation and, therefore, costs. Initial experimentation with this approach would suggest that as people are more capable and more flexible, the increased compensation given to these workers is balanced by allowing the organization to operate leaner staffing models than traditional organizations because the employees are more productive and are better able to meet the variety of work demands and work fluctuations (Belcher, 1989).

Pay-for-Performance

Organizations are struggling with rediscovering a true merit increase system. Linking an individual's salary increase to performance makes sense and is critical in the current financially challenging environment for health care and other businesses. Merit increases for many hospitals have simply meant an across-the-board/cost-of-living adjustment or annual increase, and have not been truly based on the performance of an individual or team. This practice has resulted in continued higher wages over the years, regardless of an employee's performance level. Separating out the merit portion of a scheduled pay increase from the market adjustment would make it clearer to the employee that this is a true merit increase and one that must be earned again each time an increase is scheduled.

Conclusion

For any of the future wage and salary methods described, as with any new initiative, careful planning is essential. Components of the planning process are to

- Understand the culture of the organization
- Study data on actual and perceived needs of nurses
- Communicate from the very beginning of considering change
- Collaborate with key departments, such as human resources, finance, executive management
- Determine a method for evaluating the outcome of the change

As organizations move away from traditional wage and salary systems, more at-risk pay practices will emerge. These will help to focus individual employee's attention on supporting the goals of the organization and the teams. Innovative wage and salary changes are clearly based on staff empowerment. With that empowerment comes increased independence and interdependence. Staff and managers alike must strive to educate and support themselves in these new behaviors so that continuing success can be insured.

THE ROLE OF THE NURSE MANAGER IN COMPENSATION

The nurse manager plays a vital role in shaping the development and implementation of the organization's compensation program. Nursing's high level of involvement is appropriate, as it is one of the largest departments in terms of both the service provided and labor costs. All staff in nursing need to be able to contribute to articulating to executive management and others their key contributions of providing quality care, ensuring patient satisfaction, and using health care resources cost effectively to assure financial viability and retain customer loyalty.

Shaping compensation for an organization must be a process in which nurse managers are actively involved rather than taking what others have determined. Four key responsibilities of the nurse manager in administering the compensation program are (1) communication, (2) confidentiality, (3) consistency, and (4) currency.

Communication

Managers need to understand the organizational philosophy around compensation to be able to communicate effectively with employees. Most organizations are open to communication on how pay policies and structures are established, and managers should avail themselves of this information. This will help to explain decisions to employees on compensation, especially when placed in the difficult position of unfavorable compensation decisions.

Confidentiality

To maintain a trusting relationship with the compensation staff in the human resources department, managers need to be cautious with information sharing around compensation until appropriate communication plans for the entire organization are implemented. Managers may be pressed to breach confidentiality regarding individual employee salary information in the face of open discussions among employee groups. However, maintaining the basic principles of confidentiality is essential.

Consistency

Management of any compensation program requires a concerted effort to be consistent in application. Inconsistency may result in unfair employee grievances, mistrust among management and staff, salary readjustments for entire groups of employees to remedy internal inequity problems that resulted from favoritism, and the undermining of the validity and reliability of the entire compensation program. Most formal compensation programs have exception processes established to address unique compensation situations that managers feel do not fit the rules.

Currency of Program

Another responsibility of the manager is to work closely with the compensation staff to collaborate about changes in job design, responsibilities and requirements, working conditions and market changes. Programs that are not maintained lead to multiple exceptions to established policy, which erode trust in management, and to employee morale issues regarding unfair compensation.

A formal annual evaluation process should be initiated by the compensation department in collaboration with nursing services. Questions that should be asked might include

1. Are the needs of staff changing? (i.e., aging workforce, many part-time employees, child care and elder care issues among the workforce)
2. Are current incentives helping to produce expected results?
3. What are the projected human resource needs for the future, and how might compensation changes affect them?

Nurse managers are placed in a highly valued position in the organization, close to the staff who provide customer service on a continual basis. This position allows them direct information on staff needs for compensation programs as well as other insights into opportunities for improvement. Nurse managers' professional networking offers additional opportunities for sharing creative solutions to compensation planning as well as other problem solving. With a national movement toward total quality management, the environment is right to test new, creative approaches to meeting the needs of a changing workforce.

References

American Hospital Association, Society for Hospital Personnel Administration. (1984). *Fair shakes: The healthcare compensation handbook*. Chicago, IL: Pluribus Press.

American Society for Personnel Administration and the American Compensation Association. (1981). *Elements of sound base pay administration*. Scottsdale, AZ: Author

Bauman, B. & Powers, E. (1988, October). *Salary compensation for variable hours worked: A strategy in support of a professional practice model*. Paper presented at Second National Symposium, Retention of Hospital Nurses: What Works, Boston, MA.

Belcher, J. (1989). Reward systems: Time for change. *Brief, 74*, 1–8.

Berman S., Markham, S., Scott, K., & Little B. (1992, March–April). Gainsharing experiments in health care. *Compensation and Benefits Review*, 57–64.

Joel, L. (1992). Nursing salaries: Recurring themes and new insights. *Journal of Nursing Administration, 22* (3), 13–17.

Johnson, J., Frederiksen, S., & Holdwick, C. (1989). A non-traditional approach to wage adjustment. *Nursing Management, 20*(11), 36–39.

Jones, D., & Hauser, M. (1991). Putting teeth into pay for performance programs. *Healthcare Financial Management, 45* (9), 32–36.

Management Science Associates. (1992). *The Annual MSA National Compensation Survey* (pp. 5–11). Independence, MO: Author.

Marc, R., Minnick, A., Ginzberg, E., & Curran, C. (1989). *A Commonwealth Fund Paper: What to do about the nursing shortage* (pp. 1–24). New York: The Commonwealth Fund.

Perry, L. (1991). Nursing supervisors continue to lead the climb up the ladder. *Modern Healthcare, 21* (21) 27–34.

Schmeckel, C. (1991). Nursing group practice: One innovative model. *AORN J 53* (5), 1223.

Sibson, R. (1990). *Compensation* (pp. 1–17). New York: American Management Association.

Strassen, L. (1992). Nursing salaries are adequate! *Journal of Nursing Administration, 22* (3), 12–18.

Vestal, K. (1989). Gainsharing: Rewarding nurse performance. *Journal of Nursing Administration, 19* (12), 10–11.

William Mercer Co. (1991). *Nursing compensation practices in Michigan* (pp. 5–8). Detroit, MI: Author.

CHAPTER 15

ORIENTING AND TRAINING OF THE NEW NURSE

BETH R. KEELY

EXECUTIVE SUMMARY

This chapter addresses the transition of an employee to a new work environment. Whether a nurse is a new graduate or an experienced veteran, the development of professional relationships, the establishment of professional practice competencies, and socialization to a new role and environment are all developmental issues. Additionally, continuing education is addressed in respect to organizational need and fiscal restraint. Suggestions regarding educational technology and academic collaboration are offered as adjuncts or alternatives to existing educational practices.

Since Kramer first described reality shock and its serious consequences for graduate nurses and the entire nursing profession (1974), numerous attempts have been made to bridge the gap between education and practice. The literature contains a myriad of articles describing the vast diversity of special orientation programs occurring before and after graduation that attempt to aid the neophyte into making the transition to the clinical work setting. Despite these efforts, both the new graduate and the experienced nurse struggle to establish professional practice. They continue to have difficulty transferring the theoretical basics into patient care situations.

Nurses want to make a difference in patient care. The neophyte comes to the work setting with an idealism that is grounded more in vision than in practical experience. Too often the experienced nurse has lost sight of this difference and holds performance expectations far beyond that which the neophyte is capable. Establishing a mentorship or preceptor program can help prepare experienced staff nurses to assume a partnership with the new graduate. Such a relationship allows both individuals to work harmoniously toward the common goal of providing a structured environment, allowing the neophyte to gain those behaviors necessary in professional practice.

Numerous studies (Highriter, 1969; Soule, 1978) have demonstrated no significant differences in technical skill perfomance between graduates of different nursing programs. However, nursing service administrators have repeatedly found that less time is needed for graduates who most nearly meet the employer's needs and expectations (Guest, 1979). Therefore, nurse administrators must have a clear vision of the goals and mission of the organization. From such a vision comes the leadership to ensure that there is a natural fit between the organization and the nurses hired to fill its professional ranks. Additionally, it provides the direction that guides nurse educators in developing staff development programs that will support the strategic plan.

HELPING THE NEW EMPLOYEE DURING ROLE TRANSITION

Three strategies are used by nurse administrators and educators to help the nurse change from the role of student to that of practitioner or to introduce the experienced nurse to a new work environment: orientation, internships, and preceptorships. The design, content, and length of these programs vary considerably, although the benefits of each are readily recognized. The unique challenge for educators is to meet the varying needs of nurses at different levels of experience without making the program remedial or boring. The most successful programs focus on unit-specific skills as well as providing a general overview. Developing such programs in collaboration with the colleges and universities that provide new graduates can assist both organizations to understand each other's programs. It further helps the nursing service educator to select content relating to the appropriate level of competency for the novice, as well as the advanced practitioner.

Orientation Programs

Orientation programs not only provide instruction about policies, procedures, and administrative reporting structures unique to the institution, but they also assist in resolving the problems that come with trying to adjust to the new work role. This is the period when the novice begins the socialization process that develops a support system within the new work environment. Additionally, orientation programs provide the opportunity for the new nurse to initiate an understanding of the mission, goals, and philosophy of the organization. Orientation programs are generally short in duration and focus on individualized learning needs (see Fig. 15–1 as an example of an orientation agreement).

Internships

The second strategy to assist the transition of a nurse from one role to another is internship. Conceptually, internship can be several things: a planned, supervised experience in an agency whereby the student nurse gains practical work experience, a supervised didactic and clinical work experience for the nurse who is cross-training from one specialty area to another, or a prolonged orien-

HOAG MEMORIAL HOSPITAL PRESBYTERIAN
NURSING ORIENTATION AGREEMENT

Name _____   Unit _____   Date _____

Head Nurse _____   Status: ☐ FT ☐ SPT ☐ PD ☐ Traveler

Start Date _____   Shift _____

The following are orientation requirements for employment at Hoag Memorial Hospital Presbyterian:

ALL NURSES

☐ BLS Certification   Current: ☐ Yes ☐ No   Exp. Date: _____

☐ Pharmacology Assessment Test   Score: _____   ☐ Pass   ☐ Fail

☐ Skills/Knowledge Checklist   ☐ Completed   ☐ Not Completed
(To be returned to Nursing Education within 90 days)

☐ General Orientation   Date to Attend: _____
(within 90 days)

☐ Nursing Orientation   Date to Attend: _____   ☐ Attended   ☐ Not Attended

MATERNAL CHILD

☐ Neonatal Resuscitation Contract   Received: ☐ Yes ☐ No

9TH FLOOR

☐ Basic EKG Assessment Test   Score: _____   ☐ Pass   ☐ Fail

☐ IV Monitored Drug Test   Score: _____   ☐ Pass   ☐ Fail

CRITICAL CARE

☐ Basic Knowledge Assessment Test   Score: _____   ☐ Pass   ☐ Fail
(Unit Specific)

☐ Emergency Protocol Signature Sheet   Signed: ☐ Yes ☐ No

☐ ACLS Certification   Current: ☐ Yes ☐ No   Exp. Date: _____
(Required for ECU RN's)

☐ Other

I have read the above, understand the requirements, and agree to the terms listed.

_____   _____
                    NAME   DATE

Cleared to Work By: _____   _____
                         ORIENTATION COORDINATOR   DATE

WHITE: TO ED. FILE   YELLOW: TO HEAD NURSE   PINK: TO EDUCATOR   GOLDENROD: TO EMPLOYEE

Figure 15–1 Nursing orientation agreement. (Courtesy of Hoag Memorial Hospital Presbyterian, Newport Beach, CA.)

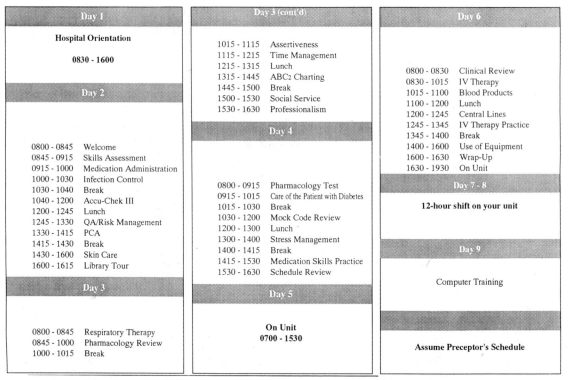

Day 1

Hospital Orientation

0830 - 1600

Day 2

0800 - 0845	Welcome
0845 - 0915	Skills Assessment
0915 - 1000	Medication Administration
1000 - 1030	Infection Control
1030 - 1040	Break
1040 - 1200	Accu-Chek III
1200 - 1245	Lunch
1245 - 1330	QA/Risk Management
1330 - 1415	PCA
1415 - 1430	Break
1430 - 1600	Skin Care
1600 - 1615	Library Tour

Day 3

0800 - 0845	Respiratory Therapy
0845 - 1000	Pharmacology Review
1000 - 1015	Break

Day 3 (cont'd)

1015 - 1115	Assertiveness
1115 - 1215	Time Management
1215 - 1315	Lunch
1315 - 1445	ABC2 Charting
1445 - 1500	Break
1500 - 1530	Social Service
1530 - 1630	Professionalism

Day 4

0800 - 0915	Pharmacology Test
0915 - 1015	Care of the Patient with Diabetes
1015 - 1030	Break
1030 - 1200	Mock Code Review
1200 - 1300	Lunch
1300 - 1400	Stress Management
1400 - 1415	Break
1415 - 1530	Medication Skills Practice
1530 - 1630	Schedule Review

Day 5

On Unit
0700 - 1530

Day 6

0800 - 0830	Clinical Review
0830 - 1015	IV Therapy
1015 - 1100	Blood Products
1100 - 1200	Lunch
1200 - 1245	Central Lines
1245 - 1345	IV Therapy Practice
1345 - 1400	Break
1400 - 1600	Use of Equipment
1600 - 1630	Wrap-Up
1630 - 1930	On Unit

Day 7 - 8

12-hour shift on your unit

Day 9

Computer Training

Assume Preceptor's Schedule

Figure 15–2   Sample new graduate nursing orientation schedule. (Courtesy of Hoag Memorial Hospital Presbyterian, Newport Beach, CA.)

tation program for the novice or graduate nurse. In all cases, the program is designed for a gradual introduction into the new work setting (Fig. 15–2). Initially, this means that the work load is reduced until the new skills are assimilated. There must be a commitment by management to allocate sufficient resources and time to maximize the learning experience. If this does not occur, the student can become frustrated and leave in search of a more supportive environment.

Internship differs from orientation in that participants may or may not be employees even though they are paid. Such payment is usually a stipend substantially below that of existing salary ranges. This creates a unique set of problems. Although they may be less costly for the institution in the long run, such programs may be less rewarding to students than straight employment. This issue is of particular significance in situations where salaries of existing employees are reduced during cross-training programs.

The institution always faces the risk of having interns leave shortly after completion of the internship, so the investment in training does not pay off. Despite this problem, hospitals across the country find internship a viable method of preparing nurses for specialty practice as well as introducing students to the reality of professional practice.

Preceptorships

The third strategy used to move newly educated nurses into the work force is the preceptorship. Although some schools associate this term with programs for novice nurses, it is applied more frequently to graduate study or formal course work in an advanced clinical specialty. Such experiences allow the student to experience the real world context of a new nursing role and to synthesize didactic knowledge for direct clinical application. Close communication and collaborative working relationships between the hospital and the academic institution can help minimize the myriad of problems that may arise from such arrangements.

In the planning of a preceptorship, the student must be intimately involved and committed to the process. Objectives and learning outcomes need to be negotiated among the student, school, and institution. If this does not occur, any one of the parties may consider its role and ideas undervalued. Such negotiations may or may not be extensive, depending on the previous relationship established by the school and health care organization and also on the maturity of the student (Alspach, 1987). Part of these negotiations must include a clarification of who is evaluating the student and who is accountable for patient interactions and interventions taken. Frequently, these issues are clarified within the framework of formal contractual agreements.

The selection of a preceptor, whether by the school, the educator, or the student, is a critical factor in the success of any preceptorship. Although preceptor roles can enhance the position and status of the nurses selected, a mismatch can threaten the entire learning experience. Selecting more than one preceptor can offer the student a wider range of experience as long as the continuity of the learning experience is not jeopardized.

MENTORING THE MENTOR

Nurses are used as mentors in orientation programs, internships, or preceptorships. These mentors must have a respect for learning and be able to communicate that to the nurses with whom he or she works. Although mentors need not know all the answers, they must be able to guide their charges to appropriate reference sources. Mentors must be flexible, articulate, and proficient clinicians, must possess good interpersonal skills, and must share a desire to help develop the new graduate or staff nurse. However, any organization that wants to maximize the mentorship role must commit to more than what the individual brings naturally to the process. Therefore, once mentors are identified, they must be developed to assume this critical role.

Nurses who assume mentoring roles should be oriented to the role just as any nurse is prepared for a new work environment. It is important that experienced nurses recognize and appreciate the skill and knowledge gaps that will occur between themselves and the neophyte. Even more experienced nurses entering the institution or transferring from another unit will function at a lower level. All nurses in new situations will experience stages of learning. The nurse new to any situation does not become a highly skilled expert overnight, yet this is often the expectation.

One strategy to prepare nurses for a mentorship role is to provide a workshop in which the mentor's role is defined. Alspach's preceptor's bill of rights (1987) provides a unique way to introduce role responsibilities. Further content should focus on communication and feedback skills, resource availability, conflict management, and problem solving.

The mentor needs to have an understanding of the entire orientation program, including her or his role in it. Role playing and presentation of case studies can help the staff nurse in learning how to respond to future situations. It is important that nurses understand that socialization to a new role is a developmental process (Table 15–1).

Benner's work (1984) describes this development process in five stages as one moves from novice to expert. Her work established a framework that integrates the Dreyfus model of skill acquisition into applied nursing practice (Table 15–2). Using this model as a framework allows experienced nurses to identify their own current clinical mastery and differentiate that from what is expected

TABLE 15–1 Becoming a Preceptor

I. Introduction	IV. Teaching strategies
II. What is a preceptor?	A. Communication
A. Characteristics	B. Demonstration
1. Role model	C. Role modeling
2. Resource	D. Feedback
3. Evaluator	E. Goal setting
B. Role expectations	F. Problem solving
1. To new nurse	G. Tips to good teaching
2. To head nurse	V. Evaluation and feedback
3. To educator	A. Descriptive vs evaluation
III. Adult learning principles	B. Specific vs general
A. Characteristics of adult learners	C. Timing
B. Facilitating learning vs teaching	D. Clarity
C. Barriers to learning	E. Meeting specific goals
D. Benner's model	F. Directed toward positive action
1. Novice	VI. Problem solving
2. Advanced beginner	A. Interpersonal
3. Competent	B. Intrapersonal
4. Proficient	C. Organizational
5. Expert	D. Reality shock
	VII. Review of forms and documentation

TABLE 15–2 Performance Characteristics of Nurses Using the Dreyfus Model

LEVEL	TEACHING IMPLICATIONS	CHARACTERISTICS
Novice	Requires policies, procedures, and rules; usually in the student role	Behavior is rule driven and inflexible; task oriented
Advanced beginner	Needs guidelines for transferring policies and procedures into practice; needs help in setting priorities New graduates or experienced nurses in new clinical settings	Has established enough experience to demonstrate marginally accepted performance; overall, global aspects of care can be identified but cannot differentiate or discriminate
Competent	Has been in the same or similar work environment for 2 to 3 years; benefits from case studies and simulating that focus on decision making	Begins to see actions in terms of long-range goals; has established the ability to prioritize and successfully manage many aspects of clinical nursing
Proficient	Has worked 3 to 5 years with similar patient populations; best taught using complex case studies; use inductive approaches where nurse contributes experiences	Perceives situations as wholes and performances as guided by maxims that reflect nuances of the situation; perceives action based on long-term outcomes; knows how to modify plans based on events; knows when the expected norm does not materialize
Expert	Has worked with a client population in excess of 5 years; seeks own education experiences	No longer relies on analytic principles; has an intuitive grasp of the situation; frequently cannot articulate why he or she does something; has a vision of what is possible; can consult with other nurses

of the new graduate. Additionally, application of the model allows integration of new employees who are experienced nurses as well as those in cross-training programs.

ESTABLISHING PROFESSIONAL PRACTICE COMPETENCIES

Nursing has evolved over the years to the point where standards of education and practice are clearly articulated. The recognized accountability nursing has to the public has mandated the establishment of competencies for all assigned roles. Each organization must define practice competencies based on established nursing roles and special patient populations. Because of the specificity of developing such competencies, nurse administrators are in the best position to provide the leadership for this process.

Competency relates to specific knowledge, skills, abilities, and personal characteristics essential for adequate practice. Competencies must be evaluated not only on employment as part of the orientation process but also on an annual basis. Various methods can be used to determine clinical competence, but it is important to evaluate both deductive and inductive reasoning skills along with technical skills. Competencies in nursing are complex because one nursing activity may be a combination of several different functions. Therefore, it is helpful to break down competency statements into subcomponents for easier evaluation. For example, a competency statement might read "Maintain good body alignment when repositioning a comatose patient." This breaks down into the following subcomponents:

1. Apply knowledge of anatomy and physiology, including skin integrity.
2. Demonstrate skills related to proper body alignment when repositioning, including use of body support apparatus.
3. Explain to family why turning is important and the rationale for maintaining proper alignment.

Since it is virtually impossible to test the entire domain of nursing knowledge, selecting critical competencies is important. Focusing on high-volume and high-risk procedures for each area can facilitate identifying the areas of greatest importance. Written examinations can supplement competency-based skills checklists. When competencies are identified for high-risk areas but patient or procedure numbers or both are low, simulation exercises can be used for evaluation (Fig. 15–3).

Competencies must be evaluated and analyzed for appropriate learning activities based on expected outcome behavior. Knowledge, comprehension, and application are in the lower level of the cognitive hierarchy, whereas evaluation, analysis, and synthesis are considered at a higher level. This leveling of learning is important not only to determine learning objectives but also to define appropriate evaluation strategies.

Competencies change over time as patient populations, technology, and treatment regimens evolve. Therefore, a mechanism of review and revision needs to be established so that the evaluation of clinical competency does not deviate from actual practice. Need for change can be identified through quality improvement activities or risk management efforts.

SOCIALIZING NEW PROFESSIONALS

Professional socialization is a very complex process. The person not only acquires the knowledge and skills of a particular job but also develops a sense of occupational and professional identity. The end product of the socialization process is an individual who develops the technical competencies inherent in the job and internalizes the values and attitudes of the group. Developing this sense of culture has benefits for both the individual and the profession.

According to Cohen (1981), professional socialization has four goals.

1. Learning the technology of the profession—the facts, skills, and theory

FIFTH FLOOR
SKILLS/KNOWLEDGE CHECKLIST

Competent	Needs Practice	Never Done	Skills and/or Knowledges	Date/Initial	Preceptor Signature	Learning Resources and References
			Self-Assessment		**Preceptor Assessment**	
			XX. Radiation Therapy, follows precautions according to policy			P&P I 1.4c/Intravaginal
			A. Care of patient with radiation implant			Cesium Implant Care Plan
			XXI. Reports pertinent information to:			
			A. The following shift			Preceptor
			B. The physician			Preceptor
			C. The Head Nurse			Preceptor/HN
			D. The Charge Nurse			
			XXII. Restraints, Demonstrates legal and safe use of			
			A. Application of vest			P&P R 1.4b
			B. Application of wrist			P&P R 1.4b
			C. Application of waist			P&P R 1.4b
			D. Mit restraints			
			E. Fall precautions			Std. Fall Precautions
			F. Documents critical elements			
			XXIII. Scales, Demonstrates use of			
			A. Bed scale			P&P W 1.0a
			XXIV. Sequential Compression Device, Demonstrates use of			
			A. Ted hose/Thromboguards			P&P T 2.0
			B. Jobst stockings			Preceptor
			XXV. Specimen collection, Demonstrattes according to policy			
			A. Clean catch - urinalysis and/or culture from voided specimen			P&P U 1.4b

Figure 15–3 Sample skills/knowledge checklist. (Courtesy of Hoag Memorial Hospital Presbyterian, Newport Beach, CA.)

2. Learning to internalize the professional culture
3. Finding a personally and professionally acceptable version of the role
4. Integrating this professional role into all the other life roles

Every individual attains these goals at his or her own rate and in his or her own way.

Cohen (1981) associates three theories in establishing a developmental model for professional socialization (Table 15–3). The first is Piaget's work on cognitive development. Piaget delineated stages of intellectual development and concept formation. He introduced the notion of knowledge transference. Kelman's theory introduces the aspect of social influence. This helps explain how students integrate the norms and values of professional culture into self-concept. Such internalization stabilizes the concept one has of oneself without eliminating the possibility of future change. Finally, Erickson's theory of human development explains the acquisition of independence and self-identity. One cannot go un-

TABLE 15–3   Cohen's Integration Model of Professional Socialization

Unilateral dependence	For 1 year or so, students focus on learning technology. They are dependent on instructors.
Negative/independence (autonomy vs shame) and doubt/willpower and initiative vs guilt/ purpose	Nurses explore those components of the professional role that are congruent with their self-concept. Begin to question knowledge and weigh importance of theory. As they gain confidence, they learn which rules are flexible and which are inviolate. This level is critical because if they remain dependent, they will not achieve true professionalism. Students begin to establish critical thinking skills.
Dependence/mutuality (industry vs inferiority/ competence)	Nurses seek avenues to make the professional role acceptable. They acquire role limits and examine self-presentations. They compromise between professional role images and their own individuality. They seek role models and professional mentors.
Interdependence (identity vs role diffusion/fidelity)	The professional role is internalized. Nurses take responsibility for their own actions. Nurses are confident in the role, have established a set of values concerning that role, and exhibit an image free of internal conflict.

changed having internalized the affective and cognitive components of a professional role into one's identity.

The successful socialization of the neophyte nurse is crucial to the advancement of the profession as a whole and the organization specifically. Much of this success is based on trust during the time the neophyte is establishing autonomy and initiative. It is during this time that the preceptor role becomes critical in supporting the neophyte in making the transition from a student role to that of practitioner. It is imperative that the preceptor understand the socialization process and provide feedback that modifies behavior without devastating the newly acquired fragile identity.

Many things can affect the socialization process outside the preceptor relationship. Cultural norms and values can be challenged by the role expectations of the nursing profession. Personal academic ability affects how each student develops and achieves. Conflict ultimately arises when the neophyte is cognitively mature yet psychologically immature. Men entering the profession may find it difficult to resolve professional role expectations with outdated social images. Additionally, the socialization process can be hampered when nurses at any stage are faced with multirole conflict. Most often, women assume many roles throughout the course of time. When the roles of wife/mother/professional nurse and more begin to demand time and energy all at once, some roles are set aside for other priorities. It is important to realize where an individual's priorities and ability lie so that expectations and goals can be established realistically. Not all nurses will achieve professional behaviors at the same time, and some nurses may never acquire them. Therefore, it is imperative that we evaluate the professionalization of nurses as well as nursing.

Nurse educators and clinical preceptors need to focus beyond the technical skill acquisition when socializing new nurses into organizational roles. Specific learning activities must be built into orientation curricula that address organizational as well as professional values. Critical thinking and decision making must be supported both in the classroom and on the nursing unit. Regular triad conferences among the preceptor, educator, and orientee can help identify problem areas and establish individualized goals. Integrating a self-evaluation process can help the orientee assess ongoing technical needs as well as establish a way to help internalize expected culture behaviors.

As difficult as the first step appears, it sets the stage for the nurse's entire career. Learning is a lifelong process, and health care demands that nursing professionals stay abreast of many technological, political, and social changes. Socialized well, the nurse will embrace change as a way to move ahead and grow with the organization. When it does not occur, nurses can become the millstones that keep nursing and health care from reaching its potential.

CONTINUING EDUCATION

The rapid advances in health care scientific and technologic knowledge, shifting social attitudes, and the expansion of nursing practice opportunities require nurses to regularly update their knowledge and skills. During the 1970s when education dollars were plentiful, there was a dramatic increase in the number and variety of educational offerings. Evaluation indices, often based on satisfaction scores, demonstrated that continuing education was worthwhile. However, these results were often based on soft data, and the hard questions were not asked (Heyerman, Phillips, & Lessner, 1987).

As cost containment has become inherent in fiscal accountability, however, the hard questions are now being tackled. The learning needs of nursing staffs are still present, but administrators are making sure that the limited dollars are being well spent. Of great concern is that continuing education cannot compete for limited resources, and in many hospitals, entire education departments have been eliminated. This is because many continuing education managers have difficulty demonstrating that their costs are justified or that they are generating acceptable returns on educational investments.

Continuing education departments can accomplish important organizational goals while being cost effective. This mandates that the objectives of the education department reflect the strategic goals and mission of the organization (Keely & Davis, 1990). When these strategic goals are addressed, a substantial contribution can be made to both the nursing staff and the organization. In addition, health care consumers gain the benefits when the nursing staff is responsive and understands the organizational goals.

Continuing education activities vary enormously in type, length, medium, and objective. There are three major target areas for providing ongoing education within a health care setting.

1. Ongoing in-service programs
2. Staff development for advancement
3. Management development

In-service education is increasingly directed at being unit specific and unit based. Content is most often diagnosis, technology, or treatment specific. Greater emphasis is being placed on environmental, safety, and risk management issues. Because of vast content areas, educators are becoming increasingly creative in how educational needs are met. Not only are interdepartmental resources being tapped, but posters, self-learning modules, gaming, and audiovisual media are being used.

Formal classroom instruction will continue to be a format used for presenting didactic material. Class content can vary widely, and this method can be most effective in reaching larger audiences. Methodologies of instruction that are not as adaptable to the nursing units can be used. Examples include simulation exercises, video vignettes, or seminar-type discussions to enhance critical thinking skills.

Unlike in-service programs that tend to target groups of nurses, staff development activities are more individualized. Developmental plans or learning contracts or both can be used to establish educational goals and outcomes. Plans can be developed on a personal level or in conjunction with the performance evaluation process. Learning activities become specific to meeting professional growth objectives and can be a combination of formal and informal options. Classes outside the organization may be sought to fulfill specific content areas. This is particularly true in cases where management training is incorporated as a component of the plan.

Staff development activities frequently place the educator in a mentorship role. As the individual grows within the organization, there is a socialization process that occurs in which the nurse begins to assume new values and attitudes. If the nurse transfers to a new department, formal training will become part of the plan. As the nurse becomes more confident within an assumed role, he or she will have greater authority to make change and influence innovation (Stoner & Wantal, 1986).

Not every employee is going to be the star who produces high-quality work, nor are there unlimited opportunities for upward mobility. Therefore, staff development activities attempt to maximize the potential of staff nurses by maintaining a sense of personal growth and achievement. Helping staff identify their potential and establishing career goals can enrich the organization because these individuals are usually more motivated. They contribute to their work environment and can more readily translate change opportunities into day-to-day reality.

Management training has become an increasingly important role for many nursing education departments. Technical, financial, human resource, and organizational skills are required of nurse managers throughout the industry. Although different managerial levels require different types of skills, all levels must balance competing goals and set priorities. Since many entry level management positions are filled from within the organization, there is a greater demand to better prepare nurses to assume management and supervisory functions. Since the best way to learn to be an effective manager is by working and observing good managers, a mentoring or preceptor relationship should be incorporated along with the didactic elements.

TEACHING VS FACILITATING

Nurses are faced with the need for lifelong learning. As with many professional groups, this has generated from technical, socioeconomic, and political influences. Staff developers are, therefore, working with an adult population of learners who have unique challenges and needs. Nurses who attend continuing education programs are no longer concerned about meeting graduation requirements. They are concerned about how any learning activity meets their own perceived need. Therefore, their readiness to learn and willingness to participate in a learning situation is directly related to how useful they perceive the information to be (Puetz & Peters, 1981).

Adult learners expect to be treated as individuals who are mature and independent persons. They have had the opportunity to gain experience in the work setting and have a strong self-concept. Although experiences may vary among individuals, they all have a common bond in dealing with people in a variety of situations. Nurses expect to be treated with dignity and will not remain in a learning situation that they perceive as threatening to their self-esteem.

Nurses, like all adult learners, seek educational opportunities where they can apply the information immediately. This here-and-now application must be a core ingredient of any continuing education program. Learners must be able to use their own past experiences to build new ones. Participants learn from each other, and they can easily relate new learning to past activities. Therefore, classroom techniques must allow for a participative style where learners can problem solve and explore new ideas and concepts.

Since adults come to a learning environment with their own set of attitudes, values, and knowledge, the educator becomes a facilitator. It is the educator's responsibility to provide a meaningful learning experience and to allow the contribution of participants. Learning is a shared process that requires collaboration between colleagues and the educator. The educator's role becomes one of assisting participants to process information and discover the meaning of the material on a personal level. This role differs greatly from a strict teaching format, where information is given without the opportunity to assimilate it and discover its meaning.

Throughout the process of nursing education and development, each individual will encounter both strategies. There is the appropriate time and place for each. The successful educator will be the one who learns when and where the best technique can be used. However, facilitation of learning can occur only when the individual nurse assumes the accountability to be responsible for his or her own learning needs.

USING INSTRUCTIONAL TECHNOLOGY

The media used in education have exploded as fast as the entertainment industry has produced new technology. Filmstrips and audiocassettes have given way to the high-tech use of computer-assisted instruction and interactive video. Learning laboratories can now become independent learning centers supported with sophisticated mannequins tied to computer systems. However, there are advantages and disadvantages to all instructional media (Table 15–4).

The cost of hardware to support computerized systems is expensive and often competes with other demands for capital dollars. In many cases, the cost may not justify the software applications available. Although software programming for health care is becoming more advanced and sophisticated, it still faces many limitations. Identifying more than one use for systems or taking advantage of lend-lease programs can help offset such difficulties.

Despite the surge in use of video and other techniques, limited resources for education may make such options unavailable. Use of any education technology must be evaluated against the learning objectives and expected outcome. Do not overlook the flexibility and variety that multimedia options provide. It is still the best policy to use the cheapest method that can get the job done.

COLLABORATION BETWEEN ACADEMIA AND SERVICE

Leaders in both academic and service settings have been attempting to come to some consensus on the effective preparation of nursing students for both present and future practice. Collaboration among educators, researchers, practitioners, and managers must occur to define the scope of nursing roles and practice as well as the scientific base on which they rest. The limitation of resources in both settings mandates that academia and service work together rather than in two separate spheres. It is no longer acceptable that the educator provide only education that develops the theoretical and scientific basis for nursing while clinicians provide effective and economic service.

Educators in both areas must be willing to work together to define those skills necessary for entry into practice. Nursing administrators must come to accept responsibility for staff development, and nursing professors must come to grips with balancing the cognitive skills with the technical skills. Neither arena has the resources to duplicate educational experiences or assume the other's role. Innovative programs to integrate education and practice have been initiated in several areas (Aydelotte, 1981). A few of these are as follows.

- Appointments of faculty to practice committees in community hospitals
- Joint planning of continuing education programs between hospitals and colleges/universities
- Advisory councils to schools of nursing containing hospital nursing representatives

TABLE 15–4 Instructional Media

Films	Use of motion pictures is good for learning visual identification, such as procedures. They have advantages in maintaining consistency of information and demonstrating relationships. They can consist of short clips or complete films, and they are adaptable to groups of all sizes. Their major disadvantages include cost of production and the changing equipment technology, which may make them obsolete.
Audiocassettes	Although easy to prepare and flexible in use, audiocassettes are better used to supplement other learning media. When used alone, they are best adapted for factual material or developing desirable attitudes. They tend to be overused as replacements for text reading.
Filmstrips	Use of filmstrips is declining, although they are compact, easy to handle, and maintain sequencing. Compared to other media, they are inexpensive and adaptable to group or individual study. They are difficult to produce outside a professional laboratory, and presentation order cannot be changed. They do not have the same visual impact that motion pictures have and are less effective in developing effective skills.

Newer Applications

Satellite networks	Access to satellite networks dedicated to health care education has increased over the past several years. Programming must be contracted, and like commercial television, scheduling is at the discretion of the network. Unless programming can be repeated, health care institutions must incur the additional cost of videotaping the program for increased flexibility. The primary advantages include adaptability to large audiences in multiple locations and the ability to have interactive response via telephone hookup. Additionally, information can be current, and live programming can be used.
Computer-assisted instruction	Although computerization has been around for many years, health care education applications have lagged behind other fields. Hardware development surpassed software for many years. Despite new software programs being released, many tend to be too basic for advanced practitioners. Computer programming is ideal for teaching factual material, principles, concepts, and rules. One difficulty is the continuous improvement in technology, which outdates hardware quickly despite major investments in capital resources.
Future modalities	Future applications of technology, such as interactive video instruction and the use of laser discs, are already being used in other industries. Although these applications have been used rarely in the health care industry, they have potential. A major reason for this is the cost of program development as well as the need to add to or replace existing hardware within the organization. Until systems are developed to a point that costs can be reduced, such media applications will find limited use.

- Educational contracting through schools of nursing to provide educational services
- Financial underwriting of a faculty position by hospitals to expand student services

Joint appointments also provide opportunities for both hospitals and schools. The increase in communication between organizations can reduce conflict among nurses as well as increase access to teaching resources. There is the potential to increase clinical research by staff as well as the students and faculty. Furthermore, faculty can maintain clinical competence and are, therefore, seen as experts who offer a contribution to the organization.

A further consideration in collaborative programs is the potential for recruitment. When a school works closely with a given health care organization, students are welcomed and supported as potential future employees for the nursing staff. Students seek those organizations for employment in which they felt comfortable in the learning role. The school can benefit from the referral of students from these same organizations.

Collaboration between service and academia additionally helps provide reality-based training. When instructors work in the health care organization, their currency in clinical practice helps provide insight into curriculum development. When curriculum reflects the reality of the work setting, shock is minimized (Kramer, 1974) as new graduates make the transition into the work place. Professional currency in faculty is a major issue in providing such educational ease and is being addressed in two ways.

1. Provision of education grants to renew clinical skills in existing knowledge areas or for cross-training
2. The requirement by accrediting bodies that faculty demonstrate clinical relevance in a specialty focus

The rapidly changing treatment modalities and health care delivery models mandate that faculty collaborate closely with health care providers so that students do not enter the work environment with obsolete ideas and outdated expectations.

Collaboration between service and academia offers many challenges, but done successfully, it provides many rewards. Nurse administrators and educators must challenge both themselves and their colleagues in academia to explore new options in better preparing nurses to face the ever changing practice modalities in the current health care environment.

CONCLUSION

Health care organizations exist to take care of patients. Their most valuable resource is the nursing staff. As administrators and educators, we cannot lose sight of the fact that this resource must be nurtured, cultivated, and managed like any other scarce commodity. The commitment and investment to develop nursing staff to achieve the optimal potential will result in better retention, higher productivity, and decreased vacancy and turnover rates.

References

Alspach, J. (1987). The preceptor's bill of rights. *Critical Care Nurse, 7*(1), 1.

Aydelotte, M.K. (1981). Approaches to conjoining nursing education and practice. In J. McCloskey and H. Grace (Eds.), *Current issues in nursing*. Boston: Blackwell Scientific Publications.

Benner P. (1984). *From novice to expert: Excellence and power in clinical nursing practice*. Menlo Park, CA: Addison-Wesley.

Cohen, H.A. (1981). *Developmental sequence of professional socialization. The nurse's quest for a professional identity*. Menlo Park, CA: Addison-Wesley.

Guest, L.B. (1979). Diploma schools foster professionalism. *Hospitals, 53*(10), 107-108.

Heyerman, K.S., Phillips, K.M., & Lessner, J.R. (1987). Collaboration: Clinical education and hospital orientation. *Nursing Management, 18*(2), 64-66.

Highriter, M.E. (1969). Nurse characteristics and patient progress. *Nursing Research, 18*(6), 484-501.

Keely, B., & Davis, K. (1990). Productivity in education. *The Journal of Continuing Education in Nursing. 21*4), 150-153.

Kramer, M. (1974). *Reality shock: Why nurses leave nursing*. Saint Louis: C.V. Mosby Company.

Puetz, B., & Peters, F. (1981). *Continuing education for nurses*.Rockville, MD: Aspen Systems Corporation.

Soules, H.M. (1978). Professional advancement and salary differentials among baccalaureate, diploma, and associate degree nurses. *Nursing Forum, 17*(2), 184-201.

Stoner, J., & Wantal, C. (1986). *Management*. Englewood Cliffs, NJ: Prentice-Hall.

Bibliography

Green, G. (1988). Relationships between role models and role perceptions of new graduate nurses. *Nursing Research, 37*(4), 245–248.

Greipp, M.E. (1989). Nursing preceptors—Looking back—Looking ahead. *Journal of Nursing Staff Development, 5*(4), 183–186.

Guinee, K.K. (1978). *Teaching and learning in nursing*. New York: Macmillan Publishing Co.

Huckaby, L.M. (1980). *Conditions of learning and instruction in nursing*. St. Louis: C.V. Mosby Company.

Keely, B. (1991). Applying standards to practice: The critical step. *Dimensions of Critical Care Nursing, 10*(5), 251–252.

Myrick, F. (1988). Preceptorships—Is it the answer to the problems in clinical teaching? *Journal of Nursing Education, 27*(3), 136–138.

Nederveld, M.E. (1990). Preceptorships: One step beyond. *Journal of Nursing Staff Development, 6*(4), 186–189.

Simms, L.M., Price, S.N., & Ervin, N.E. (1985). *Developing human potential. The professional practice of nursing administration*. New York: John Wiley & Sons.

Statewide Nursing Program. (1985). *Reference guide: Instructional strategies*. Dominguez Hills, CA: California State University.

The benefits of preceptorship. (1986). *Journal of Nursing Administration, 16*(6), 4.

Ulschak, F.S. (1988). *Creating the future of health care education*. Chicago: American Hospital Publishing, Inc.

CHAPTER 16 • • • • • •

STAFF DEVELOPMENT AND MENTORING

SUSAN H. CUMMINGS

EXECUTIVE SUMMARY

Staff development facilitates professional growth of clinical staff at all levels of expertise within an organization and supports attainment of organizational outcomes related to quality cost-effective care. Successful staff development programs clearly articulate learner and organizational objectives and delineate strategies to effect learning. An educational model best developed by nursing staff in collaboration with those responsible for education and supported by nursing leadership provides a unifying focus and common reference point around which education programs and services can be developed. Mentoring and precepting are strategies to facilitate one-to-one professional and career development of staff at all levels within the organization. They facilitate the transfer of professional standards and enhancement of the profession as qualified nurses and leaders are developed. Practical strategies for preceptor and mentor development and program evaluation are discussed within the context of decentralizing education to the point of service. A cost-effective staff development program is a powerful tool not only to support individual growth but also to facilitate health care outcomes in the 1990s.

A cornerstone of health care organizations in an era of paradigm shifts is the professional development of the clinical staff. Professional development of nurses, whether at the novice or expert level of nursing practice, and achievement of organizational outcomes related to quality cost-effective care can be supported through active staff development programs in the clinical practice setting. Effective staff development can support an organization's beliefs about the importance of lifelong learning within a professional practice framework.

OUTCOMES OF STAFF DEVELOPMENT

Critical to the ongoing success of staff development programs is a clear identification of learner and organizational goals and the development of strategies to effect learning for nurses within a clinical practice setting. Outcomes of staff development for individual nurses include

- Ongoing competency development
- Professional growth
- Preparation for career advancement
- Enhanced job satisfaction

Outcomes of staff development for organizations include

- Operationalizing the mission statement, values, and philosophy
- Meeting compliance with regulatory and accrediting body requirements
- Providing quality cost-effective care
- Creating a positive recruitment and retention strategy
- Marketing internal expertise in the community

EFFECTIVE STRATEGIES OF STAFF DEVELOPMENT

Effective staff development strategies must match teaching and learning activities with expected individual and organizational outcomes and usually take the form of problem solving, decision making, critical thinking, skill competency, or role development. Fuzzard (1989) identifies multiple interactive teaching–learning strategies for staff development. They include feedback lectures, performance-based instruction, role playing, case method, in-basket, gaming, scenarios, and portable patient packs as well as computer-assisted and video-assisted instruction. All of these strategies provide nurses with simulated opportunities to learn and develop competencies related to their own professional development. Ultimately, effective staff development programs must prepare nurses for current and future practice situations, many of which are significantly different from those they have experienced previously. As postulated in *The Futurist,* learners must begin to think like dolphins. "When dolphins don't get the results they expect, they almost immediately begin to invent new behaviors that appear based on new points of view" (Think like, 1988, p. 54).

EDUCATION MODEL BUILDING

Creating a framework for nursing staff development is critical to the successful development of a nursing organization. Frameworks are best developed by nursing staff in collaboration with those responsible for education and supported by those who will be using educational services to support their staff's development. These educational models should reflect the nursing philosophy and identified standards of practice within the context of the organization's mission, values, and philosophy. Key issues to be addressed during development of the educational model include

- Beliefs about education and professional role development
- Articulation of beliefs with the nursing philosophy, nursing conceptual framework, defined standards of practice, and the mission, values, and philosophy of the organization

- Components of nursing professional development related to remedial education, standards development and application, clinical skills, and professional role development
- Purposes of educational model
- Education outcomes for individual learners and the oganization
- Identification of learners
- Definition of levels of competency
- Assessment of learning needs
- Application of learning theories
- Identification of strategies for cognitive, affective, and psychomotor learning as well as development of critical thinking
- Clarification of the role of the provider/facilitator of education
- Fit of learning activities with the intended outcomes
- Development of systems and tools to support staff development programs
- Determination of learning outcomes
- Maintenance of competency levels
- Use of evaluation data

PRECEPTORS AND MENTORS IN STAFF DEVELOPMENT

One of the most effective models for facilitating professional development is the use of preceptors and mentors, who in their one-to-one relationships can facilitate development of nurses at all levels of practice within an organization. Preceptors often have been associated with the orientation of new graduates and staff. They may be equally effective in ongoing staff development of clinical nurses as well as managers. Although the preceptor role is multifaceted and includes consultant, teacher, researcher, and practice roles (Morrow, 1984), its primary role focus is one of facilitation. In this role, the preceptor is a learning resource and guide, providing education at the point of service. The preceptor may demonstrate competencies, emphasize organizational culture and values, encourage risk taking in exploring new alternatives, and ask the "what if" questions that will facilitate the learner's ability to think and practice. These interactions facilitate thorough integration of learning and critical thinking.

Mentors facilitate professional development of nurses and their potential advancement in multiple roles within the organization. Mentorship usually involves a high investment of psychologic and interpersonal energy. Mentor-mentee relationships usually evolve over a longer period of time and exist outside a formal educational program, where the focus is usually on less clearly specified outcomes than those attained during a preceptor–learner relationship. Mentors and mentees select each other, whereas preceptors and learners are selected for each other. It is my hypothesis that succesful mentors develop as a result of participation in a successful mentor–mentee relationship or an educational program, and preceptors' development is best facilitated through a structured educational program. Preceptor and mentor development and evaluation strategies to determine program effectiveness in an organization are the primary focus of this chapter.

TRAINING PRECEPTORS

Once an organization has made the commitment to decentralize some aspects of staff development by using preceptors to assist staff in translating theory into practice, several key questions must be addressed.

* When should preceptors be used?
* What decisions need to be made related to program planning?
* What resources are necessary to support such a program?
* How should preceptors be selected?
* How should preceptors be trained and developed?
* How should preceptors be supported and evaluated?

Program Development

Preceptor programs are extremely effective when numbers of nursing staff are to be socialized to new or expanded roles over a defined period of time. They are less effective for one-time education due primarily to efficiency and financial resource use issues. Obviously, preceptors are also less effective if the ratio of learners to preceptors is unmanageable for the desired outcomes. This ratio is based on identified needs of the organization as well as the learners.

The basic processes of program development also apply to establishing a preceptor program. After goals for the educational program have been clearly defined, a review of literature and formal and informal consultation with other organizations can be helpful in developing a preliminary program proposal. Organizational commitment for the change and a commitment of resources must be attained before implementation plans can be finalized. Contingent on the organization's experiences with implementing major organizational change and time frames, a preceptor program may be implemented either with or without a pilot preceding full-scale implementation. The planning group defining the program development process must focus on clearly articulating the performance standards for preceptors, the educational program for preceptor development, the role of preceptors within the organization, an implementation plan, and a plan to evaluate the program's success.

Participant Selection

Selection of participants is a threefold process in implementing a successful preceptorship program. Obviously, selection of learners who have the potential for success within a preceptor–learner relationship is essential. A program coordinator is vital, at least initially, to facilitate coordination and integration of the preceptorship program. Attributes to consider in selection of a coordinator include commitment to the program, leadership abilities, and expert practitioner skills. In addition, educational skills, program development, and evaluation skills are critical attributes. Preceptors may be selected by interview, through peer review processes, or through administrative processes. Selection focuses on assessing the candidate's potential for development, level of current skills and competencies related to precepting, professional values and behaviors, and ability to meet program outcomes. Selection in many organizations is considered a career advancement opportunity.

Initial and Ongoing Development

Initial and ongoing preceptor development will facilitate program success. In concert with current adult education philosophies is the concept that individuals learn differently and can be accountable for their own learning and acquisition of preceptor skills. Learning of these skills can be enhanced through multiple teaching–learning strategies. An assessment of preceptor needs can provide the foundation for ongoing program development for preceptors and should be formulated using performance evaluation data and self-identified learning deficits of participants. Often, these needs assessments focus on the need for information or skill enhancement related to adult learning theory, teaching–learning strategies, preceptor–learner relationships, goal setting, giving and receiving performance feedback, evaluation and development plans, and documentation. Strategies that can provide adequate initial and ongoing learning opportunities include workshops, self-learning, and interactive feedback sessions.

The focus of preceptor education is on developing competencies related to the role performance standards. Content that can be incorporated in preceptor workshops is outlined in Table 15-2. A role development model originally designed for precepting clinical nurse specialist students that focuses on advanced clinical skills, communication skills, leadership skills, and group skills (Hill, 1989) can provide a structure for workshops for preceptors who will be precepting those in expanded clincial or educational roles. These templates for preceptor education provide the basic learning maps to assist novice preceptors to sharpen their competencies related to designing adult learning experiences, providing evaluation feedback, and using such tools as skills checklists and learning contracts. They also promote development of experienced preceptors so they can efficiently and effectively meet performance standards for their roles.

Factors That Facilitate Success

Positive outcomes of preceptor programs depend on the motivation of both the preceptor and learner. The selection and development of preceptors and learners in concert with development of systems and tools facilitates the learning of both and ensures ongoing program success. Tools should cue the preceptor and learner about key learning activities and streamline documentation of competency attainment. Communication to nursing staff within the organization and ongoing leadership support also affect positive outcomes.

Reinforcement of preceptor behaviors, interactive problem solving, and update sessions based on program and self-evaluation must be incorporated into the ongoing implementation phase of preceptor programs. Benner's levels of clinical nursing practice (1982), novice, advanced beginner, competent, proficient, and expert, can provide a template for ongoing preceptor education that incorporates differing levels of competency. As preceptors develop within a nursing organization, it is usually possible to match preceptors with learners so they are more expert than those they are precepting. Nederveld's model (1990) for a successful advanced preceptor workshop incorporated three distinct content areas.

1. Redefinition of the preceptor's role
2. Development of interpersonal skills
3. Clarification of precepting processes

Advanced workshops (Nederveld, 1990) and preceptor updates provide opportunities to review role responsibilities, build competencies, provide a forum for interactive problem solving, and recognize the preceptor contributions to the organization. Role playing, scenarios, and small group interaction allow participants to explore unit-based problems associated with preceptorships and develop creative strategies to enhance effectiveness and competency development. Brief updates can assist preceptors in the role-clarification process, reframing responsibilities, and synergistic problem solving. Concepts discussed in a survival skills for preceptors update 3 months after initiation of a preceptorship program by the author focused on continued development of teacher skills, emulating characteristics of superior teachers, bringing individual styles and strengths to the preceptor–learner relationship, continuing self-learning, and facilitating and acting as a resource to learners. The discussion of evaluation strategies focused on eliciting evaluative feedback about performance as a preceptor and observing development of learner competencies.

Scenarios and role-playing situations were used to explore affective content focusing on coping with the preceptor role vs peer perception of the role and effectively coping with feelings in the teaching–learning process. "What ifs" for common situations defined by preceptors and problems in preceptorship role implementation can be simulated in small group interactive exercises. Usually, nominal group technique (Hunsaker & Cook, 1986) provides group identification of possible scenarios. Facilitators can prepare scenarios for problem solving based on managerial input or previously experienced preceptor–learner situations.

Program Evaluation

It is critical to develop the program evaluation during the program-planning stage of a preceptorship program. Irrespective of the model, program evaluation must focus on evaluation of individuals as well as organizational outcomes. Evaluation of individuals is completed through the organization's performance evaluation system and associated assessment of competencies related to role development. Program evaluation serves as a basis for evaluating the ongoing success of the program. In addition, it may serve as a database for termination of an unsuccessful program and can identify opportunities to improve exisitng programs. Renzulli's key features model (Munro, 1983), which measures key variables of success identified by vested interest groups over time, provides a relatively simple framework for program planning and evaluation. Benchmarks of this model include

TABLE 16–1 Preceptor Program Evaluation Model: Vested Interest Groups and Key Variables

VESTED INTEREST GROUPS	KEY VARIABLES
Nursing administration/ managers/program coordinator	Cost of program
	Recruitment and retention data
	Qualitative and quantitative improvement in clinical outcomes
	Performance evaluation/competency assessment results
Learners	Competency/performance evaluation feedback
	Enrichment/professional development
	Values and behaviors support organization's mission
	Satisfaction with preceptorship program
	Job satisfaction
Preceptors	Enrichment/professional development
	Role satisfaction/job satisfaction
	Effectiveness/efficiency of preceptor program
	Competency/performance evaluation feedback

- Identification of stakeholders
- Indicators or criteria that signify success
- Frequency of measurement to facilitate evaluation and capitalize on opportunities for improvement

Vested interest groups and key variables for implementation of this model for a preceptor program evaluation are shown in Table 16–1.

Preceptors provide an invaluable resource to support and validate competency development in a decentralized staff development program. The design, implementation, and ongoing evaluation of all facets of a preceptor program facilitate the ongoing positive contribution to organizational outcomes related to quality, cost-effective, and efficient patient care.

TRAINING MENTORS

Preparation for mentoring often focuses on using previous successful experiences as a mentee as a basis for self-development of the mentor role. Mentors may be trained through participation in formal management and role development programs. Growth of mentors evolves within the confines of the continuum of a mentor–mentee relationship in a supportive organizational environment. Knowledge of expected outcomes of the mentoring relationship and understanding role functions of mentors provides a self-assessment framework for development of oneself as a mentor as well as for planning formal educational programs.

Role Definitions

Multiple definitions of mentoring provide us with helpful insights about the role of mentoring. Mentoring (Kram, 1985b), a key component of the leadership role, is defined in general terms as the development and advancement of talented subordinates. Mentoring has also been defined by Anderson and Shannon (1988, p. 40) as a

> Nurturing process is which a more skilled or more experienced person, serving as a role model teaches, sponsors, encourages, controls and befriends a less skilled or less experienced person for the purpose of promoting the latter's professional and/or personal development. Mentoring functions are carried out within the context of an ongoing, caring relationship between the mentor and protege.

Bowen (1985, p. 31) views mentoring in this way.

> Mentoring occurs when a senior person (the mentor) in terms of age and experience undertakes to provide information, advice and emotional support for a junior person (the protege) in a relationship lasting over an extended period of time and marked by substantial emotional commitment of both parties. If the opportunity presents itself the mentor also uses both formal and informal forms of influence to further the career of the protege.

Mentoring functions, as defined by Kram (1983), include sponsorship, exposure and visibility, coaching, protection, and challenging assignments. These functions need to be coupled with role modeling, acceptance and confirmation, counseling, and friendship.

Mentors (Levinson, 1978) act as teachers, sponsors, hosts and guides, exemplars, and counselors as well as visionaries who untap the human potential of proteges. Inherent in the mentoring relationship, mentors (Vance, 1982) provide career advice, professional role modeling, intellectual and scholarly stimulation, inspiration and idealism, teaching, advising and tutoring, and emotional support.

Organizational Culture

Critical to success in training mentors is an organizational culture that supports the mentoring process, as evidenced by sanctioning of formal or informal mentoring relationships. A culture supportive of mentorships must value

- Coaching
- Encouraging and praising mentees
- Promoting others' strengths
- Career counseling

The literature hypothesizes (Kanter, 1984) that organizations that wish to achieve excellence should encourage managers to become mentors. In many organizations, managers are evaluated on their ability to mentor or develop subordinates. Levinson (1979) has stated

- All managers should be mentors
- Performance appraisals should measure effectiveness of mentoring
- Each manager/protege should be knowledgeable about mentoring and modeling behavior and required to teach it
- Mentoring should be part of all management education

Mentor–Mentee Relationships

Organizations (Fagan & Fagan, 1983) can effectively use mentoring relationships to enhance professional development by teaching the value and importance of mentoring to potential mentors and mentees. Providing rewards to nurses who show an interest in mentees and creating an environment that is conducive to allowing social interactions between novice and expert nurses at all levels of the organization facilitates mentor–mentee relationships.

Human resource literature offers some guidelines related to positive mentor relationships. Gastein (1985, p. 157) advises

- Ensure the voluntary participation of mentors
- Minimize the rules and maximize the mentor's personal freedom
- Create networking possibilities for mentors
- Share and negotiate expectations between mentor and protege
- Reward mentors and increase their visibility
- Include the managers of proteges

Intense interpersonal interactions (Kram, 1983) occur throughout the phases of the mentoring relationship—initiation, cultivation, separation, and redefinition—that usually last for 8 to 10 years. Understanding the interactions between the mentor and mentee during the four phases serves as a learning opportunity for the mentor before facilitating a mentoring relationship. Initiation, the first phase, lasts 6 to 12 months and focuses on establishing relationships. The mentor is viewed as competent and as having the ability to guide the mentee, and the mentor views the mentee as someone with potential who will benefit from the relationship.

Cultivation, lasting 2 to 5 years, involves testing of the positive expectations of the initiation phase against the reality of the relationship. The work of the mentoring–mentee relationship related to the development of the mentee is accomplished. Separation accomplishes the work of terminating the intensiveness of the relationship. As the mentee becomes more autonomous, the relationship becomes less important and necessary. Successful separation is followed by a redefinition phase when mentor and mentee are peers and colleagues. If their termination and anxiety of separation have been effectively resolved, redefinition is successful.

In establishing relationships, mentors look for mentees who are intelligent, ambitious, risk takers, able to use power, loyal, have the potential to perform the mentor's role, and are committed to the organization. The ideal mentee would also have the ability to be perceived positively within the organization and be able to network and establish alliances. On the other hand, mentees (Zey, 1984) want mentors who are competent, powerful, good teachers and motivators, are secure in their roles, and are perceived positively within the organization. Both the mentor and mentee may benefit from the functions of the relationship, with the mentee often supporting the mentor with important data and technologic expertise in exchange for development of organizational and management skills.

Although development of skills is necessary to a successful mentoring relationship, Darling (1983) clearly identified certain attributes required for successful mentoring relationships: attraction, action, and affect. Attraction refers to the connection that occurs between two people based on admiration or respect, action refers to guidance within the relationship, and affect refers to the feelings that support individuals' self-esteem in the mentoring process.

Role Development

Formal or informal developmental activities for mentors should focus on a conceptual framework developed for mentoring within the institution. Such conceptual foundations may be derived from definitions of mentoring and specific behaviors or role functions that need to be identified in the operationalization of mentoring.

Understanding the role functions of mentors and mentees and the phases of the mentoring relationship, as well as participating in a mentoring relationship, provides the foundation for developing successful mentoring relationships with another professional. Self-review of critical role functions and competencies can serve as the blueprint for continued self-development of mentoring skills. These concepts can provide the blueprint for development of other expert nurses as mentors within an organizational culture that supports leadership development.

Concrete strategies (Kram, 1985a) for organizational development aimed at developing and improving the mentoring process include

1. Definition of objectives
2. Identification of individual organizational circumstances enhancing or interfering with effective mentoring
3. Implementation of educational programs, reward systems, and task designs
4. Modification of programs based on ongoing evaluation

Mentoring with its high emphasis on development of social processes can be effectively learned through observation and imitation. Bolton (1980) cites the impossibility of identifying all the specialized behaviors that can be developed via planned and unplanned social processes and cites the implication that some aspects of learning can not be reduced to a book or formal setting.

It becomes strikingly apparent that mentoring relationships involve learning and teaching psychomotor, cognitive, and affective behaviors. Techniques effective in preceptor education, such as role playing, observation, active participation, and discussion of situations, are positive adjuncts to the learning process related to mentoring. Mentoring relationships transcend precepting and apprenticeship relationships because of the strong interpersonal bond that develops in effective mentor–mentee relationships. This interpersonal relationship facilitates sharing of affective data critical to the protege's growth in the organizational setting. Mentorships also strengthen the participants' views toward professionalism and facilitates the transmission of these views to future generations of nurses.

Inherent in the training of mentors is the concept of risk. These risks (Prestholdt, 1990) may take a variety of forms, including the risk of being wrong in giving counsel or in selection of a mentee and the risk of rejection by the mentee Mentees also are subject to risk through bad advice that may damage their careers and the dependencies associated with the relationship. Mentors must learn, often by experience, that although caring is at the core of the mentoring relationship, mentees control the relationship, receiving wisdom only when they seek it and are able to assimilate it. Mentees can value insights on how to attract mentors and interact effectively within a mentoring relationship.

Preparation for mentoring should include an analysis of toxic mentoring styles (Darling, 1985), that is, styles that are actually detrimental to the growth of others. Darling describes avoiders as mentors who are generally unapproachable and who ignore situations where guidance would be beneficial. Dumpers create opportunities and experience, but they provide inadequate support for mentee role development. Blockers are mentors who actively impede mentee progress by withholding information, providing too close supervision, or actively refusing to help mentees because of their unavailability. The last category of toxic mentor is the mentor who destroys or criticizes the mentee, endangering the mentee's ability to grow and develop self-confidence.

Ongoing role development of mentors, whether formal or informal, focuses on assuring application of basic management skills related to role functions. Effective deployment of these skills is reflected in behaviors that do not stifle creativity. Ongoing discussion of situations where mentoring has been successful enhances ongoing development of actual and potential mentors as well as facilitating the organizational and individual benefits of the role.

Program Evaluation

Mentors, mentees, and organizations all benefit from formal or informal mentoring programs. Mentees benefit in terms of career development, professional development, and personal development, and mentors benefit from intrinsic satisfaction associated with developing a mentee, a task of the developmental phase of generativity identified by Erickson. Gifts of mentoring (Edlin & Haenshey, 1985) have been identified by mentors as completion of their own work, stimulation of ideas, personal satisfaction, and establishment of long-term relationships. Organizations benefit with increased numbers of qualified personnel who can continue to develop the organization.

The literature is replete with studies reflecting the value of the mentor–mentee relationship on staff developmental outcomes. Roche (1979) surveyed subscribers to the *Harvard Business Review* and found that executives who had a mentor were 2 years younger than those who did not, earned more money, were better educated, had defined a career path, and perceived themselves more successful and satisfied than their peers without mentors. In a study of nurses (Larson, 1986), both mentor and mentees job satisfaction scores were higher than for a group who had not participated in a mentor–mentees relationship. Burke's study (1984) examining mentoring in organizations as experienced by mentees early in their careers reflects mentees' learning related to human interactions, increased confidence, increased skill levels, insight into themselves, new approaches to work and problems, and a greater understanding of their organizations.

Other researchers present opposing evidence related to staff progress as a result of mentoring. Spengler (1982) noted that nurses without mentors in her study viewed themselves as self-starters. Several researchers (May et al., 1982) have postulated that mentors may have negative effects on orientees, such as encouraging too early a career focus, developing clones, and promoting risk avoidance.

COACHING: A KEY SKILL OF PRECEPTORS AND MENTORS

Successful preceptors and mentors have incorporated the skill of coaching into their professional behaviors. Coaching skills are best developed in an organizational climate that values the process by individuals who are willing to risk the time and practice necessary to become proficient coaches. Performance evaluation and coaching are not to be confused: coaching involves support and feedback. Coaching is probably one of the most difficult skills in management. It encapsulates needs assessment, interviewing, decision making, problem solving, analytic thinking, active listening, motivation, and communication.

The Process of Coaching

Coaches (Orth et al., 1990) must monitor performance and identify opportunities for employees to develop new skills and enhance performance. Observational data may be acquired from direct observations, peer and subordinate observations, employee interviews, and review of outcomes. Observation and analytic skills enable the coach to identify opportunities for employee improvement and determine if coaching is an appropriate developmental strategy or if education, counseling, or a change in role may be more appropriate. Interviewing focusing on an array of techniques, including open, closed, and reflective questions, coupled with active listening facilitates the coaching process. Feedback that is specific, descriptive, behaviorally focused, appropriately timed, and clearly understood fosters employee improvement.

Coaching Model

A simple coaching model is based on interactive problem solving. Before the coaching meeting, it is important to plan for and identify an intended outcome of the coaching session. The next step is to clearly identify performance standards and provide the employee with accurate observations about performance and opportunities for improvement. Effective development plans are created jointly, with the employee's input. Employee progress is monitored after the employee has agreed to the plan and identified action steps have been implemented. It is important to provide both positive and negative feedback and rewards or recognition based on performance outcomes. The coaching process should be documented according to organizational policies.

Key Success Factors

Key success factors of a good coach include a sincere desire to help employees improve. This can be accomplished by having a thorough knowledge of job requirements and performance criteria and providing recognition of individual differences through creation of a progressive development plan.

Constructive Feedback

Behaviors that support receiving and valuing feedback in a coaching relationship include

- Eliciting feedback
- Assessing emotional readiness
- Active listening
- Asking for clarification
- Summarizing what was said
- Setting goals for change

Constructive feedback should motivate the receiver to continue or improve effective behavior, minimize the negative effects of ineffective behavior, and provide information and guidance to facilitate problem solving and individual effectiveness. Successful coaching requires patience, energy, and close attention to employee needs and occurs routinely rather than infrequently.

MONITORING STAFF PROGRESS

Formative and summative program evaluation strategies are vital to ensuring attainment of staff and organizational outcomes of preceptor and mentor programs. Several specific examples of effectiveness of staff development can be measured through ongoing assessment of competency development.

- Successful participation in career advancement programs
- Evidence of increased ratings on employee performance evaluations
- Employee job satisfaction surveys

Organizational effectiveness of staff development may in part be measured by

- Increased productivity
- Decreased turnover rates
- Satisfaction of patients and physicians with patient care
- Attainment of organizational outcomes related to quality cost-effective care

Effectiveness of staff development external to the organization is often evidenced through sharing of individual and organizational expertise through professional publications, presentations, and participation in health care forums.

References

Anderson, E.M., & Shannon, A.L. (1988). Toward a conceptualization of mentoring. *Journal of Teacher Education, 39*(1), 38–42.

Benner, P. (1982). From novice to expert. *American Journal of Nursing, 82*(3), 402–407.

Bolton, E.B. (1980). A conceptual analysis of the mentor relationship in the career development of women. *Adult Education, 30*(4), 195–207.

Bowen, C. (1985). Were men meant to mentor women? *Training and Development, 39*(1), 30–34.

Burke, R.J. (1984). Mentors in organizations. *Group and Organizational Studies, 9*(3), 353–372.

Darling, L. (1983). So you've never had a mentor . . . not to worry. *Journal of Nursing Administration, 13*(12), 38–39.

Darling, L. (1985). What to do about toxic mentors. *Journal of Nursing Administration, 15*(5), 43–44.

Edlin, D. & Haenshey, D. (1985). Gifts for mentorship. *Gifted Child Quarterly, 29*(2), 55–59.

Fagan M.M., & Fagan, P.D. (1983). Mentoring among nurses. *Nursing and Health Care, 4*(2), 77–82.

Fuzzard, B. (1989). *Innovative teaching strategies in nursing*. Gaithersburg, MD: Aspen Publishers.

Gastein, M. (1985). Mentoring, an age-old practice in a knowledge-based society. *Journal of Counseling and Development, 64*(2), 157.

Hill, A. (1989). Precepting the clinical nurse specialist student. *Clinical Nurse Specialist, 3*(2), 71–75.

Hunsaker, P., & Cook, C. (1986). *Managing organizational behavior*. Reading, Mass: Addison Wesley.

Kanter, R. (1984). *Change masters*. New York: Simon & Schuster.

Kram, K.E. (1983). Phases of the mentor relationship. *Academy of Management Journal, 26*, 608–625.

Kram, K. (1985a). Improving the mentoring process. *Training and Development Journal, 39*(4), 40.

Kram, K. (1985b). *Mentoring at work: Developmental relationships in organizational life*. Glenview IL: Scott Foresman.

Larson, B.A. (1986). Job satisfaction of nursing leaders with mentor relationships. *Nursing Administration Quarterly, 11*(1), 53–56.

Levinson, H. (1978). *The seasons of a man's life*. New York: Knopf.

Levinson, H. (1979, August). Mentoring socialization of leadership. Paper presented at the 1979 annual meeting of the Academy of Management, Atlanta, GA.

May, K.M., et al. (1982). Mentorship for scholarliness: Opportunities and dilemmas. *Nursing Outlook, 30*(1), 22–25.

Morrow, K. (1984). *Preceptorships in nursing staff development*. Rockville, MD: Aspen Publishers.

Munro, B. (1983). A useful model for program evaluation. *Journal of Nursing Administration, 13*(3), 23–26.

Nederveld, M. (1990). Preceptorship one step beyond. *Journal of Nursing Staff Development, 6*(4), 186–189, 194.

Orth, C.D., et al. (1990). The manager's role as coach and mentor. *Journal of Nursing Administration, 20*(9), 11–15.

Prestholdt, C. (1990) Modern mentoring strategies for developing contemporary nursing leadership. *Nursing Administration Quarterly, 15*(1), 20–27.

Roche, G. (1979). Much ado about mentors. *Harvard Business Review, 57*(1), 14–16.

Spengler, C. (1982). *Mentor–protege relationships: A study of career development among female doctorates*. Unpublished doctoral dissertation, University of Missouri, Columbia, MO.

Think like a dolphin. (1988). *The Futurist, 22*(2), 52.

Vance, C. (1982). The mentor connection. *Journal of Nursing Administration, 12*(4), 7–13.

Zey, M. (1984). *The mentor connection*. Homeward, IL: Irwin.

CHAPTER 17   •   •   •   •   •   •

PRODUCTIVITY AND COST PER UNIT OF SERVICE

JANET BARRON

EXECUTIVE SUMMARY

For many years, productivity in health care has been measured by such methods as hours per patient day (HPPD) or full-time equivalents per adjusted occupied bed (FTE/AOB). Unfortunately, these measurements can show that hours are in line while costs are over budget in terms of dollars. This chapter reviews the HPPD method and offers an alternative for measuring productivity based on cost per unit of service.

The chapter points out how standard productivity measurements affect nursing care. For example, HPPD assumes that certain tasks are done the same way in the same amount of time. This idea leaves little space for innovation or technologic change. In addition, staffing schedules often are developed based on the HPPD approach. Since not all hours are equal—for example, an agency RN on overtime vs a staff RN—staffing needs are not accurately reflected in budget numbers. In short, this narrow focus stifles creative staffing efforts and, more importantly, prevents us from clearly defining the problem.

As an alternative, converting productivity to cost per unit of service ($/UoS) is introduced. The chapter provides information on $/UoS software and discusses how this concept can be coupled with computer simulation to determine an effective and efficient staff mix. Cost-reduction strategies based on the concept are provided.

Using a cost per unit of service measurement decentralizes financial decision making and improves productivity by allowing nurses to respond quickly to their changing environment. The real proof of this system may be in what happens when managers and staff are held to dollars rather than hours. Nurse managers using $/UoS report a sense of choice in financial cutbacks rather than a feeling of helplessness. With choice, can creativity and innovation be far behind?

H ealth care journals are filled with reports such as this: A recent panel of 28 heath care experts predicted continued decline in the financial performance of hospitals through 1995. Their solution was to suggest further improvements in productivity, although they expressed pessimism that current efforts would be successful in reducing cost (Healthcare Financial Management Association [HFMA], 1992).

There is a growing concern that health care professionals have no notion of how to control costs. This appears justified given that the way health care professionals think, even the terms we use, boxes us into cost-insensitive decisions. Changing deeply imbedded behaviors will require breaking the mental models that limit our actions (Senge, 1990). These mental models are the internal images of how the world works, beliefs that limit us to familiar ways of acting and thinking, actions that have led to cost-insensitive decisions, and spiraling health care expenditures.

DEFINING PRODUCTIVITY

A flaw is our basic belief about what constitutes productivity in health care. Although desperately concerned about financial viability, hospitals persist in holding onto productivity measurements, such as hours per patient day (HPPD) or full-time equivalents per adjusted occupied bed (FTE/AOB) that are poor substitutes for true financial indicators. Every organization can show examples of being in line with HPPD and over budget in dollars, a fact that should force us to examine our basic definition of productivity. Productivity can be measured by the equation

$$\text{Productivity} = \text{input/output}$$

In the health care industry, that commonly translates into

$$\text{Total hours worked in a day/number of patients}$$

Dividing hours worked by patient days results in HPPD, which can be used to compare units within and across facilities. By design, the HPPD productivity measure eliminates cost factors from affecting this statistic. Managers think in HPPD and even make value judgments based on a unit's budgeted HPPD. A unit's HPPD often includes only those staff who are giving hands-on care. Terms used to designate staff providing patient care as direct in contrast to indirect staff, such as clerks and managers who work in other capacities, have led to the belief that certain staff do not count in costs. In reality, anyone who gets paid counts.

Budgets have been divided into fixed for positions that do not vary based on census and flex or variable for positions that vary according to the number of patients on the unit. By viewing fixed staff as constants, managers may overlook their sometimes substantial impact, particularly when patient volume or length of stay drops.

Managers concentrate on productive time or worked hours, those hours when staff are being paid to work. Often, little notice is taken of nonproductive time when staff are being paid for sick time, vacation, and holidays. Although paid hours include all productive and nonproductive time, managers often brush aside nonproductive time with the justification that those hours and dollars are out of their control.

WORK MEASUREMENTS

Nursing tasks have been broken down and measured by time and motion studies to determine the average time required to start an IV or give a bed bath. As long as nursing tasks remained relatively stable, such time and motion studies could be used across units. Nurses often resent this static view of nursing as defined by tasks and question the validity of conventional management engineering measurement techniques for capturing the art of nursing.

A weakness in the industrial approach to workload measurement is the assumption that tasks should continue to be done in the same way, taking the same time, even though the task could be performed differently or by another care provider. Perhaps the task does not need to be done at all. Staying current on the minutes required for each nursing task becomes problematic with the rapid evolution of technology and nursing practice.

PATIENT ACUITY

Clearly, nursing workload is significantly affected by patient acuity. Substantial effort is being put into quantifying severity of illness and patient dependence on nursing care (Buckle & Horn, 1989). To meet the requirements of the Joint Commission on Accreditation of Healthcare Organizations (JCAHO), patient classification systems (PCS) have been used to translate patient acuity into the number of nurses required. Some PCSs indicate the total number of people needed, whereas others show the breakdown by skill mix but fail to incorporate the cost differences of an agency nurse or overtime shift. By focusing on the minutes attached to each task, PCSs have perpetuated the belief that the higher the acuity, the more staff a unit deserves. This approach has led to acuity creep and units running over budget on a regular basis. When hospitals are unable to add more personnel to staff, nurses often feel that they are not being treated fairly.

A dilemma for nursing and hospital administrators is this: *Just because patients are sicker does not mean that the hospital is getting more money to care for them.* We are rapidly approaching the point when we will be forced to acknowledge that patients would benefit from a level of care that is beyond the human and financial resources available in today's reimbursement structure.

There was a time when excessive labor expenses could be justified merely by showing patient acuity figures. We are moving into an era when it is no longer acceptable to explain away budget excesses. Managers and administrators are finding their jobs on the line if they fail to keep their units or departments at or below budget.

Although JCAHO sets the broad boundaries within which U.S. hospitals must function, many managers' beliefs about these federal regulations restrict their thinking even more than intended. As a result, most hospitals' PCSs are much more formal and rigid than is required by JCAHO. In fact, the 1992 JCAHO requirements provide greater latitude in managing care and costs than in the past. Table 17–1 highlights the JCAHO regulations on managing the staffing, scheduling, and cost of care in all settings within the hospitals.

TABLE 17-1 1992 JCAHO Standards of Nursing Care

NC.1	Patients receive nursing care based on a documented assessment of their needs.
NC.1.1	Each patient's need for nursing care related to his/her admission is assessed by a registered nurse.
NC.1.1.1	The assessment is conducted either at the time of admission or within a time frame preceding or following admission that is specified in hospital policy.
NC.1.1.2	Aspects of data collection may be delegated by the registered nurse.
NC.1.1.3	Needs are reassessed when warranted by the patient's condition.
NC.2.1.2	Nursing care responsibilities are assigned to a nursing staff member in accordance with
NC.2.1.2.1	the degree of supervision needed by the individual and its availability, and
NC.2.1.2.2	the complexity and dynamics of the condition of each patient to whom the individual is to provide services and the complexity of the assessment required by each patient, including
NC.2.1.2.2.1	the factors that must be considered to make appropriate decisions regarding the provision of nursing care, and
NC.2.1.2.2.2	the type of technology employed in providing nursing care.
NC.2.2	The determination of a nursing staff member's current clinical competence and the assignment of nursing care responsibilities are the responsibility of registered nurses who have the clinical and managerial knowledge and experience necessary to competently make these decisions.
NC.3.3.1.1	In making the decision when or where to admit and/or transfer a patient, consideration is given to the ability of the nursing staff to assess and meet the patient's nursing care needs.
NC.3.4	Policies and procedures describe the mechanism used to assign nursing staff members to meet patient care needs.
NC.3.4.1	There are sufficient qualified nursing staff members to meet the nursing care needs of patients throughout the hospital.
NC.3.4.1.1	The criteria for employment, deployment, and assignment of nursing staff members are approved by the nurse executive.
NC.3.4.2	Nurse staffing plans for each unit define the number and mix of nursing personnel in accordance with current patient care needs.
NC.3.4.2.1	In designing and assessing nurse staffing plans, the hospital gives appropriate consideration to the utilization of registered nurses, licensed practical/vocational nurses, nursing assistants, and other nursing personnel, and to the potential contribution these personnel can make to the delivery of efficient and effective patient care.
NC.3.4.2.2	The staffing schedules are reviewed and adjusted as necessary to meet defined patient needs and unusual occurrences.

Table continued on following page

TABLE 17–1 1992 JCAHO Standards of Nursing Care—*continued*

NC.3.4.2.3	Appropriate and sufficient support services are available to allow nursing staff members to meet the nursing care needs of patients and their significant other(s).
NC.3.4.2.4	Staffing levels are adequate to support participation of nursing staff members, as assigned, in committees/meetings, and in educational and quality assessment and improvement activities.
NC.4	The hospital's plan for providing nursing care is designed to support improvement and innovation in nursing practice and is based on both the needs of the patients to be served and the hospital's mission.
NC.4.1	The plan for nurse staffing and the provision of nursing care is reviewed in detail on an annual basis and receives periodic attention as warranted by changing patient care needs and outcomes.
NC.4.1.1	Registered nurses prescribe, delegate, and coordinate the nursing care provided throughout the hospital.
NC.4.1.2	Consistent standards for the provision of nursing care within the hospital are used to monitor and evaluate the quality of nursing care provided throughout the hospital.
NC.4.2	The appropriateness of the hospital's plan for providing nursing care to meet patient needs is reviewed as part of the established budget review process.
NC.4.2.1	The review includes
NC.4.2.1.1	an analysis of actual staffing patterns, and
NC.4.2.1.2	findings from quality assessment and improvement activities.
NC.4.2.2	The allocation of financial and other resources is assessed to determine whether nursing care is provided appropriately, efficiently, and effectively.
NC.4.2.2.1	The allocation of financial and other resources is designed to support improvement and innovation in nursing practice.
NC.5.2	The nurse executive or a designee(s) participates with leaders from the governing body, management, medical staff, and clinical areas in developing the hospital's mission, strategic plans, budgets, resource allocation, operation plans, and policies.
NC.5.2.1	The nurse executive develops the nursing budget in collaboration with other nursing leaders and other hospital personnel.
NC.5.3.1	Registered nurses evaluate current nursing practice and patient care delivery models to improve the quality and efficiency of patient care.
NC.5.5	The nurse executive or a designee(s) participates in evaluating, selecting, and integrating health care technology and information management systems that support patient care needs and the efficient utilization of nursing resources.

From Joint Commission on Accreditation of Healthcare Organizations, 1992.

HPPD-BASED STAFFING AND SCHEDULING

In most hospitals, a staffing matrix has been developed for each unit to show how many of each category of staff are budgeted for each census level. Although this HPPD approach worked when the staff cost remained fairly stable, hospitals may now experience a tenfold difference in the cost of an hour of care from an inhouse nursing assistant to an agency RN on overtime. Even the same nurse can cost more on Tuesday than Wednesday with the bonus plans that proliferated during the last nurse shortage, yet hospitals take a cost-insensitive stance by counting HPPD as if all hours were equal.

Early computerized systems were designed to automate existing practices, and as a result, they perpetuate all the inefficiencies of HPPD decision making. These staffing systems have kept managers thinking in HPPD by measuring productivity as the difference between actual and budgeted hours. As recently as 1991, hospitals still found the chief benefits of these systems to be speed and time savings in creating schedules and staffing worksheets or tracking license renewals (Warner, Keller, & Martel, 1991). Managers could make the cost-insensitive decisions more quickly, and the result has been escalating costs. As Senge (1990, p. 57) pointed out, "Today's problems come from yesterday's solutions." The traditional automated staffing office systems have boxed managers into HPPD thinking.

UNITS OF SERVICE

Using hours worked as the numerator of input/output is fraught with problems, and the denominator has difficulties as well. Output in health care has been measured as the volume of service provided. For example, inpatient service commonly has been measured in patient days and labor and delivery output in deliveries. Surgical cases/hours/minutes may be used in the operating room. Outside nursing, the units of service may vary from cleanable square feet to pounds of laundry or from procedures to filled prescriptions. The unit of service may be dictated by uniform accounting and reporting requirements in states having such programs. Some departments have attempted to track workload statistics based on relative consumption of resources needed to provide a service. College of American Pathologists (CAP) units in the laboratory and relative value units in a variety of departments are attempts to standardize workload statistics. Efforts to translate nursing resource requirements into relative intensity measures have been underway for years (Grimaldi & Micheletti, 1984), but the dynamic nature of nursing practice makes this a formidable task.

In the absence of alternatives, the patient day as a measure of workload has been used throughout inpatient areas and is generally measured once a day at midnight. In the past when patients came into the hospital the night before surgery and stayed until they were well on their way to recovery, the number of patients in a midnight census may have averaged out to accurately reflect workload. Now, as lengths of stay have shortened and patients are requiring significant nursing intervention during their brief hospitalizations, measuring workload at one point in time has made it difficult to grasp the variability of patient activity over 24 hours.

Another problem arises when outpatient procedures are performed on inpatient units with staffing that reflects only patients in bed at midnight. Outpatient chemotherapy, limited observations, or recoveries from outpatient procedures are common outpatient activities on inpatient units. Attempts have been made to adjust the patient day figures to compensate for equivalent outpatient activity, resulting in such measurements as an adjusted occupied bed. In areas such as labor and delivery, where normal deliveries are on their way to becoming outpatient procedures, it has become quite complex to determine equivalent workload of the mother and baby components of a mother-baby couplet given the mix of outpatient stress tests, the varied intensity of stages within a delivery, or a cesarean section vs vaginal delivery.

Although the adjusted occupied bed or patient days are commonly used for units of service in nursing, problems arise as hospitals shift to patient-centered units where housekeeping, phlebotomy, and other clinical functions are absorbed into the HPPD. It is not possible to add a housekeeping unit of service, such as cleanable square feet, or the laboratory's measurement of CAP units to HPPD without a common denominator. As a result, hospitals are struggling with an equitable way to measure the units of service delivered across diverse clinical and support areas.

TRADITIONAL COST-REDUCTION STRATEGIES

When the U.S. automobile industry complains that it cannot compete effectively with the Japanese because it has to pay more for health care than for steel, health care leaders must take notice. People and businesses in this country are making strong statements that they no longer accept double-digit inflation in health care and that the health care industry already consumes enough (or too much) of the gross national product. Revenue enhancement strategies will not solve hospitals' financial problems when our society is demanding greater emphasis on cost control in health care.

Often when faced with reducing their expenses, managers look to their supply budgets. As described elsewhere in this book, managing material resources is a critical component of a manager's job. However, in most departments, far more significant cost control opportunities can be found in labor dollars than in supply costs.

The traditional approach to labor cost reduction has been to reduce FTEs. Consultants are notorious for spending a few days (or hours) in a unit and then proclaiming that the manager should be able to live with five fewer FTEs. When the consultant walks away, the manager is faced with questions about how to get the work done with fewer staff.

A narrow focus on FTEs or HPPD has hurt morale and inhibited efforts to explore creative staffing patterns. In an HPPD approach to staffing, there is no difference in the 8 hours delivered by an agency RN on overtime (at $60/hour) and the 8 hours delivered by a nursing assistant (at $6/hour). When faced with a limit on the number of personnel, managers and staff consistently pushed for a rich RN mix. This created a vicious downward spiral. With decreased HPPD, there was a demand for more RNs even when they came from costly sources, so costs rose, leading to further pressure to reduce HPPD and eliminate positions.

In the past, reducing the workforce was something organizations did once based on changes in practice patterns or demographics. Management struggled with the most compassionate way to downsize, usually based on the premise that amputating by inches was more painful than making broad cuts once and getting on with life. Now, major cost reductions may be followed by additional cuts the next year. Rallying the troops to generate cost-saving ideas gets more challenging the second or third year in a row (Barron, Flynn-Hollander, & Smith, 1992).

Controlling costs has been complicated by information systems that box managers into cost-insensitive behaviors by their lack of timely information. For example, although most nursing cost reduction strategies include plans to reduce agency nurses, managers often do not receive daily reports of the agency cost. Many have to wait until the monthly revenue and expenses reports are issued by the finance department to see the dollars spent on agencies. In some organizations, agency costs show up as expenses when the bill is paid—weeks or months after the work was performed—making it difficult, if not impossible, for managers to tie costs to workload. The overall cost-insensitive focus on HPPD has led to negative outcomes for health care (Table 17–2).

WHY THE OLD VIEWS OF PRODUCTIVITY PERSIST

With all the problems created by a limited HPPD/FTE view, why does health care still hold so tightly to an antiquated notion? Until recently there were no systems available that could capture cost data in a timely fashion. Payroll reports were often run a week after the payroll period, and monthly revenue and expense reports from finance might be produced several weeks after the reported month. Managers needed a measurement that could (1) be used prospectively to allocate staff and (2) be easily calculated manually or with the first generation of computerized staffing office systems. Hours met both requirements. Hours could be compared easily within and across facilities. Nursing executives and managers could discuss their HPPD with distant colleagues, occasionally explaining who was counted or excluded from the HPPD.

Although nursing executives and managers were responsible for departments

TABLE 17–2 Outcomes of HPPD Thinking

Hospital budgets that are out of control
A lack of credibility that nurses can control dollars
Resistance to skill mix changes
Failure to explore or initiate new ways of delivering care
Patient acuity data that are unreliable because they have been padded in an
    attempt to obtain more staff
Frustration at all levels as costs continue to rise

with multimillion dollar budgets, there was a time when neither finance nor nursing really expected nursing to meet its budget. There was tacit approval that if the justification for being over budget was credible, nursing leaders were excused. Managers were hired for their clinical expertise and their abilities to work with staff and physicians, not their financial skills. In an economically constrained environment, it is unacceptable for nursing executives or managers to abdicate responsibility for the financial health of their units or departments. If nursing as a profession does not take control of its pursestrings, someone else will. So what is the alternative to the HPPD/FTEs limited view?

A NEW VIEW OF PRODUCTIVITY: COST PER UNIT OF SERVICE ($/UoS)

Nursing leaders, such as Spitzer-Lehmann (1986) and Strasen (1988), for years have been advocating the need to rethink productivity and convert to cost per unit of service. This shift requires that organizations have the tools to hold managers accountable on a daily and year-to-date basis for the money spent delivering care.

Letting go of the traditional HPPD or FTE approach to measuring productivity in health care is critical to survival in a resource-contrained world. The first step is becoming aware of the limitations. In order to shift an organization to thinking in $/UoS, it will be necessary to put in place a process to surface, test, refine, and recreate mental models. In Ackoff's words: "Proactive planning consists of designing a desirable future and finding ways of moving toward it as effectively as possible" (1978, p. 26). The following process has been successful in moving organizations into a future where nursing departments come in under budget because managers control their cost per unit of service.

A Process to Convert to $/UoS

PolyOptimum, an international software firm with its headquarters in San Francisco, has converted health care organizations to $/UoS decision making, using a process captured in its $/UoS Loop (Fig. 17–1).

Setting $/UoS Targets

The first step in the process is to determine $/UoS targets that are reasonable and equitable. Setting $/UoS targets can be as simple as dividing the annual budgeted dollars by the projected units of service or as complex as incorporating midyear fiscal adjustments to a shrinking revenue base, variable patient volumes, and a restructured skill mix. Targets should reflect economic reality and may well move downward each year.

Nurse executives have a considerable history in determining the fairness of budgeted HPPD but often have little or no experience in the equitable distribution of $/UoS across units. In the past, costs may have increased without an accompanying change in programs or case mix that would support the increase. Basing allocation of dollars on actual costs spent in prior years may penalize creative or efficient managers and reward those who have resisted change. As more

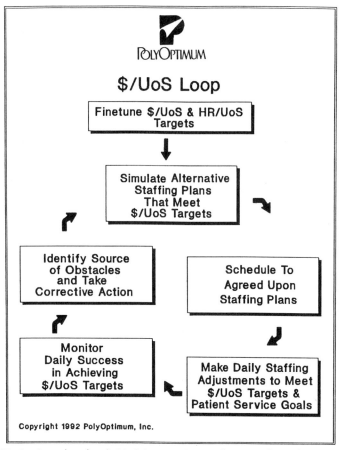

Figure 17–1   Sample of a $/UoS Loop. (Copyright 1992 by PolyOptimum, San Francisco, CA.)

hospitals convert to $/UoS, their experiences are creating a valuable database for comparison of $/UoS targets across facilities.

Making a Vision Come Alive Through Computer Simulation

In both health care and the world at large, people have struggled to imagine what does not exist. As "reality-bound mortals" (Emery, 1991), our attempts to imagine ways of delivering care with fewer or less costly resources may require envisioning the unknown or untried. Although leaders may be able to articulate their vision, not all managers have equal ability to visualize the alternative ways of working needed to make the vision come alive. Often managers need to see the changes in their units before they fully commit. Computer simulation tools provide managers with the ability to improvise reality (Flynn-Hollander, Smith, & Barron, 1992).

Using traditional systems, managers were held to HPPD targets that provided little incentive to explore creative, cost-effective staffing alternatives. $/UoS simulation tools stimulate change as managers explore cost reduction alternatives in a nonthreatening way. Through computer simulation, a range of possibilities can be examined that vary delivery modes, the mix of licensed and nonlicensed staff, shift lengths and starting times, shift rotation, weekend options, workload shifting, and the use of relief staff and bonus pay plans. The traditional walls of disciplines and departments can disappear in computer simulation, allowing managers to see a very different approach to care.

Simulation can be used in merging hospitals or units to spark discussions on the makeup of new units and the issues that need to be faced in merging services. Opening a new hospital or service is another excellent time to simulate what exists only in the mind so that all stakeholders can gain a shared understanding of what the new unit/hospital will be.

The best state of mind when embarking on simulation may be amnesia, forgetting all that is known about patient care delivery and the limitations of staff. To create new ways of delivering care requires imagination and letting go of the mental models and assumptions that we hold regarding how, where, when, and by whom care should be delivered. As Einstein once noted, "I never discovered anything with my rational mind." Leaving rationality behind and imagining a new future for health care may be the best starting point from which to create that future. Then, the future view can be checked against the organization's most valued standards.

Scheduling with an Eye on $/UoS

The way managers and staff think about schedules will change under $/UoS decision making. To illustrate, perhaps the standard staffing plan calls for four RNs, plus LPNs, nursing assistants, and unit secretaries, but the schedule has five RNs on duty. Do you float your own RN out and float in an LPN?—not a very popular approach. Why not simulate an alternative staffing plan that has five RNs but meets the $/UoS target (obviously by having fewer support staff)? Then staff can see ahead of time how they will have to work if five RNs are scheduled. If the standard plan calls for four RNs on the weekend but the manager consistently posts a schedule with three, the weekend supervisor does not have to struggle to find another costly relief RN but shifts to the staffing plan for three RNs.

$/UoS Staffing Practices

One of the outcomes of simulation would be a staffing matrix at each census level that provides a variety of acceptable choices to staff a unit, all within budgeted $/UoS. From these options, managers, charge nurses, or staff use their nursing judgment to select a plan that matches patient needs with the available staff. Alternative staffing plans can accommodate differences in patient acuity while requiring that all plans meet dollar targets.

Clearly, there are minimum levels of licensed staff dictated by state and federal regulations as well as professional standards. Although the legal scope of practice places restrictions on what care providers can do, far greater limitations are placed by the mental models we hold in nursing about our roles and the roles of others. How an organization conceptualizes the role of the professional nurse dictates the price tag and becomes the plan for care delivery (O'Rourke, 1989). When staff at the unit level are assisted in understanding the scope of practice of all providers and can plan ahead for different ways of working, they can move in and out of delivery modes with far less strain.

As Manthey (1992) so clearly states, if you have only one choice, there is no choice. If you can see two possibilities, you have a dilemma. If you can see three or more choices, you have the ability to respond to any change. Almost every staffing office in this country has a staffing matrix with only one plan per unit that assumes one fixed skill mix in spite of the widespread awareness that we need to be more flexible with skill mix. In contrast, a $/UoS system recognizes that there are and should be many choices within the budgeted dollars.

Monitoring Success in Achieving $/UoS Targets

Spitzer-Lehmann (1986) makes a strong argument for decentralizing financial decision making as a way to improve productivity by allowing nurses to respond quickly to changing circumstances. Before administrators will delegate any of their authority for financial decisions, they must be assured that nurses will closely monitor and control costs. A $/UoS-based system provides managers with daily monitoring of where they stand relative to dollar targets. Even before finalizing staffing decisions, managers can see the financial impact of their options. When managers and staff are faced with the daily cost of bonus pay practices, overtime, or expensive relief staff, they make different staffing decisions.

Managers cannot be held to both dollar and hour limits. Either they manage the hours and watch what happens to the dollars, as is the common practice, or they manage the dollars and watch what happens to the hours. Past practice has led to tightly controlled hours and escalating dollars. A $/UoS system tightly controls dollars while allowing flexible hours.

Simpson (1992) articulates the need for immediate access to information on key indicators of hospital performance. For today's hospitals, $/UoS has to be one of those critical indicators. However, it is not enough to get reports that merely multiply hours by the average wage and divide by the number of patient days. Organizations have to change the thinking that created the HPPD-based problems in the first place. Each step in the process of allocating labor resources should include the monitoring of $/UoS. Traditional systems that have been updated to include cost data usually force the manager to make decisions in terms of the desired number of staff for scheduling and daily staffing, and only at the end of the process do they show results in dollars. If managers continue to make decisions in hours all along the way, their outcomes will reflect the desired HPPD and not the dollars necessary to stay within budget.

Identifying Obstacles to Managing $/UoS

Confucius recognized the need to seek truth from the facts. Such wisdom has particular relevance in an age when computers can generate reams of facts from which managers must seek the truth. A good $/UoS-based nursing executive information system will help managers discover the source of problems that can be hiding in the numbers.

Senge (1990) vividly describes the learning organization that is necessary to thrive in turbulent times. For Senge, learning is not synonymous with acquiring more information but with expanding our capacity to produce the desired results. An organization and its people have to live in a continual learning mode, questioning, challenging, exploring new paths. Nursing and financial information systems have to provide more than data on actual vs budgeted parameters. They have to lead managers to the source of the problems and stimulate ideas that challenge old thinking. If, for example, excessive dollars are being spent for relief, managers should be shown the pattern of relief staff use by shift and day of the week. If sick-time dollars exceed budget expectations, managers should be able to distinguish individual behaviors from system problems that are reflected in sick-time use.

$/UoS Cost-Reduction Strategies

Cost reduction looks quite different when an organization thinks in $/UoS, namely, in the role of the leader, the process used (such as the $/UoS Loop), and the outcomes achieved.

The Leader in a $/UoS Organization

Tolstoy, in his novel *War and Peace* (1889), proposed that the real genius of leadership lay not in what leaders did themselves but in their abilities to explain events to their followers in ways that made sense of the world. A level of genius will be required as nursing leaders attempt to make sense of the rapid, often disjointed, changes in expectations of health care providers (Table 17–3).

The challenge facing nursing leaders is worldwide. Biscoe (1989) highlighted the global uncertainty that plagues those responsible for resource planning in health care. Gilmore (1990) points out the difficulty leaders face in managing uncertainty while fostering sufficient stability to get the work done. His analogy of riding a bicycle while building it depicts the awkward balancing act for

TABLE 17–3 The Leader's Role Under $/UoS

Articulate the vision of where the organization is headed
Establish the framework and boundaries within which managers and staff can act
Set resource targets based on what the organization can afford
Provide $/UoS tools
Then get out of the way

---

managers who are building new vehicles for delivering care while they travel rocky roads at hair-raising speeds. No wonder we look so frazzled at the end of a day.

Managers and staff are in the best position to make staffing choices that meet the needs of their patients but can still be held to $/UoS financial constraints. Their choices may include changes in skill mix, starting times, shift lengths, weekend or bonus plans, workload shifting, or a host of other options. When managers and staff are held to dollars rather than hours, their creativity is unleashed and the results are refreshing.

Real innovation happens when managers and staff let go of rigid, compartmentalized views of what can be done by nursing and by other departments. Fortunately, nursing leaders, such as Spinella at Vanderbilt University Hospital, are breaking down the walls that compartmentalize care. By broadening job categories and expanding sharable skills, Vanderbilt is challenging the traditional assumptions about how care is structured (Spinella, 1992).

The need for flexibility has never been greater. One delivery mode will never work for all units or all census levels. Rather than getting stuck on one delivery mode for all situations, staff should learn to match the mode to the census, acuity, and available resources. The unit's culture may lend itself to one delivery

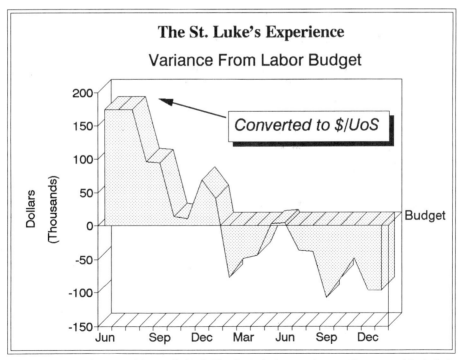

Figure 17–2 Transition to $/UoS: The St. Luke's experience. (Courtesy of St. Luke's Hospital, San Francisco, CA.)

mode over another, but staff should be comfortable adjusting their predominant mode on short notice.

Outcomes of $/UoS Thinking

The financial outcomes of shifting to $/UoS are impressive, as evidenced by a graph of the cost savings derived by St. Luke's Hospital in San Francisco (Fig. 17–2). The savings are both immediate and sustainable over time. In addition, intangible results occur from the shift to $/UoS as managers experience a sense of choice in financial cutbacks rather than feelings of hopelessness that cost reductions are out of their control.

As nursing professionals seek to implement a variety of forms of differentiated practice, they often meet resistance from administrators who fear that costs will further escalate. Cleland (1991) was able to demonstrate with her Differentiated Pay Structure Model that it is possible to reward differentiated practice while maintaining budget neutrality. Nursing leaders can gain acceptance from even the most dollar-driven CEO or CFO by shifting to $/UoS and proving that professionally based decisions can be made within cost constraints (Barron, 1991).

A Test of an Organization's $/UoS Thinking

Enthoven (1988) and Buerhaus (1992) both speak to a health care system that is cost-unconscious. In spite of all the pressure to control costs, the nursing profession remains predominantly cost-unconscious. Those who disagree and are currently receiving data in $/UoS or believe their managers are considering cost in their staffing decisions should try the following test in the next management meeting.

Without warning or preparation, ask each manager to write the following information from memory without referring to any reports: budgeted and actual year-to-date HPPD on each unit for which they are responsible. Next, ask them to write the budgeted and actual year-to-date $/UoS for each of their units. If managers know their HPPD but would have to look up their dollars, they still think in hours. If they think in hours, they will control hours, not dollars.

An Organization That Thinks in $/UoS

In contrast, an organization that thinks in $/UoS acts quite differently. Perhaps the best way to understand the difference is to hear from people who made the transition to $/UoS in their organization.

St. Luke's Hospital is a 250-bed not-for-profit, community hospital in San Francisco, California, delivering primary care in an innercity setting. For 120 years, its mission has been service to one of San Francisco's poorest communities. Their payor mix is 78% Medicare, Medicaid, and charity, with the remaining 22% in contract, insurance, and private pay. This payor mix creates significant challenges for the management team and demands efficient control of expenses.

The shift to $/UoS was orchestrated by Marie Smith, RN, MS, the vice president of patient care services. Smith abandoned the traditional HPPD-based system, which provided no incentive to rethink RN intensive staffing practices. She encouraged her management team to use computer simulation to make changes in their delivery systems and then to decide the appropriate skill mix.

With a reimbursement picture such as St. Luke's faced, there was precious little cushion for financial surprises. Using a $/UoS-based computer system, units were kept informed of their daily costs, resulting in no uncertainty waiting for budgets reports to be run. Mary Coulton, RN, MS, director of medical surgical services, highlighted the accountability and control she gained when managing dollars on a daily basis. She acknowledged the education needed so that nurses would think of the budget as their own, like their own checkbooks, and given such education, staff understood $/UoS and staff mix more readily than they did HPPD. Nursing worked with their financial analysts to determine $/UoS targets. Then managers planned their staffing to meet the targets by using computer simulation. As the hospital restructured operations and expanded the nursing units to focus on all patient services delivered at the bedside, thinking expanded to include the labor cost of services, such as phlebotomy and housekeeping, in what had been nursing budgets.

The idea of fixed positions changed as well. In the psychiatric services, fixed salaries of management, social workers, and therapists previously had not been included in the HPPD. The shift to a focus on the labor cost necessary to provide services to psychiatric patients altered the perceptions of fixed costs. Cecilia Smith, RN, MS, director of psychiatric services, gained more control and had the rationale to request that salaried staff take time off with census fluctuations. Now the whole team flexes to patient needs.

Although units of service vary in departments, such as surgical services, the concepts of managing $/UoS are equally relevant. As director of nine surgical services, Pat Babcock used $/UoS computer simulation to explore her ideas and to determine when it made sense to have someone on-site rather than on-call.

Managing costs in critical care can be challenging within the narrow confines of 1 : 1 or 1 : 2 nurse/patient ratios, yet Linda Houlihan, RN, MS, director of critical care, found that she was able to have more people than she would have had with the old HPPD approach to staffing. She could make skill mix changes and immediately see the impact on dollars spent. Given the short stays in critical care and the daily turnover of patients, she watched fluctuations in daily $/UoS but managed primarily to the year-to-date figures.

Even when new managers were hired, they were able to get the feel for controlling dollars quickly. Martha Vrana, director of maternal child services, found it easier to track and understand $/UoS reports. As director of education and training, Maryann Cutone, RN, MEd, was surprised by how quickly managers grasped the concepts of controlling dollars even in a period of speedy and unrelenting change.

A shift to $/UoS had an impact on staff positions as well as line managers. As nurse recruiter, Candis Haley, RN, MPA, had to shift recruiting efforts as staffing decisions changed under $/UoS. By understanding the dollar impact of orientation, she was able to plan innovative solutions.

Tools That Make a Difference

Although St. Luke's had a sophisticated computerized staffing and scheduling system in place, the system was serving to perpetuate HPPD-based decision making. They replaced their traditional automated staffing office system with PolyOptimum's $/UoS-based system and, as a result, were able to break the cycle of budget excesses that was crippling their organization.

Eva Laraya, staffing coordinator, now talks to the clinical directors in dollars and cents. The staffing office found that even their image was altered by converting to $/UoS. Sandra Alfaro, assistant staffing coordinator, noted that the esteem in the staffing office improved when they were able to produce daily cost reports that the management team wanted and needed to make complex decisions.

The patient care management team does not even think in hours anymore. To illustrate the point, in a management meeting with a new financial analyst when asked about their current HPPD, not one of the managers had an answer. They would have to look up HPPD because they now think in dollars instead.

The following scenario demonstrates how far the nursing management has come under $/UoS-based decision making. When the CEO of another hospital came to visit St. Luke's to find out how they were able to achieve such dramatic decreases in expenses, he asked about FTEs, only to be softly nudged by the St. Luke's nurse executive: "You know that really isn't the focus any more. What matters is the bottom line."

SUMMARY

The time has passed when hospitals can measure their performance solely in HPPD or FTEs. For survival in a cost-constrained environment, the health care industry must shift from a narrow focus on HPPD or FTEs to prospective decision making based on cost per unit of service.

Manthey (1992) notes that only by changing our focus of attention can we make a true paradigm shift. If the nursing profession wants to control costs rather than allow others to do so for us, we have to change the focus to $/UoS. That means more than looking at costs. We have to make our decisions based on the dollars spent for the outcomes produced. The power of the nursing profession will grow stronger as each leader accepts the challenge of managing cost per unit of service.

References

Ackoff, R.L. (1978). *The art of problem solving*. New York: John Wiley & Sons.

Barron, J. (1991). Persuading the CEO/CFO to try differentiated practice. In I.E. Goertzen (Ed.), *Differentiating nursing practice into the twenty-first century* (pp. 271–275). Kansas City, MO: American Academy of Nursing.

Barron, J., Flynn-Hollander, S., & Smith, M. (1992). Cost reductions. Part 2: An organizational culture perspective. *Nursing Economic$, 10*, 402–405.

Biscoe, G. (1989). The future: Planning, reformation, uncertainty. In G. Gray & R. Pratt (Eds.), *Issues in Australian nursing 2* (pp. 83–97). Melbourne, Australia: Churchill Livingstone.

Buckle, J.M., & Horn, S.D. (1989). Severity indices: Potential uses in quality measurement. *Topics in Health Record Management, 10*(2), 45–55.

Buerhaus, P.J. (1992). Nursing, competition, and quality. *Nursing Economic$, 10,* 21–29.

Cleland, V. (1991). A differentiated pay structure model for nursing. In I.E. Goertzen (Ed.), *Differentiating nursing practice into the twenty-first century* (pp. 243–259). Kansas City, MO: American Academy of Nursing.

Emery, G. (1991, January 7). Close encounters of a virtual kind. *Insight,* 30–31.

Enthoven, A.C. (1988). Managed competition: An agenda for action. *Health Affairs, 7*(3), 25–47.

Flynn-Hollander, S., Smith, M., & Barron, J. (1992). Cost reductions. Part 1: An operations improvement process. *Nursing Economic$ 10,* 325–330, 364.

Gilmore, T.N. (1990). Effective leadership during organizational transitions. *Nursing Economic$, 8,* 135–141.

Grimaldi, P.L., & Micheletti, J.A. (1984). RIMs and the cost of nursing care. In L.L. Curtin & C. Zurlage (Eds.), *DRGs: The reorganization of health* (pp. 219–237). Chicago: S-N Publications.

Healthcare Financial Management Association (HFMA). (1992, March 20). *Hospitals,* 82.

Manthey, M. (1992). The art of "breaking set." *Nursing Management, 23*(2), 20–21.

O'Rourke, M.W. (1989). Generic professional behaviors: Implications for the clinical nurse specialist role. *Clinical Nurse Specialist, 3*(3), 128–132.

PolyOptimum, Inc. (1992). *$/UoS Loop.* Copyrighted Figure of PolyOptimum, Inc., 188 The Embarcadero, San Francisco, CA.

Senge, P.M. (1990). *The fifth discipline: The art and practice of the learning organization.* New York: Doubleday.

Simpson, R.L. (1992). Why executive information systems are important, *Nursing Management, 23*(2), 1–19.

Spinella, J. (1992, February). *A horse of a different color: Innovation in inpatient care delivery through operations restructuring.* Paper presented at the meeting of the Organization of Nurse Executives-California, Palm Springs, CA.

Spitzer, R. (1986). *Nursing productivity: The hospital's key to survival and profit.* Chicago: S-N Publications.

Strasen, L. (1988). Implementing salary cost per unit of service productivity standards. *Journal of Nursing Administration, 20*(3), 6–10.

Tolstoy, L. (1889). *War and peace.* New York: Cromwell.

Warner, M., Keller, B.J., & Martel, S.H. (1991). *Journal of the Society for Health Systems, 2*(2), 66–80.

CHAPTER 18 • • • • • •

MANAGING THE DIFFICULT EMPLOYEE

MARGARET MURPHY VOSBURGH

EXECUTIVE SUMMARY

No one ever said that leadership was easy. We only know that it is necessary to fulfill our mission in caring for the sick.

No manual can provide you with step-by-step directions for every situation involving an employee problem. This chapter is intended to give you a sense of your own leadership strength and provide you with a few management tools. You are encouraged to discuss complex personnel issues with the experts in human resources and to never lose sight of their importance as advisors. Ultimately, you must shoulder responsibility for how your unit is run. Human resources can be a great reference for the institution's policies and procedures, state and national regulations, hospital precedent, and just plain work experience. It is always best to consult with them very early and generally proves to be rewarding, especially when you work collaboratively with them in fulfilling the institution's mission. You might want to consider assisting human resources and become involved in reviewing hospitalwide human resource policies. The nurse manager, more than anyone, must live with these policies on a regular basis and should take a leadership role in developing the guidelines that will govern personnel practices.

TODAY'S NURSE MANAGER

Who is it who has contact, on average, with over 100 people a day and manages a million dollar budget in an industry that is both capital intensive and labor intensive? Who is it who must recruit from a shrinking work force into a work environment that is chaotic and influenced by at least 160 regulatory agencies? Who is it who must create a positive work environment when very often the work involves unpleasant sights and smells, human loneliness, and death? Picture an ad that describes the job at hand.

Wanted: Nurse manager with excellent clinical skills; sound foundation in human physiology and nursing science; working knowledge of hospital economics, accounting principles, and inventory control, human resource techniques, and labor laws. Must be available 24 hours a day to allay the fears of seriously ill patients and nursing, medical, and support staff. Should be able to create a sense of direction and vision for the department. Must be innovative, yet conform to regulatory standards.

The amazing fact is that nurse managers easily meet those varied challenges, but when asked to name the most difficult part of their job, the majority of managers cite problems dealing with employees. It seems that the heroes of the health care industry can conquer complex data with relative ease and spend most of their time and energy dealing with human dynamics.

This chapter presents some management techniques that will enhance the manager's repertoire when dealing with problem employees. It does not label aberrant behavior or describe personality traits that contribute to problem behaviors. The intention is to differentiate between the organizational champion and the employee whose behavior has become dysfunctional. This chapter demonstrates how strong nursing leadership and an organizational vision can equip employees to function as champions. It reviews several theories that attempt to explain aggressive behavior and provides some checklists and operational plans that can channel the employee's energy into purposeful outcomes. Finally, it reviews examples and offers suggestions on how nurse managers might approach complex management problems.

PROBLEM EMPLOYEE OR ORGANIZATIONAL CHAMPION?

By definition, a problem employee is an individual whose needs conflict with the goals or values of an organization. Unfortunately, this definition does not differentiate a champion from the problem employee. The business literature is replete with the notion that innovation is our leading competitive advantage. To remain competitive, we must find new ways of doing our work. We must shift paradigms and view the world through fresh eyes.

To encourage innovation, managers must develop a high tolerance for diversity and create environments that do not stifle creativity—environments that allow for mistakes and encourage risk taking. Champions are generally individuals who take creative ideas and make them come alive in a finished product called innovation.

Innovation, then, is the initiation, adoption, and implementation of new ideas into an existing system. It seems that all ideas need a champion to define, nurture, and make them come alive. Champions must enthusiastically promote innovation, build coalitions of support for their position, wear down resistance, and see their innovation through to completion. When champions are successful, they are heroes. When champions are seeking endorsement for their ideas, they may be perceived to be problem employees. Generally, champions are risk takers. They are convinced of the rightness of their idea and are characterized by extremely high self-confidence, persistence, and energy. They are not opposed to breaking the rules and frequently fail to follow the chain of command in favor of more expedient results. They have unfaltering vitality and tend to question the tried-and-true method. On any given day, we may love them or avoid them. However they affect us, we know that they are necessary to help us prepare for an uncertain future. We have no proven solutions for today's complex problems, and there are no historically correct answers to fall back on. For example, change in the Medicare reimbursement methodology, which introduced diagnosis-related groups (DRGs), created a ripple effect that has us grappling with case management, work redesign, and myriad other strategies to enhance our competitive positions. Our only certainty is that we need new solutions for these new challenges. In this setting, champions are individuals who see the world differently and help us formulate new solutions.

The difficulty facing nurse managers is how to separate the champion from the problem employee. There is no proven formula to identify these people, but the following questions should help you analyze the motivation and direction of a nonconformist. You must then decide how the consequences of the nonconformist's actions will affect your other staff and the goals you have established for the unit.

IDENTIFYING A PROBLEM EMPLOYEE VS A PROBLEM SOLVER

Several questions may be asked to identify a problem employee.

1. Does the employee's nonconformity disrupt the unit?
2. Does the behavior jeopardize patient care?
3. Is the morale of the unit suffering because of the employee's behavior?
4. Is the productivity of the unit disrupted?
5. Is the reduction in productivity temporary and will greater gains be realized in the future?
6. Are other departments hindered from meeting their goals?
7. Is the disruptive behavior a violation of the organization's value system?
8. Does the employee have a vision that is in concert with the unit's ultimate goal?
9. Does the employee possess the persuasive abilities to create the innovation?
10. Is the employee's vision consistent with your belief system?

Asking these questions will quantify the risk ratio and help predict the probable outcome. If, after analysis, you believe that the nonconformist has the potential to innovate, your approach will be to nurture, guide, and encourage the employee. Articulating the nonconformist's goals at a staff meeting might serve to build a team that can support the champion and, perhaps, offer them useful suggestions. On the other hand, if your analysis uncovers behaviors that jeopardize patient care or unit morale, you must realize that you are facing a situation that requires a different management response.

THE PROBLEM EMPLOYEE

It is not uncommon to see popular literature categorizing problem behaviors according to personality types or behavioral traits. Titles, such as "bootlickers," "blockers," and "passive aggressive behavior," serve to describe certain responses and allow us to segment those behaviors so we can understand and deal with them. I am reluctant, however, to use those categories because they tend to view behavior from a myopic vantage point. These titles suggest that the traits are clear-cut and based on developmental deficiencies that surface regularly. Instead, I would like to explore the origin of aggressive tendencies through the work of several major theorists, describe specific behaviors without labels, and offer suggestions on how to handle complex employee problems. This approach shifts emphasis from managing the difficult employees to managing difficult employee problems.

ORIGINS OF AGGRESSION

None of us are at a loss to describe employee behaviors that grate on our nerves. We can recite behaviors and attitudes that evoke machiavellian tendencies in us and prompt us to explore the management techniques of Attila the Hun. We know the type of behaviors that evoke aggression in us far better than we understand aggression itself.

Social scientists tend to agree that behavioral problems arise as a response to internal frustration. Behavior is generally goal directed. Therefore, people behave in a manner that serves to satisfy their needs. Frustration distorts goal-directed behavior, and the individual's reactions often appear to be illogical. Troubled employees seem erratic at times because they are reacting to frustration rather than proceeding in an organized fashion toward a specific goal (Maier, 1961). The list of reactive behaviors employees use to deal with frustration is limitless, and many are not disruptive. Disruptive behaviors that concern managers are those categorized as aggression and include physical or verbal assaults, rumor generation, negativism, unproductive work habits, withdrawal, avoidance, and regression.

The origin of aggression is not truly understood. Adler (1968) described aggression as a distinct instinct, one that arose in an attempt to master inferiority. Freud (1920) theorized that aggression arose due to the frustration of libidinal instincts in the id. Other psychoanalytic theorists contend that aggression arises when desires are frustrated (Fenichel, 1945).

Biologic studies examine genetic factors, the endocrine system, and brain structure to understand the phenomenon of aggression. In 1981, Valzelli identified a correlation between aggressive behavior and changes in an individual's serotonin level. Animal studies reveal rage reactions when the hypothalamus is subjected to electrical stimulation (Egger & Flynn, 1963), and other studies suggest that aggressive behavior has its origin in coded neural pathways (Boelkins & Heiser, 1970).

Learning theorists contend that humans are born with the cognitive and morphologic potential to act aggressively. Whether humans choose to act aggressively depends on events and situations in their environment (Lewis Lanza, 1983). Another school of learning theory contends that aggression is learned rather than innate (Hayes, Rincover, & Volosin, 1980).

Field theorists take yet another position. Lewin (1935) describes a conflict situation that disrupts the energy in two forcefields, causing tension and, finally, aggression. Dembo, another field theorist, postulates that frustration does not always lead to anger. She contends that the individual always has the potential to move away from the cause of the frustration. She maintains that in order for frustration to lead to aggression, the individual must become entrapped in the barrier causing the frustration. Therefore, aggressive acts cannot manifest themselves without a special event that changes latent animosity into overt aggression (Dembo, 1931).

Galbraith (1971) takes an organizational approach to explain aggression and suggests that aggression arises when organizational power impinges on the individual's autonomy.

The only thing certain about the origin of aggression is that there are speculation and many opinions to explain aggressive behavior. The commonality among all of the theorists is the belief that all people have the capacity to be aggressive, that aggression can be manifested in several ways, including anger and withdrawal, and that external forces can exacerbate aggression.

ROLE OF NURSE MANAGER IN MANAGING DIFFICULT EMPLOYEE PROBLEMS

How can we deal with aggressive behavior if its origin is uncertain and if it manifests several forms? Is it possible to approach aggressive behavior without having a proven theory of behavior or a set of generalizations that explain why people behave as they do? One possible solution might be to confront complex behavioral problems with a clear, concise leadership direction that describes the behaviors we want to see and the consequences for behaviors that are disruptive. A relevant quote is: "Patients go without care for the lack of someone in charge" (Florence Nightingale).

The nurse manager is unquestionably the primary leadership person responsible for the provision of nursing care. The role of nurse manager is the most influential role in the hospital. It is the nurse manager who ensures that the product of the hospital, patient care, satisfies consumer expectations in a way that is cost effective. To accomplish the work of the hospital, the nurse manager must emerge as a leader and create an effective, patient-focused team.

Bennis and Vanus (1985) contend that failing organizations tend to be overmanaged and underled. "To manage" means "to bring about, to accomplish, to have charge of or responsibility for, to conduct." "Leading" is "influencing, guiding in direction, course, action, opinion." Managers are people who do things right, and leaders are people who do the right thing.

United Technologies published a message in the *Wall Street Journal* in 1985 entitled "Let's Get Rid of Management." It contends that people want to be led, not managed, and makes the statement, "You can *lead* your horse to water, but you can't *manage* him to drink."

Developing a Vision

Leadership involves bringing a unifying vision to purposeful work. It includes setting a course, defining an outcome, and articulating expected behaviors to achieve the vision. The Taoists tell a story of Yen Ho, a tutor in ancient China, who was assigned to teach a man with an aggressive disposition. He sought the advice of a sage, who responded, "I am glad that you asked the question. . . . The first thing you must do is not improve him, but to improve yourself" (Thai merchant, 19th Century).

To improve ourselves, it might be helpful at this point to explore some building blocks for developing a vision. A vision is both a road map for the future and a philosophy. It should be lofty enough to inspire people and realistic enough to be understood and achieved. In developing a vision, you must be painfully clear about what business you are in. You must have a sense of the importance of nursing within that business, as well as an unfaltering pride in the work of nursing.

To formulate your vision, you must reflect on how, in an ideal world, you would like your unit to run. How would patient care be delivered? What behaviors would you require from your staff to achieve these goals? How would you interact with physicians, support services, and your boss? How would you need to look, sound, and behave to achieve your vision? Once you have painted your ideal world, you may sharpen or mute some of the colors within your vision to conform with realities of the present and the challenges of tomorrow. Avoid the tendency to add gray, nonspecific concepts to your slate. Remember what Walt Disney said, "If you can dream it, you can do it" (Bennis & Vanus, 1985). Dare to hope. The next step is to commit your vision to paper in the form of a vision statement and, finally, establish benchmarks to achieve this picture. Your road map should be detailed and contain long-range plans against which results can be measured. Be certain to promote the solidarity and growth of your employees along the way.

Table 18–1 should assist you in painting a vision that is unique to you and your unit.

The final step is to articulate your vision and make it common knowledge. If possible, design a symbol to dramatize and market your plan, which will allow everyone to know that something new is happening. Speak of your vision frequently and with conviction. Remember, leaders lead because their constituents trust them and have confidence in them. Martin Luther King did not say, "I have a pretty good idea." He said loudly and clearly, "I have a dream." With that dream and conviction, he forever changed the fiber of American society.

Establishing Behavioral Expectations for Implementation of the Vision

Let us assume that you have a clearly articulated vision. How do you establish behavioral expectations for your staff that will bring your vision to completion? (See Appendix 18-A for an example of how this can be done.)

Job Description

The job description is generally the first place to start. Job descriptions are, by nature, generic and broad enough to cover people in job categories throughout the institution. To convey your values and provide specific direction, it is generally wise to provide performance expectations specific to your staff and patient population. Performance expectations allow your staff to know exactly what is expected of them. It elaborates the job description. Appendix 18-A contains an example of long-range goals for a surgical nursing service and lists the perfor-

TABLE 18–1 To Formulate a Vision

Consider
- The business you are in
- The work of the nurse
- The contribution of nursing to the organization
- The mission statement of the organization
- The executive management's strategic plan
- The commonly held values within the organization
- The skills, systems, style, and staff within the organization
- The financial health of the organization
- The predominant management style within the organization
- Your strengths
- The internal strengths and weaknesses of your organization
- The external opportunities and threats facing your organization
- The culture of the organization
- What you believe about nursing
- What you need to be great

Define
- The unit's purpose, objectives, and goals
- Mutual expectations of staff
- Priorities to achieve unit's goals
- Allies within the staff and among colleagues, including medical staff, support services, and your boss

Construct
- Innovative work environments
- A system that nurtures champions
- Implement strategies to achieve both short-term and long-term goals
- Measurable outcomes
- Regular monitors that evaluate progress toward the goals and communicate successes to the staff
- Clear behavioral expectations
- Meaningful work
- Learning experiences for everyone

Control
- Exert authority
- Assume responsibility for decisions within your sphere of control
- Influence the acceptance of your ideas
- Take calculated risks
- Assume accountability for your decisions and stick with them

mance expectations for the nurse manager, the RN, the nursing assistant, and the unit receptionist. Note how the performance expectations support the overall goals and bring unity of purpose to the team.

Operational Plan

An operational plan was devised by the nurse manager on the ENT service to focus new graduates on his unit (Table 18-A1 in the Appendix). This plan elaborates the job description and further defines the direction he wanted his staff to take. Note that the operational plan includes target dates and has a column to summarize accomplishments that can be filled in during a joint session between the employee and the head nurse. The operational plan had a relatively short time span and was successful in helping focus the energies of novice practitioners.

Responsibility Charting

Responsibility charting is another technique that often is helpful in clarifying communication and enhancing teamwork. Responsibility charting is a management tool that identifies a participant's involvement in a project or plan and describes in clear language what he or she must accomplish (Vosburgh, 1988). This interactive process is useful for problems or projects that involve a number of players. Appendix 18-A lists the six steps of responsibility charting and applies these principles to a clinical situation.

The key to effective leadership is the articulation of a realistic vision and the establishment and communication of expected behaviors for all members of the team. It is always wise to focus on behavior, rather than values, because only behaviors have been shown to respond to praise and criticism. Values are much more elusive and difficult to influence.

HOW TO DEAL WITH EMPLOYEES WHO FAIL TO MEET PERFORMANCE EXPECTATIONS

We all have known colleagues and employees who failed to meet performance expectations. How does the enlightened leader manage this situation?

Most employees want to do a good job and will comply if the expectations are clear, reasonable, and achievable. The operational plan is a good way to frame a conversation with an employee who is falling short of expectations. Together you can define a goal and outline specific behaviors and time frames in which to achieve the goal. This is a good teaching tool as well as a vehicle for timely follow-up. It can serve as a contract if both parties sign it at the end of the counseling session. Clear direction and stated confidence in the employee's ability to do the job are generally enough to reach the outcome both parties want.

If at the completion of this session the employee still has difficulty performing, the leader must begin the formal counseling process.

Remember

1. *To avoid meetings when you are angry* or when the employee is so upset that she or he is unable to discuss her or his position. Anger is a common reaction, but it is the least effective emotion when problem solving, so if possible, wait to get past it.
2. *To get all the facts.* Has this problem happened before? Is there a pattern? Was the behavior documented in the past? Was corrective action instituted? How was it handled?
3. *To consider background information.* Was the material covered in orientation? Did the employee receive education on the institution's policies and procedures? Did ineffective systems cause the problem? Were there extenuating circumstances, such as two codes on the unit at once?
4. *To be consistent.* How were similar situations handled in the past? What is the human resource policy? What are the consequences of the problem? Who was harmed?
5. *To focus on job performance.* Avoid the tendency to explore and solve emotional problems. Focus on the behavior and the consequences of the action.
6. *To articulate the consequences of the behavior.* Follow up with written documentation and have the employee sign that he or she understands the infraction and the consequences. Be clear in stating the next stage if the behavior continues, including suspension and termination. Progressive discipline usually involves (1) verbal counseling, (2) written follow-up, including a description of the incident, outcome of the behavior, the reason the action is considered irregular (violation of policy and procedure), consequence if the behavior is repeated, and a statement of concern and encouragement that the problem can be solved, (3) suspension, and (4) termination.
7. *To conduct the counseling session in private and maintain the individual's dignity.*

Some phrases that might set the stage for open discussion and mutual respect include
- "Please let me know how I can help you solve this problem."
- "I am here to ensure your success."
- "Please feel free to discuss this with me. I am here to help you."
- "I know that this must be upsetting for you."
- "You are a valuable team member. We want you to feel good about your work."
- "What would you do if the roles were reversed and you were in my chair?"

COMMON SITUATIONS AND POTENTIAL ACTION STEPS

The last part of this chapter deals with common employee problems and suggests action steps to deal with these problems. You will see that aggressive behaviors are manifested in several forms, including avoidance and anger, but behaviors and not values are addressed. In all cases, operational plans that include clear, strong directions should be used along with progressive disciplinary activities.

Problem: Absenteeism and Insubordination

An experienced team member asks for time off at the last moment, and the request cannot be honored because of patient needs and staffing requirements. She calls in sick on the request day.

Action Steps

1. Avoid responding to circumstantial evidence. She may have had a car accident on the way to work.
2. Check her overall attendance history.
3. Examine the institution's absenteeism policy and their policy on insubordination. Explore how these problems have been handled in the past.
4. Talk with the employee and listen to her interpretation of the event. If it is warranted, begin disciplinary action. The employee will be better informed and the institution protected should this go to court if there is evidence of progressive disciplinary action (verbal and written counseling, suspension, discharge).
5. Ensure that all steps in the process are well documented and that your human resource representative is brought into the picture early.
6. If the employee has not intentionally taken an unauthorized day off, ask how you can be assured that this situation will not happen again. Emphasize that you expect her to adhere to the policy for requested time off and that you will work with her to meet her need. If, however, patient care needs prevent you from granting her request, you expect her to support your decision and report to work.
7. Reiterate the importance of her contribution to patient care. Review the request policy with her to ensure that she understands it and the behaviors you expect.
8. Reinforce the consequences of her action if this behavior is repeated.
9. Establish a written document of the behaviors you expect with time frames.
10. Follow up on time.

Leadership Prerogative

1. To reduce the total number of callins, establish a guideline that requires employees to talk directly with their supervisor. No relayed messages should be accepted.
2. Discuss the absenteeism policy at a staff meeting, stressing how sick calls affect patient care and staff morale. Emphasize how poor attendance affects performance appraisals, raises, and promotions.

Problem: Drug Use

After several months and many unreconciled narcotic counts, you discover that the only common denominator in all cases of missing narcotics is your night nurse.

Action Steps

1. Ensure that the facts are correct. Review the staffing sheets, incident reports, and narcotic sheets yourself.
2. Review the employee's past record. Are there unwarranted absentee patterns? Has there been a change in the employee's job performance? Has her appearance become unkempt? Does she seem more withdrawn than she has in the past? Do you sense a change in her affect?
3. Alert security and the pharmacy. If the evidence is sketchy, check her shift narcotic count on a regular basis.
4. Randomly send sample narcotics to the laboratory for purity testing. It is not uncommon for drug users to replace narcotics with normal saline. Some are even clever enough to add a little albumin so the solutions foam like narcotics when shaken.
5. Alert the employee's supervisor. The supervisor should closely monitor the patient's response to pain after the employee medicates them to ensure that the drugs are not being diverted and the patient is not being left in pain.
6. Review the institution's policy on drug diversion and drug testing. Become familiar with your state's position on preemployment and random drug testing. Be familiar with how the Board of Registered Nurses handles these cases and what your responsibilities are.
7. Talk with the employee. Let her or him know the findings of your investigation. Such comments as "You are such an important person, Jane. I want to help you with this problem," allow the employee to know that you value her. If your investigation leaves little doubt that the person is abusing drugs, be very direct. "All the evidence points to the fact that you are diverting drugs."
8. If you can establish reasonable suspicion, you can require a drug test. It is essential that you follow the steps outlined in your policy. Bring human resources and your boss into the process early.
9. Follow the institution's policy and document each step. Most policies on drug abuse in the hospital setting require that the drug abuser be removed from the patient care setting immediately. Very often, the institution will assist the addicted nurse in finding a suitable rehabilitation program.
10. Avoid the temptation to explore the events that led to the employee's dependence on drugs. Focus only on the behaviors. Remember that we are a long way from understanding aggression in humans. The best we can hope to achieve is a humanistic, caring approach focused on performance expectation and our vision for safe patient care. The tragedy of this situation is overwhelming. Since you are dealing with a colleague

in pain, show how affected you are but maintain your responsibility to protect the patients, the institution, and the employee.

11. Document all steps in the disciplinary process and review with human resources. If you must discharge the employee, notify the person you report to and determine if you will need security to support you while you deal with the employee.

12. Make a referral to the Employee Assistance Program (EAP) or a rehabilitation program.

13. Maintain the employee's confidentiality.

Leadership Prerogative

1. Do you have the right to control an employee's drug problem when the employee is not working? The answer lies in the job responsibilities. You can take disciplinary action if the employee's off-duty activities affect his or her ability to perform the tasks at work.

Problem: HIV or AIDS in the Work Force

An employee with direct patient care responsibilities is rumored to be HIV positive.

Action Steps

1. AIDS is one of the conditions protected by the Americans with Disabilities Act (ADA). Many states have passed statutes forbidding HIV testing and have restricted employers from asking about HIV exposure on applications. Rumors about an employee's exposure to HIV must be handled very delicately to avoid incurring an invasion of privacy lawsuit. The courts generally will rule in favor of protecting the rights of high-risk individuals unless there is a genuine threat to public safety. In the case of a health care worker, the health and safety of the public usually outweigh the employee's right to avoid self-incrimination, and the employee is, therefore, bound to submit to HIV testing (Alexander Hamilton Institute, 1991). Always remember that if the results of a positive HIV test become public knowledge and breach of confidentiality is traced back to your institution, there is every likelihood of your sustaining a defamation suit. It is, therefore, essential that the rumor mill be controlled. Be aware that most states ban discrimination based on sexual preference.

2. An employee with a diagnosis of AIDS is treated like any other employee with an illness.

3. AIDS is a protected handicap, so we have a legal obligation to provide reasonable accommodation when the employee is qualified to perform the expected duties. Reasonable accommodation might include

   - Job restructuring
   - Change in duties
   - Part-time work

- Modification in work schedule
- Time off for medical treatment
- Medical leave

4. Review your institution's policies and procedures and confer with human resources and the person to whom you report in order to provide administrative consistency. Most states restrict employers from inquiring about high-risk behaviors and prohibit HIV testing. Hospitals, however, generally fall under another set of considerations in which the courts are concerned with reducing the risk of communicable disease. It is, therefore, in the purview of the hospital to establish a policy that requires HIV testing when there is a threat to public safety.

5. Once you, as the nurse manager, are notified that the employee is being treated for AIDS, you should sit down with the employee and determine if he or she is capable of performing the required job responsibilities. This is the time to explore alternatives that will accommodate the employee's health needs while protecting the rights of the public. Most employees will be relieved to learn that you have their best interest at heart and will work with you to determine a suitable course of action.

6. You can always request that the employee submit a written medical statement outlining any limitations. It is perfectly acceptable to request a second medical opinion if your concerns are not satisfied.

7. The employee who is unable to satisfy the requirements of the job should be treated under the normal procedures for a medical leave. This is the time to offer compassionate support to a colleague. Inform the employee of appropriate support groups, and encourage the employee to contact EAP.

8. Questions from co-workers should be handled carefully with the protection of the infected employee's confidentiality foremost in your mind. It might be useful to ask the employee how you should handle inquiries. This is also a good time to ask the employee how you can be of assistance.

9. Employees with a confidential diagnosis of AIDS should be treated like any employee with a serious illness. Once you have established that the employee's work poses no threat to the safety of patients or co-workers, your obligation is to assist the employee in matching capabilities with the workload. Be flexible and allow for part-time work, job restructuring, time off for medical treatment, and other modifications in the work schedule.

Thus far, we have dealt with complex problems that are concrete in nature. What is the best way to deal with an employee who is very subtle in aggression but is having a negative impact on the morale of the unit?

Employees who are more obtuse in their behavior can, at times, seem too elusive to counsel. So often, we see good managers drowning in a sea of innuendo and near-broken rules. Some employees delight in walking just up to the line of insubordination but never over it, so the manager feels helpless in dealing with them. Consider the following situation.

Problem: Disgruntled Employee

An employee provides basic, safe care but is always complaining, making snide remarks, and disrupting unit morale.

Action Steps

1. Employees have an obligation to the institution that goes beyond the basic tasks of their job. They have a responsibility to maintain the institution's standard on customer relations and team building. It is not acceptable to just perform tasks. Employees must take responsibility for how their actions affect patients, co-workers, and other departments.

2. We have all known employees who do their jobs but make everyone else miserable. You, as nurse manager, have an obligation to provide your staff with a healthy, safe work environment. Do not let one person's approach ruin your entire team. If attitudes and small innuendoes disrupt your department, bring it to the employee's attention. An operational plan stating expected behaviors and responses to requests is an effective tool to provide the direction and support the employee might need.

3. Do not hesitate to address situations that, when viewed alone, might seem petty. In context, they will paint a picture of a disruptive employee who probably needs to reevaluate career plans. Most employees want to be accepted and valued for their contributions. A person who is constantly acting out probably needs time to reflect on his or her suitability for the job, but, above all else, he or she simply cannot ruin the morale of the unit.

4. As the nurse manager, you are charged with the complex problem of nurturing champions, breaking down barriers that frustrate your staff and lead to aggressive behaviors, while at the same time preserving the sanity of your department.

The Alexander Hamilton Institute (1991) suggests the following format to help you assess if your decision to counsel an employee is defensible.

- Have you set standards of performance and behavior that are not only in line with company policies but also appear reasonable to an outside observer?
- Has the employee been judged by measures he or she has helped set, or at least agreed to—in writing?
- Are other factors involved that you should take into account before laying down the law—anything that is beyond the control of the employee?
- Is your course in this case in line with past experience, both your own and that of other company managers, and can you pinpoint those procedures and practices?
- Before you get to the "last chance," have there been other chances for the employee to alter behavior or improve performance, and did you offer a helping hand to ameliorate the situation?

TABLE 18–2 Operational Plan

Objective	Action Steps	Target
Excellent patient care supported by a work environment that is collegial and supportive	1. A communication pattern that is positive and supportive of management and co-workers	Immediate
	2. Problem solving that is timely and follows the chain of command	Immediate
	3. A personal demeanor that mirrors the values of the unit and communicates respect, caring, and concern for patients and employees	Immediate
	4. Interpersonal relationships that avoid antagonism, reduce conflict, and prevent undue patient anxiety	Immediate

If, after reviewing these points, you believe that you have satisfied them, it is time to engage in the progressive disciplinary process. You will probably find that the employee is relieved. No one, after all, wants to face a work environment that does not fulfill their needs. Your job as a leader is to set the tone in your department that nurtures champions and keeps the vision alive. An operational plan will make your intentions known (Table 18–2).

You should illustrate which behaviors you have seen in the employee that fail to meet your objectives and suggest alternatives. You might say, "Mary, rather than making negative comments at the staff meeting, such as 'No one ever listens to us,' I'd like you to provide a clear statement of the problem, such as, 'Housekeeping doesn't pick up the trash every day.' Together, we can solve problems. Snide remarks defeat our purpose and will not be tolerated." Set a date for follow-up to review the employee's progress. If the employee impinges on one of the action steps, discuss it in private immediately. If the employee shows sustained improvement, write a memo illustrating the progress you have seen and express thanks for the effort.

References

Adler, A. (1964). *Superiority and social interest*. Evanston, IL: Northwestern University Press.

Alexander Hamilton Institute. (1991). *The employee problem solver*, D3-7. Maywood, NJ: Modern Business Reports.

Bennis, W., & Vanus, B. (1985). *Leaders: The strategies for taking charge* (p. 21). New York: Harper & Row Publishers.

Boelkins, F. C., & Heiser, J. F. (1970). *Biological bases of aggression, violence and the struggle for existence* (pp. 15–22). Boston: Little, Brown and Co.

Dembo, T. (1931). *Dynamics of anger, field theory as human science* (pp. 324–422).

Egger, M. D., & Flynn, J. P. (1963). Effects of electrical stimulation of the amygdala on hypothalamically elicited attack behavior in cats. *Journal of Neurophysiology, 26,* 705–720.

Fenichel, O. (1945). *Psychoanalytic theory of neurosis.* New York: W. W. Norton.

Freud, S. (1920). *Beyond the pleasure principal.* London: Hogarth Press.

Galbraith, J. K. (1971). *Economics, peace & laughter.* Boston: Houghton Mifflin Co.

Hayes, S., Rincover, A., & Volosin, D. (1980). Variables influencing the acquisition and maintenance of aggressive behavior, modeling theory vs. sensory reinforcement. *Journal of Abnormal Psychology, 89,* 254–262.

Lewin, K. (1935). *Dynamic theory of personality.* New York: McGraw-Hill.

Lewis Lanza, M. (1983). Origins of aggression. *Journal of Psychosocial Nursing Mental Health Services, 21*(6), XX.

Maier, N. R. (1961). *Frustration: The study of behavior without a goal.* Ann Arbor, MI: University of Michigan Press.

Thai merchant (19th century). Story told in Ching Mai.

United Technologies Corporation. (1985). *Wall Street Journal.*

Valzelli, L. (1981). *Physiological basis for aggression.* New York: Raven Press.

Vosburgh, M. M. (1988). Responsibility charting: A tool for team building. *Journal of Pediatric Nursing, 3*(2), 118–122.

Example Behavioral Expectations*

SURGICAL NURSING SERVICE GOALS: April 1993–June 1994

I. **Implement an action-oriented approach to ensure excellence in nursing care.**
  A. Use ANA Standards to implement and evaluate nursing care.
    1. All patients will have a pertinent plan of care 4 hours after admission.
    2. All patients will have accurate documentation of their response to therapy.
    3. All patients will have a discharge plan based on the realistic needs of the patients in their community settings.
  B. Develop strategies to implement and sustain a professional practice model.
    1. Monitor patient care needs correlating patient acuity and NHPPD.
    2. Devise staffing patterns that meet standards of care.
    3. Maintain accurate master rotations.
    4. Evaluate use and mix of personnel.
  C. Conduct weekly patient-centered conferences to provide an interdisciplinary approach to patient care.

II. **Base management decisions on a philosophy of excellence and clarity of purpose.**
  A. Open communication to encourage input from patients and staff.
    1. Review minutes from head nurse meeting at biweekly staff meetings.
    2. Conduct biweekly staff meetings in order to
      a. Communicate the institution's current position.
      b. Discuss patient's compliments and complaints.
      c. Encourage innovative approaches to patient and unit challenges.
      d. Review appropriate educational content based on staff learning needs.
    3. Establish and use clear, concise performance expectations for all job categories.
  B. Define the role of the assistant head nurse.
    1. Assist with transitions from staff to management positions.
      a. Provide direction to actualize management principles.
      b. Construct operational plans and review every 3 months with new assistant head nurses.

III. **Communicate a culture of pride to the community.**

IV. **Continue to reduce financial expenditures in the area of personnel and supplies by 5%.**

PERFORMANCE EXPECTATIONS
Head Nurse
Knowledge of Work
> • Demonstrates commitment to professional growth by
>   • Ensuring that daily patient-centered conferences occur on each module.

*From Vosburgh, M.M. (1988). Responsibility charting: A tool for team building. *Journal of Pediatric Nursing,* 3(2), 118-122.

- Identifying staff learning needs.
- Coordinating educational programs with nursing education to meet the staff's learning needs.
- Coordinating attendance at educational programs.
- Plans, implements, and evaluates a master staffing rotation that is based on the patient's acuity level, the patient's need for continuity of nursing care, and sound staff retention principles.
- Submits an updated patient staffing plan every 3 months.
- Follows the master staffing plan when hiring new employees.

Leadership

- Makes daily rounds to provide direction in the application of the nursing process, quality assurance standards, organizational and departmental goals, and the Nurse Practice Act.
- Writes quarterly operational plans for all staff members identifying learning needs and direction for the achievement of divisional and unit goals. (See Table 18–A1.)
- Collaborates with nursing education to coordinate a unit orientation program based on the specific learning needs of the individual staff member and the unique nursing care requirements of the unit's patient population.
- Meets with inservice personnel and unit orientation preceptor monthly to evaluate the effectiveness of the program.

Judgment

- Assists with patient care at least 2 days per month in order to maintain clinical skills, serve as a clinical role model, assess particular patient requirements, and provide support to staff.
- Serves as a resource to other units in area of specialization.
- Employs principles of group dynamics, problem-solving strategies, and conflict resolution to negotiate inter- and intra-unit discrepancies.

Administrative Activities

- Develops, administers, and reconciles a fiscally sound budget for the unit, including salaries, capital expense items, and nonwage.
- Offers cost-effective approaches to achieve the necessary level of patient care.
- Monitors the use of overtime and institutes plans to reduce it 10% by February.
- Hires staff within budgeted position guidelines.

Initiative

- Designs a specific career development plan for nurses interested in the clinical or managerial track in order to provide a cadre of prepared practitioners to assume leadership roles.
- Makes rounds every 2 months and as necessary with support services to establish effective communication and to provide a safe, clean environment for patients, staff, and visitors.

TABLE 18–A1 Operational Plans*

OBJECTIVES	ACTIONS AND ACCOUNTABILITY	TARGET DATES	ACCOMPLISHMENTS AND DATES
Complies with role of the Registered Professional Nurse	1. Uses the nursing process to assess/diagnose/plan/implement and evaluate care on every client.		
	2. Uses the nursing process to evaluate the newly admitted patient within 8 hours of admission.		
	3. Uses the nursing process to communicate client's condition to other health professionals as stated in unit guidelines.		
	4. Evaluates care given by LPNs, NAs, and unit secretaries.		
	5. Documents nursing process—includes nursing diagnosis and patient's responses.		
	6. Cooperates with other health professionals in attaining the highest quality care. a. Other nurses b. Medical profession c. Family counseling (social service) d. VNA liaison nurse/other outside agencies e. Pharmacy f. Respiratory care g. Dietitians/dietary department h. Other in-hospital departments		
	7. Uses grievance procedure appropriately.		
	8. Uses unit-specific nursing protocols.		
	9. Accepts/calls nursing consultations.		
	10. Participates in continuing education by giving a patient-centered conference once monthly and by attending required number of continuing education hours.		
	11. Demonstrates professional responsibility/accountability of the registered nurse by signing the nurse-peer contract.		
	12. Participates in defining nursing duties and nonnursing duties. *Example:* 1. a. Bed making = nonnursing b. Potential for contamination RT linen = nursing		

*Courtesy William Whitehead, Albany Medical Center, Albany, NY.

TABLE 18–A1 Operational Plans *Continued*

Objectives	Actions and Accountability	Target Dates	Accomplishments and Dates

	2. a. Bath = nonnursing
	   b. Potential for breakdown of skin integrity = nursing
	3. a. Passing fluids (H_2O, juices, etc.) = nonnursing
	   b. Potential for fluid volume deficient = nursing
	13. Participates in regular self-evaluation by using the performance expectations of the Registered Nurse.		

Ensures professional dependability	1. Use 6 unscheduled days off or less per year. 2. Use scheduled time off within unit's policies/parameters.		

- Establishes and evaluates written use standards for facilities and equipment and posts these in the standards orientation manual.
- Meets with the assistant director quarterly to review and revise operation plans that
  - Identify personal learning needs.
  - Outline steps to build a theoretically sound clinical and managerial framework.
  - Provide clear direction to meet organizational goals.
- Establishes annual unit goals and personal goals that conform with and support the division of nursing's philosophy and submits a copy to the assistant director in July.
- Sits on a nursing committee and reports progress at monthly joint head nurse/assistant head nurse/clinical nurse specialist/surgical nurse clinician/enterostomal therapist meeting.

Cooperation

- Assists in recruitment efforts.
  - Keeps the recruitment office apprised of available positions.
  - Coordinates interviews with minimum time lapse.
  - Notifies prospective employees of the decision regarding hire and provides rationale if the employee could profit from improved interview skills.
  - Notifies staffing office of the decision to hire/not hire.
- Reviews performance appraisals.
- Institutes disciplinary actions in accordance with established policies and procedures.

- Reviews position control weekly with administrative assistant.
- Attends bimonthly nurse manager meetings and weekly head nurse meetings in order to develop patient care policies and procedures.
- Adjusts personal schedule in order to
  - Conduct staff meetings with all three shifts.
  - Meet patient care needs.
  - Spend a minimum of 6 hours per month on the off shifts to evaluate patient care and talk with the staff.
- Meets each semester with clinical instructors to plan, implement, and evaluate student nurses' clinical experience.
- Conducts weekly conferences with the clinical nurse specialist, liaison nurse, and modular leader to evaluate the patient teaching program and make recommendation when necessary to assure the optimal level of patient/family preparation and posthospital care.

Planning, Organizing, and Ability to Attain Goals

- Provides calm, rational direction to staff during stressful times.
- Conducts regularly scheduled performance evaluations for the unit staff based on clear, measurable performance expectations.
- Makes daily rounds to evaluate nursing activities and assure continuity of nursing care.
- Submits a written evaluation of patient care and the patient care environment bimonthly to assistant director using the two existing forms.

Communication

- Communicates nursing's professional posture and its unique contribution to the health care team.
- Makes daily rounds to collaborate with medical and support staff and to coordinate patient care activities.
- Communicates and interprets the philosophy of the surgical nursing service to patients, staff, colleagues, and other departments.
- Interviews each patient on the unit twice a week to evaluate their concept of nursing care and interpret hospital policies and procedures.
- Conducts staff meetings twice a month that communicate pertinent information to the staff and provide a forum for them to voice concerns and participate in management decisions.

Staff Nurse
Job Knowledge

- Provides written assessment of patient on admission.
- Documents specific nursing orders, develops short-term and long-term goals, specifying expected outcome and evaluation dates.
- Summarizes assessment data and makes a nursing diagnosis that is charted and communicated to staff in report.

- Reviews, evaluates, and updates patient care plan based on a continuing assessment of the patient.
- Follows care plans/nursing prescription of other nurses. Implements clinical and technical aspects of care in accordance with established policies, procedures, and medical plan of care.
- Develops an effective discharge plan that uses community resources appropriately.
- Participates in daily team conference.
- Acts as a clinical and professional role model for students and orients and contributes to their evaluation.

Cooperation

- Complies with hire rotation agreement.
- Shares knowledge and expertise with staff through team conferences, orientation, and inservice programs.
- Uses factual data for problem solving and resolution of patient/staff-related conflicts.
- Approaches interpersonal relationships in a manner that avoids antagonism, reduces conflict, and prevents undue patient anxiety.

Initiative

- Identifies personal learning needs and seeks opportunities for self-growth.
- Maintains inservice records.
- Provides direction and leadership in nursing care through collaboration, delegation, and follow-up.
- Attends mandated programs and complies with the unit's continuing education policy.
- Maintains a clean, safe environment.
- Maintains equipment and reports malfunctions to maintenance and biomedical engineering.
- Involves the patient and family/significant others in determining the goals of their care.
- Assumes the role of patient advocate by supporting the patient from opposition, abuse, neglect, or physical harm.
- Regularly communicates with patient, family, and significant others regarding the patient's progress.
- Encourages colleagues to meet their individual learning needs by assisting with co-workers' patient assignments.

Accuracy

- Communicates pertinent information regarding patients' status at shift report.
- Shares pertinent information in staff meetings, patient conferences, and nursing and medical rounds.
- Offers theoretically sound rationale for nursing actions.

Dependability

- Consults with and advises appropriate personnel of situations requiring follow-up.
- Provides proper notification for absence.
- Is punctual for shift report.
- Plans scheduled time off to meet organization, divisional, and unit goals.
- Encourages the patients to achieve their maximum health potential through health teaching and the support of independent functioning.
- Challenges inappropriate decisions by other health care professionals.

Productivity

- Establishes priorities that allow adaptation to changing workload without compromising quality nursing care.
- Completes assignments within the prescribed time frame.
- Achieves assignments and arranges time for inservice education, unit meetings, and professional conferences.

Adaptability

- Demonstrates ability to adjust work activities to meet the changing needs of the patient and institution.
- Performs in a manner consistent with the protocol outlined in the ANA Code for Nurses.
- Identifies unit problems and suggests potential solutions.
- Complies with organizational and divisional changes.

Nursing Assistant
Knowledge of Work

- Is familiar with performance expectations and job description.
- Performs tasks accurately.
- Follows care plans and observes established policies and procedures to ensure proper treatment and care of patients.
- In collaboration with a registered nurse, participates in the identification of physical, emotional, spiritual, cultural, and overt learning needs of patients by collecting specific data.
- Assists in the orientation of new personnel to the unit, as directed.
- Uses policy, procedure, and laboratory manuals and other reference materials as necessary to ensure proper action.
- Demonstrates knowledge of emergency procedures, fire drills, evacuation procedures, and internal and external disaster drills and procedures.

Productivity

- Establishes priorities that allow adaptation to changing workload without compromising care.
- Completes responsibilities within a prescribed time frame.

- Communicates the need for additional collegial support in order to fulfill responsibilities.

Quality of Work

- Under the direction of a registered nurse
  - Performs treatments and procedures, such as enemas, surgical skin preparations, and applications of ice packs and heat.
  - Provides specific morning and evening care routines.
  - Takes and records vital signs (TPR, BP), height, weight (and other measurements as appropriate) in an accurate manner.
  - Prepares patients for meals, assists in feeding patients, distributes nourishment/water as appropriate.
  - Provides postmortem care and transport of the body to the morgue.
  - Collects specimens, labels them properly, and provides for appropriate mode of transport to laboratory.
  - Assists with or performs duties as specified by unit policy/standards.
  - Performs all patient record activities and charting transcriptions with great attention to detail and accuracy as specified by unit policy.
  - Responds to call lights promptly.
  - Remains calm, reassuring, and able to provide direction during emergency situations and Stat. requested treatments.

Initiative

- Identifies personal learning needs and seeks opportunities for self-growth.
- Maintains inservice records.
- Attends mandated programs and meetings. Complies with unit's continuing education requirements and maintains inservice records.
- Maintains a neat, safe environment.
- Maintains equipment and reports malfunctions to module leader.
- Assists peers to meet individual learning needs by providing instruction or by covering their assignment when requested by head nurse.
- Seeks guidance and direction, as necessary, for performance of duties.
- Contributes to team effort by recognizing and meeting the needs of the unit.

Dependability

- Complies with hire/rotation agreement.
- Provides proper notification for absence.
- Is punctual for shift report.
- Plans scheduled time off to meet organization, divisional, service, and unit needs.

Interpersonal Relations

- Approaches interpersonal relationships in a manner that avoids antagonism, reduces conflict, and prevents undue anxiety.

- Establishes a cooperative working relationship with peers, nursing personnel, physicians, and supervisory and other department staff.
- Accepts peers and other staff into the work group.
- Observes uniform and dress code standards and wears name pin and I.D. badge.
- Is able to perform job functions in a calm manner during emergency and crisis situations.

Adaptability

- Demonstrates the ability to adjust work activities to meet the changing needs of the patients and the institution, including reassignment.
- Identifies unit problems and suggests potential solutions.
- Participates in organizational and divisional changes.

Judgment

- Reports any changes observed in condition or behavior of the patient to the registered nurse.
- Protects the patient's and staff's right to confidentiality.
- Uses grievance procedure appropriately.
- Seeks guidance and direction, as necessary, for the performance of job responsibilities, particularly when they involve legal/ethical matters.

Unit Receptionist
Knowledge of Work

- Uses policy, procedures, and laboratory manuals and other reference materials to ensure appropriate action.
- Provides accurate and timely information using discretion and protects confidentiality.
- Demonstrates awareness of hospital systems and procedures, locations of departments, treatment areas, and other patient services.
- Assists in orientation of new nursing and medical personnel and other unit receptionists.
- Demonstrates knowledge of emergency procedures, fire drills, evacuation procedures, and internal and external disaster drills and procedures.

Productivity

- Records and communicates messages accurately.
- Receives and accurately distributes items for patients.
- Meets the changing patient census by maintaining an appropriate level of forms and requisitions, materials, and supplies.
- Maintains bulletin boards, reference materials, and policy and procedure manuals, ensuring accuracy and timeliness of information.
- Maintains patient records by filing tests and reports appropriately and sequentially.

- Complies information as requested in a detailed and precise manner.
- Assumes responsibility for communicating pertinent information to appropriate personnel throughout the shift and at change of shift.
- Attends mandatory inservice programs and meetings and maintains personal inservice record of attendance.
- Maintains equipment assigned to the unit and reports broken, malfunctioning equipment, orders service, and follows up on its return as necessary.

Quality of Work

- Receives, greets, and directs patients, visitors, and hospital personnel, providing accurate responses in a positive, courteous manner.
- Receives, places, and transfers telephone calls using appropriate telephone etiquette.
- Remains calm, reassuring, and able to provide direction during emergency situations and Stat. requests.
- Maintains accurate assignment sheet, including patient's name, staff, patient acuity, census, and transfer information.
- Performs appropriate client recording activities and charting transcriptions with great attention to detail and accuracy.
- Transcribes physician prescriptions, completing necessary forms and requisitions, and communicates requests to registered nurses completely and accurately.

Initiative

- Identifies personal learning needs and seeks opportunities for self-growth.
- Assists peers to meet their individual learning needs by providing instruction or by covering their assignments when requested by head nurse.
- Recognizes and anticipates the needs of the unit.
- Intervenes to meet the changing needs of the unit. Contributes to a team effort by performing duties as requested.

Dependability

- Complies with hire rotations.
- Provides proper notification for absence.
- Punctual for shift report.
- Plans scheduled time off to meet unit, departmental, divisional, and organizational goals.
- Is aware of patient location at all times, especially when patient is off the unit.
- Is aware of head nurse location at all times in order to refer messages to appropriate person in head nurse's absence.
- Performs and completes assignments and provides follow-through on assignments while maintaining consistent quality and quantity of work.

Interpersonal Relations

- Accepts peers and other new personnel into work group.
- Establishes good rapport and working relationships to foster the interdepartmental communications necessary for delivery of patient care.
- Observes uniform and dress code standards, wears name pin and I.D. badge.

Adaptability

- Maintains a neat, hazard-free, and responsive work station that is service oriented.
- Is able to set priorities in workload, separating emergency or Stat. prescriptions and requests from regular work flow.
- Participates in unit, departmental, divisional, and organizational change.

Judgment

- Protects the patient's and staff's rights to confidentiality.
- Uses grievance procedure appropriately.
- Seeks guidance and direction as necessary for the performance of job responsibilities, particularly when involving legal or ethical matters.
- Advises appropriate personnel of situations requiring follow-up.

RESPONSIBILITY CHARTING
The Process

The six steps of responsibility charting are as follows:

1. Define the problem or project and assemble participants who will influence the outcome.
2. Break the project down into outcome-oriented goals.
3. Construct a list of necessary activities to achieve the goals.
4. Determine the level of involvement for each participant.
5. Record the participant's name next to specific activities.
6. Establish a time frame for the accomplishment of each activity and define a feedback mechanism.

Step 1 in responsibility charting focuses the attention of the group on a specific topic. Participants should include those people who can influence the project as well as those who might be influenced by the outcome and, therefore, need to be consulted.

Step 2 involves breaking the project down into measurable components following a logical sequence.

Step 3 clarifies the activities necessary to achieve the goals. It provides a checklist of things to do.

Step 4 clarifies language and determines the necessary levels of involvement for each participant. Distinctions should be drawn between those who have approval power and those who can offer recommendations.

Step 5 encourages participants to assume responsibility for activities. It is extremely important for participants to volunteer for specific activities and to have group consensus on which member will become involved in each activity.

Step 6 defines the framework in which each activity should be accomplished. Time frames ought to be realistic and have group support. A feedback session should be provided so the group can evaluate that outcome and discuss what they liked and what they would change with the process.

Application

The following plan simulates how responsibility charting can clarify communication in a clinical setting.

Linda Rudik, RN, pediatric intensive care unit nurse manager, notes tension between Mrs. Elrod and the staff. The medical record indicates that Mrs. Elrod's daughter, Catherine, had been a healthy, active 10-year-old until she developed the sudden onset of a severe headache. She subsequently lapsed into coma and, after neurologic and radiographic examination, was taken to the OR for evacuation of a cerebellar hematoma. Catherine is presently in her eighth postoperative day. She remains comatose on ventilatory support. She has developed an occipital decubitus and an elevated temperature and is receiving 150 ml of Ensure per nasogastric tube every 4 hours.

Mrs. Elrod has expressed anger, stating, "No one is talking to me. No one knows what's going on. The doctors can't get their stories straight." After talking with Mrs. Elrod, the nurse manager learns that Mrs. Elrod is fearful that her boyfriend may have hurt Catherine. Mrs. Elrod perceives that the neurosurgeon is optimistic about Catherine's outcome but finds the pediatric neurologist guarded. The nursing staff finds Mrs. Elrod to be difficult to deal with and critical of Catherine's care. They also suspect Mrs. Elrod's boyfriend may have been responsible for Catherine's condition. Dr. Holmes, Catherine's neurosurgeon, expresses frustration over the confusing information given to the patient's family but has no control over what the pediatric neurologist tells Mrs. Elrod. Dr. Holmes and Ms. Rudik agree to discuss better care coordination.

Ms. Rudik arranges the meeting and includes B. Holmes, MD, neurosurgeon; K. Collar, MD, neurologist; S. Murray, RN, primary nurse; R. Johnson, RD, dietician; and B. Barry, MSW. At the meeting, Ms. Rudik reviews the process of responsibility charting, and the group agrees to focus both on Catherine's immediate care and on support for Mrs. Elrod. They devise the following plan (Table 18–A2) which illustrates how responsibility charting can be used to fix responsibilities even when natural crossovers occur among consultants and disciplines.

TABLE 18–A2 Clinical Situation: Caring for Catherine and Family, with Follow-Up

PROCESS	ACTIVITIES	PLAYERS AND RESPONSIBILITY*
All disciplines will evaluate Catherine's present status and update their plan of care	Evaluate Catherine's present neurologic status	B. Holmes, MD, *A* K. Collar, MD, *C* S. Murray, RN, *C*
	Devise a plan of care considering her present LOC and long-term rehabilitation needs	B. Holmes, MD, *A* K. Collar, MD, *C* S. Murray, RN, *C*
	Choose one MD to communicate with Mrs. Elrod	B. Holmes, MD, *A*
	Evaluate Catherine's nutritional status Revise the caloric intake Initiate an ongoing evaluation	B. Holmes, MD, *A* K. Johnson, RD, *I/C* S. Murray, RN, *C*
	Evaluate Catherine's occipital breakdown Consult with ET	B. Holmes, MD, *A* ET, RN, *C/I* S. Murray, RN, *C/N*
	Evaluate Catherine's pulmonary status Consult with pulmonary physician	B. Holmes, MD, *A* Pulmonary consult MD, *C/I* S. Murray, RN, *C/N*
	Evaluate Catherine's elevated temperature Consult with infectious disease MD	B. Holmes, MD, *C/A* Infectious disease MD, *C/I* S. Murray, RN, *C/N*
	Evaluate Mrs. Elrod's need for emotional support. Social work consult to evaluate the suspected child abuse and Mrs. Elrod's need for emotional support	B. Holmes, MD, *C/A* B. Barry, MSW, *C/I* S. Murray, RN, *C/N*
Reevaluate PRN in 1 week Date _____	Implement plans and evaluate for team discussion	B. Holmes, MD, *I* K. Collar, MD, *I* S. Murray, RN, *I* R. Johnson, RD, *I* B. Barry, MSW, *I*

*Defining responsibilities: A (approves) final authority to accept or reject a decision; C (consults) provides expert advice; I (initiates) defines issues for a specific project, develops alternatives, analyzes options, and makes recommendations; N (notified) kept informed of decisions after they are made but before they are publicly announced.

CHAPTER 19

MANAGING CHEMICAL DEPENDENCY IN THE WORKPLACE

JOANNE MARKY SUPPLES

EXECUTIVE SUMMARY

Although nursing has done a great deal of work to assist and understand the chemically dependent professional, there is more to be done. Nurses need to increase research efforts to learn what the special and specific treatment and recovery needs of nurses are. Nurses are valuable and scarce resources that deserve to be conserved. Most importantly, nurses are valuable human beings whose lives need to be preserved and enhanced. It is hoped that this overview of the issue of chemical dependence will assist the nurse manager in managing collegial chemical dependency by suggesting means aimed at prevention, early recognition, and facilitation of effective treatment.

T his chapter addresses the problem of chemical dependency at work. Other terminology has been used to characterize the often painful dependence on chemicals from which some nurses suffer. The term "chemical dependency" was chosen because it allows a more precise conceptual progression to discussions of chemical dependence as a disease or as a moral, legal, or ethical issue. A distinction we wish to draw is that a person can be chemically dependent without being impaired. In the discussion that follows, chemical dependency refers to the habitual or excessive use of alcohol, the illegal use of legal drugs, and the use of illegal drugs.

THE SCOPE OF THE PROBLEM

Alcohol and drug dependency are significant problems in this country. Trends indicate a rise in the known prevalence of addiction to drugs and alcohol among professionals that is similar to the increase occurring in the general population. Naegle's survey (1988) found that 3% of America's 1.7 million nurses (51,000) regularly use drugs. The American Nurses Association estimates that 8% to 10% (136,000–170,000) of American nurses have serious problems with drugs or alcohol (Elliott & Heins, 1987; Green, 1989). In 1987 alone, the National Council of State Boards of Nursing reported that 2026 registered nurses had actions brought against their license because of problems involving drugs or alcohol. Despite the widespread use of diversion programs by many state boards of nursing, the actions against licenses are not decreasing. Simultaneously, diversion into medical treatment systems has the effect of removing these nurses from publicly known prevalence data by shielding their records from public purview. There is convincing evidence that in addition to the known numbers of nurses with addiction problems, unknown numbers of nurse addicts never come to the attention of either state boards of nursing or diversion programs (Hutchinson, 1986; Supples, 1988).

Based on these prevalence data, it is highly likely that the nurse manager will encounter one or more nurses with a chemical dependency, to drugs or to alcohol or to both, in the course of her career as a nurse. Identifying and intervening with a chemically dependent nurse can be daunting. In addition to acquiring knowledge and skills about etiology, recognition, and intervention, it is necessary to be cognizant of one's personal philosophy and beliefs about chemical dependency, since nurse managers will be designing and implementing policies. Staff nurses who worked with the chemically dependent nurse will need the assistance of the nurse manager in resolving their conflicted feelings (Supples, 1990). This chapter is designed to provide an overview of the current literature and offer for consideration some of the issues and questions that are raised by chemically dependent nurses in the workplace.

SELF-REGULATORY OBLIGATION

Not unlike other professions, nurses are both legally and ethically obligated to pursue self-regulation, principally to protect the public from harm. Nurses also are ethically bound to dignify their calling by offering effective care for nurse colleagues who may have or may develop chemical dependence in the course of their lifetime. Other professional groups, such as pharmacists, dentists, and physicians, in response to similar problems, have begun efforts to assist chemically dependent professionals in their own ranks.

ETIOLOGY OF CHEMICAL DEPENDENCY AMONG NURSES

Increasing numbers of nurses are reported to be chemically addicted and often functionally impaired. There is speculation in the literature that persons who choose the so-called helping professions, such as nursing, have an increased risk for the development of substance abuse problems because of shared differences, i.e., dysfunctional psychosocial history, educational deficits, and work environment (Black, 1981).

Dysfunctional Psychosocial History

The first of these shared differences is the common presence among nurses of a dysfunctional psychosocial history, e.g., sexual abuse, physical abuse, or addictions present in the nurses' families of origin. Research indicates that these factors lead to the development of caretaking behaviors learned in childhood as an aberrant way of coping with feelings of inadequacy and the need for belonging in the family. These caretaking behaviors are carried over into adult life as codependency and thus influence the choice of profession. The issue of co-dependency is a frequent theme in the literature on addictions in the nursing profession (Black, 1981; Crosby & Bissell, 1989; Haack & Hughes, 1989). In Sullivan's study (1987a), 61% of addicted nurses reported alcoholism or drug addiction in their families. In contrast, only 37% of nondrug-addicted nurses reported substance abuse in their families. The nurses in Sullivan's study also reported more problems related to sexuality, e.g., incest, molestation, out-of-wedlock pregnancy, miscarriage, and abortion. A genetic factor is cited increasingly as a predisposition to drug and alcohol addiction (Sullivan, 1990).

Educational Deficits

Deficits in the education of professionals is the second commonly cited shared difference associated with nurses' risk for developing addictive disease (Bissell, Sullivan, 1991). It is posited that a lack of knowledge in individual nurses about the process of becoming an addict—going from casual therapeutic use of drugs (perhaps at one time legitimately prescribed for the nurse) to drug dependency—results in a naivete about drugs. Although nurses may learn a great deal about the pharmacologic action of drugs, they learn little or nothing about the seductive nature of addictive substances. Studies by Hoffman and Heinemann (1987) found that information about the process of becoming an addict and the treatment of addiction is provided in only 57% of nursing schools in the United States.

There is a prevalent belief among nurses and other health care professionals that pharmacologic knowledge confers a certain immunity to addictive disease. This belief results in the development of pharmacologic optimism or pharma-ceutical coping in some professionals, which is the conviction that chemicals are safe and therapeutic and that because of the pharmacology knowledge gained in nursing school, these chemicals can be self-prescribed with impunity (Sullivan, 1991; Supples, 1988).

Work Environment

The work environment, a third commonly shared factor contributing to the development of addiction, has a two-pronged etiologic effect: (1) ready access to drugs and (2) high stress resulting from frustration with the health care system. Ready access to drugs is just emerging as a serious contributing factor that has been underestimated as a force aiding causality. Peer nurse assistance programs report that lax accounting for controlled substances within many institutions is aiding illegal drug access from institutional supplies (Pace, 1990; Supples, 1991). Second, the stress of facing the illnesses, pain, and death of people in the nurse's care can produce feelings of powerlessness, especially for those who tend toward codependency. Stress is experienced in many life situations, however, and researchers point to a web of causality rather than to a single etiologic factor. The literature indicates that in addition to stress, this causal web includes the previously cited factors of drug accessibility, pharmacologic optimism, psychosocial circumstances, and the life history of the individual (Sullivan, Bissell, & Williams, 1988).

REVIEW OF THE LITERATURE
Profiles of Chemically Dependent Nurses

Much of the literature dealing with chemical dependency in the nursing profession is descriptive and includes profiles of chemically dependent nurses (Abbott, 1987; Bissell & Haberman, 1984; Bissell & Jones, 1981; Green, 1984; Haack, 1988; Hutchinson, 1987; Sandroff, 1982; Sullivan, 1987, 1990; Summers, 1991) and collegial and ethical concerns (Kaab, 1984; Supples, 1988, 1990). The classic studies by Hutchinson (1987a, b) on addiction in the nursing profession describe the process of addiction (self-annihilation) and recovery (reintegration). Hutchinson used record reviews, interviews with recovering nurse addicts ($n = 20$), and participant observation in recovering nurses' groups to describe the stages of addiction and recovery in nurses. These studies have some important findings for nurse managers and executives, the first of which is that nurses do get hooked on drugs accidentally. Second, Hutchinson showed conclusively that recovery is a self-integration process that is cyclical, having ups and downs and never ending. These landmark studies define recovery from chemical dependency as more than abstinence from the chemical of choice. The notion of recovery is expanded to encompass the reintegration of the person in a holistic sense rather than the narrower notion of abstinence. We still need to learn if there are other models of recovery, what organizational and occupational climates are conducive to recovery, and what intervention strategies are successful at each stage in recovery (Hutchinson, 1987a, p. 343) if we are to assist chemically dependent colleagues effectively.

Sullivan, Bissell, and Leffler (1990) surveyed 300 nurses recovering from alcohol and other drug dependency to determine the disciplinary and job-related issues that surround this phenomenon. These researchers found that nurses begin drug and alcohol use at a young age, often even before entry into nursing school, with chemical dependency occurring soon after. This means that some nurses are already using chemicals before they are hired for their first nursing position.

Recovery Rates

Except for the study by Sullivan (1987b), which found that 67% of nurses ($n = 139$) had not relapsed since they began recovery, little is known about the recovery rates of nurses. In a small sample of physicians ($n = 73$), Morse, Martin, Swenson, and Niven (1984) found that 83% of the physicians were abstinent at a 2-year telephone follow-up compared to 62% of the general population group. These authors speculate that the threat of loss of license is a strong motivator for continued recovery. No comparable study pertaining to nurses appears in the literature.

Professional Self-Regulation: Helping Employees

Supples (1988) found that significant efforts are made by colleagues and employers to gain conformity from nurses who are unable or unwilling to do their work according to standards of care. This includes nurses who are chemically dependent. Findings indicate that self-regulation in nursing is institutionalized under the rubric of "help." Further, in order to receive help from either peers or supervisors, the nurses had to be viewed as workable and worthy colleagues and employees. Typically, the worthy nurse was defined as one who was a fairly long term employee, had been flexible in meeting the needs of both the institution and the work group, and was seen as a willing and loyal worker. A workable nurse was defined as one who had problem recognition, saw her or his fault in the problem, and was willing to comply with the directives of the superior in regard to improving performance or, in the case of chemical dependence, was compliant in following the treatment regimen designed by the institution. It was commonly found that a workable, worthy nurse received significant offers of help in the workplace and that the chemically dependent nurse often was able to obtain treatment and to maintain a recovery program stimulated by employer intervention alone, without any report to or involvement with the regulatory board. The addiction problem that institutions were willing to handle internally could involve the theft of narcotics from agency stocks or patient supplies. Nurses who were reported to the regulatory board were either nurses who did not fit the pattern of worthy and workable or nurses who failed to comply with the treatment regimen designed by the institution. A subsequent review of records of nurses who were reported to the state board of nursing in Colorado indicated that a majority of the chemically dependent nurses who came before the state board of nurses had previously received significant offers of help in their workplace.

EXAMINING THE DIFFERING VIEWS OF CHEMICAL DEPENDENCY

Since philosophical beliefs about chemical dependency will influence the policy of the institution and the response of the nurse managers and co-workers, exploring the various views of this condition is in order. Because chemical dependency has both physiologic and behavioral manifestations and a stigmatized history often associated with nonproductive members of society or criminals, sorting through one's beliefs about chemical dependency and consciously choosing a comfortable stance may not be easy. The history of alcoholism over the past 200 years is a case in point. In the United States, alcoholism has been viewed as a problem of will and morals, an illness, a crime, and a chronic disease. This section of the chapter reviews chemical dependency from several commonly held perspectives: that of an addictive disease, a moral issue, and a crime.

Addictive Disease

Chemical dependency is increasingly, though not unilaterally, being viewed as a disease process that emanates from a causal web. As was evident in the literature review, predisposition and genetic factors are major etiologic considerations. Many writers agree that maladaptation to environmental and physiologic stressors is a precipitating factor. In order to handle the stress and to calm down or cheer up, people use chemicals. In other words, chemicals are used to alter moods. In mild forms of chemical dependency, the chemical of choice could be food or caffeine. One binges on chocolate, for instance, in response to worry or a bad day. This sort of addiction does not cause the cognitive functional impairment that addictive substances, such as drugs and alcohol, can cause. However, no single theory has been promulgated to adequately explain this complex phenomenon. Some proponents of the medical disease model of chemical dependency assert that this condition arises in persons whose genetic makeup and body chemistry make them susceptible. The most persuasive evidence of a gene-linked predisposition to alcoholism comes from the adoption and twin studies in which adopted sons of alcoholic birth parents were found to have three times the likelihood of becoming alcoholics as adopted sons of nonalcoholic birth parents (Goodwin, 1976).

Regardless of the view of etiology that is adopted for the disease model, viewing addiction as a chronic disease removes it from the domain of the justice system and puts the nurse manager in the role of a therapeutic agent, although not therapist. Under this philosophy, the manager's task is defined as early recognition of the disease and facilitation of diagnosis and treatment for an ill colleague.

Americans with Disabilities Act

Emanating from the disease perspective of chemical dependency, the notion that persons with addictive disease are handicapped is relatively new. The Americans with Disabilities Act applies to any employer of 25 or more employees and became effective on July 26, 1992. This law prohibits discrimination in hiring and firing policies and other employment-related activities if a person has a qualifying disability. Illegal use of legal drugs and use of illegal drugs are specifically not covered under this law. However, some authorities interpret this law to cover persons recovering from addictive disease in much the same way it covers a condition like Crohn's disease or arthritis. This has important applications to personnel policy.

Some interpretations of this law say that the same consideration must be given to the nurse addict as the nurse diabetic. In other words, providing sick leave and treatment opportunity and making reasonable job readjustments are legally mandated. An example of a job readjustment might be to reassign the recovering nurse addict to a unit in which administration of narcotics is not a requirement of the position. Exempting a recovering nurse from shift rotation is another possible concession that might be expected. How this law will address the issue of relapse or multiple relapses is not clear and is yet to be tested in case law. Competent legal advice is always prudent when issues of discrimination might arise. Although it is clear that a handicapped person is held to the same standard of performance as a well person, it is easier to speculate what this means when the disability is physical rather than a cognitive impairment of judgment by drugs or alcohol. At the time of this writing, the accumulation of case law is insufficient for comment. For easy reference, a brief overview of the Americans with Disabilities Act is presented in Appendix 19-A. Careful reading and understanding of this act is vital to policy development, especially in regard to hiring and firing the recovering addict.

The Moral Perspective

Some people view chemical dependency as a problem emanating from a failure of will and equate such weak will with sin or immorality. The entire responsibility for the chemical dependency is thus placed on the person. In a diverse society such as ours, drinking is allowed, although too much drinking is frowned on. In some subcultures, recreational drug use (e.g., marijuana and cocaine) is not considered deviant. The dominant view in the United States remains one of disdain for drug users, and this sentiment is likely to grow because of the linkage of illicit intravenous drug use with transmission of the AIDS virus. In addition, illicit drug use has been linked to increases in thefts carried out to support the chemical dependency. The overall problem in this country is seen as one that is attacking the moral fabric of youth, as we are reminded almost daily by media stories about teen addict mothers and crack babies. Whenever victims of chemical addiction are not just the users, but innocent newborns, it will be increasingly difficult for people to develop and hold to a disease model of chemical dependency.

Legal View

The legal view develops in part from the moral view, since societies traditionally have expressed their moral stance in law. The law against drugs will persist as a deterrent to crime committed to support the habit of chemical dependency. There is a societal sense of powerlessness over the problem of chemical addiction, which is increasing in epidemic proportions. Even Alcoholics Anonymous uses strong references to the idea that some persons are powerless in the face of drugs/alcohol and that drugs and alcohol are "cunning and baffling," requiring a higher power to overcome. This implicates the will of the user as part of the etiology along with the seductive power of the substance in question.

Legal/Ethical Perspective

Statutes against the use of certain drugs are likely to remain in force. Some institutions have a policy of reporting to law enforcement authorities (either federal or local) drug theft, drug diversion, and discrepancies in record keeping of controlled narcotics. The nurse manager must be cognizant of the standards in the community when addressing issues of theft or diversion of controlled drugs. The institution's policy may clearly stipulate that any kind of theft is cause for summary dismissal. An institution is not prevented from having this as a policy, nor is it prevented from having a policy imposing dismissal on users of illegal drugs. This, of course, would not preclude other concomitant action on the part of the institution, such as therapetuic intervention and referral of the chemically dependent nurse.

Nurse practice acts in every state and territory proscribe against habitual and intemperate use of drugs and alcohol. The various practice acts are far from uniform in detailing conditions for reporting, however. Researchers assert that in spite of mandates to report chemically dependent nurses, this does not necessarily occur with any regularity.

Firing a chemically dependent nurse, especially one who is a long-term employee, is not a risk-free enterprise. Courts have been inclined to view chemical dependency and alcoholism as a treatable disease or, in the case of a nurse in recovery, a handicap to which workplace adjustments can be made. A clear understanding of the Americans with Disabilities Act must form one basis of the institutional policy (see Appendix 19-B for a sample institutional policy). The workplace adjustments mandated by this law may vary significantly according to location and size of the institution. For example, a recovering nurse addict could be assigned to a unit in a hospital where narcotic administration would not be a required task. At smaller institutions, especially in rural areas where multiple skills are required from one nurse, such an adjustment might not be feasible.

Nothing can replace a fair and consistently applied personnel policy regarding chemical dependency in the workplace (Table 19–1). This means that two employees with the same background involved in the same breach of standards must receive the same penalty or help. If, for instance, your institution has allowed a nurse simply to be taken home when found to be under the influence of alcohol, another employee cannot be dismissed for the same offense, even if the second employee is problematic in other employment areas. If practice is substandard, the practice issues must be addressed regardless of etiology. If chemical dependency is a major etiologic factor in the substandard practice issues, both problems can be addressed simultaneously. Most authorities assert that practice standards are the last to be affected by chemical dependency, since the nurse protects the job as the way to obtain the chemical either by diversion or purchase. In the latter case, the salary is vital to support the dependence.

INVESTIGATING POSSIBLE CHEMICAL DEPENDENCY: THE NURSING PROCESS

Addictive disease frequently can go unrecognized for long periods of time. Therefore, by the time signs of addiction are apparent in the workplace, the nurse may already be seriously ill. This delay in diagnosis is a function of both the elaborate system of concealment by the nurse addict, which is a feature of addictive disease, and a reluctance on the part of nurse colleagues to consider the stigmatizing diagnosis of addiction or alcoholism in another nurse. In addition, Crosby and Bissell (1989) found that nurses' work groups function in many ways like families and that by "hiding the family secret" (p. 36) an enabling process is set in motion that delays effective intervention and treatment for the ill nurse. The persistence of stigmatized thinking among nurse addicts and colleagues alike reinforces denial and coverup by all parties.

Early recognition of the symptoms of chemical dependency in a nurse colleague often will depend largely on the staff nurse who is in close enough contact with the nurse addict to notice behavioral changes or fluctuations. Whether staff

TABLE 19–1 Some Essential Elements of an Institutional Policy for Chemical Dependency

---

- Clear investigatory procedure
- Procedure for drug/alcohol screening; can be required for everyone, randomly carried out or done in response to probable cause. Employee consent is usually asked for. The laboratory that is used for the test should be able to specify the drug accurately. Many over-the-counter drugs can give false positive results. Some drugs, such as Fentanyl, are so rapidly excreted by the body that a false negative result can occur
- Process of employee notification
- Issues of transport of a potentially impaired employee to place of residence
- Type of institutional response: suspension, dismissal, sick leave, leave without pay, and so on
- To whom will the problem be reported? Police, district attorney, state Regulatory Board, internal administrators?
- How and by whom will records be kept? It is ideal to designate a nurse specially trained for this task
- Are you willing to rehabilitate the nurse?
- If so, you will want a back-to-work agreement that will stipulate conditions of reemployment
- How will relapse episodes be treated?
- Under what conditions can an employee be dismissed?
- What help will the work group need to process their feelings about their co-worker?

---

nurses are capable of recognizing early cues and subsequently passing them on to the nurse manager will depend on several factors:

- His or her knowledge and experience with addiction
- The effective promulgation of a humane agency policy and procedure for addressing addictive disease
- A history of even-handed treatment of nurse addicts or alcoholics within the employment setting in the past

These factors are present in direct proportion to the opportunity afforded staff nurses to learn about addictive disease and the presence of and knowledge about a humane institutional policy. Opportunities to learn about addictive disease will not automatically come for staff nurses, and as noted earlier in the chapter, nursing schools do not provide extensive content about addiction, particularly as it pertains to nurse colleagues. Therefore, this responsibility falls to employers. Orientation for new employees presents an ideal opportunity to begin the education process and for the institution to create an atmosphere of openness and acceptance toward helping employees with chemical dependency.

ROLE OF NURSE MANAGERS

Once the nurse manager has been alerted to a potential problem, the steps in the nursing process are operationalized.

- The nurse manager must begin to gather subjective and objective data about the person as well as about the circumstances that have aroused suspicion.
- Accurate and detailed notes will be needed with both times and dates recorded.
- The confidential assistance of the pharmacist will be needed should drug theft or drug diversion be a concern.
- The ethical obligation of confidentiality that is owed to the employee at every point in the process must be kept in mind. Should the suspicion of the nurse's addiction become widely known in the institution, treatment and subsequent recovery can be complicated further.
- Disclosure of the chemical dependency, which is a common step in recovery, should be made at the discretion of the nurse addict.

Data Collection

Some of the behavioral indicators of chemical dependency include

- Repeated absences, with the patterns of absence following holidays and weekends
- Elaborate excuses for absences or tardiness
- Disappearances during the shift, long periods spent in rest room
- Behavior change, erratic behavior, mood swings, and unpredictability
- Exercising poor judgment
- Decline in work quality or quantity
- Changes in handwriting as the shift progresses
- Complaints from clients, staff, or visitors, especially complaints about poor pain relief on certain shifts
- Discrepant narcotic counts
- Evidence of drug or alcohol intoxication: slurred speech, dilated pupils, alcohol on breath
- Laboratory data

Objective data can include laboratory confirmation and should be carried out according to the guidelines of the institution. It is common for employment policies to stipulate that an employee may be asked to submit to a drug or alcohol screen when there is probable cause. At this time, there appears to be increasing movement toward drug testing on demand policies and even random drug testing in some settings. Some of this reaction comes as a result of reports in the media of chemically impaired truck drivers, airplane pilots, and railroad engineers, some of whom have allegedly caused deaths as a result of their impaired state. Other objective data will include such documents as narcotic signout sheets, patient records that correspond to the narcotic records, and patient records that show evidence of deteriorating handwriting or illogical recording.

Preparing for the Confrontation

While collecting data and moving toward a diagnosis, the nurse manager also should begin to gauge the workability of the nurse. By workability is meant the ability of the nurse to recognize his or her own part in the problem and to be willing to remediate the situation, that is, to participate in treatment. The nurse manager also will want to have a clear idea of the available options in terms of plan of treatment and institutional sanctions in the event that the process proceeds faster than anticipated. Should the nurse addict act on a suspicion that there is an investigation being conducted, the nurse manager will need to be prepared for an encounter precipitated by the nurse addict. It is unadvisable to proceed with sensitive encounters, however, without at least one other administrator as well as a mental health or employee assistance person in attendance.

Although it is not unheard of for a nurse with a chemical dependency to admit to the problem during the investigatory process because she suspects it is no longer a secret, often an intervention on behalf of the nurse that requires confrontational elements is necessary. The classic confrontation with a chemically dependent person requires the attendance of the nurse manager, an administrator, staff colleagues, and family members or friends. These persons attend in order to assist with the breakdown of the elaborate denial system that dependent persons have constructed for themselves.

Consultation with an Expert

In addition to careful data gathering and documentation, the nurse manager will find it helpful to consult with an expert who has experience with this problem and who perhaps can lead the confrontation session. Confidential sharing is the hallmark of such a consultation and must be assured. If there is an internal employee assistance program, consultative help might be sought there. State nurse associations can be of assistance, as can peer employee assistance programs that are operated by nurses. Community mental health centers and other psychiatric providers are valuable resources. A good resource for persons who will be participating in such a confrontation is The Johnson Institute book, *To Care Enough,* by Crosby and Bissell (1989).

It is essential that all participants rehearse the confrontation. This idea of preparing and role rehearsal is useful in any confrontational situation, but it is especially needed in a session where chemical dependency is an issue, since denial and confabulation on the part of the chemically dependent nurse are such prominent features of this condition. The session itself includes the presentation of the gathered evidence with the expectation that those in attendance will affirm the facts that they can truthfully verify. It cannot be overly stressed that the defense mechanisms of the nurse addict are very highly developed.

In some cases, it will be necessary to administer medical assistance to the nurse who has overdosed on drugs or alcohol or both during the shift. Usually, the emergency room is the place where this is done. In less clear-cut cases of possible impairment due to chemical use, it is still prudent to take special care not to institute or carry out the commonly written policy of sending the drunk or drugged employee home. The nurse manager must assume that the nurse who is unfit to work is unfit to drive and should be transported home, preferably accompanied by two other supervisory level employees. This event may well be replayed later, possibly in court.

Reporting to State Regulatory Agency

All states have nurse practice acts that address habituation to or intemperate use of chemicals and addictive or illegal substances. The nurse manager should be cognizant of the requirements in the particular state as regards reporting. A confidential inquiry can be made to a nurse practice consultant at the state board of nursing for clarification of the requirements. He or she can readily supply the stipulations of the law in the state.

Some states have diversion programs for chemically dependent nurses if the nurse is willing to self-report and is participating in treatment. These diversion programs remove the offending nurse from the criminal justice system, although the nurse in most cases will have to comply with probationary stipulations against her license. Probation typically lasts 2 years and requires random drug screens and quarterly reports from the employer and the therapist. It usually is necessary that the nurse be in an employment situation for which the RN license is required.

Many state nurses associations have implemented peer assistance programs that are designed explicitly to assist chemically dependent nurses and that give advice to employers as well. Sometimes, these groups can provide direct assistance with the intervention process. Nurse managers practicing in nonurban centers may find that calling the state nurses association will provide them with the particular confidential help and direction they need. There are also peer assistance programs throughout the United States that are external to the state nurses associations and not affiliated with the regulatory board. The advantage of talking with either the state nurses association or the peer assistance program is being able to discuss the particular aspects of the situation and getting help with processing the solution from experienced people.

Peer assistance programs are also a good place to obtain a referral for an attorney should that be desired. Lawyers, like nurses and physicians, have areas of experience and competence, and nurses seeking defense for chemical dependency–employment–licensure issues are advised to seek out a lawyer with the appropriate experience. The family lawyer will not suffice in this situation. The nurse practice act falls in the domain of regulatory law.

It is true that regardless of legal mandate, some employers go to great lengths to assist employees in recovering from chemical dependency without reporting them to the regulatory agency. Views on the advisability of this are divided. Some assert that the delay in imposition of sanctions can also delay effective treatment for some nurses. Others say that effective therapeutic interventions can be carried out in the workplace. Persons who hold to the last view also point out that if practice has not been affected by chemical misuse, there is no need to report. It will be the task of each nurse manager to decide this issue.

In contrast to this view, staff at the state regulatory agency, while defining their principal role as protection of the public, feel this protective role does not preclude the assumption of a therapeutic stance vis-a-vis the impaired nurse (Supples, 1990). They view the threatened or actual licensure revocation as the precipitating factor in getting the nurse to recognize and confront the fact of his or her chemical dependency and addiction. Some states, in response to charges of "undue harshness" in addressing chemically dependent nurses, as well as in consideration of a shifting belief that chemical dependency is a disease requiring medical attention, have structured their intervention so as to divert nurses out of the justice system into a therapeutic milieu. One result of this diversion is the postponement of certain licensure sanctions.

Some regulatory staff people have raised questions about what diversion might mean for nurses who are very resistent to treatment. These regulatory professionals theorize that diversion and the resultant postponement of sanctions against the license may delay effective intervention and treatment for some nurses with addictive disease by avoiding, if only for a time, the creation of a sufficiently motivating crisis situation for the nurse addict. Although it is conceded that not all nurses need threats to their license to engage in successful treatment, there is a feeling that there are some nurses who can respond to intervention and treatment only when their livelihood is threatened. Some regulatory staff have observed that nurses who have had threats against their license have a course of recovery that is more free from relapse than that of nurses who have had lesser actions or no actions against their license.

Monitoring the Recovering Nurse

Just as the nurse manager is likely to be in the position of discovering and intervening with a chemically dependent nurse, she or he also is increasingly likely to be in the position of monitoring a nurse who is in recovery. In support of this enterprise are reports of successful recovery of the nurse and literature on the cost effectiveness of such an effort to the employer (LaGodna & Hendrix, 1989). If the nurse has been reported to the board of nursing, generally there are formal reports that must be produced for the regulatory agency or the state's diversion program. These quarterly reports typically ask the nurse manager to testify to the performance, regularity of attendance, and lack of evidence of chemical use of the nurse who is on probation. Concomitantly, reports are required from treatment providers, drug screening laboratories, and AA sponsors, among others. The usual period of probation is 2 years. The actual stipulations of the probation are usually provided to the nurse manager as a matter of law by the nurse who is on probation. These stipulations spell out the conditions for probation for that particular nurse. The nurse manager can greatly help the recovering nurse by completing the reports willingly, without the recovering nurse having to repeatedly request them. The regulatory board places the onus for the timely receipt of progress reports on the recovering nurse. If the reports are late or not done at all, the sanctions are imposed not on the employer but on the nurse who is on probation.

It does no service to the recovering nurse if, suspecting that a relapse is

TABLE 19–2 Elements of a Back-to-Work Agreement

Purpose: to stipulate contractual agreement by all parties, i.e., the employer, the nurse, and the treatment provider. This agreement should be drawn up and signed by both parties before the nurse returns to work. The usual duration of the agreement is 2 years. The nurse agrees to comply with the following

1. Elements of the rehabilitation program include
   - Attendance at regular AA/NA meetings, 1–2 times a week
   - Attendance at nurse recovery group if available
   - Attendance at prescribed therapy sessions
2. Documentation of these stipulations should be provided to the employer on a weekly basis. The nurse should provide permission for employer to contact treatment provider, drug screening provider, and AA sponsor as needed.
   Other standard clauses are
3. A section that expresses the promise of the nurse to abstain from mind-altering substances, including alcohol, stimulants, soporifics, narcotics, and over-the-counter medications except on the specific advice of a physician
4. Provision for random urine and blood samples in the presence of a qualified witness
5. A statement indicating what sanctions will be imposed in the case of noncompliance with this contract.

occurring, the nurse manager denies it. In general, the worst that will happen in the event of a relapse is that the regulatory board will order that treatment be intensified and the probationary stipulations extended for a longer period. Revocation of licenses is rarely carried out unless the nurse shows lack of good faith participation in a recovery program by repetitive noncompliance. As an employer of recovering nurses, the nurse manager must consider what action to take in the case of relapse. For example, some recovery programs allow for one self-reported relapse, with a resultant extension of the treatment time. Such decisions can best be made in each particular circumstance and should be specified in the back-to-work agreement (Table 19–2).

NURSING'S ROLE IN PREVENTION

Nurses in all settings need to be attuned to the seductive nature of drugs and be warned against self-medication from the very outset of their career. Pocketing a Tylenol No. 3 that was refused by a patient and diverting it to one's own use when working a long grueling night shift is not such a far-fetched probability. Using substances to dull the frustration of dealing with a complex health care system is not remote. Downing a substantial amount of bourbon or schnapps after a 12 hour shift in a long-term care facility where the care provided did not come close to one's standard of care or the death of a beloved client all add up to pain. We also call this frustration, sadness, fatigue, unhappiness, and stress. This pain can and does lead to the chemical solution.

Since these stresses comprise the normal circumstances of a nurse's day-to-day life, it is the task of nurse educators and nurse managers to mount an effort at prevention of chemical coping. The literature supports that addiction happens early in one's career and can happen by accident. Therefore, early intervention must take its place with education and stress reduction as primary and secondary prevention measures. Nurse managers can be alert to nurse behaviors that reveal a propensity toward pharmacologic optimism. As part of nurses' yearly evaluation, diagnostic questions should be asked about each nurse that a manager supervises. Has the nurse's behavior changed recently? Has the drug count been wrong? Is the nurse's absence rate higher? The same symptoms sought in data gathering when there is a report of chemical dependence can guide the nurse manager to early detection and intervention. Inservices about the seductive nature of drugs as well as sessions addressing the professional response to chemical dependence can help. In addition, a caring dialogue in the workplace is a valuable adjunct to prevention and early intervention.

THE ANA RESPONDS

In 1984, the American Nurses Association was prompted by the Ohio State Assembly of nurses to address the problem of chemically dependent nurses, which they hesitantly labeled the impaired professional. As we refined our language in this regard, we have come to know that chemical use and even chemical dependence does not necessarily equal impairment. Furthermore, the ANA (1984, p. iv) correctly notes

> A term that has been used to refer to individuals with psychological dysfunctions and chemical dependency is "impaired professional." The task force views this term with reservations. Although impairment results from these problems, it is an impairment of function rather than of the person that occurs.

The ANA admonishes further that with continued treatment, wellness increases in the nurse, and patient care improves. They conclude by advising that this condition can be arrested and need not be considered an unalterable condition (1984, p. iv). Recovering nurses agree.

RECOVERING NURSES RESPOND

When a small group of recovering nurses was interviewed to learn about their experience, they said that the current modes of intervention, treatment, and rehabilitation often are neither effective nor sufficient to promote and maintain sobriety or a drug-free state. The recovering nurses said that the regulatory agency and the bureaucratized profession of nursing itself militate against successful recovery and reentry into practice. The following comments illustrate the views of the recovering nurses.

1. Recovering nurse addicts reported that intervention attempts by colleagues and supervisors were inadequate and naive. They said that colleagues and su-

pervisors were easily bluffed out of their suspicions by the addict, with the result that intervention and treatment were delayed. They said that the lying, cheating, and stealing to get their drug, which is a prominent feature of the disease, is so highly developed that they can and do "bullshit their way out of anything."

2. Recovering nurses reported feeling isolated in AA and Narcotics Anonymous groups that were integrated with persons from other occupational groups and that the integrated AA/NA group was not a safe haven for them to either identify themselves as nurses or to candidly air their particular concerns about adaptation to sobriety. Small communities will find this a difficult problem to overcome.

3. The nurse addicts said that the workplace can conspire against the recovering addict by failing to view the nurse as chronically ill. Recovering nurses say that employers often are unable or unwilling to provide scheduling and assignments that would promote recovery by eliminating assignments with unsupervised drug access and eliminating the stress of night and rotating shifts. They also said that employers are unable to view relapse as a feature of chronic disease and are apt to see it as failing rather than as a minor setback.

4. There is a persistent stigma applied to addictive disease whereby some nurse colleagues continue to view addiction as a crime, a moral weakness, or moral failure. Recovering nurse addicts said that the profession, schools of nursing, and employers have not done enough to dispel this stigma.

References

Abbott, C. (1987). The impaired nurse. *AORN Journal, 46*(5), 870–876.

American Nurses Association. (1984). *Addictions and psychological dysfunctions in nursing: The profession's response to the problem.* Kansas City, MO: American Nurses Association.

Bissell, L, & Haberman, P.W. (1984). *Alcoholism in the professions.* New York: Oxford University Press.

Bissell, L., & Jones, R.W. (1981). The alcoholic nurse. *Nursing Outlook, 29*(2), 96–100.

Black, C. (1981). *It can never happen to me.* Denver: MAC Publishing.

Clemmer, J. (1987, October). When an addicted nurse comes back to work. *RN,* pp. 62–63.

Crosby, L., & Bissell, L. (1989). *To care enough.* Minneapolis: Johnson Institute.

Elliott, R., & Heins, M. (1987). *Disciplinary data bank: A longitudinal study.* A monograph presented to the National Council of State Boards of Nursing. Chicago: National Council of State Boards of Nursing.

Goodwin, D.W. (1976). *Is alcoholism hereditary?* New York: Oxford University Press.

Green, P. (1989, March). The chemically dependent nurse. *Nursing Clinics of North America,* pp. 81–94.

Haack, M., & Hughes, T. (1989). *Addiction in the nursing profession.* New York: Springer.

Hoffman, A., & Heinemann, M.E. (1987). Substance abuse education in schools of nursing: A national survey. *Journal of Nursing Education, 26*(7), 282–287.

Hutchinson, S. (1986). The chemically dependent nurse: Trajectory toward self-annihilation. *Nursing Research, 35*(4), 196–201.

Hutchinson, S. (1987a). Toward self-integration: The recovery process of chemically dependent nurses. *Nursing Research, 36*(6), 339–343.

Hutchinson, S. (1987b). Chemically dependent nurses: Implications for nurse executives. *Journal of Nursing Administration, 17*(9), 23–28.

Kaab, G. (1984). Chemical dependency: Helping your staff. *Journal of Nursing Administration, 14*(11), 18–23.

LaGodna, G., & Hendrix, M.J. (1989). Impaired nurses: A cost analysis. *Journal of Nursing Administration, 19*(9), 13–18.

Morse, R., Martin, M., Swenson, W., & Niven,

R. (1984). Prognosis of physicians treated for alcoholism and drug dependence. Journal of the American Medical Association, *251*(6), 743–746.

Naegle, M.A. (1988 January–February). Drug and alcohol abuse in nursing: An occupational hazard? *Nursing Life,* pp. 42–53.

Pace, E. (1990, October). Peer employee assistance programs for nurses. *Perspectives on Addictions in Nursing, 1*(4), 3–7.

Sullivan, E.J. (1987a). A descriptive study of nurses recovering from chemical dependency. *Archives of Psychiatric Nursing, 1*(3), 194–200.

Sullivan, E.J. (1987b). Comparison of chemically dependent and nondependent nurses on familial, personal and professional characteristics. *Journal of Studies on Alcohol, 48*(6).

Sullivan, E.J. (1991). Impaired health professional. In E.G. Bennett & D. Woolf (Eds.), *Substance abuse* (2nd ed.) (pp. 293–304). Albany, NY: Delmar.

Sullivan, E.J., Bissell, L., & Leffler, D. (1990). Drug use and disciplinary actions among 300 nurses. *The International Journal of the Addictions, 25*(4), 375–391.

Sullivan, E.J., Bissell, L., & Williams, E. (1988). *Chemical dependency in nursing: The deadly diversion.* Menlo Park, CA: Addison-Wesley.

Supples, J.M. (1988). *Self-regulation within the nursing profession.* Ann Arbor, MI: University of Michigan Press.

Supples, J.M. (1990, August). My colleague, my friend: The impaired nurse. *Nursing Management, 21*(8).

Trachtenburg, M. (1990). *Journeys to recovery.* New York: Springer.

United States Equal Employment Opportunities Commission (1992). *Americans with Disabilities Act* (EEOC Publication #M-1A), Washington, D.C.: U.S. Government Printing Office.

Facts about the Americans with Disabilities Act

Title I of the Americans with Disabilities Act of 1990, which took effect July 26, 1992, prohibits private employers, state and local governments, employment agencies and labor unions from discriminating against qualified individuals with disabilities in job application procedures, hiring, firing, advancement, compensation, job training, and other terms, conditions and privileges of employment. An individual with a disability is a person who:

- Has a physical or mental impairment that substantially limits one or more major life activities;
- Has a record of such an impairment; or
- Is regarded as having such an impairment.

A qualified employee or applicant with a disability is an individual who, with or without reasonable accommodation, can perform the essential functions of the job in question. Reasonable accommodation may include, but is not limited to:

- Making existing facilities used by employees readily accessible to and usable by persons with disabilities;
- Job restructuring, modifying work schedules, reassignment to a vacant position;
- Acquiring or modifying equipment or devices, adjusting or modifying examinations, training materials, or policies, and providing qualified readers or interpreters.

An employer is required to make an accommodation to the known disability of a qualified applicant or employee if it would not impose an "undue hardship" on the operation of the employer's business. Undue hardship is defined as an action requiring significant difficulty or expense when considered in light of factors such as an employer's size, financial resources and the nature and structure of its operation.

An employer is not required to lower quality or production standards to make an accommodation, nor is an employer obligated to provide personal use items such as glasses or hearing aids.

PRE-EMPLOYMENT INQUIRIES AND MEDICAL EXAMINATIONS

Employers may not ask job applicants about the existence, nature or severity of a disability. Applicants may be asked about their ability to perform specific job functions. A job offer may be conditioned on the results of a medical examination, but only if the examination is required for all entering employees in similar jobs. Medical examinations of employees must be job related and consistent with the employer's business needs.

DRUG AND ALCOHOL ABUSE

Employees and applicants currently engaging in the illegal use of drugs are not covered by the ADA, when an employer acts on the basis of such use. Tests for illegal drugs are not subject to the ADA's restrictions on medical examinations. Employers may hold illegal drug users and alcoholics to the same performance standards as other employees.

EEOC ENFORCEMENT OF THE ADA

The U.S. Equal Employment Opportunity Commission will issue regulations to enforce the provisions of Title I of the ADA on or before July 26, 1991. The provisions take effect on July 26, 1992, and will cover employers with 25 or more employees. On July 26, 1994, employers with 15 or more employees will be covered.

FILING A CHARGE

Charges of employment discrimination on the basis of disability, based on actions occurring on or after July 26, 1992, may be filed at any field office of the U.S. Equal Employment Opportunity Commission. Field offices are located in 50 cities throughout the United States and are listed in most telephone directories under U.S. Government. Information on all EEOC-enforced laws may be obtained by calling toll free (800) 669-3362. EEOC's toll-free TDD number is (800) 800-3302. For TDD calls from the Washington, DC, Metropolitan Area, dial (202) 663-4494. (U.S. Government Printing Office, 1991).

Sample Institutional Policy

STATEMENT OF PHILOSOPHY AND BELIEF RE THE PREVENTION, ETIOLOGY, TREATMENT, AND INTERVENTION FOR ADDICTIVE DISEASE AMONG EMPLOYEES

Employees in high-stress job situations have been found to be at increased risk for the illegal use and abuse of substances, such as drugs and alcohol. This is due in part to the need to decrease the unpleasant effects and feelings resulting from workplace and life event-caused stress. Stress often results from life situations about which we often can do little. Employees need to anticipate stress as a part of life and further anticipate the possible temptation to use drugs and alcohol as a solution to problems and to alter unpleasant moods. Using drugs and alcohol for these purposes can and often does result in a condition known as addictive disease, which ultimately can and does have adverse effects on patient care and nursing practice.

This institution believes that addictive disease is treatable, and it is our sincere intention to assist employees who have substance abuse problems, hopefully before the problem becomes too severe and before patient care and professional standards are compromised. To do this, we will need the help of all staff if we are to succeed in early intervention. With this in mind, the following policy is instituted.

TITLE: POLICY RE SUBSTANCE ABUSE AND ADDICTIVE DISEASE

Purpose: *To assure patient safety and to provide assistance to staff in the case of addictive disease and/or chemical dependency.*

Policy: *Prescription and over the counter medications:* Staff need to be cognizant of the possibility of impairment of safe performance when using certain substances, such as alcohol and prescription and over-the-counter medications. We need to depend on your discretion in not reporting for work should you find yourself in such a situation. It would facilitate staffing patterns if you do anticipate such an occurrence that you notify your supervisor in advance, as in the case of planned dental work for instance. This would allow time for appropriate work assignments. If a condition arises in which the long-term use of potentially impairing drugs is prescribed, you may be asked to verify that condition with the physician's statement or the prescription as a legal safeguard for the institution and the employee.

Addictive disease: Because people with addictive disease problems are usually powerless to intervene on their own behalf, we need to rely on alert staff persons to be cognizant of the signs and symptoms of possible chemical dependence/addictive disease resulting from drug or alcohol abuse and to report such concerns to their supervisor or the designated person on the staff who has been appointed to be responsible for further evaluation and intervention with the potentially ill staff person. It is not necessary to be certain of a problem, but only to suspect a problem may exist.

Possible signs and symptoms can include but are not limited to

1. Increased absenteeism, absent after weekends
2. Unusual affect, mood swings
3. Inappropriate responses, behavior that seems "hyper"
4. Dilated or constricted pupils, reddened eyes, tearing eyes
5. Perpetual/chronic cold symptoms, sniffles
6. Slurred speech, ataxic gait, changes in legibility of handwriting
7. Odor of alcohol on breath

Confrontation

1. The supervisor will have the responsibility to confront the staff person (with another supervisory or administrative staff person in attendance).

2. Make an estimate of the validity of the report and arrange for relief staffing if indicated.

3. Employees acceding to their need for assistance will be counseled and then referred for evaluation and treatment, with great care taken to monitor confidentiality on behalf of the staff person in question.

4. Employees who are reported to supervisors within the institution may, under some circumstances, be asked to submit to a drug/alcohol screening test (blood, breath, urine, or hair).

5. Employees judged to be impaired at work, whether or not such impairment is confirmed by laboratory data, will be assisted in safe return to their residence. (Never send a person judged to be impaired home from work in his or her own auto as the driver. This opens the possibility of all kinds of problems.)

6. It is the responsibility of the supervisor and administrator involved to document the incident in writing and to communicate this information to the director of nursing at the earliest convenience.

• • • • • •

CHAPTER 20

LABOR RELATIONS AND THE LAW

JANINE FIESTA

EXECUTIVE SUMMARY

A nurse manager is in the unique position of being both employer and employee. Because of this dual status, the nurse manager must be aware of labor laws to protect her or his own rights and to ensure proper actions in dealing with others. Labor law includes such things as wrongful termination, negligent hiring, sexual harassment, discrimination, and worker's compensation. This chapter provides a primer on which to base actions in regard to these sensitive areas.

The chapter begins with an overview of procedure and substance, the meaning of which is essential to understanding labor laws. In brief, procedure refers to any attempt to provide an employee with notice, whereas substance involves proving that an employee did or did not do what is claimed. Substantive problems include refusal of assignment, ethical beliefs, and the duty to communicate.

Helpful, concise guidelines are provided for such things as how to avoid antidiscriminatory language, contract disclaimers, using the proper language in an employee handbook, hiring, performance reviews, promotions, and dealing with termination and discharge. In addition, an in-depth review of the recently enacted Americans with Disabilities Act is provided, along with timely examples.

Statutory regulations including unionization attempts, worker's compensation rules, and the occupational safety and health act or "right to know" are reviewed. The section on sexual harassment reviews the Equal Employment Opportunity Commission's guidelines and outlines the two types of workplace sexual harassment: quid pro quo and hostile environment.

A section on licensure and how the law deals with the chemically dependent nurse round out the information. Excellent examples and court cases are sprinkled throughout this informative chapter to bring the message home: Be prepared.

E mployment law is a maze of common law doctrines, statutes, contract-established rules, judicial pronouncements, and administrative agency findings (Decker, 1987). The employment area presents many situations in which a nurse may be either a plaintiff or a defendant, since the nurse is both employee and employer. The nurse defendant may be a nurse functioning in a management capacity and acting as an agent of the employer.

EMPLOYMENT LAW LITIGATION

Employment law litigation involving health care providers has included cases about wrongful termination or discharge, negligent hiring and retention, defamation, invasion of privacy, sexual harassment, discrimination, workers' compensation and unemployment claims. Of particular interest to health care providers are the cases involving loss of licensure. Although perhaps not technically considered within the realm of labor law, these cases do involve the loss of ability to earn a livelihood or practice a profession.

LABOR RELATIONS AND THE LAW

As the nature of the American economy has changed over the last 40 years, so has the field of labor relations. The service sector of the economy has grown significantly. With the decline of organized labor, the average worker is not as likely to seek the assistance of co-workers in achieving an economic objective or redressing personal grievances.

Employees seek better pay and more rewarding work by enhancing their education and skills. If the system does not provide opportunities for advancement on a fair basis, employees have access to a host of statutory and common law remedies. The authority of unions has diminished for a variety of reasons, not the least of which is employers' attempts to compete with unions by providing comparable benefits and wages to nonunionized employees. In the health care delivery system, the substantial increase in wages during the last 5 years provided to nurses is an example of this pattern.

The basic theoretical underpinnings of most labor relations statutes are not complex. However, the application of legal theory to substantive employment practices may be both complex and unpredictable. Theory becomes meaningful when applied to actual situations, and answers to specific questions contribute to the general understanding of the law.

PROCEDURE AND SUBSTANCE

Because the nurse manager is both employer and employee, the nurse manager needs to be aware of labor laws to protect his or her own rights and to defend actions taken as a nurse manager. One attorney has suggested that managers should be evaluated on their ability to prevent unnecessary litigation (Henry, 1984).

A manager's decision-making ability must be developed and conformed to the procedural and substantive requirements imposed on employers. Procedure means that one must consider whether all of the notice or due process preconditions to supervisory action have been met. Substance involves whether the manager and employer can prove that the employee did or did not do whatever the claim alleges (Hollander, 1978).

Procedural Requirements

Procedural requirements, regardless of the specific form taken, such as progressive discipline, communicating with employees, performance evaluations, investigatory steps prior to discipline, and documentation, represent an attempt to provide employees with notice. Disciplinary decisions of employers who fail to provide employees with adequate and timely notice are rarely upheld. Proof of compliance with procedural requirements is protection against claims of termination because of discrimination. Providing an employee with appropriate notice also encourages voluntary improvement.

Termination is the final step of progressive discipline and the most severe. Procedural safeguards should be applied before the action is taken. These safeguards should include evaluation of facts and the sequence of progressive discipline, full investigation of the current incident and verification, compliance with internal requirements stated in policies and procedures, appropriate documentation, and careful preparation of the termination notice and the statement of cause. Policies and procedures should never state that progressive discipline must be followed in all instances or imply that the absence of progressive discipline will void the disciplinary action taken.

Substantive Problems

Substantive problems may involve conduct when the employee has acted improperly or performance when the employee's work product is below standard. Performance problems are generally managed through the progressive disciplinary process. Employee misconduct can involve a variety of examples and must be specifically identified. Examples include insubordination, theft of employer's property, fighting on the premises, and attendance problems.

If procedural safeguards are consistently followed, the courts are not as likely to question the employer's judgment as it relates to the substantive issue.

Refusal of Assignment

One substantive issue that the courts have considered is whether the nurse may refuse a work assignment. With the nursing shortage, one scenario dealing with this issue is a nurse's refusal to accept an assignment to float to a specialty area in which the nurse does not feel qualified to render care.

In a New Mexico case, a nurse was employed to work in the intensive care unit. Some time later, his supervisor told him to take temporary charge duty on the orthopedic unit. Even though floating was a hospital policy, he refused the assignment because he was unfamiliar with procedures on the unit and would jeopardize patient safety. He was suspended indefinitely. He refused an offer to be oriented to the other unit. The court ruled for the hospital, holding that the hospital's floating policy was valid (*Francis v. Memorial General Hospital,* 1986).

As a general rule, the nurse is not permitted to refuse a patient care assignment. If the nurse feels that he or she is not qualified to perform the assignment, this should be put in writing and submitted to the supervisor with emphasis on the potential harm to patients that may occur through acceptance of the assignment. If the supervisor continues to insist that the nurse must accept the assignment because there is no other alternative for patient care, the nurse should accept the assignment.

In New Jersey, a registered nurse refused to dialyze a terminally ill patient because of her moral and ethical personal beliefs. She was terminated from employment and sued for reinstatement. Guidelines from the American Nurses Association Code of Ethics were presented into evidence. The court rejected the nurse's argument and held that to allow an individual health care provider to impose his or her own values would lead to chaos in the health care delivery system [*488 A. 2d 229* (N.J. 1985)].

In accordance with state conscience laws, in many jurisdictions, a nurse cannot be required to participate in an abortion procedure. Some states have added sterilization procedures to these laws. This is apparently the only exception to the general rule.

Refusal to care for a patient suffering from acquired immune deficiency syndrome (AIDS) has not been accepted as a reasonable refusal by the courts (*Dept. of Health & Hospitals v. Jeffries,* 1991).

With the nursing shortage, the use of agency nurses frequently is a management issue. Guidelines for minimizing risks with agency employees emphasize the importance of orientation programs, verification of credentials, and communication with the agency regarding all positive and negative observations about agency employees (Nelson, 1989).

Duty to Communicate and Corporate Liability

Another substantive issue for the nurse manager centers around the staff nurse's most important legal duty—the duty to communicate. With the emergence of corporate liability (Politis, 1983), it is clear that the hospital, as a corporate entity, has assumed responsibility for the quality of care given to all patients. Corporate liability cases have included liability for short staffing, equipment, security, environmental safety, lack of policy implementation and monitoring, and liability for the actions of physicians who are not employees (*Thompson v. Nason,* 1991).

In the corporate liability analysis, it becomes the nurse manager's responsibility to continue the chain of communication initiated by the staff nurse in the clinical area. When the staff nurse communicates to the nurse manager, it becomes the manager's role to either solve the problem or continue the line of communication to upper management. In addition to the corporate liability issue, the nurse manager may assume direct liability for clinical care issues. In a specific patient care example, the staff nurse frequently calls the nursing supervisor when an unusual problem with a patient exists. For example, the nurse may be having difficulty in notifying a physician as the patient's condition is worsening. The staff nurse appropriately notifies the nursing supervisor, documents on the patient's medical record "nursing supervisor notified," and also tells the supervisor that this documentation is on the chart to allow the supervisor to respond. The supervisor has now assumed accountability for the resolution of the patient care issue. Chain of command protocols should clearly define the staff nurse's and nurse manager's responsibilities (Fiesta, 1990).

RECRUITMENT AND HIRING

Selecting employees from a pool of persons who apply for work raises the potential of legal liability. The most frequently asserted claims are contentions that specific recruiting policies or practices have had a disproportionate adverse impact on those protected by antidiscrimination statutes. Application of the recruitment policy in a disparate manner may also be a basis for claim.

Avoiding Antidiscriminatory Language and Job Misrepresentation

To prevent these claims, employers should avoid language that explicitly or implicitly suggests a preference for a particular race, religion, national origin, sex, or age group. The employer should include a statement that it is an equal opportunity employer.

Representations about the job made during the recruiting stage may lead to a breach of an implied or expressed contract claim. Such representations usually occur during prehire interviews or contract negotiations or in offer letters, application forms, or employee handbooks. Typical problems include promises of future wage or benefit increases, moving expenses, term of employment, or a for-cause termination standard.

Employee Handbook Statements

Employee handbooks may create enforceable rights to specific disciplinary procedures (Decker, 1984). A handbook statement that "three warning notices within a twelve month period are required before dismissal" created liability for a hospital that failed to follow their own requirement (*Touissant v. Blue Cross/Shield of Michigan,* 1990).

Contract Disclaimers

To prevent this problem, employers are advised to include contract disclaimers in all literature, asserting that no statements made for the company should be interpreted to be binding contractual promises. Reasonable recruitment and screening procedures should include

1. An inspection of the information provided by the applicant—look for gaps in employment and other suspicious or unusual entries or omissions.
2. Contacting each previous employer and personal reference listed on the application—if the information provided by the applicant is insufficient, obtain further information such as forwarding addresses.
3. Asking all former employers if they have any reason to doubt that the applicant is reliable, trustworthy, and honest, or if they are aware if the applicant has engaged in any violent, criminal, improper, or harassing conduct.
4. Obtaining the applicant's consent to get information from former employers, personal references, past and present landlords, credit bureaus, and other sources, together with a waiver and release from liability in connection with the reference check.

Avoiding Claims of Fraud and Misrepresentation

To avoid claims of fraud and misrepresentation the employer should

1. Avoid making promises regarding career opportunities, future compensation, or expected job duties.
2. Use words such as "possible," "potential," and "maybe" when describing career opportunities.
3. Not predict future pay raises or bonuses, and refer to past increases or bonuses as "purely a guide."
4. Use words such as "currently," "at present," or "now" when describing benefits, and note that all employee benefit plans are "subject to change."

Federal Laws and Regulations

An employer's selection procedures are regulated by several federal laws and regulations, including Title VII, the Civil Rights Acts of 1866 and 1871, the Age Discrimination in Employment Act, the Americans with Disabilities Act of 1990, the Rehabilitation Act of 1973, Executive Order n. 11246, and state fair employment practices statutes.

Rehabilitation Act of 1973

The Rehabilitation Act of 1973 (Rehabilitation Act) forbids employers receiving federal financial assistance or those having contracts with the federal government from improper discrimination against employees with a drug or alcohol problem that meets the definition of a handicap (*29 U.S.C. s701*, 1986). However, the Rehabilitation Act clearly states that although an employee cannot be fired for those handicaps alone, if the employee who has a drug or alcohol problem "cannot perform the duties of the job in question or whose employment, by reason of such current alcohol use or drug abuse, would constitute a direct threat to property or the safety of others," the employee may be disciplined by the employer. Such appropriate discipline includes, but is not limited to, suspension or termination (Brent, 1991).

Americans with Disabilities Act of 1990

A second federal law that is far more sweeping than the Rehabilitation Act is the recently passed Americans with Disabilities Act of 1990) (ADA) (*42 U.S.C.A., s12,* 1991). Effective July 26, 1992, the ADA prohibits discrimination by employers whether or not they receive federal funds in, among other things, the discharge of qualified employees because of a handicap. The illegal use of drugs or alcohol is not included in the ADA's definition of a disability. However, an employee is considered handicapped and receives protection by the ADA if he or she

- Has successfully completed a drug rehabilitation program and is no longer engaging in the illegal use of drugs
- Is participating in a supervised rehabilitation program and is no longer engaging in such use

- Is erroneously regarded as engaging in such use but is not engaging in such use (*42 U.S.C.A. s12,* 1991).

These and similar state laws mandate that the employer discharging an employee involved in drug diversion or drug use, abuse, or impairment do so because patient or employee safety is threatened, property may be diverted or stolen, or the employee has violated the established employee conduct code. Sample conduct violations include working under the influence of a drug or alcohol, theft of hospital or agency property, and alteration of patient records or other records kept in the course of providing care, including narcotics records and patient charts.

In an Illinois case, the court held that plaintiff, who suffered from uncontrollable epilepsy, was not, despite her epilepsy, otherwise qualified to work in defendant's burn unit. The hospital hired plaintiff to work in the burn unit knowing she suffered from idiopathic epilepsy. Subsequently, defendant received reliable reports showing plaintiff suffered unpredictable seizures while on duty. During these seizures, plaintiff injured herself, compromised staffing levels and patient care, and was generally a danger to patients. Both defendant and plaintiff agreed that an examination by an expert at another hospital would be desirable. After the examination, the expert informed plaintiff that the seizures were not controllable and it was dangerous for her to work in the burn unit. Plaintiff knew the results of the examination were not favorable and refused to inform defendant. Defendant placed plaintiff on leave because she failed to provide defendant with the examination results.

The court held, in light of the undisputed facts, that the plaintiff's forced leave did not violate the Rehabilitation Act. The court ruled plaintiff did not meet her position requirements and defendant did not act with prejudice or unfairly in removing her from her duties (*Gault v. University of Chicago Hosp.,* 1991).

Under the ADA of 1990, an employer may require a preemployment medical examination only after extending an offer of employment and only if all entering employees in the same job category are subjected to such an examination regardless of disability. A test to determine illegal drug use is not considered a medical examination under the ADA.

The heart of ADA is its requirement—its affirmative mandate—that employers make reasonable accommodations to the known disabilities of applicants and employees (Schurgin & Rowland, 1991). The Act is specific in requiring reasonable accommodation not only to permit applicants and employees to perform essential job functions but also to permit applicants to comply with testing and application procedures and to permit disabled employees to enjoy the same benefits and privileges of employment as other similarly situated employees. Furthermore, unlike many state handicap statutes, the ADA lists many important accommodations employers must consider in making employment decisions. "Reasonable accommodations" under the ADA include (Schurgin & Rowland, 1991) the following:

- Making existing facilities accessible to individuals with disabilities

- Job restructuring
- Job reassignment
- Part-time or modified work schedules
- Granting unpaid leave
- Acquisition or modification of equipment
- Providing qualified readers or interpreters
- Adjustment or modifications of examinations, training materials or policies
- A catch-all—other similar accommodations for individuals with disabilities

NEGLIGENT HIRING
Legal Obligations of an Employer

An employer is legally obligated to protect its employees, patients, and visitors from injury at the hands of a dangerous employee. To satisfy its obligations, the employer must reasonably investigate prospective employees' backgrounds before hiring them. Additionally, an employer is expected to properly train its employees. A cause of action for negligent hiring asserts that an employee was unfit for his or her employment and thereby caused injury to another. The standard of fitness will vary depending on the position the employee holds. Employers should conduct more thorough investigations of employees hired to work in positions requiring higher standards of fitness.

The employment application should include a statement that termination of employment will occur on discovery of dishonest answers on the application.

The plaintiff must prove not only that the employee was unfit but also that the employer proximately caused the injuries by hiring or retaining the unfit employee. To show causation, the plaintiff must submit evidence that had it not been for the employment relationship, the plaintiff would not have been exposed to injury. Also, evidence must be offered to show that the employer knew, or should have known, that the employee was unfit. This element usually depends on establishing that a reasonable person would have investigated the employee's background and that a reasonable investigation would have disclosed the employee's lack of fitness. If the claim is for negligent retention rather than negligent hiring, the employer may be expected to have actual knowledge of the employee's lack of fitness. Even if an employer follows its customary hiring procedures, a plaintiff may argue that those procedures were inadequate. More frequently, however, problems arise when an employer neglects to verify background information, contact references, or notice apparent problems in an employee's work history (McCandless & Cortez, 1990).

Negligence Litigation and the Health Care Environment

The health care environment is tailormade for such litigation. The hospital's duties to its patients include a duty to provide quality care, to provide qualified employees, and to provide a safe environment (Fiesta, 1988). Health care providers have a special obligation to their patients because of the vulnerability of the hospitalized or ill patient and his or her nearly total dependence on the hospital staff for safety and well-being (Husson & Bond, 1991). Few employment environments give employees more opportunity to commit violent, criminal, or otherwise wrongful acts against the person or property of often helpless individuals (McCandless & Cortez, 1990).

Reference Checks to Prevent Negligence Litigation

In *Deerings West Nursing Center v. Scott* (1990), the court assessed actual damages of $35,000 and punitive damages of $200,000 against a nursing home that hired an unlicensed nurse and placed him in a supervisory position. In this case, the defendant male nurse (who was 6 feet 4 inches tall and 36 years old) assaulted an 80-year-old woman who was attempting to visit her brother. If the employer had insisted on proof of licensure, it would have found 56 prior convictions for theft and other offenses.

In *Wilson N. Jones Memorial Hospital v. Davis* (1977), a patient suffered injuries when an improperly trained orderly negligently removed a Foley catheter. The orderly was hired before any reference check because the hospital had a critical need for orderlies. The hospital checked only one employment reference after the orderly was hired, and that reference failed to provide the hospital with answers to critical questions about the orderly's job suitability. The hospital failed to check the employee's reference with the United States Navy. It would have learned that the orderly was expelled after only 1 month training and that he had a serious drug problem, as well as a criminal record. The hospital failed to follow its own hiring policies. The court awarded the patient punitive damages. The theory of negligent hiring allows for the recovery of punitive damages more readily than in an ordinary negligence case.

It is only a matter of time before a court holds an employer liable for failure to disclose adverse information about a former employee where the previous employer should have reasonably foreseen that such a failure to disclose could lead to monetary loss or physical harm to others (Husson & Bond, 1991). The Georgia Bureau of Investigation is examining a nurse's role in about 15 suspicious code blue emergencies at an Atlanta hospital in 1990. The same nurse has been charged with murder by police in Alabama. The hospitals that employed the nurse also are named, with one $5 million suit claiming the hospital "knew or should have known that the nurse posed a continuing danger to patients." Despite an investigation of his connection to the mysterious deaths and being fired by four hospitals within a year, he was able to continue working as a nurse (Brown, 1991).

Limited Disclosure

Employers should follow a limited disclosure policy. In situations where it is reasonably foreseeable that a risk of physical or monetary harm to others could occur as a result of hiring the individual in question, any factual information concerning the employee should be provided by the employer. Employers can take precautions to protect themselves from the threat of future employee reference lawsuits by keeping opinions about the employee out of any references (Decker, 1984).

PERFORMANCE EVALUATIONS

It is vital to maintain uniform operating procedures for all performance evaluations. Performance evaluation documentation should reflect the reasons that the employee's performance is deemed deficient, the performance standards that will be applied in the future, and the consequences of the employee's failure to meet those standards. The employee whose performance is being reviewed should have an opportunity to examine the documentation and to indicate his or her agreement or disagreement with particular criticisms and comments. Each supervisor's evaluations should be monitored to ensure consistent ratings throughout the hospital. Education should be provided to minimize deviations.

Employees should be provided with time to correct deficiencies. The employer should set a realistic schedule for the employee to follow and also ensure that any goals set are fair and attainable by the employee. This obviously means that the employer will have to accept an additional period of marginal performance until it becomes clear that the employee is truly incapable of satisfying the employer's performance standards. No matter how improbable it may seem that an employee will be able to overcome deficiencies and retain the job, it is important that no documentation indicates or suggests that the employee's failure was a foregone conclusion by the employer. Where the employer documents that belief, no matter how sincerely, the employer provides the employee with an opportunity to raise a claim that the probationary period was merely a pretext in furtherance of the employer's unlawful plan to terminate the employee.

The employee should be provided with periodic progress reviews during the period of time in which he or she is expected to improve work performance. These reviews should be looked on by the employer as an opportunity to further document any performance deficiencies that were ignored previously. Subsequent reviews will provide a more balanced and complete picture of the exact nature of the performance problems in the event a lawsuit is brought after the employee has been terminated. It is important that the documentation be accurate and clear and not appear to be self-serving.

DISCIPLINE AND DISCHARGE

Because of the great potential for litigation associated with the implementation of discipline and termination policies and the possibility for large damage awards, employer procedures in this area should be of special concern to all management.

Disciplinary Standards and Procedures

Guidelines should be applied consistently, uniformly, and in good faith. An employer that advises employees that it will use certain disciplinary standards and procedures and then fails to apply them uniformly is probably in a weaker position, from a legal standpoint, than an employer that advises its employees that they may be terminated for good cause, for bad cause, or for no cause at all.

Lifestyle Regulation

There should be a connection between each work rule and a recognizable and valid business concern. Regulation of off-duty conduct is an issue in this area. Generally, an employee's private activities at and outside the workplace are not open to employer scrutiny or regulation. Yet in certain areas directly affecting the employer's business affairs, the employer may attempt to regulate the employee's lifestyle. This may result in employee disciplinary actions, including termination, where employee lifestyle actions adversely affect the employer's business.

Lifestyle regulation may include dress and grooming standards, spousal employment, consumption of alcohol, smoking, and drug use. The regulation should be reasonable and directly related to the employee's job. Outside the workplace, limits may include other employment opportunities that may directly conflict with the employer's business and activities that may injure the employer's image in the community.

Posted and Printed Work Regulations

Employees should be provided with notice of employer work rules. The rules, standards, and associated penalties should be posted within the employer's facility and set forth in an employee handbook. The employee should sign a written form indicating that he or she has read and understood the rules or standards.

Employers should be consistent in the application of work rules. One means of enhancing uniformity in disciplinary actions is to limit the number of persons who conduct disciplinary investigations. A human resources manager and legal counsel should review investigations where termination is contemplated. Personnel file documents should record similar violations in the same terminology.

Termination and Discharge

Suspected infractions of work rules must be investigated properly. The employer should ascertain whether the employee was or should have been aware of the rule or standard, whether the infractions were recorded accurately, and whether there were mitigating circumstances that had been accepted previously as excuses in similar cases involving other employees. A proper investigation should not be based on the presumption that the individual in question is guilty. In evaluating whether an investigation has been conducted fairly, the employer should always apply an objective third-party point of view. It is unwise to terminate an employee on the spot. It is preferable to suspend pending further investigation.

Investigation and Objective Evidence

Disciplinary actions should be based on objective evidence. In discipline and termination cases, witnesses often disagree about important facts, based on their preconceptions, physical vantage points, or personal biases. Where incongruities in witnesses' observations arise, the hospital should attempt to determine whether a particular version is consistent with any objective evidence. The employer should seek out additional witnesses by canvassing other employees.

Prompt, Appropriate Disciplinary Actions

Disciplinary actions should be administered promptly and in accordance with established company policy. The disciplinary measure should be appropriate to the infraction. It is preferable that a hospital's written personnel policy not state a strict delineation of what penalty should attach to each form of misconduct. Even where an employee's misconduct is sufficient to warrant immediate termination, the employer should consider an employee's outstanding work record and long tenure as a mitigating factor. A termination decision may be made because the infraction is the culmination of an extended history of prior violations of policy rather than a single incident of misconduct. These cases should be supported by adequate documentation of previous related offenses.

Private Discussion of Disciplinary Action

To minimize potential liability for defamation, employers should discuss discipline in private, be honest with employees about the reasons for the termination, limit publication of statements to those who have a need to know, and consider obtaining a waiver from terminated employees to allow for a substantive letter of reference. When references are requested, the information requested should be documented as well as the response. All calls for references should be handled through one central office in the human resources department.

Wrongful Discharge and Intentional Infliction of Emotional Distress

An emerging area of labor litigation is the employee's lawsuit for intentional infliction of emotional distress. This suit is based on the employer's extreme and outrageous conduct.

To state a cause of action for the tort of intentional infliction of emotional distress, a plaintiff must allege facts establishing *(52 ALR 4th 853)*:

- That the conduct of the defendant was extreme and outrageous
- That the emotional distress suffered by the plaintiff was severe
- That the defendant's conduct was such that the defendant knew that severe emotional distress would be certain or substantially certain to result

In a Texas case, a former head nurse in a hospital's labor and delivery unit stated a cause of action for intentional infliction of emotional distress by alleging that following her refusal to assist a physician in the performance of an unauthorized continuous epidural anesthesia procedure, the physician, the hospital's director of nursing, and the hospital had engaged in a course of conduct to harass, humiliate, and degrade her good name, which eventually resulted in her willful, malicious, and unlawful termination. The court held that the nurse's failure to pursue her wrongful discharge claim did not mandate dismissal of her emotional distress claims where such claims were based on harsh treatment and rumors circulated about her before her discharge, not only by her employer but also by the physician and nursing director individually (*Havens v. Tomball Community Hospital*, 1990).

Another basis for claim is interference with a business relationship. In an Alabama case, a nurse's aide alleged that the facility intentionally interfered with her business when after it terminated her employment for arguing with a patient, it refused to permit her to continue serving as a private duty sitter for its patients. The nursing home was justified, as a matter of law, in adopting a policy that would not permit discharged employees to be employed by patients as private duty sitters, and that policy served as a defense to the aide's suit (*Finley v. Beverly Enterprises*, 1986).

In the United States, under the employment-at-will doctrine, employers had the authority to fire employees for any reason or no reason. Recently, state legislatures and the courts have limited this broad right. For example, employers may not discriminate on the basis of race, sex, religion, or place of origin or because of an employee's union activity *(29 U.S.C. s794-794a)*.

A bargaining agreement in a unionized hospital may limit management's ability to fire employees. Many union contracts require "just cause" for disciplining or discharging an employee. Furthermore, if an employer states that an employee can be fired only "for cause" in a personnel handbook, this constitutes an implicit contract that takes precedence over the common law employment-at-will doctrine. Just cause may include breach of confidentiality or failure to follow hospital policy.

A psychiatric nurse was discharged because of unacceptable and inappropriate conduct, which included negative comments about the hospital and its staff and instructions to new employees to ignore violations of hospital policy. For example, petitioner stated that one half of the administration should be fired and that orientees should "turn their heads" when confronted with patients engaged in sexual activities. The latter directly contradicted the hospital's policy. Before her discharge, petitioner had been instructed by her supervisor to improve her negative attitude.

The court determined there was just cause for petitioner's removal. The court interpreted just cause to require removal actions be taken only for reasons relating to a state employee's job performance and ability to perform competently. The court found that petitioner's job performance was impaired based on her conduct with new employees at orientation sessions, her advice to ignore violations of hospital policy, and her negative comments about the hospital and its staff. The court held that those factors went to the essence of job performance and met the criteria of just cause (*Kachmar v. Pennsylvania*, 1989).

The Supreme Court of North Dakota has affirmed a lower court's dismissal of a claim brought by a nurses' aide against a county hospital and nursing home for wrongful termination of employment and defamation. The nurses' aide, who had made offensive and derogatory remarks about her supervisor and the hospital in general in the presence of residents of the facility and visitors, was terminated for "breach of confidentiality of both patient-specific and facility-specific information" (*Caroline Eli v. Griggs County Hospital*, 1986).

Public Policy Exceptions

In April 1981, through the Whistleblowers Protection Acts, Michigan became the first state to protect employees who expose illegal or dangerous employee activity *[42 U.S.C. 2000e; 29 U.S.C. 158(a)(1)(4)]*. This law provides that employees will be protected for exposing such activity.

More recently, applications of a public policy exception have attempted to limit the employment-at-will doctrine. If the nurse can demonstrate that the termination violates a clear and significant public policy, a legal action for wrongful discharge may be successful. Some activities protected by the public policy exception have included union membership, filing a worker's compensation claim, or serving on a jury.

The Arizona Supreme Court held that an employer may fire an employee-at-will for good cause or for no cause but not for "bad cause," such as in violation of public policy. In this case, the nurse claimed that she was discharged in part because she disapproved of her supervisors' and other employees' behavior, which violated the state's indecent exposure law (*Wagenseller v. Scottsdale Memorial Hospital,* 1984).

In *Seery v. Yale-New Haven Hospital* (1989), a nurse anesthetist and anesthesiologist sued the hospital for wrongful discharge. They alleged that the hospital forced them to work with an impaired physician and that the hospital violated public policy by failing to report the physician to the Connecticut Department of Health. In this case, the court discussed the concept of constructive discharge. Constructive discharge occurs when an employer renders an employee's working conditions so difficult and intolerable that a reasonable person would feel forced to resign. A claim of constructive discharge must be supported by more than the employee's subjective opinion that the job conditions have become so intolerable that he or she was forced to resign. The court stated (*Seery v. Yale-New Haven Hospital,* 1989), "Normally, an employee who resigns is not regarded as having been discharged, and thus would have no right for action for abusive discharge. Through the use of [the term] constructive discharge, the law recognizes that an employee's "voluntary" resignation may be, in reality, a dismissal by the employer. . . . [H]owever . . . the employee must still prove that the dismissal, in whatever form, occurred for a reason violating public policy."

Patient advocacy is not yet considered a public policy exception. Those claims of wrongful discharge based on the public policy exception but supported only by personnel, moral, or ethical standards have not defeated the employer's right to fire under the at-will doctrine. In Colorado, a head nurse was fired for her inability to follow staffing patterns and stay within budget. She sued the hospital for wrongful discharge. She claimed that the preamble to the Nurse Practice Act required that she safeguard the patients' health and welfare. Her refusal to reduce her staff's overtime work was based on the belief that reducing the staff would jeopardize the health of the patients. The court refused to recognize the preamble to the Colorado Nurse Practice Act as a basis for the public policy exception to the employee-at-will doctrine (*Lampe v. Presbyterian Medical Center,* 1978).

The First Amendment right to freedom of speech may offer some protection. To be entitled to constitutional protection, speech must relate to matters of "political, social, or other concern to the community" (*Wheelers v. Manning*, 1987).

In *Jones v. Memorial Hospital System* (1984), Nurse Jones, who worked in the intensive care unit, wrote an article describing conflicts between the wishes of terminally ill patients and their families and the orders of attending physicians. She signed her name to the article but did not implicate any specific physician or the hospital. Subsequently, she was fired and brought action against the hospital. The hospital argued that there was a legitimate basis for her termination other than the publication of her article. The court was not persuaded by this argument and focused on whether her free speech right had been infringed. The court held that she was entitled to constitutional protection because the article was written on her own time, did not interfere with her work performance or with her employer's business, and was intended to inform the public on a controversial public issue.

The First Amendment protected the comments of a municipal hospital employee expressed in a letter to a hospital board and to an individual board member where the employee's statements, although they cited specific concerns over certain hospital employees, had addressed public issues involving alleged waste, inefficiency, and favoritism at the hospital and had been directed to public officials charged with overseeing the hospital's financial stability. The employee had not encouraged other employees to take action against the hospital. The employee's right to freedom of association and right to petition for redress of grievances were inseparable from her right to speak (*Schalk v. Gallemore*, 1990).

A former director of nursing at a psychiatric hospital failed to state a cause of action for wrongful discharge under the "public policy" exception to the Missouri doctrine of employment-at-will, even though her petition alleged that the criminal act of forgery had been committed when "bogus minutes" of "meetings" for a nonexistent infection control committee had been prepared for an inspection by the Joint Commission on Accreditation of Healthcare Organizations (JCAHO). She alleged that she had been fired because she told JCAHO investigators that there had been no committee meetings and that her employer had not implemented a patient classification system. Even if the preparation of "bogus minutes" constituted the crime of forgery, the public policy exception was not applicable where there was no allegation that the director herself had been directed to prepare such minutes or that she had been fired because of her refusal to do so (*Crockett v. Mid-America Health Services*, 1989).

Although remedies remain somewhat limited, recent judicial opinions indicate significant movement toward protecting employees who question employer's actions or policies. They show some recognition that an employee who puts the public's interest and welfare before that of the employer deserves society's support (Gornik, 1992).

Before deciding to take an issue outside the agency or institution, the nurse should consider these questions. Is there sufficient evidence to warrant action? A nurse making a serious accusation must have sufficient documentation to ensure fairness to the accused and to help maintain his or her own credibility. Has the nurse used all possible internal mechanisms? Following the usual channels of communication may not be sufficient. Consideration should be given to providing information to the risk management and quality assurance departments also.

The decision to blow the whistle should not be made lightly. The disclosure will have serious ramifications for both the individual disclosing and the organization.

Right to Privacy

In addition to actions based on wrongful discharge and defamation, the employee may also sue to protect the right to privacy. The Fourth Amendment protects the privacy interest from unreasonable searches and seizures. To determine whether a particular intrusion is reasonable, it must be balanced against the individual's Fourth Amendment interests and its promotion of legitimate governmental interests. The reality of the workplace may make some employee privacy expectations unreasonable when an intrusion is by a supervisor rather than by a law enforcement official. Privacy expectations in offices, desks, file cabinets, or lockers may be limited by employer practices, procedures, policies, or legitimate regulation (Decker, 1987).

Generally, searches by employers have been based on a probable cause standard. The employer interest in justifying work-related intrusions is the efficient and proper operation of the workplace.

If the employer believes that employees should be searched for the protection of third parties, such as patients, the courts will not deny the right to perform such searches as long as they are reasonable. A policy should be developed to deal with this issue. The policy should also address the indications for patient and visitor searches.

The administration of workplace drug tests and other searches also may generate claims of assault and battery and false imprisonment. False imprisonment is the intentional restraint of the physical liberty of another (*Restatement*, s35). This restraint may be imposed by actual physical conduct or by verbal threats or coercion. In the employment context, claims for false imprisonment usually arise in connection with the detention of an employee to investigate workplace theft or other wrongdoing. Such claims may also arise in connection with administration of polygraph and drug tests. Employees should not be confined or restrained against their will. Neither mental nor physical coercion should be used. Assault and battery, also intentional torts, lie where the plaintiff is subjected to an unwanted offensive contract with his or her person or the reasonable apprehension of such contact (*Restatement*, s18).

PROMOTIONS AND DISCRIMINATION

Title VII mandates that minorities be able to compete equally with nonminorities for promotions. A plaintiff establishes a case of discrimination when he or she can prove that he or she belonged to a protected group, qualified for and applied for a promotion and did not receive it, and other employees, usually outside the protected group, with similar qualifications were promoted.

Age discrimination also may be claimed in a promotions case. An employer may present business reasons for selecting one candidate over another, and the plaintiff must prove that the proffered reasons were pretextual and that age discrimination was a determinative factor in the decision. Relevant evidence may include prior treatment of the plaintiff, defendant's policy and practice with respect to older employees, procedural irregularities, and the use of subjective criteria in the decision-making process.

As in most employment discrimination cases, statistics can raise an inference of unlawful conduct. Without evidence of pretext, a trial court ordinarily will accept the employer's reason why it chose the person it thought best qualified for the job. Seniority may be used for promotion decisions if all other factors are relatively equal. An employer is entitled to rely on such things as experience, productivity, cooperation, ability to work with others, attendance and lateness record, and other barometers of reliability and leadership.

Title VII provides for back pay and reinstatement and in cases of promotion, front pay may be awarded. This is pay that reaches beyond that date the remedy is awarded and continues to run until the employee receives a comparable position.

As with any other issue, a policy need not be in writing but can be established by past practice. If a policy or past practice exists, it must be applied uniformly.

Work situations that have been problematic include giving front-line supervisors too much discretion to judge candidates subjectively, giving evaluators no written instructions as to qualifications for promotion, having excessively vague standards for qualification, and having no centralized overview of companywide policies and procedures with respect to promotion.

Each individual performing promotion interviews should have a checklist or worksheet listing uniform questions. The interviewing personnel must avoid excessively abstract or elastic standards that can too easily mask pretextual motives. For example, "poor attitude" or "lack of cooperation" are imprecise and less effective than providing specific examples.

STATUTORY REGULATIONS
National Labor Relations Act

In both public and private employment, familiarity with the National Labor Relations Act (NLRA) is important knowledge for the nurse manager. Although the NLRA covers only private employers, its provisions have been adopted by public employment entities. Even if the facility has no union contracts, provisions of the act may apply. For example, the Act may require that nonsupervised employees be reinstated if they have been terminated because of union activity. A manager is considered an agent of the employer. Therefore, a finding of an unfair labor practice will be against the employer because of the manager's actions.

Management and Union Organizing

The National Labor Relations Act is very specific on what actions management may or may not take during a union organizing campaign. The actions taken could have severe implications. Inappropriate actions by managers could legally bind the hospital and cause the Labor Board to require the hospital to recognize and bargain with the union without actually holding the election.

The scope of the bargaining unit—who will and will not vote in the election and be represented by the union if it wins—is the most important single issue to be resolved before the voting takes place. What is an appropriate bargaining unit is a difficult and complex subject.

As a general rule there can be no threat of reprisal, promise of benefits, or similar action during the campaign period. Taking disciplinary action against employees because of their union activities is prohibited.

In *Hubbard Regional Hospital v. NLRA* (1978), four union organizing nurses were terminated for the bizarre fashion in which they prepared a sedated patient for transportation to surgery. The patient was isolated before surgery because of possible infectious hepatitis. He was the husband of a nursing supervisor at the hospital. One of the nurses dressed him in a disposable yellow gown on which she had lettered the words "Yellow Bird Express." Another nurse placed a brown plastic bag over the patient's feet, a surgical mask over his face, and a plastic shower cap on his head. The patient's wife complained to the director of nursing about this conduct. The nurses were subsequently discharged from employment. The nurses filed a grievance with the NLRB and complained that they were fired because of union activities. The court held that proof was insufficient to show that antiunion feelings were the primary motive for discharge of the nurses. The bizarre treatment of the patient raised doubts with patients and other hospital personnel about the quality of nursing care at the hospital.

Grievance Process

Among the most important provisions of the collective bargaining contract is the section dealing with the grievance process. Adoption of a grievance process frequently occurs in a nonunionized environment also. This discourages the arbitrary and capricious handling of employee complaints and encourages fair and prompt settlements. The grievance procedure imposes the order in which the dispute will be examined and resolved and a time limit determining each step of the process.

Collective bargaining contracts often state that the employer may not discharge or discipline an employee except for "just cause." As noted previously, this is one of the exceptions to the traditional employee-at-will principle. Nurses who exercise their right to bargain collectively by joining a union or by working in a hospital that is unionized lose the opportunity to personally negotiate their wages, hours, and working conditions with their employer.

In *Mock v. LaGuardia Hospital* (1980), supervisory nurses were discharged for labor union activity. The court stated that management personnel owed a duty of loyalty to their employer.

Workers' Compensation

State-established workers' compensation laws replace the employee's right to sue the employer for work-related injuries. At the time of injury, the employee must provide notice of the injury to the employer. The scope of definition for a work-related injury is frequently a topic for litigation.

In *Elwood v. State Accident Insurance Fund Corp.* (1984), a nurse was assistant director of nurses for 9 years and had served as director when the need arose. Although the nurse had received average to outstanding performance ratings, there was evidence that her performance had begun to decline. She testified that there was a movement to force her to quit, and the employer requested and received her resignation a short time later. About 4 years after her termination, she filed a workers' compensation case based on her depression. The Workers' Compensation Board affirmed the insurance company's denial of her claim, and the nurse appealed. The court reversed and remanded the case and held that stressful events and conditions of the nurse's employment, including her termination, were the major contributing causes of her mental disorder.

If an employee of the hospital is unable to work because of a work-related injury or illness, the issue of whether this employee is entitled to workers' compensation becomes significant.

In *Kahn v. State of Minnesota* (1980), a nurse was asked by the director of research at the school of nursing to assist in developing a proposal for obtaining funds to study home care of children with terminal cancer. She orally agreed to a lump sum of 10 dollars per hour to be paid on completion of the project. She was 6 months pregnant and worked on the project at home. While returning home from delivering a final draft of the proposal, she was involved in a car accident that rendered her a quadriplegic. The university appealed a workers' compensation award to the nurse. The court ruled that the nurse was an employee of the university and that the injury arose in the course of her employment. The award was affirmed.

A hospital supply room manager who was unable to work because of headaches and depression caused by work-related stress was eligible for workers' compensation benefits, a Louisiana appellate court ruled. The plaintiff developed symptoms after being harassed by employees she had observed using illicit drugs in the hospital supply room. She left her job after being threatened and having personal property stolen and destroyed. The court held that compensable mental health disabilities included those precipitated by the cumulative effects of several stressful incidents (*Sparks v. Tulane*, 1988).

The New Mexico Supreme Court awarded workers' compensation benefits to the spouse of a nurse who died of a myocardial infarction during a period of employment-related stress. Even though the nurse had a history of smoking, high cholesterol, high blood pressure, diabetes, and heart disease, the court stated that the requirement that the injury be job related is satisfied if a preexisting condition was aggravated by employment-related stress (*Herman v. Miners' Hospital*, 1991).

In Arkansas, an appeals court upheld denial of workers' compensation to a nursing home employee who gave false answers on a preemployment application. The nurses' aide had previous back surgery, which she did not disclose. At the nursing home, she again injured her back and sought workers' compensation benefits (*O'Leary v. Methodist Nursing Home,* 1991).

Workers' compensation is intended to be an exclusive remedy for work-related injuries. Sometimes, an employee will attempt to sue for negligence rather than to accept the standard financial award allowed under the state workers' compensation laws. In *Johns v. State Department of Health* (1985), an employee arrived at her hospital approximately 30 minutes before the beginning of her shift. As she waited in the lobby for her shift to begin, she was assaulted by a patient. She sued her employer for negligence, and the court held that her exclusive remedy was under the workers' compensation law because the employee was not outside the course and scope of her employment.

However, a contrary result was reached by a Michigan Court. In *Jarvis v. Providence Hospital* (1989), the court ruled that an employer may be held liable for damages when the death of a fetus results from a disease contracted by the mother in the workplace. A medical technician, who cut herself while working at the hospital, submitted an accident report and advised her supervisor that she was 3 months pregnant. The hospital failed to advise the employee to obtain a gamma globulin injection, which could have prevented hepatitis from developing, and also assured the employee that there was no risk of hepatitis. The employee subsequently developed hepatitis, and her child was stillborn. Although workers' compensation laws prevented the employee from suing her employer, the employee's husband sued the hospital on behalf of the fetus. The jury awarded $400,000, and the appeals court upheld the award.

In some cases, employees have successfully sued patients for injuries sustained in the workplace. In *Widlowski v. Durkee Foods* (1989), a nurse sued a patient and his employer for working conditions that caused the patient to become delirious and bite the nurse. The patient was overcome by nitrogen gas while cleaning an industrial tank and became delirious and incoherent. He was taken to a hospital, where he bit off the tip of the finger of a nurse caring for him. The court held that the injury to the nurse was reasonably foreseeable from the employer's negligence in allowing the patient to enter the tank without proper equipment.

In a Pennsylvania decision, an intoxicated patient struck a nurse in the stomach, causing a premature delivery and death of her baby. The verdict in favor of the hospital and against the patient for $40,000 was upheld even though the nurse had an opportunity to call for help when the patient began to get violent (*Warusz et al. v. Warminster General Hospital,* 1983).

Sexual Harassment

In 1986, in *Meritor Savings Bank v. Vinson,* the United States Supreme court approved sexual harassment as sex discrimination under Title VII of the Civil Rights Act. The court found that a supervisor's sexually harassing behavior may create a hostile environment.

Sexual harassment is a form of sex discrimination and is prohibited under Title VII of the Civil Rights Act of 1964. The costs of sexual harassment can be staggering. Poor productivity, excessive absenteeism, high turnover, and exorbitant litigation expenses underscore the need for correct, effective management of the problem (Horty, 1987).

The Equal Employment Opportunity Commission's (EEOC) guidelines on sexual harassment define two types of sexual harassment: quid pro quo and hostile environment. Quid pro quo harassment occurs when submission to or rejection of unwelcome sexual conduct by an individual is used as the basis for employment decisions affecting the individual. Unwelcome sexual conduct that interferes with an individual's job performance or creates an intimidating, hostile, or offensive working environment is considered hostile environment harassment. Title VII does not proscribe all conduct of a sexual nature in the workplace, only unwelcome sexual conduct. Unfortunately, the distinction between invited, uninvited but welcomed, offensive but tolerated, and flatly rejected sexual advances or conduct is often difficult to discern. The EEOC, however, offers some guidance on this issue. The challenged conduct must be unwelcome in the sense that the employee did not solicit or incite it and in the sense that the employee regarded the conduct as undesirable or offensive. Often, the question of whether the conduct is welcome or unwelcome will come down to a question of credibility, as was the case in the Clarence Thomas hearings. The EEOC states that when credibility is the sole issue, the claim of the employee charging harassment will be considerably strengthened if he or she made a contemporaneous complaint or protest to the alleged harasser, higher management, co-workers, or others. The EEOC is quick to point out, however, that although a complaint of protest is helpful to the charging employee's case, it is not a necessary element of the claim, especially in light of many employee's legitimate fears of repercussion.

Sexual harassment in the employment setting remains an ongoing problem that can expose employers to substantial liability. Increasingly, employees are ready and willing to formally complain about incidents of sexual harassment and to pursue their complaints through formal procedures. Employers must be prepared to respond with specific policies and review mechanisms (Duldt, 1982).

Employers often claim that they are not liable for acts of sexual harassment because they did not know that the harassment was occurring. Although it is clear that employers are not automatically liable for all acts of their supervisors and other employees, mere absence of notice to the employer does not necessarily insolate the employer from liability. Employers are liable for the wrongful acts of their employees if the employees had actual or apparent authority to perform the act or if the employer actually or apparently condoned the misconduct.

In a study of registered nurses, over 60% acknowledged that they had experienced some sort of sexual harassment on the job during the previous year (Editorial, 1989).

Under the common law doctrine of respondeat superior, employers generally are responsible for the negligent and, sometimes, intentional acts or omissions of employees acting in the course and within the scope of their employment.

Courts in many states, however, have struggled with the question of whether this rule should extend to illegal acts of an employee, such as sexual misconduct, committed while ostensibly on the job but without the employer's knowledge or consent. Most courts considering this issue have declined to extend the rule. However, these cases leave open the possibility that an employer could still be liable if there is evidence that the employer was negligent in hiring or monitoring its employees or had inadequate safety and security procedures (*Szczenbaniuk v. Memorial Hospital,* 1989).

In *G.L. v. Kaiser Foundation Hospitals, Inc.,* the court addressed the issue in the context of a sexual assault of a hospital patient by a hospital employee. The court noted that three requirements must be met to find an employer liable for an employee's acts under a respondeat superior theory under Oregon common law.

1. The employee's act must have occurred substantially within the time and space limits authorized by his employment.
2. The employee's motivation in performing the act, at least in part, must have been to serve the employer.
3. The act must have been of a kind that falls within the employee's specified duties.

A cause of action for negligence, however, may lie against a provider that fails to use due care in hiring, monitoring, and evaluating employees.

The hospital is an ideal environment for sexual harassment claims. Whereas the management and medical staff are substantially male, the entire workforce is predominantly female. Management has a special responsibility to establish an environment where sexual harassment is inhibited. This duty includes the education of employees and the prompt and thoughtful investigation of sexual harassment claims. The presence of a hostile environment may impose liability on the employer.

A physician brought action against a hospital administrator for the termination of his exclusive contract for the provision of radiology services. He had been discharged based on allegations of sexual harassment made by several hospital employees (*Walton v. Jennings Community Hospital,* 1989).

In an Indiana case, the court held that the public policy represented by the Indiana Peer Review Act was violated by a contract under which, in exchange for a physician's surrender of his medical staff privileges at a hospital, the institution agreed that it would not reveal that he had been under investigation for sexual harassment of the nursing staff.

In *Moire v. Temple University School of Medicine* (1985), a female physician brought action alleging that she had been sexually harassed by a professor and that she had received a failing grade requiring her to repeat her third year of medical school because she was female. The court held in favor of the defendants.

In *Estate of Scott v. deLeon* (1985), a pharmacy assistant at a university hospital committed suicide allegedly based on a lengthy period of sexual harassment by her supervisor that was allegedly ignored by those she reported to.

The court held that sexual harassment could violate the equal protection clause and section 1983 of the Civil Rights Act.

In *Fisher v. San Pedro Peninsula Hospital* (1989), the California Court of Appeals explored the question of whether a nurse can recover for sexual harassment when offensive comments and conduct of a sexual nature occur in her presence even if she is not the intended victim of the conduct. The court found that offensive sexual conduct not directed at the nurse could still create a hostile work environment and thus form the basis of a claim for sexual harassment. The conduct allegedly consisted of pulling nurses onto his lap, hugging and kissing them while wiggling, making offensive statements of a sexual nature, moving his hands in the direction of a woman's vaginal area, grabbing women from the back with his hands on their breasts or in the area of their breasts, picking up women and swinging them around, throwing a woman on a gurney, walking up closely behind a woman with movements of his pelvic area, and making lewd remarks about the breasts of anesthetized female patients. All of this conduct occurred in the hospital.

In *Lipsett v. University of Puerto Rico* (1988) a female participant in the university medical school surgical residency program established a quid pro quo sexual harassment case against the director of the program.

Occupational Safety and Health Act

In addition to other legislation described in this chapter, the Occupational Safety and Health Act (OSHA) and right-to-know laws have been enacted to protect the worker.

The OSHA of the 1970s was an attempt to reduce work-related injuries and illness that impose substantial burden on commerce through lost production, wage loss, medical expenses, and disability compensation payments.

OSHA grants employees the right to question unsafe conditions and request a federal inspection. Employees have the right to refuse to perform hazardous job activities where they reasonably believe there is a real danger of death or injury and there is no time to request administrative action to remedy the danger. However, employees risk termination if it is subsequently determined that they acted unreasonably or in bad faith *(29 CFR ch. XVII s1901)*.

Worker right-to-know laws have been enacted by many states. These statutes require employers to notify employees when they are working with specific toxic or hazardous substances *[Fed. Reg. 52(163): 31852-86]*.

LICENSURE

Any discussion of the legal implication of labor law would be incomplete without addressing the loss of nursing license. Loss of licensure terminates the nurse's ability to practice the profession. The nurse manager is frequently involved in identification and reporting of problems that may lead to the individual nurse's licensure restrictions. The nurse manager, faced with this situation, is frequently in conflict because of the desire to provide for safe, quality patient care and the realization that to achieve this primary goal, a nurse may lose his or her livelihood.

Nurse Practice Act

The legal basis for licensure rests on the government's responsibility to protect the health, safety, and welfare of the public. Licensure establishes standards for entry into practice, defines a scope of practice, and allows for disciplinary action (Cushing, 1986). The Nurse Practice Act defines and limits the practice of nursing and thereby determines what constitutes unauthorized practice or practice that exceeds the scope of authority. In addition to the Act, rules, regulations, board rulings, and advisory opinions offer some guidance.

Grounds for disciplinary action are enumerated in the Nurse Practice Act. Although these reasons differ somewhat from state to state, the general categories usually include fraud and deceit, criminal acts, incompetence, substance abuse, mental incompetence, and unprofessional conduct. As with any legislative enactment, the courts must determine on a case by case basis how these laws should be interpreted. In *Tuma v. Board of Nursing of the State of Idaho* (1979), the court held that responding to a patient's request for information regarding the use of Laetrile was not unprofessional conduct. In *Leukhardt v. Commonwealth of Pennsylvania State Board of Nurse Examiners* (1979), the court held that a nurse should not have been reprimanded for unprofessional conduct because she slapped a patient to make him release his grasp on another nurse's arm.

If the state board has received a complaint, they must investigate and decide whether to discipline. Notice must be given to the nurse, stating the charges as well as the time and place of the hearing. Due process requirements include this as well as the right to cross-examine witnesses, the right to produce witnesses, the right to appear with counsel, the right to a record of the proceeding, and the right to a judicial review.

Nurses frequently express concern regarding the possibility of loss of licensure. For the most part, the situations on which the questions are based do not deal with licensure issues. For example, a hospital may decide to ask nurses to participate in a new procedure, e.g., a policy requiring obstetric nurses to perform vaginal examinations on women in labor. Nurses, faced with this new policy, may be concerned about a perceived threat to their nursing licenses. In reality, situations like this rarely affect nurses' licenses. Nurse Practice Acts usually have a great deal of flexibility to allow for changes and growth within the nursing profession. Although some nurses would like more specific direction and guidance from the state board, it is often an advantage to the nursing profession to have this degree of flexibility. This allows the profession to develop from within as the customary standards of nursing evolve to match the evolution of health care delivery.

If the hospital or a physician insists that a nurse perform an activity that is clearly contraindicated in a particular state's law, it is important to understand that the nurse cannot be protected from a possible loss of license by a third party. The third party does not have the ability to infringe on the licensing authority of the state. For example, if a state has determined that licensed practical nurses are not permitted to administer injections to children in doctors' offices, no physician can require a nurse to perform this action.

The quote, "My license is on the line," frequently indicates a nurse's misunderstanding of the issue. What is more likely to be a valid concern is the issue of malpractice liability. As a general rule, the health care institution or agency can insure or indemnify its nurses for any activity that is not clearly proscribed by law. As long as the hospital authorizes the procedure or activity, insurance coverage or indemnification will be provided (Northrup, 1987).

The Chemically Dependent Nurse and the Law

The Board of Nursing properly suspended a registered nurse's license indefinitely when he admitted that while working for a hospital, he had misappropriated Demerol and morphine sulfate for his own use and had replaced them with water or saline solution. Although such conduct might not evidence habitual intemperance or addiction to drugs, suspension was appropriate because such actions demonstrated that the nurse was unfit or incompetent and that he had engaged in behavior that created an undue risk of harm to others (*Matter of Mostrom*, 1986).

One of the most difficult issues facing the health care delivery system today is the issue of the impaired health care provider. This issue reflects a basic societal problem. The prevalence of chemical abuse permeates all levels of society. Although impairment may technically refer to physical as well as emotional impairment, most cases today deal with impairment due to drug or alcohol abuse.

Many state boards of nursing report chemical dependency as the leading cause of disciplinary proceedings. Since addiction often goes untreated and undetected, the reported prevalence may be low. Nevertheless the number of nurses addicted is reported to be 10% to 12%. This means that among every 15 nurses employed in the hospital, at least 1 will have a serious alcohol or drug-related problem (Horty, 1990).

Identification of the impaired nurse is critical if the hospital is to protect patients from harm and itself against liability. The hospital's authority to deal with a nurse's impairment derives from its legal responsibilities, both as the nurse's employer (vicarious liability) and as a corporation that owes a duty to patients for the quality of care received under the doctrine of corporate liability. The way a hospital intervenes when there is reasonable evidence that a nurse is addicted may determine whether other nurses request help or decide to hide their problems.

If the price of requesting help is loss of job or professional license or both, the impaired nurse will seldom seek help. A disciplinary response to addiction also makes it difficult for peers to deal with the problem. Haack and Hughes (1989) write about this common problem of mutual denial among professionals.

> Chemically dependent nurses do not fit the commonly held image of an alcoholic or drug addict, and co-workers can easily attribute signs and symptoms of a progressing addiction to the impaired colleague's stressful work or home environment. Furthermore, even when chemical dependency is strongly suspected, nurses are reluctant to report their suspicions. While failure to intervene may reflect a desire to protect a

colleague from punitive sanctions, such "enabling" responses deny the chemically impaired nurse much needed assistance and place at continued risk those patients for whom the nurse is responsible.

In 1985, the National Nurses Society on Addictions (NNSA) published model legislation, the Statement of Model Diversion Legislation for Chemically Impaired Nurses. This statement is not law but is intended to serve as a model for states seeking to enact their own statutory diversion programs. It establishes one or more board-appointed committees that screen nurse applicants for diversion, review treatment regimens, monitor the progress of individual nurses, and make determinations as to the reentry of those nurses into practice. Direct intervention, treatment, and follow-up of the nurses is conducted through approved regional peer assistance programs and employee assistance programs, subject to the terms of contracts with the state committees. The model law also provides

- An optional increase of licensure fees to cover the cost of the program
- Mandatory advisement to impaired nurses appearing before the board of nursing of the opportunity for diversion
- Development of written diversion agreements between the nurse and the committee
- Confidentiality with respect to all program treatment records
- Immunity from civil damages for defamation for individuals making reports "in good faith and with some reasonable basis in fact"
- Purging of diversion records on request of the nurse after 5 years of successful recovery

The model requires that a nurse's "failure to cooperate and comply (with the program) shall be reported to the Board by the committee and may result in termination of the diversion procedure." The model statement includes a significant provision granting qualified immunity from civil damages resulting from subsequent professional negligence of a nurse diversionee to all persons responsible for administering the diversion, providing treatment, and performing follow-up supervision of the nurse (NNSA, 1985).

The nurse returning to the workplace following treatment for chemical dependency is protected by the Rehabilitation Act of 1973. In a Kansas case, the court held that the hospital violated the Act through its refusal to hire a nurse who had been free of drugs for over 9 months to work in the ICU only because of her handicap—drug addiction (*Wallace v. VA, 1988*).

Because of the unique responsibility to care for a patient's life, health, and well-being, hospitals are well advised to evaluate and develop a substance abuse program. A hospital that intends to screen applicants should determine whether all applicants will be screened or only applicants for certain high-risk drug-access positions. An employer concerned with the risk to patients or others presented by an impaired employee improperly performing his or her job might determine that testing of applicants for certain nonhigh-risk jobs, such as clerical positions, is not necessary. However, where the employer's objective is to eliminate or reduce employee impairment, testing of applicants for all positions would accomplish this objective. Preemployment screening of applicants for positions in which an impaired employee constitutes a threat to patient safety may be particularly appropriate and advisable (Olson & Husson, 1990).

In *Jensen v. Mary Lanning Memorial Hospital* (1986), the Supreme Court of Nebraska upheld a hospital's action in terminating a nurses' aide from employment when she reported to work with alcohol on her breath. The aide had received two prior written warnings. In addition, the court held that the aide's "misconduct" disqualified her from unemployment benefits. The court said

> Jensen, as a nursing assistant, necessarily came into close personal contact with hospital patients. Whether she was intoxicated or not, the Hospital was not unreasonable in requiring such an employee to report to work without the odor of alcohol on her breath. Such an odor, detected at close range by a hospital patient, could well cause personal distress to the patient and weaken the patient's confidence in the abilities of the hospital's employees to properly care for patients entrusted to the hospital for treatment.

Confidential reporting within the hospital by co-workers should be encouraged. Proof of an addiction is not necessary for such a report. Factual information resulting in a belief that a problem exists should be communicated as objectively as possible. The identity of the employee bringing forward the information should be protected from discovery. The nurse manager's investigation either will confirm or deny the initial information. If confirmed, hospital policy will then determine appropriate action.

Nurses may fear a defamation lawsuit for filing such reports if the report turns out to be unsupported. As long as the nurse follows the rules and does not knowingly make false statements or intentionally intend to be malicious, a defamation lawsuit based on the report will not be successful (Stickler & Nelson, 1988).

In a Mississippi case (*Kemp v. Claiborne County Hospital,* 1991), the hospital's drug-testing program was both reasonable and not violative of plaintiff employee's Fourth Amendment rights. The court determined that plaintiff, a purchasing agent and operating room scrub technician, held a safety-sensitive position and was therefore subject to defendant's nonindividualized drug-testing program.

After learning of possible substance abuse in the workplace, defendant instituted a hospitalwide drug-testing program. Defendant gave all employees written notice of the test, which required employees to give blood and urine samples. The test required employees to undress completely and change into a hospital gown before providing a urine sample to prevent tampering with the specimen. The employees were allowed to undress in privacy behind a partition.

All employees, including plaintiff, gave written consent before the test. Despite providing such consent, plaintiff refused to comply with defendant's testing program because she was reluctant to undress. Plaintiff suggested an alternate method for producing a specimen, but defendant refused, stating it was more intrusive of plaintiff's privacy than the standard procedure and could possibly prejudice the overall testing results.

The reasonableness of the search was calculated by weighing the governmental interest in protecting the public from immediate threats to physical safety against plaintiff's rights to privacy. The court also noted that testing without individualized suspicion was permissible for individuals holding safety-sensitive positions, and the degree of safety sensitivity was an important factor in determining the reasonableness of the test.

In finding plaintiff's position as a scrub technician was safety sensitive, the court noted that plaintiff might allow a patient to fall from a gurney or operating table, bump into a surgeon during surgery, or fail to account for all of the sponges if she was impaired by drugs or alcohol. Furthermore, the court cited case law that held that a nurse was a safety-sensitive employee. The court concluded that the government's compelling interest in protecting the public from such potential harm outweighed plaintiff's expectation of privacy.

References

29 CFR ch. XVII s1901.

29 U.S.C. s701 (1986).

29 U.S.C. s794-794a.

42 U.S.C.2000e; 29 U.S.C. 158 (a)(1)(4).

42 U.S.C.A. s12, 101-12,213 (West Supp. 1991).

52 ALR4th 853.

488 A.2d 229 (N.J. 1985).

Brent, N.J. (19912). The impaired nurse: Assisting treatment to achieve continued employment. *Journal of Health and Hospital Law, 24*(4), 113.

Brown, C. (1991). Background checks questioned: Nurse and hospitals are sued. *Hospital Risk Management, 13*(10), 130.

Crockett v. Mid-America Health Services, 780 S.W.2d 656 (Mo.App. 1989).

Cushing, M. (1986). How courts look at nurse practice acts. *American Journal of Nursing, 86*(2), 131–132.

Decker, K.H. (1987). *Employee privacy: Law and practice.* New York: John Wiley & Sons.

Decker, K.H. (1984). *Handbook and employment policies—Employer beware.* 20 U.Pitt. L. Commerce 207.

Deering West Nursing Center v. Scott, 787 S.W.2d 484 (Texas App.1990).

Duldt, B.W. (1982). Sexual harassment in nursing. *Nursing Outlook, 30*(6), 336–337.

Editorial. (1989, July). Sexual harrassment. *Hospital Risk Control, 3*(8), 1–7.

Caroline Eli v. Griggs County Hospital and Nursing Home et al., Supreme Court of North Dakota, Civil No. 11, 011, April 10, 1986.

Elwood v. State Accident Insurance Fund Corp., 676 P.2d 922 (1984).

Fed. Reg. 52(163): 31852-86.

Fiesta, J. (1988). *The law and liability: A guide for nurses* (2nd ed.). New York: Delmar Publishers.

Fiesta, J. (1990). The nursing shortage: Whose liability problem. *Nursing Management, 21* (2).

Fiesta, J. (1994). *20 Legal pitfalls for nurses to avoid.* New York: Delmar Publishers.

Finley v. Beverly Enterprises, Inc., 499 So.2d 1366 (Alabama 1986).

Fisher v. San Pedro Peninsula Hospital, 262 Cal.Rptr.842 (Calif.Ct. of App., Oct. 2, 1989 as modified, Oct. 16, 1989).

Francis v. Memorial General Hospital (N.M. 1986).

Gault v. University of Chicago Hosp. No.90 c0321 (U.S.Distr.Ct., March 18, 1991).

Gornik, S. R. (1992) Note: An exception to the employment-at-will doctrine for nurses. *Health Matrix, 2*(89), 111.

Haack, M.R., & Hughes, T.L. (1989). *Addiction in the nursing profession.* New York: Springer.

Havens v. Tomball Community Hospital, 793 S.W.2d 690 (Texas App. 1990).

Henry, K.H. (1984). *The health care supervisor's legal guide.* Gaithersburg, MD: Aspen Publications.

Herman v. Miners, Hospital, No. 19, 488, New Mexico Sup.Ct., Feb. 28, 1991.

Hollander, P.A. (1978). *Legal handbook for educators.* Boulder, CO: Westview Press.

Horty, J. (1987). Hospitals can be liable when supervisors are linked to sexual harassment incidents. *Modern Healthcare, 17*(23), 142.

Horty, J. (1990, June–July). Chapter 4: Helping the addicted nurse—Legal alternatives. *Patient Care Law,* An Action-Kit publication, 2.

Hubbard Regional Hospital v. National Labor Relations Act, 579 F.2d 1251 (Calif. 1978).

Husson, J.J., & Bond, R.F. (1991). Health care providers can avoid negligent hiring claims. *HealthSpan, 8*(2) 3–8.

Jarvis v. Providence Hospital, 178 Mich.App. 586 (1989).

Jensen v. Mary Lanning Memorial Hospital, 357 N.W.2d 144 (Neb. 1986).

Johns v. state Department of Health, 485 So.2d 857 (Fl 1985).

Jones v. Memorial Hospital System, 677 S.W.2d 221 (Texas 1984).

Kachmar v. Pennsylvania, 559 A.2d 606 (Pa.Commonwealth 1989).

Kahn v. State of Minnesota, 289 N.W.2d 737 (Minn. 1980).

Kemp v. Claiborne County Hospital, no. W89-0076 (b) (U.S.Dist.Ct.S.D.Miss., June 4, 1991).

Lampe v. Presbyterian Medical Center, 590 P.2d 53 (Colorado 1978).

Leukhardt v. Commonwealth of Pennsylvania State Board of Nurse Examiners, July 1979.

Lipsett v. Univ. of Puerto Rico, 864 F.2d 881 (1st Cir. 1988).

Louisiana Department of Health & Hospitals v. Jeffress, 593 So.2d 680 (La. 1991).

Matter of Mostrom, 390 N.W.2d 893 (Minn. App. 1986).

McCandless, S.R., & Cortez, P.J. (1990, winter). Employer–employee relations: Managing workplace issues in the 90s. *Tort and Insurance Law Journal, 25* (2), 258.

Meritor Savings Bank v. Vinson, 477 U.S.,57,106 S.Ct.2399 (1986).

Mock v. LaGuardia Hospital, Michigan Comp. Laws 15.3615.369 (1980).

Moire v. Temple University School of Medicine, 613 F.Supp. 1360 (1985).

National Nurses Society on Addictions. (1985). Statement on model diversion legislation for chemically impaired nurses.

Nelson, K.L. (1989). Agency nurses pose growing liability. *Forum, 10*(1), 6.

Northrup, C.A. (1987). *Legal issues in nursing*. St. Louis, MO: C. V. Mosby Company.

O'Leary v. Methodist Nursing Home, No. CA 90-357, Arkansas Court of Appeals, May 8, 1991.

Olson, S.M. & Husson, J.J. (1990). Hospital obligations toward recovering addicted employees. *HealthSpan, 7*(4), 3.

Politis, E. K. (1983, fall). Nurses' legal dilemma when hospital staffing compromises professional standards. *University of San Francisco Law Review, 18*, 112.

Restatement (Second) of Tort s18.

Restatement (Second) of Tort s35.

Schalk v. Gallemore, 906 F.2d 491, (C.A. 10, Kansas 1990).

Schurgin, W. P., & Rowland, D.J. (1991). Disability discrimination in the 1990s. An overview of the employment provisions of the Americans with Disabilities Act. *Journal of Health and Hospital Law, 244*(9), 278.

Scott, Estate of, v. deLeon, 603 F.Supp 1328, (1985).

Seery v. Yale-New Haven Hospital, 554 A2d 757 (Conn.Ct.App. 1989).

Sparks v. Tulane Medical Center Hospital, 537 So2d 276 (La. 1988).

Stickler, B.K. & Nelson, M.D. (1988). Defamation in the workplace: Employer rights, risks and responsibilities. *Journal of Health and Hospital Law, 21* (3), 97.

Szczenbaniuk v. Memorial Hospital for McHenry County, 536 N.E.2d 138 (IND.1989).

Thompson v. Nason, 591 A.2d 703 (Pa. 1991).

Touissant v. Blue Cross/Shield of Michigan, 292 N.W.2d 880 (1990).

Tuma v. Board of Nursing of the State of Idaho, 593 P.2d 711 (1979).

Wagenseller v. Scottsdale Memorial Hospital, 74 P.2d 412 (Ariz. 1984).

Wallace v. Veterans Administration, 683 F.Supp. 758 (Kansas 1988).

Walton v. Jennings Community Hospital, Inc., 875 F.2d 1317 (7th Cir. 1989).

Warusz et al. v. Warminster General Hospital, No. 27-12302-12 (Pa. 1983).

Wheelers v. Manning, 682 F.Supp. 869 (S.D. Miss. 1987).

Widlowski v. Durbec Foods, 546 N.E.2d 770 (Ill. 1989).

Wilson N. Jones Memorial Hospital v. Davis, 553 S.W.2d 180 (Texas App.1977).

CHAPTER 21

COLLABORATIVE PRACTICE IN A UNION ENVIRONMENT

NANCY STEIGER
ROBIN HAGENSTAD
SUSAN GADBOIS

EXECUTIVE SUMMARY

Empowerment may be the theme of the 1990s, but can it work in a union setting? According to the staff of Santa Rosa Memorial Hospital in northern California, the answer is a resounding Yes. This chapter examines collaborative practice and reviews the activities of the Staff Nurses' Association at Santa Rosa in collaboration with Nursing administration in implementing a professional practice model.

At its core, collaborative practice (also called self-governance, shared governance, or professional practice) gives nurses a voice and allows them to make decisions about their practice. The chapter defines governance and management and moves on to a brief discussion of labor relations. It then chronicles the events that led to the development of the Santa Rosa Professional Practice Model. DRGs, escalating costs, and downsizing led to a reorganization of hospital administration. Work previously done by management was redistributed to councils made up of managers and staff. This action decreased costs and increased opportunities for nurses to participate in decision making. In 1989, members of nursing management and the Staff Nurses' Association board decided to develop a professional practice model.

Details of the model are provided in the chapter and its appendix. A decision by the National Labor Relations Board at Yeshiva University, New York, also is reviewed for its impact on registered nurse unions in regard to employees' decision-making power and the role of the union in governance activities.

The councils and the professional practice model of Santa Rosa Memorial Hospital are alive and well. One of the most significant results: previously unsolvable problems are now solved by those vested in the solution.

E mpowerment, the theme of the 1990s, is the ability to change and influence others in nursing to exercise control over nursing practice. Recently, a variety of strategies have been employed to empower nurses. Collaborative practice models have been used as vehicles to help empower nurses and shape nursing practice. Although these models have gained popularity in their effectiveness over the last 10 years, it has been said that such models cannot be implemented in the presence of a union. This chapter describes how to overcome the obstacles of implementing a professional practice model in a union setting. We compare and contrast traditional and bureaucratic models as a basis for the professional practice model at Santa Rosa Memorial Hospital and describe the necessary structure and relationship to implement a collaborative practice model in a union environment. Although we are still journeying toward our goals, we experienced a cultural change that has elements of magic. Our goals have become clear, but the road map is still evolving. Thus, this is not the end of our story.

Santa Rosa Memorial Hospital is a 225-bed full-service, not-for-profit hospital in Northern California, sponsored by the Sisters of St. Joseph of Orange through the St. Joseph Health System. We who are associated with Santa Rosa Memorial Hospital are committed to four core values: dignity, service, excellence, and justice. These values are a foundation on which the model is constructed, and they support the continuing evolution of our professional practice model.

COLLABORATIVE PRACTICE DEFINED

Nurses want a voice. They want to participate in decisions about their practice. This desire is appropriate in that quality care, professional satisfaction, and individual values all dictate that practitioners must be directly involved in decisions about how they practice. Four of the many different models that have been developed in an effort to enhance nurses' participation in the governance of nursing are (1) self-governance, (2) shared governance, (3) collaborative practice, and (4) professional practice.

These models suggest a new way of governing nursing, a different philosophy for thinking and practicing. According to McDonough (1990), governance in its most generic sense refers to the operations or structure through which a governing body exercises its authority and performs its function. In contrast to management, which directs or controls specific functions or groups, governance is broader and describes the entire structure and process by which a professional group functions.

The bureaucratic models employed in many hospitals and health care organizations are designed to control and centralize to increase efficiency. The autonomy and control over practice that nurses are so interested in frequently are not possible or are not integrated into institutions relying on these bureaucratic, top–down communication, task-oriented systems. Perhaps it was partially for this reason that in 1988, the Secretary's Commission on Nursing, established to address the critical shortage of registered nurses, recommended that models be developed to enhance nurses' decision-making ability.

Nursing's goal is to meet the needs of those they serve. As well, nurses have an obligation to the public and the profession of nursing. This is accomplished when nurses in all roles and settings share the conviction that responsibility and accountability are shared and that the wholeness of the profession is preserved. It is incumbent upon us to develop models that allow nurses and nursing to grow and develop and serve this vital role.

LABOR RELATIONS HISTORY

Registered nurse participation in labor unions may have developed, at least partially, as an effort to exert influence over the conditions of their practice of nursing. In the past, those registered nurses in California who wished to be represented by a union have chosen two major routes—professional associations or unions with a more traditional industrial union perspective. Within the last 20 years, those choices have expanded to independent associations or unions—of which the Staff Nurses' Association of Santa Rosa Memorial Hospital is one—and such unions as UNAC (affiliated with AFSCME) and Local 250 (AFL-CIO), which have extensive histories representing employees outside the industrial arena. The relationships between labor organizations and management have sometimes been strained and polarized.

To explore creative and less adversarial ways to govern institutions, new relationships between employees and employers are being developed collaboratively.

A variety of companies and unions outside of health care have moved from the more traditional labor–management relationship to innovative approaches to the governance of their institutions. During the 1980s, perhaps driven by the need of some American industries to survive foreign competition, there was some success in forming relationships between labor and management. These relationships were formed to identify and achieve common goals accomplished by employee participation in decision making about the product and the production process (Deming, 1951).

In part, these relationships are based on a recognition of certain positive aspects of the Japanese model and Deming's principles (1951) of involving all of one's resources, including all employees' brains, in product quality and improvement. Many companies that have instituted cooperative programs have experienced a higher overall operating performance.

The most well-known example of this trend is the American auto industry and the United Auto Workers, who have reached some common understandings that assist in putting the industry in the best position to compete. Quality Circles have been used to a great extent. Also, in some cases, policy dictates that assembly line workers have the right to stop the assembly line to correct a problem in production.

Other examples of innovative approaches to labor–management relations include Dayton Power and Light, where the 14-page compact negotiated by union and management is a philosophy statement about the common understanding of the rights and responsibilities of employees and employers, with a system for resolving disputes based on trust and common sense. It also contains a joint vision of the future (Labor–Management Cooperation, 1989).

Northwestern Power and Light is another example of a company in which management and union leadership have made concerted efforts at team building and mutual respect and understanding of each other's point of view.

The U.S. Department of Labor actively supports, with grants and speakers, the development of new conflict resolution strategies among union and management leaders.

SANTA ROSA MEMORIAL HOSPITAL BEFORE THE PROFESSIONAL PRACTICE MODEL
Organization of the Staff Nurses' Association

The Staff Nurses' Association (SNA) at Santa Rosa Memorial Hospital was first organized by the California Nurse's Association (CNA) in 1974. The staff nurses decided 1 year later to decertify CNA and to form their own, independent association. From SNA's perspective, contract negotiations between 1975 and 1977 were characterized by brief discussions between the staff nurses and the administrator of the hospital.

Strained Relations Between the Staff Nurses' Association and the Hospital Administration

Whether or not it was a casual factor, SNA viewed adversity between the parties as escalating in 1977 when contract negotiations were for the first time conducted with spokespersons representing the hospital and SNA. The staff nurses were unprepared for the tenor of those negotiations.

From 1980 to 1988 relationships between the SNA and the Santa Rosa Memorial Hospital administration frequently were strained, with greater intensity during contract negotiations. Staff nurses and the SNA Board (elected staff nurses) were convinced that the hospital's intent was to destroy their power to have any control over their working environment and practice of nursing. Discussions were periodically characterized by rancorous debate, with neither side willing to regard the other as equally empowered, each party coming to the table with widely divergent agendas and points of view. Under these circumstances, common ground could be extremely difficult to find, and options for resolution were limited.

Bureaucracy Inhibits Communication and Slows Decision Making

In the early to mid-1980s, Santa Rosa Memorial Hospital's nursing division was typical of bureaucratic administrative structures. Four nursing directors reported to the vice president of nursing. There was a total of 20 nurse managers reporting to the nursing directors. The directors and managers were grouped and organized around specialties.

Decision making could be slow and tedious as problems were shunted up to the top of the organization. When this happened, frustration would mount as both manager and staff waited for the decisions to trickle back down. An example of this occurred when the newly developed standards committee began to implement the Marker Model. Starting with the structure standards for the nursing division, the committee labored industriously for several months to organize existing written and unwritten policy into standards. The committee members found that they were unable to continue because they did not have the authority to make the decisions necessary to complete the standards. The structure standards were given to the nursing directors and vice president for their completion and approval. Because of the heavy workload and multiple responsibilities of these individuals, the standards were never completed by the committee.

The administrative structure also made it difficult for one section (e.g., medical–surgical) to make a decision that would affect another section (e.g., critical care). The individual sections met once a week, but the entire nursing management team met only once a month. This led to a lack of consistency in communication between the nursing departments, which had an impact on contract implementation.

The communication problems led to mistrust and confusion. The staff nurses thought that decisions were unilateral, autocratic, and untraceable. Each department acted independently and without regard for the impact of its actions on the whole.

There were overlapping responsibilities between the manager and the director roles, which caused some managers to feel powerless, frustrated, and unsupported. Additionally, the staff believed that they had minimal opportunities to participate in decision making or committee work. The exception to this was the standards committee, which after its experience with the structure standards, focused solely on clinical procedures and protocols. Like the structure standards, the clinical procedures and protocols also required approval from the administrative nursing group. This structure encumbered the process.

DRGs, Escalating Costs, and Declining Reimbursement

At the same time, the implementation of the DRGs was being felt, and like many other hospitals in the United States, Santa Rosa Memorial Hospital was trying to cope with escalating costs and declining reimbursement. In 1987, the hospital tried numerous cost-containment plans and projects without success. By early 1988, it was necessary to undertake a major downsizing to achieve fiscal stability.

A New Administrative Team is Assigned

Concurrently, the CEO and vice president of nursing resigned. The health system assigned a new administrative team (CEO, COO, and CFO) to Santa Rosa Memorial Hospital. At that time, there were several vacant positions on the nursing management team, and those managers remaining were frustrated with the current structure and began researching different ways of organizing the work of the nursing division to cut costs and FTEs. The structure they developed led to downsizing the management team by decreasing the director positions from 4 to 1 and the manager positions from 20 to 8 and to eliminate 2.4 FTEs in the education department (for a total reduction of 17.4 FTEs in nursing administration). Also, in the model proposed by the nursing management council, the workload previously done at the management level would be distributed to councils composed of managers and staff. This would serve a dual purpose, decreasing costs and increasing the opportunities for nurse participation and decision making.

Negotiation and Problem Solving

In early 1988, the new administrative team approached the SNA's leadership regarding their concerns about the 1988 contract negotiations. The SNA Board indicated its support for a new approach by both parties negotiating without counsel at the table. Because of the fiscal instability of the institution, both parties also agreed to bring a minimal number of proposals to the table and to be as reasonable as possible about the wage proposal. This approach led to actual discussion and problem solving of issues at the table and an atmosphere of mutual respect. Most notable was that the negotiations were completed 2 weeks early, and for the first time in their negotiation history, the SNA leadership did not feel it was necessary to hold a strike vote.

The positive experience at the negotiating table led to the establishment of trust and a willingness on the part of both management and staff to work together to develop the professional practice model.

Development of the Model

The model evolved during 1988 and 1989 as changes were made to meet the needs of the staff and the hospital. It was a very pragmatic beginning. The councils began by developing a purpose statement and a list of responsibilities for each council. For example, in its 1987 JCAHO survey, the hospital had numerous contingencies, and thus each council focused its efforts toward improving patient care and assuring that the nursing division was in compliance with JCAHO standards.

Each council's early focus was very basic and primarily aimed at establishing fiscal stability, nursing standards of care, and implementation of the Ten-Step Model in the Quality Assurance Program. Councils were composed of managers and staff who began to develop mutual trust and respect as they worked together to solve problems.

As time went on, the councils became cohesive as they discussed issues and shared responsibility for making decisions and as clinical nurses were involved in decision making and in identifying opportunities to improve care and control costs.

During the first year, limited time and resources limited education for staff and managers about shared governance. No formal analysis of the model was done during this period. The workload was tremendous, but the councils rolled up their sleeves and got to work. There were advantages to this pragmatic approach as we began demonstrating early success of the model. The nurses participating in the councils had a positive experience in that their council did not just talk about issues; they took action to solve problems. The members of each council were learning about their responsibilities as they worked, a concept substantiated by Knowles' adult learning theory (1978). For example, the Nursing Quality Assurance Council members studied the Ten-Step QA Model and developed a quality assurance program. The Nursing Education Council membership learned how to coordinate classes, write objectives and evaluate programs, and plan the annual education calendar.

Success of the Councils

During the first year and a half, the amount of work accomplished by the councils was phenomenal. In March of 1990, for example, the JCAHO survey led to accreditation with substantial compliance, and the hospital was in the 10% of hospitals that received a letter of commendation from JCAHO. We believe that the councils' work was a significant factor in this JCAHO result.

Role of the Assistant Nurse Manager

At the same time, the management team was becoming more cohesive. The flatter, consolidated management structure improved communication between nursing departments and managers. Issues of inconsistent policies and supervision were unearthed and resolved. The managers were more autonomous and accountable for their performance. The assistant nurse manager role, established in 1986, became a vital link in the management team. The role of the assistant nurse manager improved communication with staff, and staff had access to their immediate supervisor, who was working side by side with them.

In the fall of 1989, the SNA board members and four members of the nursing management team attended an excellent conference, "Collaborative Governance: Innovation in Action," sponsored by Roseville Hospital, Roseville, California. When we returned, we were motivated to frame our own model. It was important to us that we were all speaking the same language and that our goals were in alignment.

Creation of a Vision Statement

To accomplish this, the group who attended the conference held a 1-day retreat in November 1989. That day we experienced tremendous synergism and created our vision statement (following page). As a group, we brainstormed together and listed the adjectives that described the environment in which we wanted to practice. Not one word is in the statement by chance. Each word was selected because it was meaningful to us. We wrote the vision first but did not completely define and make explicit our expectations, and the principles were developed to further articulate our goals. Although this was not a road map for implementation of the model, it became a framework of guiding principles.

At Santa Rosa Memorial Hospital, managers and union leaders worked together to assure that each group's point of view was considered in designing the model. In a setting where employees are represented by a union, it is important to involve union leadership in the discussion and formation of the model from the start.

- Management must avoid the appearance of establishing their own labor organizations—councils or committees—without union participation or agreement.
- Management must not sidestep the union while negotiating issues that are subject to collective bargaining—wages, hours, and terms and conditions of employment. These issues, should they arise in a council or committee discussion, should be referred to union and hospital leadership and contract forums.
- The level or type of staff nurse participation and decision making must be determined so that staff nurses maintain their distinction from management,

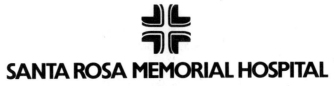

SANTA ROSA MEMORIAL HOSPITAL

A Sisters of St. Joseph of Orange Corporation

DIVISION OF NURSING

VISION STATEMENT

The vision and commitment of nurses at Santa Rosa Memorial Hospital has created a Professional Practice Model which empowers them to practice in a dynamic, collaborative environment. This supportive atmosphere promotes relationships based on trust, acceptance and equity. Nursing practice is characterized by autonomy, accountability and clinical expertise. We recognize that this is an evolving process toward continued growth and excellence. The following principles articulate the Professional Practice Model.

1. We recognize that integrity is the foundation of the Professional Practice Model.

2. We recognize the unique contribution of each individual.

3. We recognize each person has the opportunity and responsibility to contribute to the success of the Professional Practice Model.

4. We recognize that communications are open, honest, direct and caring.

5. We recognize that risk taking in a supportive environment facilitates growth and development.

6. We recognize that knowledge empowers decision making.

7. We recognize the changing health care environment requires flexibility and adaptability.

8. We recognize that quality health care is best accomplished through an interdisciplinary team approach.

9. We recognize decisions will acknowledge federal and state regulations and reasonable economic restraints.

10. We recognize that the Professional Practice Model reflects the values of the Sisters of St. Joseph of Orange.

1165 Montgomery Drive/P.O. Box 522, Santa Rosa, California 95402   (707) 546-3210

Figure 21–1   Santa Rosa Memorial Hospital Division of Nursing Professional Practice Model.

reassuring the union that implementation of the model will not jeopardize its ability to continue its status as a collective bargaining representative.

INFLUENCE OF THE NATIONAL LABOR RELATIONS DECISION

A decision made by the National Labor Relations Board in the early 1980s certainly has influenced the development of collaborative governance in union settings.

Professors at Yeshiva University in New York were denied their petition for union representation because the NLRB ruled that by virtue of their participation in faculty senates and tenure board, the professors were so intimately involved in the governance of the university that they exercised managerial functions and were not statutory employees entitled to union representation (NLRB v. Yeshiva University, 1980). As a result, leaders and members of unions who were participating or contemplating participating in a collaborative governance model were concerned by this decision. Some unions have chosen to withdraw their support and participation.

Therefore, for registered nurse unions, the Yeshiva decision illustrated the need to carefully define employees' decision-making power and the role of the union in governance activities. More recently, the NLRB ruled that the Electromation, Inc., Action Committee comprised of employees and management, violated federal labor laws as an employer-dominated labor organization (1992). According to hospital attorney Arthur Beck of Milwaukee, hospitals with employee committees, whether or not there is union representation, are advised to have their lawyers review all existing articles and bylaws creating the committees. These should spell out what the committees can address, and employment conditions normally subject to collective bargaining should not be included. Beck goes on to say that hospitals are particularly vulnerable to unfair labor practice charges if their nurses can deal with wages, shift times, flexible hours, or staffing ratio (Mayer, 1992).

Although our efforts to do so have meant that restrictions must be placed on the degree to which nurses would otherwise participate in decision making under a professional practice model, we believe that Santa Rosa Memorial Hospital's definition and delineation of management and staff roles have avoided conflict with the NLRB ruling. As an example, the clinical ladder board changed the promotion process from a committee decision to a committee recommendation to the vice president for patient care services.

DESCRIPTION OF THE PROFESSIONAL PRACTICE MODEL

Today, there are seven councils in Santa Rosa Memorial Hospital's professional practice model (Fig. 21–1). All activities within the councils are conducted within the parameters of the vision and principles of the Model. The membership of the divisionwide councils is composed of staff and management. With the exception of the coordinating council, each department has representation to each council.

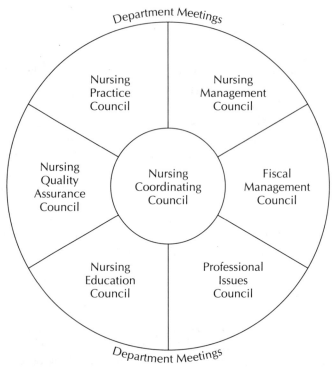

Figure 21–1 Santa Rosa Memorial Hospital Division of Nursing Professional Practice Model.

Staff nurses participate in the councils and committees of the professional practice model and contribute their expertise, knowledge and experience to the decision-making process. The responsibility and authority for management decisions (e.g., personnel actions, fiscal expenditures, policy development) rest with the hospital's management team.

To assure that the professional practice model does not conflict with the responsibilities of the union, issues concerning wages, hours, and terms and conditions of employment for registered staff nurses that are subject to the collective bargaining agreement or to the collective bargaining process are referred to the parties or to collective bargaining forums. The professional practice model in its functioning does not supersede or abrogate the collective bargaining process. Similarly, with the exception of pay for attendance at council meetings, the professional practice model is not subject to the collective bargaining process or governed by the collective bargaining agreement.

Council actions cannot be in violation of the collective bargaining agreement or Santa Rosa Memorial hospital policies. Wages, hours, and terms and conditions of employment and contract interpretation can only be discussed at the coordinating council, but any decision making concerning such issues that are unresolved can be handled only by hospital and SNA representatives, in accordance with procedures under the collective bargaining agreement and the National Labor Relations Act. This structure is essential to assure the viability of such a model in a union environment.

Detailed purpose statements and meeting schedules for each council can be found in Appendix 21–A, Addenda 1 to 7. A brief synopsis of each council follows:

Nursing Coordinating Council: develops, guides and facilitates the evolution of the professional practice model and assures integration and communication between the councils. The chairperson of the six other councils provide quarterly updates on their activities. Issues which arise in these councils regarding wages, hours and terms and conditions of employment and contract interpretation are referred to the coordinating council.

Nursing Management Council: Makes management decisions after considering council and departments' input and recommendations, and implements the decisions of the other councils into the operational activities of the nursing division.

Fiscal Management Council: Coordinates the development, implementation, monitoring and evaluation of the nursing division budget submitted for Administrative and Health System approval.

Nursing Quality Assurance Council: Coordinates and evaluates the nursing quality assurance program.

Nursing Practice Council: Develops and approves all clinical standards.

Nursing Education Council: Coordinates and evaluates department and divisional educational programs.

Professional Issues Council: Develops and monitors standards governing professional behavior. This council serves as a forum to address staff nurses' clinical and professional issues such as scope of practice, state and federal regulations and legislation, staffing, retention and recruitment issues.

Each department is represented by membership on the councils. The department representatives act as liaisons between their department and the council they attend. The council representatives report on council activities at their department staff meetings. Each department conducts its business through the department staff meeting. The development, coordination, and implementation of all departmental practice decisions occur through staff meetings. The decision making and activities within the staff meeting are in accordance with the vision and principles of the professional practice model.

REFINING THE MODEL

Since early 1990, the nursing division achieved some equilibrium, and we were able to begin to review the model. This was accomplished through education, staff development, and extensive communication. It is our firm belief that one cannot overcommunicate about the model and how it works. The vision statement provides an excellent framework to ensure a clear direction.

To accomplish our review and communication goals, an all day continuing education workshop was coordinated by the Professional Issues Council and Nursing Education Council. The workshop was offered three times. It included

TABLE 21–1   A Professional Practice Model, Evolution and Process: Shared Governance in a Union Setting

---

Objectives
- Describe the process of change to a professional practice model.
- Discuss the guidelines of implementing shared governance in a union setting.
- Describe effective methods nurses can use to participate in decisions that affect their practice.

Outline
  I. Introduction
  II. Decision Making at Santa Rosa Memorial Hospital Today
  III. Back to the Future
  IV. Model Description
  V. Why Bother?

---

content on leadership, shared governance models, staff nurse evolution and involvement in the professional practice model at Santa Rosa Memorial Hospital, assertive communication, and a description of how the councils function in our model. See Table 21–1 for class objectives and course outline.

Inservices on the professional practice model also were held at the department level. These inservices led to discussions on how to increase staff participation in problem solving and decision making at the department level as well as how to encourage staff participation in the councils. A presentation on the professional practice model and the role of staff nurses occurs monthly at nursing orientation.

To educate staff about the purpose and function of each council, continuing education programs or independent study modules or both were developed. Members became knowledgeable about the responsibilities and activities of their council and about their accountability for decisions that are made.

Our implementation of shared governance to date has been a lengthy process requiring time, commitment, and patience. It has involved both cultural and organizational change and continual communication of the vision. At the same time, it was essential to focus on the process of shared decision making. New ideas were discussed thoroughly with as many people as possible before a decision was made. This took more time initially, in the assessment and planning phases, but the implementation then proceeded more quickly and expeditiously. An example was our purchase of foam mattresses for all the beds and elimination of eggcrate mattresses. Nearly every department participated in the evaluation of the foam mattresses. The project was discussed in several councils and at staff meetings. When the new mattresses arrived, the switch was not a surprise to anyone. The nurses were aware of the benefits of the mattress and welcomed the change.

IMPACT ON NURSING MANAGEMENT

Nurse managers and assistant nurse managers experienced a change in their responsibilities under the model. The manager's role has changed from one of controller and decision maker to one of coach and facilitator. The members of the management team have been very supportive of the professional practice model and are more satisfied with their role of coaching rather than policing. However, this role change also required a great deal of communication and education to develop new skills. To assist the managers and assistant nurse managers in developing these skills, classes were offered in communication, conflict management, group process, and codependency issues for managers, among others. It is essential for the managers to develop excellent communication skills, to be less controlling and autocratic, and to put their trust in the process and the people. Additionally, an orientation plan and mentorship program for new assistant nurse managers and managers were developed.

In most settings, new nurse managers look for ways to create positive results immediately. However, new managers are advised to proceed slowly with changes and to involve as many of their staff as possible in the discussion of problems and action plans for resolution. We coach managers not to take credit for results or say, "I did this" but rather to be responsible for assisting the work group as it analyzes the problems and develops action plans.

ACCOMPLISHMENTS OF THE COUNCILS IN THE SANTA ROSA MEMORIAL HOSPITAL PROFESSIONAL PRACTICE MODEL

The amount of work accomplished in and through the professional practice model is far greater than what could have been accomplished with our limited resources in a more traditional structure. Serendipitous benefits include more creative solutions from staff involvement. As more people have input, new ideas are generated and previously unsolvable problems are solved by those now vested in the solution. Leadership skills are developed and modeled at all levels of the organization. One example is a nurses' aide on the skin care committee giving meaningful feedback and recommendations on skin care to licensed personnel. In the past, management positions were open for extended lengths of time, and there was no interest internally in promotional opportunities. Now the number of interested and qualified internal candidates for management and leadership promotional opportunities exceeds the opportunities available. Although nurses are paid for 2 hours each month for council meetings, the model actually enhances commitment and a professionalism and is fiscally responsible. Probably the most significant benefit is that staff are vested in the workplace, and job satisfaction and morale are significantly and meaningfully enhanced.

Following are some of the council accomplishments and benefits.

Nursing Practice Council
- Implemented an adaptation of the Marker Model for standards
- Evaluates new products and develops procedures
- Assures that new products are not implemented until the nurses have been inserviced

- Evaluates clinical procedures/protocols to reflect the latest research and advances in practice
- Maintains cost-effective use of material and human resources

Nursing Coordinating Council

- Provides a venue for union and management collaboration
- Discusses issues regarding contract interpretation
- Developed a counseling standard consistent with the contract that defines the philosophy and process for counseling and roles of nursing employees in the counseling process
- Developed consistent standards for signing up for extra work shifts and reduction of hours
- Participated concurrently with the nursing management council in the formulation of annual goals and objectives for the nursing division (Appendix 21–A, Addendum 8)
- Researched, selected, and will implement a theory for practice and developed a philosophy of nursing

Nursing Education Council

- Educates members about how to develop and coordinate continuing education classes
- Conducts an annual educational needs assessment
- Offers divisionwide and department-specific inservice educational classes
- Develops educational classes in response to identified needs from the quality assurance studies and new or revised clinical standards from the Nursing Practice Council
- Developed a plan for accomplishing the annual required JCAHO safety inservices, which included developing forms for documentation of the employees' participation in educational programs
- Developed department specific crosstraining plans and checklists
- Expanded participation in staff development through formulating educational programs or teaching, to any nurse who is interested. Through this approach, there is minimal overhead for the coordination of classes, which allows the council to offer classes at a nominal fee to the employee

Nursing Quality Assurance Council

- Implemented the Ten Step Model for quality assurance
- Implemented numerous changes to improve patient care (e.g., justification for purchase of new IV pumps, changes in IV protocol, revised forms for documentation of the nursing process) and assured accreditation by JCAHO

Fiscal Management Council

- Assisted in recruitment of staff nurses to a previously unpopular council
- Developed the annual salary and supply budgets through joint participation of staff nurses, assistant nurse managers, and their managers
- Developed and implemented a format for cost benefits analysis of Staff Nurse III (clinical ladder) projects
- Advises departments having problems meeting their budget targets

- Increases staff nurse awareness of the fiscal constraints and declining reimbursement in health care
- Offered educational programs for nurses on fiscal aspects of health care

Professional Issues Council
- Reviewed and revised scope of practice and job descriptions for RNs, LVNs, and CNAs
- Designed, through a recruitment subcommittee, a recruitment table display, brochure, selected the recruitment materials for career days. Nurses on the committee take turns representing the hospital at college career days, and they are the ones best able to discuss with new applicants what it is like to be a nurse at Santa Rosa Memorial Hospital.
- Designed and coordinated activities to celebrate nursing during Nurses' Week
- Regularly deals with such conflict-laden issues as staffing and has grown in its ability to deal with conflict constructively

Nursing Management Council
- Implements the decisions of other councils
- Coordinated the development of the nursing division Mission Statement, describing the values implementation in nursing practice
- Facilitated discussions about the values at department staff meetings using a prescribed set of questions. A synthesis of these led to a mission statement (Appendix 21–A, Addendum 10.)

Issues that we had to address included the need to replace one bureaucratic structure with another. It was critical to provide structure and framework so that each council clearly understood its responsibility, accountability, and parameters. There was no way around it; decision making is slower. However, implementation is faster and smoother. The role of the manager is a key role, and although education can assist in skill building, some managers feel threatened by the loss of control. After a certain point, people have a decision to make.

Staff, like managers, do not always buy into the process. Some want to come to work, do their jobs, and leave. We choose not to be discouraged by those electing not to participate but to invest our energies in those who choose to be part of the process.

Finally, articulating the model requires work and more work—and continual communication—both within and outside the nursing division.

Our experiences indicates our bias—that a professional practice model can work, even in a union environment. The advantages and disadvantages are as follows:

- Professional practice model has as its basic tenet that staff nurses participate in decision making about issues that affect their practice.
- Professional practice model works best if all participants have a basis for their own power and a nurse's individual knowledge and contributions can serve as that basis.

- The contract may legislate the number of staff nurse members on committees and negotiates for conditions of employment, such as wages and benefits, but can never truly assure staff nurses a meaningful voice in governance.
- The professional practice model provides staff nurses a means to forge partnerships with management on professional issues.
- Staff nurse leaders are a vital resource in the cultural change from bureaucracy to collaboration. In a union setting, these leaders must include elected union representatives.

Professional practice models in union settings provide the opportunity for employees and administration to work together on common issues to form a foundation of strength. The value of conflict and the exploration of options that conflict generates is self-evident and, to a certain degree, sanctioned. As we are dedicated to seeking the third, or synergistic, solution together, each party's entitlement is fully recognized by the other (Covey, 1989).

The relationships built among the leaders of nursing administration and the SNA are the cornerstone of the model. The dedication to working through issues to mutual satisfaction recognizes that we come to the discussion with very different points of view and interest.

While living with the model that was created with great care, energy, and excitement, we have discovered that the process of how we resolve issues—the recognition of individual truths and mutual investment—is as important as the resolution.

References

Bernstein, H. (1988, March 13). *Los Angeles Times*. NLRB shouldn't take strife in workplace for granted.

Covey, S. (1989). *The seven habits of highly effective people*. New York: Simon & Schuster.

Dayton Power & Light and members of Local 175, UWUA, AFL/CIO (1990). Labor compact.

Deming, W.E. (1951). *The elementary principles of the statistical control of quality. A series of lectures*. Tokyo: Nippon.

Electromation, Inc. (1992), 309 NLRB No. 163, 142 LRRM 1001.

Knowles, M. (1978). *The adult learner: A neglected species*. Houston, TX: Gulf Publishing Co.

Labor–Management Cooperation. (1989). 1989 state of the art symposium: US Department of Labor, Bureau of Labor–Management Relations and Cooperative Programs.

Mayer, D. (1992, January 13). NLRB may open nurse panels to union attack. *Healthweek*, 6(1).

McDonagh, K.J. (1990). Introducing the concept of nursing shared governance. In *Nursing shared governance: Restructuring the future*. Atlanta: K.J. McDonagh & Assoc.

NLRB v. Yeshiva University (1980), 444V S-672, 103 LRRM 2526.

Secretary's Commission on Nursing (1988, December) Department of Health and Human Services, Office of the Secretary, Washington, D.C.

Santa Rosa Memorial Hospital Division of Nursing Structure Standards

ADDENDUM 1: NURSING COORDINATING COUNCIL

Purpose

To develop, guide, and facilitate the evolution of the Professional Practice Model, inclusive of the relationship of the Model with the contractual agreement with the Staff Nurses' Association.

Responsibilities

1. Discuss implementation of the Staff Nurses' Association (SNA)/Santa Rosa Memorial Hospital agreement, e.g., wages, benefits, and working conditions
2. Develop standards to assure consistency in the administration of the provisions of the SNA contract (e.g., ROH, counseling)
3. Facilitate communication and integration of activities between nursing councils and nursing departments
4. Act as a resource in clarification of each council's responsibilities
5. Direct implementation of a theory-based practice model
6. Direct issues to appropriate councils or departments

Membership

Members of the SNA Board, Director of Nursing Operations, Vice President of Patient Care Services, one Critical Care Manager, one·Medical–Surgical Manager and the Vice President of Human Resources and Development. Guests are welcome by invitation. The chairs of other councils attend semiannually.

Chair: Cochaired by Vice President of Patient Care Services and the President of the SNA Board
Secretary: Rotates annually
Meets monthly on the third Tuesday from 1:00 to 3:00 PM

ADDENDUM 2: NURSING MANAGEMENT COUNCIL

Purpose

To provide appropriate administrative, financial, material, and personnel to carry out the business of the Nursing Division within budgetary resources and according to the values of the Sisters of St. Joseph of Orange. Nursing Management Council (NMC) is responsible for making management decisions that consider council and department input. NMC is responsible for carrying out and implementing decisions into the operational activities for the nursing division. To assure ongoing communication from each council to NMC, at least one manager acts as a liaison from each council to NMC. NMC has a responsibility to educate staff and to direct activities to other councils as appropriate. Decisions not in the domain of the other councils are referred to NMC.

Responsibilities

1. Information dissemination
2. Implement decisions from other councils
3. Operational issues
4. Fiscal accountability
5. Medical staff relations
6. Structure standard development and approval

Membership

Vice President for Patient Care Services, Director of Nursing Operations, Nurse Managers and Nursing Administrators (one representative meet weekly). Assistant Nurse Managers attend monthly (fourth week of the month). One staff nurse representing PRNC attends monthly (fourth week of the month) to facilitate communication.

Chair.   Rotating chair—rotates weekly
Secretary.   Rotates weekly

Meeting Frequency

Weekly on Tuesday, 9:00 to 11:30 AM. No meeting on the second Tuesday of the month. Assistant Nurse Managers attend monthly.

ADDENDUM 3: FISCAL MANAGEMENT COUNCIL
Purpose

To coordinate the development, implementation, monitoring and evaluation of departmental and divisional units of service, salary, nonsalary, and capital budgets for administrative and health system approval. To serve as an advisory body to the nursing management team in fiscal management.

Responsibilities

1. Evaluate and make recommendations to NMC and Administrative Staff regarding the fiscal components of new and/or existing divisional programs [e.g., productivity monitoring, patient classification system, staffing system (ANSOS), purchasing, salary, and nonsalary budget]
2. Assist managers, ANMs, and staff in working toward productivity and fiscal goals in their departments, as required
3. Assist in the education of staff and management team about budgetary principles and process as it relates to fiscal goals and nursing practice

Accountability

The Fiscal Management Council reports findings and/or recommendations to the Nursing Management Council and Administrative Staff. Since recommendations of this Council have an impact on either departmental or divisional budgets, recommendations are reported to NMC so adequate feedback and input can be received from all managers. The chairperson reports on FMC activities on a semiannual basis to Coordinating Council.

Membership

Members represent a wide range of nursing services, and the goal will be to have an equal number of staff and management members.

The Director of Nursing Operations and/or Vice President of Patient Care Services and all Nurse Managers are permanent members of this Council.

Process/Communication

FMC meetings are held the second Thursday of each month from 1:00 to 2:30 PM. Recorder of minutes rotates and minutes of meetings are sent monthly to all Nursing Management Council members, Nursing Shift Administrators, and FMC members.

ADDENDUM 4: NURSING QUALITY IMPROVEMENT COUNCIL
Purpose

To oversee the development and maintenance of nursing quality improvement programs and systems. The Nursing Quality Improvement Council (NQI) provides a planned and systematic process for monitoring, evaluating, and promoting the quality and appropriateness of patient care. The NQI Council promotes resolution of identified problems, monitors compliance with Nursing Standards, and ultimately improves patient care.

Responsibilities

1. Maintains an ongoing quality improvement program in the Nursing Division
2. Reviews and updates and provides systems and methods used in the QI program
3. Identifies Nursing Division indicators and criteria for divisionwide studies to assure the same level of care is given throughout the division
4. Approves each nursing department QI program to assure the plan demonstrates the actual level of care given
5. Coordinates Nursing Division QI activities
6. Analyzes QI data, recommends further action, and reevaluates
7. Evaluates Nursing Department QI programs
8. Integrates NQI activities with hospitalwide and medical staff of quality improvement activities
9. Preliminary review and approval of Nursing Research Proposals
10. Acts as a consultant to managers and department QI committees to assure compliance with regulatory agencies

Meeting Time

The council will meet the first Thursday of the month from 3:30 to 4:30 PM.

Communication

1. Chairperson will report on NQI Council activities to Nursing Management Council, Nursing Coordinating Council, and Vice President of Patient Care Services.
2. Managers report to the hospital QA Committee on their department's QI activities on a quarterly basis.
3. Minutes will be maintained in the Medical Staff Office.
4. The secretary will write articles about NQI activities for the Professional Practice Model newsletter.
5. NQI members report QI activities to department staff at monthly staff meetings.

Membership

1. All nursing departments will have one representative on the NQI Council. If this representative is unable to attend, a nurse who is active on this department QI committee may substitute at the Council meeting. Only one staff nurse from each department is reimbursed for attendance, per contract.
2. Selection is done at the department level. The representative to the NQI Council is a member of the department QI committee. If more than one staff nurse volunteers, the department selects the representative.
3. No more than half the membership will change at any one time. Membership tenure is 2 years.

Responsibilities and Expectations

1. Chair
   - Develop the agenda for each meeting
   - Chair the meeting
   - In conjunction with the Director of Nursing Operations, write a quarterly report summary for Medical Staff QA, write an annual QI summary report, develop annual goals for approval by council members, review and revise QI structure standard as necessary, on an annual basis
   - Orient new managers to the QI process
   - Serve as a resource to nursing departments QI representatives, and/or committees
   - Provide feedback to nursing departments on their quarterly reports
   - Communicate to other council chairpersons when QI has identified a problem that requires the assistance of their council to resolve
2. Secretary
   - Take Minutes
   - Maintain records in the Medical Staff Office
   - Compile the monthly report for the newsletter

3. Members
   • Compile the quarterly report for department
   • Provide manager with verbal report and 3 copies for the hospitalwide QA committee
   • Present oral report to NQI on a quarterly basis
   • Annually, assist in reviewing scope of service, important aspects of care, and indicators for department and division
   • Bring to the monthly NQI Council any special problems identified that may need divisionwide problem solving
   • Report every month at the department staff meeting regarding QI activities
   • Work with department QI committee to provide opportunities for staff to participate in QI studies
   • Correlate department educational offerings with QI findings
4. Subcommittees
   The following committees report to the Nursing Quality Improvement Council.
   • Skin Care Committee
   • Nursing Pharmacy Committee
   • Nursing Laboratory Committee

ADDENDUM 5: NURSING PRACTICE COUNCIL
Purpose

To delineate, develop, and approve all clinical standards that describe and guide the nursing care provided, consistent with national standards of practice promulgated by nursing specialty organizations and regulatory agencies.

The Vice President of Patient Care Services is responsible for assuring that the clinical standards (protocols, procedures, and guidelines) describe and serve as guidelines for providing nursing care to patients brought to the hospital. The Vice President for Patient Care Services participates in the development of clinical standards when necessary. However, she has delegated the authority for approval of the clinical standards to the Nursing Practice Council.

Process

1. The need to develop or revise standards can be identified by any member of the nursing staff.
2. The person identifying the need for the standard consults with the Nursing Practice Council or chair. The purpose of consultation is
   • To determine the best method of meeting need: Structure Standard, Protocol, Procedure, Guideline or Teaching Protocol
   • Instruct author in correct format
   • Avoid duplication of effort
   • Identify and instruct author in approval process
3. In developing the draft, the author gets input from nurses in his or her department to assure the standard is realistic in defining safe and appropriate care.

4. A draft of the standard is sent to the Nursing Practice Council for critique. The Nursing Practice Council assists, as needed, in revising and rewriting.
5. The Nursing Practice Council may recommend the author collaborate with appropriate clinical disciplines, administrative groups, expert resources, other nursing personnel, or medical staff for content and input when appropriate.
6. After the standard has been approved by Nursing Practice Council, the author will take the standard to other persons or committees required for approval. All new/revised standards are reviewed by Vice President of Patient Care Services, who is responsible for assuring that standards describe and guide the nursing care required for patients treated at Santa Rosa Memorial Hospital. If the standard is to be presented at a medical staff meeting for approval or information, the Vice President of Patient Care Services is notified before the meeting and given a copy, and a copy is taken to medical staff office.
7. If disagreement occurs between two approving bodies, the author will work between them to reach a compromise. In the event a compromise cannot be reached, the author can refer back to the Nursing Practice Council for assistance.
8. If any further changes are made, the author brings the completed standard back to the Nursing Practice Council. If all required persons or committees have approved, the Nursing Practice Council gives final approval.

Implementation

1. New standards are not implemented until final approval by Nursing Practice Council.
2. To facilitate communication, the new or revised standard is sent for information to the Nursing Management Council.
3. It is the responsibility of the Nurse Manager and Assistant Nurse Manager to ensure that all nursing staff is informed of all new standards.
4. New or revised standards are sent to each department, via the Nurse Manager, with a cover memo outlining placement of the standard (e.g., manual, title to be added to index, standard to be inserted into manual, and any standards that are to be removed).

Council Responsibilities

1. Determine the approval process for standards.
   - Determine when the draft standard is ready to be submitted for approval.
   - Recommend author's collaboration with other individuals, expert resources, or nursing or medical committees for content and input.
   - Assure all structure standards are approved by Nursing Management Council.
   - Assure all standardized procedures/protocols are approved by the Interdisciplinary Practice Committee.
2. Track the standard until it is approved and implemented.

Development, Review, and Revision

1. The members of Nursing Practice Council are responsible to review and revise the protocols, procedures, and guidelines at least every 3 years. The date of review/revision is reflected on each clinical standard. The old clinical standard is retained in Nursing Administration. The Nursing Practice Council minutes reflect which standards were reviewed, revised, or deleted. When clinical standards are developed or reviewed, the following is taken into consideration and recorded on the standard evaluation tool (see attached).
   - Appropriateness
   - Changes in practice
   - Current/new research findings
   - Relevant ethical and legal concerns
   - Findings from quality improvement studies/risk management
   - Staff performance problems

Membership

Drawn from professional nursing staff. Ideally, one member from each department. Members may be nominated, elected, or volunteer. Minimum term of membership: 2 years.

Membership Responsibilities

1. Consultation with author from own department, includes instructing author in correct format and in approval process.
2. Attend council meetings the second Monday of every month, 1:00 to 2:30 PM.
3. Critique all standards submitted for approval. Review focuses on
   - Format
   - Content
   - Scope of practice
   - Changes in practice
   - New QI or research findings
   - Relevant legal and ethical concerns
   - Consistent with Nursing Division philosophy and values
4. Facilitate ongoing evaluation of nursing practice by bringing appropriate department practice issues to the council meetings.

Committees

1. The Nursing Practice Council collaborates with other councils and nursing committees and task forces in the development of procedures, protocols, and guidelines.
2. The following nursing committees report to NPC.
   - Licensed Vocational Nurse Committee
   - IV Therapy Committee
   - Clinical Support Subcommittee of Resource Analysis Committee
   - Any other task forces as developed to address specific problems

Chair Responsibilities

1. Chair NPC meetings
2. Serve as resource to all councils and nursing staff
3. Coordinate approval process
4. Record and submit minutes of meetings to members of NPC and NMC

Nursing Practice Council Membership Rotation

Rotation of membership occurs as follows.

1. For even numbered years (e.g., 90, 92, 94), the following departments elect or volunteer a representative.

First East	Third East
CVU	Three North
Second East	Four West

2. For odd numbered years (e.g., 91, 93, 95), the following departments elect or volunteer a representative:

Two West	Four North
Critical Care	Rohnert Park Healthcare Center
Operating Room	Cardiac Cath Lab
Three West	

ADDENDUM 6: NURSING EDUCATION COUNCIL
Purpose

To assure that department and divisional educational programs are available to nursing staff on an ongoing basis and are designed to maintain current competence and augment the nurses' knowledge of pertinent new developments in patient care.

Responsibilities

1. Develop a needs assessment tool and coordinate the completion of the needs assessment by each department on a yearly basis
2. Integrate findings from QI/monitoring and evaluation activities into nursing education programs on an ongoing basis
3. Assure that required programs (CPR, fire, disaster, safety, infection control, radiation safety, body mechanics) are available for inservice on an annual basis
4. Assure nursing orientation is current
5. Coordinate department education activities to prevent duplication and inform staff of classes
6. Approve department-specific education programs that are offered for CE credit
7. Coordinate divisionwide nursing education programs
8. Assure evaluation of educational programs

- Program objectives are used as criteria for evaluation of program content
- Participants evaluate speakers' presentation effectiveness
9. Nursing Education Council develops annual objectives for council activities and evaluates whether objectives were met

Responsibilities for Department of Nursing Education Representative

1. Complete educational needs assessment for his or her department through utilization of the needs assessment tool
2. Assure that findings from department quality improvement monitoring and evaluation activities are used in determining needs for educational programs on an ongoing basis
3. Assure availability of teaching tools for annual required programs (e.g., CPR, infection control, electrical/equipment, disaster, fire, employee safety, radiation safety, department-specific equipment and procedures)
4. Plan and submit to Nursing Administration Secretary department specific educational offerings by the 25th of every month for inclusion in the monthly Nursing Education Calendar
5. Coordinate department-specific educational programs; assist staff in completion of required documentation for CE credit to assure it meets BRN requirements
6. Use an evaluation tool for each department's classes
7. Assure that Council objectives are met on a department level

Membership

One representative from each nursing department, who is elected or appointed by the department. The Council is chaired by a nurse knowledgeable in educational methods. A minimum of 50% of the members are staff nurses. Membership term is for a minimum of 2 years. No more than half of the members will rotate annually. All members are eligible for appointment to the Chairperson or Cochairperson position.

Meeting Time

The Council will meet the 2nd Wednesday of each month from 3:30 to 4:30 PM.

Communication

1. Chairperson or Cochairperson will report to Nursing Management Council at least monthly and to Coordinating Council quarterly.
2. Minutes will be distributed to
   - Nursing Education Council members
   - Vice President for Patient Care Services
   - Nurse Managers

ADDENDUM 7: PROFESSIONAL ISSUES COUNCIL (PIC)
Goal

The goal of the Professional Issues Council is to develop, implement, and keep abreast of standards governing professional behavior. This council serves as a forum to address staff nurses' clinical and professional issues, such as scope of practice, state and federal regulations and legislation, staffing, retention, and recruitment.

Membership

The membership consists of representatives from the Professional Registered Nurse Council (PRNC) and members of the management team. The PRNC is a contractual staff nurses' committee, and remains so. The purpose of PIC is to involve staff nurses and managers in a Professional Practice Model. New members may be nominated, elected, or volunteered from professional staff. Each department has representation. Ad hoc members may be brought in for specific projects and consultation. The chairperson is designated annually. The chairperson communicates activities to the Nursing Coordinating Council (NCC) and the Nursing Management Council (NMC). Council task forces are formed to address specific issues (e.g., retention, practice, recruitment, clinical ladder).

Meetings

PIC meets monthly for 1½ hours. PRNC meets monthly for 3 hours and paid for 2 hours per month, as contractually stated. These meetings are usually held on the same day and consecutively.

Council Subcommittees/Task Forces

Clinical Ladder Board
Recruitment
Retention
Scope of Practice
Staffing

ADDENDUM 8: GOALS AND OBJECTIVES
Goal

To provide expert, professional, and distinctive nursing services meriting Santa Rosa Memorial Hospital as a leading innovative Catholic health care facility for patients, nurses, and physicians.

Annual Objectives

A. Operationalize values of the Sisters of St. Joseph of Orange in all Nursing Division activities
B. Assure compliance with state and JCAHO accreditation standards
C. Create an empowering environment that fosters staff interdependence and collegiality

D. Balance resources to provide quality, cost-effective care
E. Continue to implement a theoretical basis for nursing practice, education, and research, combining Rogers' caring theories and self care
F. Enhance the broaden professional practice for nurses at Santa Rosa Memorial Hospital

ADDENDUM 9: PHILOSOPHY AND GOALS OF THE NURSING DIVISION
Philosophy

The art and science of nursing at Santa Rosa Memorial Hospital is shaped by the courage, commitment, competence, and compassion of the nursing staff. Our concerns are focused on the whole person and to assist people to achieve the maximum health potential. We believe that each person is unique and is characterized by his or her own life pattern.

We believe that individuals interact with their environment, and as such, the relationship between nurses and the people they care for is dynamic and complementary.

We believe that individuals create their reality and are accountable for it. Individuals have the ability to influence their health and the right to participate in health care. The experience of illness and choice of self-care is shaped by the individual's health status, culture, and health beliefs. Evaluating an individual's ability to care for self is the basis for nurse's health assessment and planning of caring strategies.

We believe that alternative healing modalities are legitimate as adjuncts to the western medical model. Used together, they address the spiritual, emotional, psychologic, sociocultural, and physical manifestations of our being, which is essential in caring for the whole person.

We believe that the need for preventive care and the occurrence of illness/ trauma existing in our life's path offer opportunities for growth and nurturance of self. In embracing another's fragile and painful health issues during our interventions, we, as nurses and healers, provide the opportunities for others to discover their own solutions and self-healing capabilities.

We believe in honoring our roles as nurses and that self-care is essential for ourselves. The choice of how we participate in this can determine our reality within the nursing profession.

We believe that caring is the essence of nursing. It is the ability to presence oneself with another individual and connect with his or her lived experience in a way that acknowledges our shared humanity. Caring also extends to our professional relationships and is articulated and operationalized through the vision statement and principles of the governance model.

We believe the values of the St. Joseph Health System—dignity, service, excellence, justice—are the roots of our model. They provide the foundation and belief from which practice can be further explored through theories. From this use of theory, nursing practice is further defined, predicted, care prescribed, and the integrity of nursing is confirmed. Collectively, the concepts of Rogers—

caring, self-care, our values—and our governance model formulate the Professional Practice Model of Santa Rosa Memorial Hospital's Nursing Division.

ADDENDUM 10: MISSION STATEMENT

The goal of the Nursing Division is to provide expert, professional, and distinctive nursing services, meriting Santa Rosa Memorial Hospital as a leading, innovative, Catholic health care facility for patients, nurses, and physicians.

Santa Rosa Memorial Hospital has created a Professional Practice Model that empowers nurses to practice in a dynamic, collaborative environment as outlined in the vision statement and principles of the Professional Practice Model.

The science and art of nursing at Santa Rosa Memorial Hospital are based on the concepts of Martha Rogers and caring and self-care theories, which have been integrated into the Nursing Division philosophy statement.

The values of dignity, service, excellence, and justice are operationalized in all Nursing Division activities and actions.

Dignity

We recognize the unique contribution of each individual by developing a trusting relationship among the patient, family, and other members of the health care team in the provision of health care. We foster this practice by

- Addressing the patient in a caring, personalized manner
- Respecting confidentiality and privacy
- Providing responsible care to the patient and family
- Encouraging participation by patient and family in plan of care as they desire or are able
- Developing care plans that recognize individual cultural and psychosocial needs
- Educating and empowering patients to be an active participant in decision making regarding their medical care, e.g., durable power of attorney for health care
- Communicating openly and in a caring manner with all members of the interdisciplinary health care team via reports, staff meetings, communication logs, patient care conferences
- Facilitating timely, honest feedback that focuses on the opportunity for personal and professional growth and development
- Recognizing and valuing individual contributions (e.g., Touch-a-Gram)
- Sharing positive feedback
- Sharing public recognition of co-workers at staff meetings (e.g., employee of the month, clinical ladder, special projects, exceptional caring, or clinical expertise)
- Encouraging family participation in hospital social events
- Fostering participation in development of staffing schedules that contribute to safe patient care

Service

The Nursing Division is dedicated to providing a service-oriented, holistic approach to meet the needs of the patients, families, and members of the health care team. We foster this approach by

- Acting as liaison between departments to provide quality patient care
- Maintaining supportive and collaborative relationships with physicians
- Sharing expertise with other departments
- Communicating and coordinating activities between departments in a courteous manner
- Allowing patient and family the opportunity to express their needs and by making every effort to meet their needs
- Active listening

Caring is the essence of nursing. We strive to foster a supportive environment characterized by hospitality, trust, acceptance, and spirit of community by

- Greeting with a warm, friendly smile
- Being sensitive to needs of others
- Being present and engaged with another, listening and learning from each other
- Acknowledging each other's special talents and contributions
- Meeting patient needs in a timely manner
- Involving patients and their family in their health care, e.g., patient care conferences
- Promoting professional demeanor in our actions and communications with patients, families, and each other

Excellence

Using the Professional Practice Model as the forum, the Nursing Division works together with other health care professionals to assure excellence. We encourage excellence by

- Providing quality patient care in a cost-effective manner
- Providing the opportunity to participate in educational offerings
- Expecting excellence in patient care, from ourselves and all others involved with the patient
- Requiring certification for various areas of expertise, e.g., ACLS, MICN, and chemotherapy
- Providing a caring, nonjudgmental environment through peer review and annual evaluation in order to ensure competency and professional development
- Assuring a safe environment for both the patients and caregivers by employing safe work practices and promoting team work among all health care providers

- Encouraging innovative ideas and research to continually improve our practice
- Participating in a dynamic quality improvement program that enhances patient care
- Developing and following written standards of care that reflect the goals of quality patient care that we wish to attain in the best of possible situations
- Making a commitment to self-growth and development

Justice

The Nursing Division promotes truthful interaction with patients, families, and the health care community, respecting each person's unique and individual needs.

With patients and families by

- Promoting honest interaction
- Coordinating a multidisciplinary team approach to patient care
- Providing quality care without regard to individual patient circumstances
- Assuring confidentiality of all patient care matters
- Offering support, education, and/or the services of the Bioethics Forum when the patient and/or family is faced with a bioethical dilemma

With health team members by

- Promoting courtesy and respect between shifts, with other departments, and with the medical staff
- Providing positive feedback, e.g., employee recognition, Touch-a-Grams, annual performance evaluations
- Educating self and others in current health care issues
- Promoting collaborative communication that is direct, specific, and non-punishing
- Encouraging nurses to volunteer needed services within the community
- Promoting awareness and action regarding health care issues in the legislative and political arenas

CHAPTER 22

MANAGING THE NURSE–PHYSICIAN LINK

JoEllen Koerner
Becky Nelson

EXECUTIVE SUMMARY

One of the most fundamental topics of consideration in the health care field today is the relationship among nursing, medical staff, and hospital administration, including the value and development of collegial relationships among health care professionals. The nurse–physician relationship is a special one, based on mutual respect and interdependence, steeped in history, and stereotyped in popular culture (Muff, 1982).

In this chapter, the authors have described the multiple facets of nurse–physician relations, including male-dominated health care system, the emergence of professional nursing, and the changing environment.

The issue of long ignored abusive communication is explored with strategies for study and intervention identified for the nurse manager.

Nursing has long been defined as both an art and a science. Florence Nightingale called it "The finest of the fine arts." Nursing is not merely a technique but a process that incorporates the elements of soul, mind, and imagination, a sensitive spirit, and the intelligent understanding that provides the foundation for effective nursing care. However, the evolution of professional nursing is a story filled with conflict, struggle, and oppression.

The healing professions were established heavily along the lines of gender. Historical religious, scientific, and educational sanctions have been held against women. Thus, class and gender issues, such as sexism and stereotyping, are pressing issues in nursing, as 96% of the 1,900,000 practicing nurses are female.

At the turn of the twentieth century, American medicine was well on its way to becoming the most male-dominated system of health care in the industrialized world. Not a single allied health profession composed primarily of women was able to practice independently of the medical profession, which was 95% to 97% male until recent years. Thus, nurses in general have limited professional independence and authority and are, in some instances, legally constrained from practicing the skills acquired in their education.

The professionalization of nursing is an intensifying paradox. Continuous pressure from within medicine and science calls for upgrading the skills and expertise of nurses. Simultaneously, it has created a desire for expanded and independent practice within the nursing discipline, placing nurses at odds with the physicians who depend on the expertise of these nurses to provide comprehensive care to their clients. Nursing's autonomy as a profession has been declared, but their independence as practitioners is controlled by multiple layers of authority: the physician, the administrator, and the payor.

Further, a significant barrier to nurses' autonomy is attitudinal. Bullough (1975, p. 229) observed that

> . . . the weight of past tradition, the subordination of nurses, the sex segregation, and the apprenticeship model in nursing education have left a mark on the attitudes of present day nurses . . . and others within the health care industry.

This same bias exists for women who are physicians. Between the years 1970 and 1986, the number of women physicians in the United States increased by 241.2% (AMA, 1987). By 1986, 86,670 women physicians were practicing. The areas most frequently chosen by females include pediatrics, internal medicine, and family practice. Less than 10% of all practicing female physicians are involved in professional activities, such as medical teaching, administration, and research. Women physicians are more than twice as likely to be employed as men physicians. In 1986, only 23.5% of men physicians were employed by another person or corporation, whereas 45.5% of women physicians were (Gonzalez & Emmons, 1986). Even though more women are present in the medical field, they are not seated in positions of power and authority to facilitate independence for each profession and interdependence for the mutual outcomes of client care.

Recent affairs, such as the civil rights movement, the feminist movement, and the rapid advances in science and technology, have had a profound impact on the role of women in society. These cultural and technical changes have redefined the work of nursing and medicine, calling for an integrated approach to meeting the total health care needs of the client.

CARING AND CURING: ROLES THAT CONFLICT AND COMPLEMENT

The most fundamental topic of consideration in the health care field today is the relationship between the person who is ill and those who profess to heal him or her—physicians and nurses.

> The physician brings knowledge and skill regarding cure; the nurse brings knowledge and skill in caring; and the patient brings his or her values and concerns for a good and healthy life. Logically, any consideration of philosophical issues, and especially ethical ones, should focus on the relationship of curing and caring. (Bishop & Skudder, 1985, p. 5)

Role theory focuses on individuals and their behaviors. Many roles are embedded within social systems, such as health care organizations. Each position is specialized and interdependent. Often, production is dependent on the sequential performance of many complex roles and tasks. Thus, individuals must learn to accommodate other specialized roles if they are to remain members of the organization.

The nurse–physician relationship is a special one, based on mutual respect and interdependence, steeped in history, and stereotyped in popular culture (Muff, 1982). The broad spectrum of these professional role relationships ranges from nonexistent to master–servant, adversarial, or collegial. Areas of conflict in male–female relationships, such as power and authority, are at stake in these interactions in both covert and overt ways. The dilemma in the current situation is twofold: practicing physicians and nurses are competent adults who are responsible for personal and professional choices and actions; the work of these health care professionals is interdependent.

The Changing Environment

The National Commission on Nursing (1981) reported that a major issue in nursing is "relationships among nursing, medical staff, and hospital administration, including nurses' ability to participate through organizational structures in decision-making as it relates to nursing care, the value and development of collegial relationships among health care professionals."

The nurse–doctor game is being altered significantly by a number of important social changes of the past two decades (Stein, 1967; Stein, Watts, & Howell, 1990). Public esteem for physicians has deteriorated from the image of selfless dedication of the fictional Dr. Kildare. Commercialization of medical care has undermined public confidence in the profession's devotion to altruistic concerns (Blendon, 1988). Physicians are more likely to be female. In 1989, 38% of freshman medical students were female, as compared with 9% two decades earlier (Relman, 1989). Although medical students are still socialized in the game, the elements that reflect stereotypical roles of male dominance and female passivity are missing.

In contrast to the glut of physicians in some areas, there is a nursing shortage that has focused attention on the value of nursing in health care. Problems inherent in the profession are widely known, causing more women in their first year of college to say that they would rather become doctors than nurses (Iglehart, 1987).

Aiken and Mullinix (1987) noted that, increasingly, nurses are being educated in degree-granting academic institutions rather than in hospitals that confer a diploma (90% received diplomas in 1967, whereas 15% received them in 1988). The image of nurses as handmaidens is giving way to that of specialty-trained and certified advanced practitioners with independent duties and responsibilities to their patients. Physicians increasingly depend on nursing expertise in select settings, such as intensive care units. Strong nursing roles in utilization review and quality assurance directly threaten physicians' authority in clinical decision making. The current scenario finds that one of the players (the nurse) has unilaterally decided to stop playing the nurse–doctor game.

An emerging trend in medical consumerism finds the typically compliant and unassertive client much more educated and articulate regarding particulars of his or her care. The increasing frequency of litigation, calls for a second opinion regarding diagnosis and treatment plans, and participation in decisions of an ethical nature reflect the emergence of an active participant role for the client. Thus, all former role behavior is glaringly obsolete for the current health care environment.

Altering Abusive Behavior

As role behavior is revised, a period of turbulence emerges. Current activities in many health care settings focus on an issue long ignored, the extensive presence of abusive communication. A recent study by Cox (1991a) demonstrated that 96.7% of staff nurses and 97.1% of nurse managers reported experiencing verbal abuse from a physician. The serious impact of this prevalent behavior produces negative and costly outcomes: high turnover, decreased productivity, increased errors, a rise in litigation activity, and ultimate deterioration in the quality of care (Cox, 1991b).

The pathology of abuse behavior must be addressed to create healthier relationships between nurses and physicians. The victim mentality experienced by many nurses must be altered so that their behavioral change disrupts the abusive chain of events (Bradford, 1989). The cycle of individuals who were abused becoming abusers must be interrupted to stop the perpetuity of an abusive culture.

Verbal abuse may be defined as a perverse form of communication that alienates people through humiliation, character assassination, or destruction of one's self-esteem. There are varying degrees of abusive communication, with some being more overt than others (Diza & McMillin, 1992; Gasparis, 1990). Five patterns of abusive communication are noted: (1) academic aggression, (2) graffiti, (3) phony verbiage, (4) sarcasm, and (5) sexual harassment.

Academic Aggression

Physicians are educated and socialized to be autonomous and singular in the management of patient care. They are the captains of the team but frequently do not include other caregivers as team members, devaluing the contributions of others to patient care by treating them as a less important member of the team. An overt manifestation may find the physician responding to a nurse's suggestion or comment by asking, "Who do you think you are? I am the doctor here," or "Here, take the chart and write all of the orders, since you think you know when it's necessary to order blood gases." More subtle behavior includes half-heartedly listening to the nurse's full description of the patient's condition. A critical exchange between both professional groups occurs during physician rounds. Both disciplines share in the responsibility of making this time productive and meaningful. The high expectations of physicians and their curtness and sometimes overt negative responses to the nurse's information and questions inhibit open dialogue and collaboration between the two disciplines. Nurses who are well versed in the patient's condition and clear on what is needed while the physician is on the unit will be less vulnerable to this behavior (Alexander, 1989).

Graffiti

This is the most overt form of verbal and physical aggression through public humiliation and temper tantrums. Cox (1991b) identified that 69% of the respondents noted this behavior following a stressful situation. Thus graffiti is used as a coping mechanism. High-acuity environments produce stressful situations and stressed caregivers, making this fertile soil for such exchanges to occur. Physicians may rant and rave in front of other health care providers, patients, or families. Charts and other items may be thrown, phones slammed, and threats such as "I'm going to have your job," or "Just who is your supervisor?" issued. Nurses may be used as scapegoats for the things that have gone wrong with the patient or the system. A "kill the messenger" phenomenon occurs when the physician explodes to a nurse reporting unstable vital signs and laboratory results of a deteriorating patient. These violent outbursts usually occur toward the more vulnerable nurse, the novice, or a part-time nurse who the physician does not know or trust. The nurse who is confident and appropriately assertive is less likely to experience this behavior from a physician. As nurses learn to respond in a positive, confident manner consistently, a change in physician behavior may occur (Alexander, 1989).

Phony Verbiage

Physicians may hypocritically commend one group of nurses at the expense of another. During patient rounds, the physician may expound on how "wonderful the nurses are on this unit. You can take care of everything, not like those incompetent nurses at hospital B." Internally, the message is more devious as the physician degrades a nursing practice on the medical–surgical unit to the staff in intensive care. Consistent with behavior of an oppressed group, the nurses being complimented internalize this praise and feel better about themselves because the dominant figure (the physician) has shown that they are better than their colleagues. However, such abusive behavior is a pattern for some physicians, and soon the nurses begin to realize that the same comments are made about them to others in the organization or to colleagues working in competing hospitals. In the end, everyone is undermined by such behavior.

Sarcasm

A common and subtle form of abuse—taunting or sneering with caustic remarks meaning the opposite of what is expressed—occurs with alarming frequency. Because of its subtlety, the statement causes confusion and hurt within the receiver, making an appropriate, assertive response difficult. The covert nature of this attack places it in a gray area, allowing the physician to go undetected or unaddressed due to lack of proof that anything irregular has occurred. This form of abuse poses unique problems for the nursing administrator and staff.

Sexual Harassment

Cox (1991a) discovered that 30% of the respondents in her study indicated an experience in the form of sexual propositioning, sexual insulting, or suggestive touching. Statements such as, "Bring your pretty little buns over here and bring me that chart," are not unfamiliar to some nurses. The intimacy resulting from a close association between a nurse and a physician over the care of a very difficult patient in the middle of the night gives some physicians the impression that because they are in control of the clinical situation they also may take liberties with the nurse involved. Obscene, offensive joke telling is common, especially in the OR. Because of this controlled setting, the nurse is unable to remove herself from the abusive situation.

The Response of Management to Abusive Behavior

The nursing administrator has the responsibility to take a lead in addressing an abusive environment. This may be a challenge because of her corporate position and the sensitivity of the issue among other administrators and the medical staff. The most effective strategy is development of a corporate approach that includes problem identification, issue resolution, and education toward prevention. Education of both disciplines is essential, recognizing abuse as an illness or pathology, a metaphor both groups know well. The etiology, symptoms, and treatment of abusive communication must be known and understood. Empowerment of the nursing staff to confront the offenders in an assertive, constructive manner is essential. Equally important is the investment of nonabusing members of the medical staff in addressing and resolving the problem.

Determining the Extent of the Problem

Initially, a *reality check* should be taken to determine the degree of the problem in the hospital environment. Nurses are an excellent source for determining the approximate percent of abusing physicians, the frequency of encounters, and which individuals or groups use abusive behavior most consistently. One hospital conducted a survey of nurses and physicians (Appendix 22–A) and determined that 10 physicians out of 350, 3.5% of all physicians in that hospital, were identified as abusers. Of that group, 3 physician's names surfaced frequently in the written responses. This objective database provided the foundation for dialogue within a committee established to address the issue.

Establishing a Bidisciplinary Verbal Abuse Committee

A *bidisciplinary verbal abuse committee,* composed of nurses and physicians, recognizes the unique working and communication relationship that exists between these two groups within the hospital setting. By limiting the membership to these two groups, other perspectives that may cloud the real issues are eliminated. Physicians may show reluctance to participate because of busy schedules and perceived personal risk. If key physicians with strong power to influence the medical staff are approached by nurses who share a strong and positive working relationship with them, there is greater potential for ongoing commitment to the committee and its work.

The initial work of the committee consists of a literature review to provide an informed, educated approach to the etiology and symptoms of the problem.

Further, it demonstrates the universal nature of the problem among professionals throughout the field. This scientific approach provides credibility for physicians who must take the work back to the medical staff because of the objective manner in which the issue is being addressed. Combining the literature findings with data generated from the reality check, a starting point for debate is created. As the dialogue between these two groups evolves, more candor arises within each group. Both nurses and physicians reflect on their practice patterns as well as those of their colleagues. In many instances, competent and caring physicians are surprised at the behavior demonstrated by aggressive colleagues, prompting such comments as, "I don't abuse nurses, and if my partners do they must be corrected." As the committee separates the problems causing stress or conflict from the behavior engaged in to cope with that problem, a blueprint for action evolves.

Educating the Medical and Nursing Staffs

Education, rather than punitive action, is the best approach to presenting the issue of verbal abuse throughout the organization. Through education of the medical and nursing staffs, awareness of the problem and ownership of the solutions begin to evolve. Medical staff leadership must demonstrate a commitment to address the issue openly through education about the etiology, symptoms, and solutions of verbal abuse. Corporate implementation of a review and a sanctioning process to address individuals identified as abusive is critical to the ultimate success of the venture.

THE ROLE OF THE NURSE MANAGER
Assisting in the Development of Assertiveness Skills

The nurse manager's primary responsibility is to assist and support staff in the development of assertiveness skills to break the cycle of abusive communication (Baggs & Ryan, 1990; Johnson, 1983; Prescott & Bowen, 1985). Nurses are given the same information as the medical staff, along with such techniques as scripting, in which the nurses develop two or three generic statements that can be used in most incidents until the nurses become more expert at individualizing their responses. A nursing leader in one hospital developed expertise in the diagnosis and symptomatology of abusive communication. She conducted seminars for interested nursing staff and managers. An active interest soon emerged in other clinical disciplines, such as pharmacy and laboratory staff, because of their experiences in dealing with abusive physicians and nurses. Thus, a heightened awareness emerged throughout the organization.

Reporting Mechanism

A reporting mechanism provides a vehicle to monitor the prevalence of the problem while minimizing personal risk to the accuser or the accused. Each incident must be investigated for accuracy, and patterns must be trended to provide information to initiate corrective action. Nursing staff often feel mis-

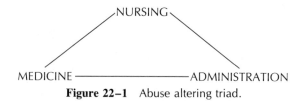

Figure 22–1 Abuse altering triad.

understood or abandoned when the nursing manager of a unit focuses on systems problems or a knowledge deficit of the nurse rather than the abusive behavior of the physician.

Collaborative Delineation of Responsibilities

Once the education has been completed, administration must develop a corporate policy to address verbal abuse (Appendix 22–B). For this process to be effective, a delineation of responsibilities must be determined collaboratively by the key departments involved: medicine, nursing, and administration (Fig. 22–1).

Mentoring

An empowering step in assisting nurses to refine assertiveness skills includes mentoring by the nurse manager. When the staff nurse reports an abusive encounter to the manager, both approach the physician together. The nurse manager is present not to determine who was right or wrong but to refocus the discussion on the behavior rather than the problem that prompted it. The nurse manager is there to support and clarify what the nurse is attempting to convey to the physician. The nurse manager who finds herself in the position of judging has not completed the preparatory work needed for intervention before the confrontation. By collaborating on the issue, both the nurse and nurse manager can clearly identify systems issues that often contribute to stressful situations encountered by both nurses and physicians working in high-acuity environments (Bohy, 1991; Makadon & Gibbs, 1985).

As the corporate environment supports reporting and intervention, a mature organization will find individuals confronting each other at the time of the incident, clarifying misunderstandings, and correcting abusive communication immediately. The resultant environment of harmony and respect will increase the quality of care for patients and the quality of life in the workplace for all.

TOWARD AN INTEGRATIVE FUTURE

In her compelling book, *Woman as Healer,* Achterberg (1990) examines the new healing consciousness emerging in the western world. Both men and women are beginning to recognize and integrate a holistic perspective into their professions and their lives. Scientific findings are validating that mind, body, and spirit each plays a vital role in the healing process. The masculine and feminine are

TABLE 22-1 The Myth of the Masculine and the Feminine

Masculine	Feminine
Intellect	Intuition
Rational	Irrational
Linear	Nonlinear
Left brain	Right brain
Knowledge	Wisdom
Power	Compassion
Analysis	Synthesis
Mastery	Mystery
Giving	Receiving
Technical	Natural
Competition	Collaboration
Objective	Subjective
Doing to	Being with
Curing	Caring
Fixing	Nurturing
Rigid	Flexible

regarded as polarities that, together, comprise the whole. Some of the identified traits are shown in Table 22–1.

Contemporary society is faced with a curing culture created by a focus on advancing knowledge and technology rather than on wisdom and honoring the earth. A healing system focused exclusively on the feminine perspective will return society to a tribal mode. Remaining strongly in the masculine will destroy the earth. The answer lies in integration of the feminine nursing and the masculine medical models.

A healing system that allows for the fuller expression of health is multifaceted—a web of health care practitioners within a sustaining environment that fosters healing. Such a model would call for healers of the mind and spirit as well as the physical body. Relationships within the web would require practitioners to be present more effectively for each other and the client (Achterberg, 1988). Characteristics of such a relationship would include honoring life and confronting the shadow.

Honoring Life

This is the essence of the healing arts, the heart of medical and nursing professional oaths. Honoring life calls for an appreciation of the richness of existence of each human being and for appreciating the beauty of diversity. It requires knowing of and honoring the many nontraditional paths that lead to wholeness as well as the traditional medical models of medicine. It calls the healer to value and facilitate a peaceful death when appropriate. Honoring life calls for each person involved in the healing process to participate and contribute in a way that enriches the client, the nurse, and the physician.

Confronting the Shadow

Recognition and eradication of the oppressive issues facing the healing community must occur if a holistic system is to be developed for the client. Women's accomplishments in the healing arts and sciences must no longer be trivialized or forgotten. The exploitation of women in the health care professions must be stopped. The unique contributions of women's professions must be freed from the direct authority of male-dominated professions and fields of endeavor. Financial and decision-making authority must be *equal* to the unique contribution of each discipline, with each receiving *direct compensation* for services rendered.

PRACTICAL APPLICATIONS

Nursing must take a proactive, rather than a reactive, stance to ensure that transformational change will occur. Deciding who we will become as a profession is the first critical step (McNutt-Devereux, 1981). As goals are redefined, the healing process will begin. Strategies that will enhance this movement include the following (Achterberg, 1990, p. 204).

- Use the differences in the nature of medical and nursing education to provide integrated, interactive health care delivery through interdisciplinary team activities.
- Facilitate a shift from the hierarchy of a power-based health system to one of more egalitarian proportions by participation in committee work and legislative and regulatory activities, with a clear vision and voice.
- Promote the elevation of women's professions to higher levels of competency. Woman's intuition must give way to a stronger educational base: collaboration will increase between roles equal in educational degrees.
- Incorporate therapists who treat the mental and spiritual aspects of health within the mainstream of health care, moving to a holistic team of care providers.
- Create a more human-centered healing system, which will be assured if the feminine nurturing voice is included.

All of this calls for significant changes in the art and science of healing. We must challenge our basic assumptions regarding the role of women, our definition of power, the effects of competition, and the place of community and collaboration in the problem-solving process. Each discipline, each gender, must value and seek some level of competence in the behaviors, skills, and attitudes of the other for an androgenous approach to critical thinking and decision making. When the balance is finally achieved, a collaborative, holistic health care system will be in place, and life will be honored in a manner befitting its creation.

References

Achterberg, J. (1988). The wounded healer: Transformational journeys in modern medicine. In G. Doore (Ed.), *Shaman's path: Healing, personal growth and empowerment.* Boston: Shamballa.

Achterberg, J. (1990). *Woman as healer.* Boston: Shamballa.

Aiken, L., & Mullinix, C.P. (1987). The nurse shortage, myth or reality? *New England Journal of Medicine, 317,* 641–646.

Alexander, C. (1989, May 18). Verbal abuse: The nurses' scalpel. *Managing Today's OR Suite*.

American Medical Association. (1987). *Physician characteristics and distributions in the U.S.* Chicago: Department of Data, American Medical Association.

Baggs, J.G., & Ryan, S.A. (1990). ICU nurse–physician collaboration and nursing satisfaction. *Nursing Economics, 8*(6), 386–392.

Blendon, R.J. (1988). The public's view of the future of health care. *Journal of the American Medical Association, 259,* 3587–3593.

Bohy, R.L. (1991, July). Defining and dealing with abusive and harassing action(s) and behavior(s). Sioux Valley Hospital.

Bradford, R. (1989). Obstacles to collaborative practice. *Nursing Management, 20*(4), 72I, 72L–72M, 72P.

Bullough, B. (1975). Barriers to the nurse practitioner movement: Problems of women in a woman's field. *International Journal of Health Services, 2*(5), 229–230.

Cox, H. (1991a). Verbal abuse nationwide, Part I: Oppressed group behavior. *Nursing Management, 22*(2), 32–35.

Cox, H. (1991b). Verbal abuse nationwide, Part II: Impact and modifications. *Nursing Management, 22*(3), 60–66.

Diaz, A.L., & McMillin, J.D. (1991). A definition and description of nurse abuse. *Western Journal of Nursing Research, 13*(1), 97–109.

Gasparis, L. (1990). *Nurse abuse.* New York: Laura Power.

Gonzalez, M.L., & Emmons, D.W. (1986). *Socioeconomic characteristics of medical practice*. Washington, DC: American Medical Association Center for Health Policy Research.

Iglehart, J.K. (1987). Problems facing the nursing profession. *New England Journal of Medicine, 317,* 646–651.

Johnson, P.F. (1983). Improving the nurse–physician relationship. *The Journal of Nursing Administration,* 19–20.

Makadon, H. & Gibbons, P. (1985). Nurses and physicians: Prospects for collaboration. *Annals of Internal Medicine, 103*(1), 134–136.

McNutt-Devereux, P. (1981). Nurse/physician collaboration: Nursing practice considerations. *The Journal of Nursing Administration, 11*(9), 37–39.

Muff, J. (1982). *Socialization, sexism and stereotyping: Women's issues in nursing.* Prospect Heights, IL: Waveland Press.

National Commission on Nursing. (1981). *Initial report and preliminary recommendations.* Chicago, IL: Hospital Research Education and Trust.

Prescott, P.A., & Bowen, S.A. (1985). Physician–nurse relationships. *Annals of Internal Medicine, 103,* 127–133.

Relman, A.S. (1989). The changing demography of the medical profession. *New England Journal of Medicine, 321,* 1540–1542.

Stein, L.I. (1967). The doctor–nurse game. *Archives of General Psychiatry, 16,* 699–703.

Stein, L.I., Watts, D.T., & Howell, T. (1990). Sounding board: The doctor-nurse game revisited. *New England Journal of Medicine, 322*(8):546-549.

Part B. Managing Material Resources

CHAPTER 23　　　•　　　•　　　•　　　•　　　•　　　•

MANAGING IN A MANAGED CARE ENVIRONMENT

RHONDA ANDERSON

EXECUTIVE SUMMARY

Over the last 5 years, many articles and books have been written about financial management in nursing. It is an important topic for all managers and nurses to study and understand. It is also imperative for managers to apply these principles when preparing their budgets, managing their units, and reviewing their monthly revenue and expense documents. This author advocates the use of these principles as each nurse manager develops a clinical enhancement proposal, a quality improvement proposal, or a new program proposal. In many health care institutions, nurse managers are excluded from the financial arena. They are not expected to be financially knowledgeable and are not included in financial decisions. It seems that institutional clinical and financial success will occur only when nurse managers are expected to understand the total picture of managing a health care facility. It is, therefore, imperative that nurse managers be expected to develop and manage their budget based on institutional assumptions, program projections, and case mix information. The finance officer and nurse executive should supply this information to each nurse manager as part of their budget packet. The nurse manager will then prepare personnel, supply, and capital budgets based on this information.

This chapter describes how clinical knowledge and the fiscal environment must be integrated for an institution to remain viable. It describes the role of the nurse executive and nurse manager in this integration and suggests a proactive approach to dealing with the rapidly evolving managed care philosophy. It details what information the nurse manager should expect for budget and monitoring purposes. Nurse managers will learn the difference in their role before the managed care evolution and in the managed care environment.

THE MANAGED CARE ENVIRONMENT

Managed care has been a heavily used term in some parts of the United States. It will continue to grow in popularity as health care reform takes shape in the 1990s. There are several definitions for managed care (see Appendix 23–A). The one used here is a system that effectively manages the health and illness continuum of an individual through efficient use of resources, i.e., controlling costs. Some nurses and nurse managers believe they have alway been using resources effectively. In this new environment, there is a need to do even better, and it must be done in conjunction with the payor's expectations.

To provide a framework for this evolution, it is important to understand cost, charges, and reimbursement as used in the health care arena.

Cost

Cost is determined by the direct and indirect dollars required to produce a unit of service. If this unit of service is provided only through human resource consumption, salary and benefits may be the only cost. If supplies and physical or technologic facility use are involved, those dollars must be applied as well.

Charges and Reimbursement

Charges are the dollars per item or unit of service that the health care institution bills a patient or an insurance company. In many cases, there is no relationship of charges to cost. There may or may not be a methodology by which these charges are developed. Charges may be based on competition or driven by regulation depending on the state in which the health care institution is located.

Reimbursement and cost are the keys to successful fiscal management for all hospitals in the 1990s. There are five major methodologies for reimbursement: (1) fee for service, (2) percent of billed charges, (3) per diem payment, (4) per case reimbursement, and (5) capitation.

Fee for Service

This has been the primary way of payment for the last 100 years. In the very early years of medicine, families paid physicians for their services by giving them food or money. Hospitals billed and patients or insurance companies paid for the service. This method has been disappearing and will soon become obsolete.

Percent of Billed Charges

This second type of reimbursement has evolved over the past 50 years. The insurer has paid a percent of charges, and the patient has paid a percent. This carries a risk to the insurer and patient, not to the provider, since the provider still collects 100%. Recently, there has been additional meaning to percent of billed charges. Third party payors are negotiating with institutions to pay only a percent of their charges for each patient to whom care is provided. That percent may decrease if the hospital experiences an increase in the patient days from all the third party payor's patients. In effect, the discount is greater as the third party guarantees an increase in the number of patients being cared for in a given institution. An example of a contract agreement for days and percent of billed charges follows.

PATIENT DAYS	BILLED CHARGES (%)
0–5,000	80
5,001–10,000	75
10,001–15,000	70
over 15,001	65

This approach begins to shift the risk to the provider and the patient if the provider by contract can bill the patient the difference. There are, however, many contracts that do not allow the hospital to bill the patient for the difference, and the hospital bears all the risk.

Per Diem Payment

The hospital is reimbursed an agreed-on amount for each day of the patient's stay. The hospital payment begins with the day of admission but does not include the day of discharge. One can easily understand the risk of this reimbursement method. Whatever costs or charges are incurred on a daily basis generally are not of concern to third party payors with this approach, since they pay a fixed amount each day. This method creates great financial risk to the institution. It behooves the institution to control the use of resources and related costs for this patient population, particularly during the discharge day, since nothing can be billed or will be paid for the last day. This method could create an adversarial relationship with physicians and employees of the institution, since the administration is focusing on decreasing resource consumption.

It is important for the institution to monitor trends, e.g., length of stay, so that it can negotiate the next contract with the physician practice pattern changes in mind. The nurse manager is instrumental in knowing and communicating to administration some of the third party changes in the clinical management of patients. The administration must establish a formal mechanism to receive this information from nurse managers so that future contracts can provide reasonable reimbursement to the institution.

Per Diem Example. Mr. Jones is admitted for a thyroidectomy. When the original contract was negotiated with the HMO, the gross charges for this procedure were reviewed and the number of days a patient stayed were analyzed. Based on the analysis, a rate of $648 per day was agreed on by the hospital and the HMO. The hospital is now losing money on gross charges on each of these patients because the medical management has changed, as has length of stay. Table 23–1 is an itemized example of what is occurring.

The charges for performing the surgical procedure and for the patient's recovery ($6174) are not even covered by the reimbursement ($2592). The cost for the surgical procedure and recovery room is approximately $4086. Assuming there is some relationship to cost and charges on each day of stay, the cost of providing the care for these patients is still not fully reimbursed. It does not take

TABLE 23–1 Example of Per Diem Reimbursement

	CHARGES	REIMBURSEMENT
Surgery	$3586	
PACU[a]	500	
Admission day	500	$ 648
PO day 1	438	648
PO day 2	375	648
PO day 3	375	648
PO day 4	400	
Total	$6174	$2592

[a]PACU, postoperative acute care unit; PO, postoperative.

many of these cases before the hospital exhibits financial instability and has no cash accumulated for capital funding replacement or new items.

Per Case Reimbursement

A hospital is paid a predetermined fixed rate to provide the inpatient care for a patient, based on the diagnosis. Outpatient services rendered as an inpatient do not qualify for reimbursement. Most health care providers can relate to this payment, since Medicare's prospective payment system (DRG) has been in effect since 1983 and is a per case reimbursement. This methodology also places the hospital at great risk. The hospital is expected to control all use of resources, but they do not have privileges to admit, discharge, or write orders. This system provides no incentive for the physicians to alter their practice or use less expensive equipment or supplies in the treatment of their patients.

As hospitals try to work with physicians to improve the hospital financial picture, adversarial situations can arise. The nurse manager must be knowledgeable about the per case patients and work with her staff and the physicians to develop an efficient plan of care for the patient and the family.

Per Case Example. A patient enters the hospital the day before having a hip replaced. A laboratory workup and chest x-ray are done. The patient is prepared for surgery. The surgical procedure is completed on day 2 of the stay. The surgeon has a choice of joint apparatus and uses one that costs the hospital $3800. The patient's postoperative course is uneventful. The surgeon begins physical therapy on postoperative day 5 and sends the patient home on postoperative day 7.

The reimbursement for this case is $9650 dollars and does not include the day before surgery or the laboratory work and x-rays done that day. The hospital has already lost a significant amount of money. The surgical procedure, recovery charges, and the prosthesis are two thirds of the reimbursement—$6426 of the $9650 for the 7 postoperative days. There are only $3224 left. It is extremely easy to understand the possible losses with this type of payment but not as easy to correct the situation.

Capitation

This is most likely the future method of financing our health care. This is the most risky financing but could be the most effective. Payment is based on a fixed monthly fee per enrollee (per member per month). This fee covers the individual's entire health care needs. The provider has total financial responsibility for the enrollee's health care. This is very risky, since it is sometimes difficult to control the public's expectations of talking to or seeing a physician whenever they choose to do so. Also, if someone has a catastrophic illness, the third party payor may never receive monthly fees comparable to the cost of the illness. An exciting aspect of this financing is that an emphasis will be placed on wellness and prevention, which could lead to a healthier American public.

It is possible for a hospital to have all five methods of reimbursement in the institution. It is very important for the nurse manager and nurse executive to know the institution's contractual arrangements and begin to influence those negotiations. The general approach used in negotiating contracts is for some finance and industrial engineering employees to be assigned to do an analysis of the patients the hospital has had the previous year from the third party payor who is requesting a contract. This group evaluates all the charges incurred from the previous year. They then initiate some assumptions. Some of these assumptions might be that the length of stay will decrease by X tenths of a day, that the use of resource consumption will decrease by a given percent, and that the hospital charges may increase by a certain percent more than the costs. They then calculate the worst case and best case scenario for their negotiations. In these contracts, there are many requirements other than price. There are expectations for outpatient care, emergency room triage, treatment approvals, and scheduling delay penalties, to name a few. Every third party payor has different requirements.

THE ROLE OF THE NURSE MANAGER

There is a major flaw in this approach to negotiating new contracts. There has been an assumption that patient care will be managed in the future as it has been in the recent past. There has been little involvement of clinicians in developing the assumptions, and consequently, there is an absence of information as part of the decision process. This is where the nurse manager must participate. The nurse manager brings knowledge of new drugs, therapies, or approaches to patient management that the doctors have discussed. The nurse manager can translate that information into the positive or negative financial impact on the hospital and communicate through the nurse executive to the negotiators. It is imperative that those negotiating understand the ramifications of the special requirements in the contracts.

It behooves the institutional negotiators to use knowledgeable nurse managers to discuss these proposed special expectations before agreeing to them in a signed contract. These requirements may be a drastic departure from how things have been done. They could lead to more costly ways of providing care, information, or paperwork to the third party payor. The nurse manager can be effective in influencing change if she or he is informed and allowed to effect the change proactively.

To prepare the nurse executive with the appropriate input for these negotiations, the nurse manager should

1. Provide the nurse executive with an analysis of the previous 6 months of patient management data
2. Provide the nurse executive with assumptions for future management
3. Provide financial and human resource projections of special contract requirements
4. Develop worst case/best case recommendations
5. Provide utilization data and quality data for the previous 6 months

To do this, one must be aware of many details of how care is directed by the physicians. One must monitor trends daily and know and understand the dynamic changes of the practice patterns. One must be able to substantiate the comments with data. Quantifying clinical knowledge is a must. The nurse manager is the key resource in the organization to successfully accomplish data collection, quantification, and change in order to meet the demands of the managed care environment.

The nurse manager must be developed into a manager who can

- Redesign how the patient care delivery system is functioning so that it is a more efficient system
- Direct the staff to be more aware of the third party payor expectations and implement them consistently
- Monitor concurrently the effectiveness of the professionals in their patient care plans and interventions
- Review with utilization management analysts and third party payor reviewers concurrently all patients and their status
- Intervene where necessary to schedule a patient's test or surgical procedure so denials of hospital days will not occur
- Help staff be comfortable with the level of care provided based on the third party payor's expectations
- Consistently understand and interpret to staff, other departments, and physicians what is expected by each patient's payor for or during hospitalization

Nurse managers in managed care environments can be the hospital's best ally or worst enemy. The environment to assure staff change or physician cooperation is critical to success. The nurse manager must understand and internalize the big picture issues while ensuring their unit's contribution to that larger picture.

PRACTICAL APPLICATIONS

There are three major components related to the managed care process in hospitals (Table 23–2). Each nurse manager must understand these and their component parts. Nurse managers must educate their staff to function in a new, more efficient way, recognizing that they can only provide the essentials of acute care and then must transfer the patients to providers outside the acute care setting, e.g., home health care.

Preadmission Process

The first area is the preadmission process. As reflected in Table 23–2, there are many components to this process.

Elective Admissions

Elective admissions require a review and screening before admission. The following are the criteria.

- Admission appropriateness
- Surgical necessity
- Level of care necessary, i.e., observation status, outpatient, ICU, general inpatient
- Precertification of the procedures to be done
- Potential discharge risk or financial risk

Generally, a new area of nursing expertise is established for a preadmission program. Nurses are involved in an outpatient setting to provide the following screening for patients.

- Laboratory and radiology results review
- Preoperative education for surgical patient
- Begin nursing history and assessment
- Social Service referral when appropriate
- Instruction on advance directives
- Answer questions and provide phone number for contact with the nurse before admission day
- Organize all chart components and give them to the unit where patient will be admitted

Along with these clinical responsibilities, financial screening is initiated to verify insurance coverage and authorization of the elective admission.

TABLE 23–2 Utilization Management Process

PROSPECTIVE REVIEW	CONCURRENT REVIEW	RETROSPECTIVE REVIEW
Preadmission screening	Case management	Delays/denials
Elective admission	Catastrophic management	Medical management information
Emergency/urgent admission	Appropriate levels of care	Health records completion
Financial assessment/verification	Discharge planning	Catatastrophic management trends
		Placement issues

Nonelective Admissions: The Emergency Department

Nonelective admissions also are screened by using the described criteria. In addition, emergency center staff must request authorization for admission and, many times, approval for treatment. In a managed care environment, the emergency center staff have to make many changes in their approach to caring for patients. The triage nurse must

- Assess the patient's physical status and complaints
- Determine what third party is the payor
- Refer to a master list with the third party payor's requirements noted
- Call the primary care provider or other designee for authorization to treat
- Triage after consulting with emergency center physician

The emergency center physicians and nurses often are in a difficult position, for they may be mandated by federal or state law to see and treat patients and then be told they are not authorized to do so by the third party payor. They may be instructed to tell patients to go to their own doctors the next working day. If they do not act appropriately, they could be violating federal statutes, yet if they treat, there may be no reimbursement for the hospital.

Nurse managers in the emergency center must be aware of all the requirements in each contract about emergent and urgent treatment. With every new contract or addendum, they should

- Establish a mechanism to provide the nursing staff with ongoing access to the current contract information
- Establish a mechanism for staff to find out which physicians are part of which health plans so specialists can be contacted if necessary
- Retrospectively review the previous day's activities to determine triage nurse effectiveness
- Review and analyze circumstances around payment denials and provide further staff education about the problem or situation

When a hospital begins to get many of these contracts, it is sometimes difficult for emergency center nurses to accept their new responsibilities in screening and seeking authorization. It takes constant education, coaching, and retrospective case review by the manager to establish compliance of the nursing staff with these new requirements.

Concurrent Review

Most hospitals have a utilization management department that employs nurses to perform daily reviews on patients and collect data on the appropriateness of services ordered, the appropriateness of level of care, and the appropriateness of continued hospitalization. These nurses work with hospital-funded physicians, i.e., physician advisors or physician reviewers, to evaluate the collected data and discuss with the attending physicians the appropriate course of medical management. These nurses and physicians know every contract and each idiosyncrasy so they can help the hospital meet its financial obligations. They review charting to make certain that physicians are documenting pertinent information. They establish discharge plans with the social workers, and they do large-dollar case review and try to influence a change in the use of resources. They have been designated as the sole conscience for appropriate use in the hospital.

Another model may be more appropriate. This model does not superimpose a new philosophy (managed care) on an old structure. It redesigns the care delivery system to meet the challenges of managed care. It builds into the RN roles and responsibilities accountability for managing the care and resources in collaboration with the physician.

The Case Management Model

This model is centered around a case manager and predetermined management of care plans designed by DRGs. An interdisciplinary team designs the care to be provided by the various health care providers for the prehospital, hospital, and immediate posthospital time frames. The process begins through an analysis of historical use of resources by payor and DRG. The interdisciplinary team then evaluates if that process is appropriate for the future or if it should be altered. After the plan of care is written, it is costed out to determine if it is within the financial guidelines of the payor. It should then be discussed with the administrative and clinical staff of the respective payor. The nurse manager and a physician (preferably chairman of the department) should colead this process. The nurse manager should have access to all the data necessary to facilitate the process. At the time of completion of the plan of care or patient management protocol, the manager needs to begin the implementation process by

- Assigning one or more case managers to be responsible for implementing the protocol on all patients with that diagnosis
- Educate nursing staff about their role when a protocol is in place
- With physician coleader, introduce protocol to the medical staff
- Redesign the quality improvement plan through use of this protocol
- Establish a mechanism for concurrent review of the effectiveness of case manager and staff
- Establish a system for case manager, social worker, and utilization management analyst to review cases, take action, and collaborate with the physician
- Be available to the case manager for guidance with high-risk cases
- Establish a system for case managers and social workers to determine what posthospital facilities are used and paid for by each payor
- Establish a mechanism to monitor cost of care per patient population, reimbursement, and denials of payment

With this model, the expectations are integrated into all providers roles and responsibilities, and everyone feels ownership and accountability for moving the patient through the acute care facility more efficiently. The case manager is providing clinical direction to all disciplines involved in the patient's care. The case manager is collaborating with the physician to determine what changes to the management protocol, if any, need to occur. The nurse manager at the point of care is coordinating all activities and holding caregivers accountable for their practice in this new environment.

Retrospective Case Review

Retrospective case review is the third area of the utilization management process. Each hospital should have medical management information that helps to monitor physician performance. This information should include

- Average length of stay (LOS) by patient type
- Average cost per case
- Outlier information, both dollars and days
- Comparison of above to other physicians and state average
- Number of delays or denied payment days for the physician's patients
- Incomplete records causing delayed billing
- Attestation compliance
- Denied presurgical days
- Adverse patient outcomes—number and type

It is recognized that all of these areas may have other variables that cause the data to be different from the average. This is where the quality improvement principles are involved. The nurse manager and physician cochairs review data and question cause and effect, i.e., systems issue, human resource issue, physician practice issue. It is more important to act on the information through one or more of the following.

- Staff continuing education
- Improving new orientation for staff
- Revision of basic patient management protocol
- Correct a systems issue
- Change process for catastrophic intervention
- If a trend of denials by a certain payor, discuss alternatives for correction with the payor
- If specific physician abuser, physician cochair to discuss with that physician

The health record can cause many problems on a retrospective basis. No matter what the payment methodology, there are generally contractual requirements for completeness of records before accepting billing. If physicians and nurses have not completed the records, documented thoroughly, or listed a discharge diagnosis, the hospital cannot bill for services rendered. It takes hours of health records employees' time and many FTEs to retrospectively read and review every chart, flag incomplete areas, and track physicians or other care providers to complete the charts. Revision of this system to meet the demands of the managed care providers seems to make sense. The unit clerk's role and responsibilities need to be modified to include a 24-hour check of every chart. Concurrent review and reminding the physicians and nurses of appropriate, complete documentation are less time consuming and allow for a completed record at the time of discharge. The nurse manager needs to support unit-based, concurrent health record functions to improve productivity and billing for the hospital.

Nurse managers have an enormous role in a managed care environment. The financial margins are so limited with most contracts that even the smallest inefficiency can cause great financial problems. It is important for the manager to impress on staff the expected changes and to help them realize that change does not equate to poor quality. The most common nursing theme, with the drastic changes required by managed care providers, is that the quality is poor. The manager has to work closely with the staff to help them recognize that they are equating quality to the process of providing care, not to the outcome. They must begin to measure outcomes.

It is imperative for acute care nurses to accept data supplied by another professional and not repeat the work. Acute care nurses formerly did all preoperative teaching and physical assessments on preoperative patients. Now, when surgical patients are admitted on the morning of surgery, those assessments have been done by preadmission nurses days before. Generally, if acute care nurses try to repeat the procedure, they are frustrated because they do not have enough time. They then bemoan the quality of care because payors will not let the patient be admitted the day before surgery. However, if a patient were tested and knows the preoperative education information, the outcome is the desired one even though the process is different from that used a few years previously. The nurse manager must redirect the acute care nurse's professional energies to appropriate concerns.

These are exciting and challenging times for nurse managers. There is an opportunity for all savvy nurse managers to effectively influence professional nurses to make valuable and noteworthy contributions to the health care team. It is an opportunity for the nurse manager to provide the hospital with a competent, efficient team of nurses who will contribute to the success of the institution. The most significant contribution, however, is the positive positioning of this efficient, quality organization to receive the next phase of managed care—health care reform.

Bibliography

Beyers, M. (1991). Editorial. *Journal of Nursing Administration Quarterly*, pp. viii–x.

Bocchino, C.A. (1990, November–December). Interview with Carol Lockhart, nurse representative of PPRC. *Nursing Economics*, pp. 371–377.

Brown, B.J. (1991). Editorial. *Journal of Nursing Administration Quarterly*, pp. v–vii.

Coile, R.C., Jr. (1990, March–April). The megatrends—and the backlash. *Healthcare Forum Journal*, pp. 37–40.

Davis, D.L., & Salmen, K.M. (1991). Nursing, planning, and marketing: From theory to practice. *Nursing Administration Quarterly, 15*(3), 66–71.

Dunston, J. (1990, October). How managed care can work for you. *Nursing 90*, pp. 56–59.

Evered, R.D., & Selman, J.C. (1989). *Organizational dynamics*. New York: AMA Publications Division, American Management Association.

Giuliano, K.K., & Poirier, C.E. (1991). Nursing case management: Critical pathways to desirable outcomes. *Nursing Management, 22*(3), 52–55.

Herrle, G.N., & Pollock, W.M. (1991, January—February). Multispecialty groups: Will they survive prepaid managed care? *MGM Journal.*

Johnson, J. (1991, October). Interview with Ben Jacobowitz, Director for Managed Care, St. Joseph Medical Center, Burbank, CA. and Donald Shubert, Director of Contracting, Mercy Hospital, Bakersfield, CA. *Hospitals,* pp. 26–30.

Jones, K.R. (1991). Maintaining quality in a changing environment. *Nursing Economics, 9*(3), 159–164.

Korenchuk, K. (1991, January–February). Negotiating and analyzing managed care contracts. *MGM Journal.*

Kouba, D.J. (1991, January–February). Primary care providers: Managing today's prepaid risk. *MGM Journal.*

LeClair, C.L. (1991). Introducing and accounting for RN case management. *Nursing Management, 22*(3), 44–49.

Lora, M.E. (1991, fall). Preserving hospitals through managed care. *Contemporary Senior Health,* pp. 17–20.

Mayberry, A. (1991). Merging nursing theories, models, and nursing practice: More than an administrative challenge. *Nursing Administration Quarterly, 15*(3), 44–53.

Miller, K., & Stepura, B.A. (1989). Converting nursing care cost to revenue. *Journal of Nursing Administration, 19*(5), 18–22.

Papenhausen, J.L. (1990). Editorial. Case management: A model of advanced pratice? *Clinical Nurse Specialist,* pp. 169–170.

Pierog, L.J. (1991). Case management: A product line. *Nursing Administration Quarterly, 15*(2), 16–20.

Raske, K.E. (1991, April/May). Interview. *AAPPO Journal,* pp. 9–13.

Schryver, D.L. (1991, January–February). Responding to managed care proposals. *MGM Journal.*

Soule, T.R. (1991). *Aspen's Advisor for Nurse Executives, 6*(8), 3–5.

Stillwagon, C.A. (1989). The impact of nurse-managed care on the cost of nurse practice and nurse satisfaction. *Journal of Nursing Administration, 19*(11), 21–27.

Vaughn, D.G., et al. (1991). Utilization and management of multiskilled health practitioners in U.S. hospitals. *Hospital and Health Services Administration, 36*(3), 397–419.

Weingart, M. (1991). Commercially managed healthcare: An experience. *Nursing Management, 22*(1), 40–41.

Zander, K. (1988). Managed care within acute settings: Design and implementation via nursing case management. *Health Care Supervisor, 6*(2), 27–43.

Zander, K. (1991, fall). Care maps: The core of cost/quality care. *The New Definition, 6*(3).

Managed Care Terminology

authorization the process of obtaining permission from the patient's insurer, or health plan, to provide services.

capitation payment for health services based on a fixed monthly amount per enrollee. Payment does not vary by the volume of services provided and shifts the risk of cost to the provider (hospitals, physician, or others).

charges the dollar amount a hospital assesses for hospital goods and services on an itemized bill (costs plus a markup).

concurrent review review of a patient's treatment plan while care is being provided for appropriate use of resources and quality concerns.

costs the expenditure made to provide a service or the outlay of dollars a hospital spends.

diagnosis-related group (DRG) payment system an approach to payment for hospital inpatient acute services that reimburses a flat rate per case based on the DRG assignment (classification determined by diagnosis, procedures, and age).

discharge planning identification of the need and provision for a patient's health care requirements after discharge from the hospital.

eligibility a process to determine if an individual meets the qualifications for covered benefits.

fee for service payment a method of payment to providers on the basis of a charge for each service rendered.

fixed price payment a payment method for a fixed price and time period. The amount of covered services provided may vary (DRG, per diem, per case).

health maintenance organization (HMO) a legal entity that provides directly or arranges for a comprehensive range of health care services to an enrolled population on a prepaid or fixed periodic prepaid basis, which assumes risk for the cost of care.

individual practice association (IPA) a type of organizational structure through which private physicians, in their own offices, participate in a prepaid medical plan.

length of stay (LOS) the number of days a patient is an inpatient per episode. The length of time a patient is hospitalized.

medically necessary covered services required to preserve and maintain the health status of a patient in accordance with the area standards of medical practice as determined by the physician.

Medicare a federal program that provides health insurance for persons 65 and older and for other specified groups.

notification a process in which the hospital contacts the health plan to inform them that a patient has presented for service.

per diem payment system   payment for inpatient hospital services based on a preestablished per day fee.

preadmission assistance program (PAAP)   preadmission testing, screening for appropriateness of admission, and nursing and social service assessment before hospital admission. If not appropriate for admission, triages to appropriate level of care, i.e., home care, short stay, observation.

preadmission testing   diagnostic test, workup, and preparation on an outpatient basis before admission to a hospital.

preauthorization/precertification   procedure whereby a health provider submits the treatment plan to the payor or its agent for approval before rendering services.

preferred provider organization (PPO)   a group of selected physicians or hospitals or both who agree to provide care to a group of individuals at a negotiated fee—often discount off charges. A PPO differs from an HMO in that the assumption of cost risk does not usually occur.

prospective review   a review of a patient's treatment plan before the provision of care for appropriate use of resources and quality concerns.

retrospective review   a review of a patient's treatment after the care has been provided for appropriate use of resources and quality concerns.

third party payor   the HMO, PPO, or insurance company that is the provider of the patient's health care and is responsible to pay the hospital bill.

utilization management (UM)   systems means for reviewing and controlling patients' use of medical care services and providers' use of medical resources. Usually involves prospective, concurrent, and retrospective activities, especially for services such as specialist referrals and emergency room use, and particularly costly services, such as hospitalization.

verification of benefits   a process of reviewing with the insurer and/or health plan the coverage of specific services required by the patient.

Source of most of the definitions is *Managed Care, Self-Directed Learning Module* by Good Samaritan Regional Medical Center, Phoenix, Arizona.

CHAPTER 24

DRGs: Their Impact on Nursing Management

Roxane Spitzer-Lehmann
Mary Ann Davivier

Executive Summary

The advent of diagnosis-related groups (DRGs) and other prospective payment systems has spawned a wide range of changes within health care organizations and in nursing departments in particular. Although one of the intents of DRGs is to reduce costs, the side effects are nothing to trifle with. This chapter explores the effects of cost-containment methods on nursing and on the quality of health care in general. The question constantly being asked is, "How can I do the job most economically while maintaining or even improving patient quality?"

Not only must RNs work more efficiently, but they must also increase their knowledge base. For example, early discharge requires many clients to return home requiring sophisticated therapies, such as IV chemotherapy. This means that the nurse must be well versed in community resources and, in some cases, may follow the patient into the home setting to provide care.

This chapter identifies several areas where cause and effect seem to rule. For example, lack of documentation can equate with lower reimbursement, so nurses must increase their skills in the area of documentation. Likewise, the use of computerized information systems requires nurses to be computer literate. Efficiency makes the day, so the need to communicate effectively with other departments, community support systems, and family members has skyrocketed.

The use of unlicensed support staff or technicians is covered, and guidelines are given for their use. The chapter closes with a look at how nursing can develop revenue-producing programs, particularly through community-based educational efforts. In this respect, innovation and marketing skills are essential in today's health care environment.

Despite the implementation of prospective payment systems (PPS), such as diagnosis-related groups (DRGs), health care costs continue to rise at a rate far in excess of the consumer price index. Efforts to explore alternative delivery systems that provide quality health care at reduced cost are continuing. The immediate focus has been on the largest expenditure, hospital care, as consumers react to reduced quality of care, early discharge, and a shortage of nurses.

Logically, one of the alternatives under scrutiny is nursing care, which has proven to produce results as good as or better in many instances than physicians achieve. Third party reimbursement is slowly manifesting itself while nurses provide new services in home care, long-term care, and skilled nursing facilities as well as private practices. This promises to change the nursing profession—the way it is practiced and the way consumers view it. This chapter explores the effects of DRGs, prospective payment systems, and other cost-containment methods on nursing practice and the quality of health care today.

CHANGES IN THE HEALTH CARE SYSTEM

The increase in patient acuity levels in acute care settings has resulted from the need to discharge patients earlier (reduced length of stay) and limiting admissions to the day of surgery or treatment. The patient population now requires a higher level of sophisticated, complex nursing care, with a shorter time in which to plan and implement it.

With this has come a shift to outpatient care, a reallocation of ancillary service and support roles, an emphasis on documentation, and great census fluctuations. These factors have all conspired to alter the acute care environment and the practice of nursing in hospitals drastically.

IMPACT ON NURSING PRACTICE
Cost Containment

Increased emphasis on finance and cost containment has placed efficiency and efficacy high in the value hierarchy. Nurses are required to avoid waste or redundancy, avoid unnecessary procedures, and assure that each treatment regimen is accomplished expeditiously with the greatest possible benefit to the patient. Multitasking has become the norm, causing RNs to do two or more tasks at once whenever possible. Many of the niceties have been eliminated or at the very least reduced to a minimum. Teaching the patient self-care as early as practical is increasingly stressed in most institutions. Furthermore, nurses are expected to look for cost savings by using less expensive substitutions, reducing the use of costly materials, and collaborating with physicians and other departments to save time and meet patient needs quickly. This is particularly difficult because nursing training historically has not included cost awareness or cost-effective practices. It places the burden directly on each professional to devise new ways to accomplish each task more efficiently without sacrificing quality or patient satisfaction. The new mind set thus required is, "How can I do the most for the least and still keep my patients happy?"

Resource Rationing

The result is a form of resource rationing, which in turn creates both legal and ethical dilemmas. Hard choices are daily concerns. Whereas the physician may remain committed to his patient's interest, the nurse at the bedside does not enjoy the luxury of avoiding decisions about who gets less care or what gets done and what is left undone. It is the nurse's responsibility to prioritize both time and resources. Nursing more and more has to juggle cost management with patient needs. Collaboration among the entire health care team is essential to support the nurse's role in the patient care process under conditions of scarcity and cost constraint.

Prioritization in Acute Care Facilities

Prioritization becomes increasingly difficult in most acute care facilities because of increased patient acuity, reduced length of stay, and early discharge. There are no less acute cases, and all patients have urgent or emergent needs. Nursing activities are intense and fast paced. Patients are admitted on the day of surgery and discharged as quickly as possible, with in-home-care aides and visiting nurses handling the convalescent period.

With no preoperative or convalescing patients, demands on nurses are far more intense. With pressures for early discharge and good discharge planning falling heavily on the nurse's shoulders as primary health care team coordinator, the work becomes yet more intense. A primary nurse with 24-hour accountability or a case manager is in the best position to expedite the patient's progress. All patient goals must be set within the DRG time frames. The case manager must facilitate patient care so as to avoid time delays or complications that might extend the length of stay (LOS).

With many nurses working part time, continuity can be a serious issue, in both planning and anticipation of patient needs.

Although technology has increased nursing's knowledge-based requirements, so has the early discharge requirement. Discharge planning for patients with IV chemotherapy, IV antibiotics, and other sophisticated therapies require knowledge of community resources and support systems not previously required. Thus, the nurse's knowledge must keep pace with both current developments in technology and the rapid expansion of community resources.

Altered Roles for Nurses

Increased emphasis on versatility, specialization, and altered roles for primary caregivers has resulted from cost-management techniques and increasing acuity under PPS.

Changing Skill Mixes

Skill mix has changed. The number of RNs in acute care settings has decreased because of the advent of multiskilled workers who perform combinations of tasks both nursing related and ancillary department related. The role, however, of those nurses who do remain in acute care as well as other settings will be cognitively based, that is, knowledge oriented versus task oriented, perfecting the skill of delegation as well as principles of advanced practice. Volunteer staff used to augment unit staff may provide another challenge to the nurse's ingenuity.

The Changing Role of Critical Care Nurses

Outpatient services provide new challenges to the nurse's role in institutional areas, such as ambulatory care, day treatment outpatient surgery, diagnostic centers, cancer treatment centers, and home care, as well as changing the way nurses in acute care settings practice. Nurses may have to be more flexible in preoperative assessment, assisting in the procedure and providing care during recovery. Telephone follow-up with patients the day after the procedure is commonplace. Nurses must be able to set up appropriate systems and methods for expeditious handling of many varied procedures, with increasingly high-risk procedures being added constantly.

New therapies not requiring overnight stay, such as lithotripsy, are prevalent. With many facilities providing home care, some acute care nurses are following their patients into their homes after discharge.

Other changes in medical care since PPS include IV antibiotic therapy, blood transfusions, and IV chemotherapies delivered in day treatment centers. Nurses knowledgeable in both inpatient acute care and outpatient treatment planning assess patients and their response to therapy, coordinate existing family and community support, and perform follow-up care as needed for patients with chronic illnesses or for the duration of a specific regimen.

Increased Emphasis on Communication Skills, Documentation, and Care Plans

Increased emphasis on communication skills, documentation, and care plans has altered nursing practice, as have nurses' educational requirements. Documentation is critical to the reimbursement for treatment under PPS. No charting of care means no reimbursement (Rutkowski, 1987).

This has led to increasing use of computerized documentation systems that capture more information at the time services are ordered or rendered. Bedside or work station computers are increasing in number rapidly, and their use requires a level of computer literacy never before seen in the profession. The use of computers frees the nurse from the excessive paperwork previously necessary and provides more time for patient care. This fact has not been lost on nurses who are sharp enough and versatile enough to learn the computer systems. The hospital without such computerized support finds itself in a most difficult position in competition for adequate, available nursing staff. Few of today's graduates wish to return to (what they perceive as antiquated) manual documentation methods. Nurse managers, too, are seeing the advantages of these new systems. Information never before available are now at their fingertips, altering management style and effectiveness.

Communication skill requirements have increased simultaneously as collaboration with other departments, health care team professionals, family members, and community support systems has become essential to promote early discharge and reduce LOS.

Increased Emphasis on Quality of Care

Increased emphasis on quality has taken two approaches: the quality of clinical outcomes and the level of patient satisfaction with care received. This is only indirectly due to PPS, however, resulting from consumer complaints that patients went home "quicker and sicker" and that quality of care had declined under DRGs. This in fact was never validated.

Service to the customer, or guest relations, is stressed in many institutions to encourage patient-centered care by all staff. Patient satisfaction surveys completed by patients postdischarge are returned to the hospital, providing feedback on all areas of the hospital experience, especially nursing care. It thus becomes essential for all nursing staff to know and understand all standards of care as guides to patient care. Further, standardized protocols have become the norm for most nursing staff.

Increased Emphasis on Patient Teaching

Increased emphasis on teaching patients has resulted from the need to reduce LOS and render the patient capable of self-care as early as possible. This becomes part of the multiteaching strategy, where nurses are required to teach and assess patients simultaneously with other interventions. Such emphasis adds to the communications skill requirement while increasing time pressures on staff.

One of the primary complaints heard from nursing staff is lack of time for appropriate patient teaching. Many institutions provide booklets or computer-produced information sheets giving patients discharge instructions or other support materials to facilitate instruction in self-care. Often, these can be generated along with care plans or at discharge, giving the patient appropriate instructions on self-care, follow-up treatment, and medications. This kind of support is essential in today's fast-paced health care environment. Ideally, information should be provided before admission.

Families often need instruction, particularly in cases of trauma or long-term illness. This further strains nurses' capabilities and adds to time constraints. Support groups and other family conference groups can be formed to support nursing staff in their area of expertise. For example, cardiac care units have found family support groups to share instructions and medical information with caregivers of patients who have experienced bypass or heart transplant surgery. This can be an extremely useful approach to improving both patient satisfaction and clinical outcomes.

Increased Emphasis on Geriatric Care Needs

An increased need for emphasis on knowledge of geriatric care has resulted from technologic advances that make it possible for people to live longer with a variety of chronic illnesses or disabilities. Thus, in most institutions, particularly the intensive care areas, a large percent of patients are of Medicare age, and many are what is referred to as "frail elderly"—85 years old or more.

Such a population requires a whole new range of skills, and with the cost and time constraints of PPS and DRGs, these skills become essential if complications and extended LOS are to be avoided. Such problems as dermal ulcers or nosocomial infections are increasingly central to quality assurance issues and clinical outcomes. Specialized geriatric care training must be included in the knowledge base of nurses if staff are to be expected to handle the problems posed by this patient population.

Census Fluctuations and Staffing Problems

Dramatic census fluctuations have accompanied the PPS, causing great difficulties for most hospitals in staffing. Census has always fluctuated with the seasons and holidays, but the fluctuations seen now are less easily explained and less predictable, and both the peaks and troughs are greater.

The result has been a day-to-day need for staffing adjustments. This, in turn, necessitates either floating among units or intermittent times off. As whole units close, open, or recombine in various ways, nurses have to cope by learning additional skills or new specialties or in other ways broaden their knowledge base.

ROLE OF THE NURSE MANAGER

The nurse manager must provide for self and staff

- Education in business and finance
- Management skills for today's health environment
- Support groups and counseling in stress management
- Cross-training to expand and enhance skills

The nurse manager must establish for units

- New skill mixes and use of multiskilled workers

If we are to shift away from the old spend-oriented system, we must educate staff to bottom-line realities and restructure the work force appropriately. Roles and functions must change; work redesign is the urgent need. For this to succeed, however, it must be patient centered, not profit centered.

Role Shifts in the Critical Care Setting

Although most ICUs are patient centered, much of the work does not require a professional nurse's knowledge-based attention. The acuity level may not be as high as the intensity, since the patient may require frequent interventions, such as turning and suctioning. The maintenance of high-tech equipment does not require professional attention, either. Many such tasks could be performed by technicians under the professional supervision of the RN. The RN then functions as care manager and overseer to assure efficacy and quality of care. Delegating tasks frees the RN to plan the care, manage patients, and communicate with family and other professionals to maximize efficiency and efficacy.

Critical elements in restructuring the ICU skills mix are

1. Maximizing and enhancing the RN's role

2. Minimizing reliance on registry personnel by developing full-time professionals and other workers and using their skills more effectively
3. Creating an environment that supports the professional in managing LOS and cost-effective resource allocation

This can be accomplished if the following conditions prevail.

1. Recognition of the contribution that nonlicensed caregivers can make.
2. Determination of the skill level needed and assurance that the characteristics of the new worker are carefully considered and selection is based on criteria.
3. Competency-based education is initiated at the start of the change and continued to assure competency long term.
4. The involved staff design the required criteria and select their new team members.
5. Evaluation systems are in place to assure appropriate patient outcomes and skill level competency of all staff.
6. The RN is enhanced, supported, and rewarded consistent with hospital goals.
7. Feedback and rewards are built in for all team members, and teamwork is encouraged and supported.
8. Patient care is planned and supervised under the RN's direction so that care is RN directed, not RN intensive.
9. Skill mix and adjustment are based not just on allocating tasks but also on identifying how those tasks relate to the patient's severity of illness.

The conclusions drawn from our experience at one hospital (with a 15-bed ICU and an 11-bed CCU) regarding the role of unlicensed caregivers in the critical care setting include the following.

1. Unlicensed caregivers can be an asset to critical care.
2. Incorporating unlicensed caregivers in routine staffing patterns is dependent on an adequate and stable census.
3. The presence of unlicensed staff enables the nursing staff to absorb increased census to some degree.
4. Support staff cross-trained to perform both clerical and clinical tasks is optimal for the night shift.
5. The turnover rate of unlicensed staff presents a challenge to management.
6. Float pools or crisis pools can be used to offset census fluctuations.
7. Computer-based care plans, order entry, and documentation using bedside, portable, or unit-based systems are essential.
8. Streamlined work and redesigned nursing units for convenience, efficiency, and stress reduction should be carried out.

Hiring Criteria for Unlicensed Caregivers

Hiring criteria must be developed that enable managers to select reliable persons. In critical care, our approach has been to recruit in-house patient care technicians (PCTs) who have demonstrated their clinical abilities, reliability, and flexibility in other units.

Crisis Pools

Crisis pools have been used for several years in large institutions. Since fluctuations in both admissions and acuity occur at various times of the year in intensive care units and in medical–surgical units, one hospital developed a hospitalwide crisis intervention nursing pool. This reduced the tendency of nurse managers in these areas to overstaff in an effort to offset the sudden surges in census or acuity. Thus, the nurse managers, knowing that a float pool of well-trained staff was available when needed, could staff on the basis of the normal census and acuity levels in their respective units.

The crisis intervention nurses are highly experienced nurses who float well and can handle fast-moving developments wherever they are called. They are not given regular patient assignments but can respond to any unforeseen situation that develops.

Unit secretaries also were included in the crisis pool, available to respond in times of emergency of short duration, often for only 2 to 3 hours a day during peak admission times. The pool was established as a separate cost center, and its staff was paid each 2 week pay period from the costs gleaned from the units using their services.

Developing a crisis team of this type reduces the cost of continuous over-staffing for emergent situations. It allows units to be staffed according to a standard based on average acuity and census and thus saves scarce dollars.

Computerized Systems

Computerized documentation, staff scheduling, order entry, results reporting, and case management are essential in today's high-paced, high-stress environment if nursing care is to keep pace with demand and at the same time be cost effective. Quality care with personalized care plans and hands-on attention to patient needs is still central to nursing care. The use of computers to streamline and expedite the paperwork and order entry and to plan care can do much to improve nursing efficiency.

Bedside computers with handheld terminals are one ideal from the standpoint of the busy nurse, moving rapidly from patient to patient, since they eliminate the need to return to the nursing station between interventions for documentation purposes. Point-of-care documentation is the preferred approach and necessitates bedside terminals, handheld portable terminals, or clinical work stations near patients for maximum effectiveness. This approach is discussed thoroughly elsewhere in this book and is not dealt with in detail here. Hospitals are studying numerous approaches to providing cost-effective nursing support computer systems and finding them beneficial to productivity, cost control, and efficiency (Lower & Nauert, 1992). In one study, savings included 8% in actual hours, or approximately 18.12 hours per day.

Redesigned Workspace and Patient Care Units

Redesigned nursing work and work environments can go far to alleviate stress, frustration, and duplication of effort and improve accuracy. Wherever possible, units should be standardized with respect to storage of materials, arrangement of the nursing station, and basic layout. This facilitates interchange of personnel when floating is required, as well as efficiency in the work environment.

If every unit places equipment and so on in the same location in the nursing station, arranges the medications and linen areas similarly, and has a physical layout that is roughly the same, moving from unit to unit can be done with a minimum of stress. Familiarizing new staff with the unit can be accomplished more quickly, and errors can be reduced significantly. While accomplishing all this, it is important to look to the ergonomics of the layout, furnishings, and placement of equipment to ensure maximum efficiency and a minimum of frustrations, errors, and redundancies.

A health care industrial designer can be instrumental in preventing serious mistakes in workplace design. Small conveniences can be major contributors to reducing job stress, increasing job satisfaction, and facilitating rapid response from nursing staff to patient requests. Placing lunchrooms, rest areas, and meeting rooms near the nursing station (which, in turn, should be central to the unit rather than at the far end of a long hall) will provide much better support for a higher productivity level in nursing staff.

DEVELOPING REVENUE-PRODUCING PROGRAMS

Beyond these efforts, nursing needs to be proactive in developing revenue-producing programs. Through the targeting of appropriate market segments, current product or service lines may be enhanced or expanded. Although efficiency and efficacy are relevant everywhere in health care, revenue production is even more important to the institution and nursing survival. Innovation and marketing skills are essential in the current health care environment. Marketing through community outreach programs, educational classes, weight control and prenatal programs, families of heart patient support groups, survivors of trauma victims, and many other programs can be instrumental in spreading the word that an institution has the well-being of the entire community at heart and is prepared to provide a wide range of services. Nursing has always been in the forefront of community outreach (i.e., marketing) programs and needs to continue these efforts. Thus, it can be seen as a revenue producer and not just another aspect of overhead. Nursing must always look to the value added as their key to enhancing revenue in the institution. Once again, this is basically a marketing approach (albeit internal within the institution), yet it is important for management fully to recognize nursing's contribution to the health care product—quality patient care, successful outcomes, and satisfied customers, both physician and patient. Nursing must never lose sight of who their customers are and what their true purpose is. It must never let management forget either. Without nursing services, hospitals have little to sell anyone. This fact should never be lost in the shuffle. Separate costing and billing of nursing would surely enhance nursing's success in focusing both customers and management on the value added they supply. However, inasmuch as few can agree on how to cost out nursing services appropriately and capitated payments are in the future, this will probably *not* occur.

To support innovation and entrepreneurship, nurse managers need to promote personal involvement in all levels of the organization through use of committees, task forces, and special projects. Empowering nurses to take the initiative in program or service development contributes to nursing satisfaction and retention, in addition to enhancing nursing's value added. Incentives in the form of recognition dinners and presentation of awards for outstanding contributions or exemplary service can further these goals.

Bibliography

Beyers, M. (1985). *Perspectives on prospective payment*. Rockville, MD: Aspen.

Block, P. (1987). *The empowered manager*. San Francisco: Jossey-Bass.

Burns, T., & Stalher, G.M. (1987). *The management of innovations*. London: Tavestock Publishers Ltd.

Cox, H.C., Harsavyi, B., & Dean, L.C. (1987). *Computers and nursing: An application to practice, education and research*. Norwalk, CT: Appleton & Lange.

Drucker, P. (1974). *Management tasks, responsibilities, practices*. New York: Harper and Row.

Lauer, M., & Novert, L. (1992, July). Charting the impact of bedside computers. *Nursing Management, 23* (7).

Porter-O'Grady, T. (1987). *Nursing finance: Budgeting strategies for a new age*. Rockville, MD: Aspen.

Rutkowski, B. (1987). *Managing for productivity in nursing*. Rockville, MD: Aspen.

Saba, V., & McCormick, K. (1990). *Essentials of computers for nurses* (pp. 203–223). Philadelphia: J.B. Lippincott.

Spitzer-Lehmann, R. (1988). *Impact of DRG's on nursing:* Report of the Western Institute of Nursing, US DHHS-PHS.

CHAPTER 25 • • • • • •

BUDGETING PRACTICES

KATHERINE R. JONES

EXECUTIVE SUMMARY

With everyone from federal government officials to the man on the street complaining about the high cost of health care, the need for a well-defined budget process is exceedingly clear. One option is to push the system of budgeting to the patient care unit level. Regardless, the nurse manager must understand and be able to document the financial impact of nursing care. This chapter presents an excellent review of budget practices and offers numerous, practical examples of the various budgetary steps.

The chapter begins with a review of budgeting philosophy, which is basically a choice between a top–down, control orientation or a bottom–up participatory effort. The current trend is bottom–up. This is followed by an explanation of the budget planning process and identifies assessing, review of organizational mission, listing of assumptions, and forecasting as major components of the process. Detailed explanations and examples are provided for determining personnel budgets, specifically FTE calculations.

The section on variance analysis, which includes controlling the direct, variable costs of a particular unit, is critical to the nurse manager. Some strategies used to reduce direct nursing costs include changing the skill mix to include more lower-paid personnel, reducing overtime, and limiting the use of agency nurses.

The final section of the chapter concentrates on budgeting methods. Definitions and examples are provided for flexible budgeting, program budgeting, and zero-base budgeting, which asks the question: Are services being delivered at present in an efficient and effective manner to meet the organization's goals and objectives?

Although budgeting is not everyone's cup of tea, in today's competitive environment it is essential that we all try to acquire a taste. The information in this chapter goes a long way toward that end.

Increased attention is being paid to financial management and budgeting in health care organizations. The driving forces behind this are the increased competition for paying patients, rising health care expenses, and increasingly restricted reimbursement for services being delivered. In response, health care organizations are hiring financial experts, upgrading the accounting, finance, and budgeting skills of their current managers, and implementing new, integrated financial and clinical management information systems. Nursing is an integral component of these changes. Nursing costs are being incorporated into hospital cost accounting systems, variable billing for nursing services is being considered, and determination of patient acuities is being incorporated into budgeting systems. Furthermore, budgeting and control systems are being pushed down to the patient care unit level. As a consequence, frontline managers now require knowledge of accounting and budgeting to meet these challenges. Nurse managers will be able, and required, to document the financial impact of nursing care and to take appropriate actions to improve productivity, efficiency, and effectiveness (Scodro, 1988).

BUDGETING PHILOSOPHY

Organizations tend to have specific philosophies of fiscal affairs. This is especially true in the area of budgeting. The amount of participation that any individual manager has in the budgeting process depends on the approach or philosophy of the organization's top management. The organization may use a top–down or a bottom–up approach to budget formation. Top–down is a centralized effort that places the whole responsibility for budgeting on one or two persons who are members of administration, are financially oriented, and have a general knowledge of department activities and needs. The budget can be generated in a short period of time under this system (Herkimer, 1988). The budget officer acquires the necessary projections of use for the departments and develops preliminary budgets, with projected staffing patterns most often based on historical information. These preliminary budgets are then reviewed by the nurse executive, who may provide more specific information, leading to modification of the projections. However, control is maintained at the top level (Finkler, 1984).

The current trend is toward increasing decentralization of the budget process (Mark and Smith, 1987). Useful budgets must be realistic. This means that those nearer the point of service need to play an active role, since they are more aware of the specific circumstances and conditions that exist in the day-to-day operations of the organization and department. A participatory philosophy presumes that an individual who is responsible for meeting a part of the overall budget must help determine the budgeted amount and must also have some control over the actual outcome. In a bottom–up environment, directors of nursing, department heads, and unit managers have much more responsibility for developing and managing the unit or department budgets. They work closely with people in finance, purchasing, personnel, and accounting in retrieving the data necessary to project utilization, staffing, and expense levels. The budgeting director provides assistance, but primary responsibility shifts downward in the organization. Increasing cost pressures in health care suggest that the decentralized approach will become more prevalent (Mark and Smith, 1987.) The health care manager of today is called upon to preserve, conserve, quantify, and manage the resources available, and the budget is one tool in this effort.

Management Control Aspects

The budget is an annual statement of the expected revenues and expenditures for the organization. It is a statement of anticipated results in financial terms (revenue and expense budgets) or in nonfinancial terms (statistics budget). A budget compares expected receipts with expected expenditures to ascertain the organization's expected financial position. Budgeting is the process by which decision makers allocate resources to support specific programs that accomplish the strategic plan of the organization for the coming year (Lusk and Lusk, 1979; Mark and Smith, 1987).

The budget is the master plan for annual operations, a control device, and an evaluation tool to determine the organization's performance over the past year or specific period of time (Strasen, 1987). The key to controlling the budget begins with preparation of the annual budget, when department managers are informed of the overall goals and direction of their organization and then must establish specific, measurable budgetary goals for their own departments or units (Esmond, 1982). The annual operating budget is based on the organization's carefully constructed strategic plan, which will identify what goals the organization wants to accomplish over the next three to five years (Strasen, 1987).

The *basic objectives of the budgeting process* are to develop a document that (Esmond, 1982; Finkler, 1983):

- Defines in monetary terms the policies, plans, and goals of the hospital
- Provides a basis for evaluating the financial performance of the plans
- Provides a useful tool for control of costs
- Provides a tool for communication and coordination within the organization

The *purposes of budgeting* are to (Scodro, 1988):

- Translate financial objectives into projected monthly spending patterns
- Improve financial planning and decision making
- Identify controllable and uncontrollable cost areas
- Provide a useful format for communicating financial objectives to all concerned parties
- Assign financial responsibility and accountability
- Provide feedback concerning the extent to which actual expenditures conform to budgeted spending
- Provide a way of measuring financial success

Preparation of the budget makes an organization plan ahead (Finkler, 1983). The budgeting process forces managers to establish goals and to forecast the future. Changes in the internal and external environment can be anticipated, and their impact on the finances of the organization predicted (Finkler, 1992). This allows for managerial actions and strategic responses that anticipate changes rather than merely respond to them after the fact (e.g., proactive rather than reactive). If money is wasted through poor budgeting practices and lax control techniques, the quality and range of services offered will be diminished. Thus, the degree of care exercised in budgeting can directly influence the quality of care delivered to patients (Finkler, 1984).

The budget also can serve to motivate managers and other employees and to provide a yardstick for evaluation (Finkler, 1992). Careful budgeting helps minimize the number of operational surprises, provides all levels of management with a set of predetermined operating standards with which to evaluate operating performances, and serves as an excellent means of educating and developing managers (Herkimer, 1988). Smeltzer and Hyland (1989) recommend using the budget as a tool to educate clinical managers about finance. They believe that managers can be held accountable for the budget only if they fully understand what they are to accomplish. Budgets should be useful for evaluation of performance of individual departments and cost centers, as well as individual managers, because they provide specific goals or end points (Finkler, 1984). Managers can tell from the budget exactly what is expected of them. However, the budget process is a motivational strategy only if appropriately used by the organization. If the organization establishes a budget or budgetary goals that are impossible to meet, it can discourage managers and cause low morale (Finkler, 1992). A reasonable budget, especially if tied to an incentive structure, can stimulate top performance by managers.

THE BUDGET PLANNING PROCESS

The budgeting process requires an organizational structure, a chart of accounts, an identified set of production units, a data collection system, a management reporting system, a budget director, a budget committee, a budget calendar, and a budget manual (Herkimer, 1988). The first step in the planning process is to conduct an environmental assessment, which is one component of the organization's strategic planning process. The environmental assessment is an analysis of the operating environment of the organization. Management analyzes the current status of the organization (its strengths and weaknesses), as well as threats and opportunities in the external environment. Evaluation of industry trends, changes in customer base, technologic changes, and so on help the organization determine where it should be going (Finkler, 1983). The environmental assessment is followed by an examination and revision or refinement, if necessary, of the organizational mission and long-term objectives. These are broad statements of primary purpose and need to be reviewed, clarified, and revised on a regular basis. These objectives are key to determining which programs and services are to be included in the operating budget (Strasen, 1987).

Completion of the environmental assessment and statement of goals and objectives are followed by management's development of a list of assumptions about the future. Several scenarios may be generated that involve assumptions about price changes, availability of staff, and case mix changes, for example. These assumptions, along with the organization's long-term objectives, are then used to develop operating objectives or department goals for the coming year.

Preparation of the budget manual is usually done by the chief financial officer (CFO) and the director of the budget (Strasen, 1987). The manual will include the necessary forms, timetables, and instructions for the department heads. Management then proceeds to preparation of forecasts. These are projections of future volumes for different services and products. For the nursing units, it usually refers to days of care and specific supplies. In the operating room or recovery room, number of surgical cases must be forecast. In the clinics or emergency room, it is number of visits. In the past, a simple forecast of days of care was sufficient. It involved historical trend analysis adjusted for predicted changes in the medical staff, facility changes, and other anticipated events. Today, more specific forecasts of days of care by diagnosis-related group (DRG), acuity/severity level, and source of payment are required.

Budget preparation then moves to the departmental or cost center level, with the department managers completing the budgets with assistance from the finance office. Budget hearings are held in either a formal or informal setting. At these hearings, department managers may negotiate with the budget officer on various items, such as new positions, new programs, salary increases, or net income targets. Final presentation of the proposed budget is made to the finance committee of the board of directors. If approved, the budget is ready for implementation. The budget is monitored on at least a monthly basis to assess how closely actual expenditures match the budgeted amounts. The department manager may need to develop specific strategies to address variances from the budget.

Budgets generally are prepared annually, with monthly projections then prepared within the annual budget. This allows evaluation and adjustment of performance throughout the year (Finkler, 1983).

TYPES OF BUDGETS
Operating Budget

The operating budget consists of the statistics or volume budget, the revenue budget, and the expense budget. In preparing the operating budget, managers must consider and identify factors that will affect activity in their area of responsibility and thus affect their operating budgets. The manager develops the budget after considering the operating goals and objectives of the parent organization and the philosophy and objectives of the nursing department. The organizational structures and nursing care delivery model must be clearly defined, since they affect the level and mix of nursing personnel required. The manager then generates specific operational goals for the unit. These may include changes in staff mix, acuity systems, or service delivery patterns (Finkler, 1984).

Statistics Budget

Developing the statistics budget is an important first step in the budgeting process, since it provides the basis for subsequent development of the revenue and expense budgets (Ward, 1988). The statistics budget translates departmental or cost center goals and objectives into usable mathematical statements. More specifically, it provides measures of workload or activity (units of service to be delivered) for each department or cost center for the budget period. In most cases, it is no longer possible to use past performance as the primary forecasting basis for the statistics budget. Hospitals have been facing decreasing length of stay (LOS), increasing acuity, decreasing admissions, and changes in case mix, making forecasting a difficult process. The projections must also incorporate seasonal variations in use, the impact of changing technology on such items as medications and supplies, and other factors (Cleverley, 1986).

At the macrolevel, forecasting is required to estimate days of care and number of outpatient visits, including the emergency room. At the microlevel, forecasting is done for utilization statistics, such as number of dialysis treatments, number of major surgeries, number of minor surgeries, number of meals served, pounds of linen laundered, and number of work orders completed (Strasen, 1987). According to Herkimer (1978), factors that need to be considered in developing the statistics budget include

1. Historical data and trends—fewer admits? more outpatient visits? change in case mix? fewer or more physicians? shorter LOS?
2. Departmental goals and strategies—increased use of disposables? contracting for food service or housekeeping?
3. Government and third party payor decisions—PPS or Medicaid policy changes? reimbursement for outpatient surgery only?
4. Outside competition—new HMOs? competitor satellite opening in market area? creation of network by competitors?
5. Other known facts as well as rumors—major employer layoffs?

Revenue Budget

The revenue budget is directly related to the volume of services delivered and the rate or charge structure. Establishment of rates or charges is based on an analysis of the direct costs, indirect costs, and desired contribution margin of each service or product. The health care organization has several major sources of revenue. Patient care services provide the single largest source of operating revenue. Other sources of operating revenue include the cafeteria, coffee shop, gift shop, parking, telephone rental, and TV rental. Sources of nonoperating revenue include interest income, donations, gifts, and governmental appropriations. Net operating income is always less than gross operating income because of multiple deductions that occur in health care organizations. These deductions from revenue include amounts for charity care, bad debt, discounted charges to PPOs/PPAs/HMOs, contractual adjustments, and free care (usually professional courtesy discounts or free care to employees or other professionals) (Esmond, 1982). As of 1990, reporting rules were changed so that charity care is excluded from gross patient revenue and deductions from revenue, and bad debts are classified as an operating expense (Finkler, 1992).

The revenue budget is thus an estimate of gross revenue to be achieved from charges for services rendered, minus allowed deductions from revenue, plus revenue from other operating and nonoperating sources. The revenue budget is not usually the responsibility of the unit or department managers (Ward, 1988). If there is an estimate of revenue for a nursing unit, revenue usually is based on room and board charges, calculated according to projected patient days. The current rate per day is multiplied by the rate adjustment factor, reflecting the new, budgeted rate per day for the coming year, and then multiplied by the projected number of patient days for that unit (Finkler, 1984). Other units may have to project number of deliveries, number of visits, or number of major operative procedures and then multiply by the newly adjusted rates or charges to determine the relevant revenue for the budget year. It is becoming common to project revenue based on major payor group. First, payor mix is forecasted for the unit (% Medicare, % Medicaid, % Blue Cross, % HMO, and so on). Next, total days per payor group are forecasted. Revenue is then estimated according to the various payment schemes particular to each payor group (DRG fixed rate, Medicaid per diems, HMO discounted charges). A change in payor mix on the unit can significantly alter total departmental revenue, even if there is no change in the number of days of care delivered.

Expense Budget

The third component of the operating budget is the expense budget. The major categories of expense budgets are the personnel budget (salary, payroll) and the supply or commodities budget.

Personnel (Salary, Payroll) Budget

The personnel budget represents the greatest single source of expenditures and the opportunity for the most control over the budget. The manager must identify full-time equivalents (FTEs), positions, and employment costs. Labor or salary costs can be divided into fixed and variable cost categories (Strasen, 1987). Fixed labor costs are those paid regardless of level of activity or volume of patients. The salaries of the nurse manager, ward secretary, clinical nurse specialist, and monitor technician may be fixed for the nursing unit (Strasen, 1987). Variable labor costs are those positions that flex or vary with patient census and acuity levels (Strasen, 1987). Staff registered nurses above minimum staffing level, licensed vocational/practical nurses, and various nurse extender positions usually are variable cost categories. Salaries can be divided by direct and indirect classifications. Direct nursing care salaries are those paid to direct caregivers. The activities of the direct care employees are traceable to the cost objective, in this case, specific patients receiving nursing care. Indirect nursing care salaries are those paid to noncaregivers, such as the nurse manager and the unit secretary. In general, the activities of indirect caregivers are not traceable to specific patients. Usually, direct costs are variable and indirect costs are fixed, over a relevant volume of patients or activity.

The personnel budget for the patient care unit is based on the forecasted level of activity or workload for that unit. Nursing workload is a function of two variables: number of patient days and hours of nursing care required per patient day. Both are key to budgeting nursing salary costs (Kirby & Wiczal, 1985). Average nursing hours per patient day are budgeted for individual patient care units and then treated as a constant unless a change in workload can be documented in an objective manner. The variation in staffing then becomes a function of patient days (Kirby & Wiczal, 1985).

For example, the nursing unit may have a total capacity of 36 beds and a projected occupancy rate of 80%. This translates into a projected average daily census (ADC) of 29 patients (36 beds × 0.80 = 29) and a projected number of patient days of 10,585 for the coming year (365 days × 29 patients = 10,585 patient days). If the nursing care unit has a projected nursing care standard of 5.2 hours per patient day (HPPD), the projected total annual nursing care hours that need to be budgeted and staffed for on the unit are 55,042 (5.2 HPPD × 10,585 patient days).

To calculate nursing hours per patient day, management collects patient classification data and calculates time spent in direct patient care activities, such as documentation, communication, and education. Factors affecting nursing hours per patient day include patient acuity, case mix, standards of care, skill mix, type of hospital, average length of stay, patient demographics, availability of hospital support services, and various physical aspects of the hospital. In addition, nursing care standards in use at comparison hospitals and the organization's own financial constraints may be considered. Multiple factors also need to be considered in the forecast of patient days. These factors include census trends, physician forecasts of admissions and surgeries, marketing projections, and program changes.

After calculating the required number of nursing care hours for the unit, it is necessary to determine the number of FTEs required to provide the projected needed patient care services as defined by the projected nursing hours of care. An FTE is a workload statistic. One FTE is equal to 2080 hours of work per year, or 40 hours of work per week. It does not equal a position or person. The distinction between a position and an FTE is an important one. A position is one job for one person regardless of the number of hours worked. An FTE is a conversion of hours to a standard base of one employee working 8 hours a day, 40 hours a week, 80 hours a pay period, 52 weeks a year. Using the FTE standard, it is possible to describe staffing patterns that include full-time and part-time employees and 8, 10, and 12 hour shifts, in a way that allows comparisons across departments and institutions and over time (Strasen, 1987).

Dividing the total required number of hours of patient care by 2080 (1 FTE) is the first, but not final, step in determining the required number of FTEs for staffing the unit. In the cited example, 26.5 productive FTEs are required (55,042 hours/2080 hours per FTE). However, a person filling a one-FTE slot does not work 2080 hours. Paid time-off is granted for vacations, holidays, sick leave, and training time, and therefore fewer hours are available for patient care activities. This must be accounted for in the determination of number of FTEs needed to meet the projected nursing care requirements. To achieve 26.5 productive FTEs, it is necessary to multiply the number of required productive FTEs by a factor that adjusts for the percentage of time an employee is paid but not available for patient care activities. If we assume that these nonproductive hours amount to 15% of productive hours, the total required number of FTEs to meet the patient care standard for the sample patient unit is 30.5 (26.5 FTEs × 1.15). We can then multiply the total required FTEs by the number of hours paid per FTE (2080) times the average salary rate for the unit staff to determine the projected annual salary expense that needs to be budgeted for the unit. If we assume that the average salary rate is $15.00, the projected salary expense for the sample unit will be $951,600. If the 5.2 HPPD standard does not include indirect caregivers on the unit, we would add to this figure the number of fixed or indirect caregiver FTEs and their associated paid hours and multiply that number by the appropriate average hourly salary rate to get an estimated annual salary expense for fixed or indirect caregivers.

A slightly different technique for estimating salary costs has been described by Smeltzer and Hyland (1989). The projected unit patient days are multiplied by the nursing care standard (10,585 × 5.2 = 55,042) to determine the required productive annual hours. This is multiplied by the nonproductive time factor (55,042 × 1.15) to determine total productive and nonproductive hours (63,298.3). To this figure are added the paid training hours on the unit (orientation, staff development) (63,298.3 + 1500 hours per year = 64,798.3) to determine required paid hours. The total paid hours are then multiplied by the weighted average wage rate to determine the salary budget for the unit.

The weighted average wage rate is the average salary of registered nurses, licensed vocational nurses, patient care assistants, and registry nurses, weighted by the percentage each is represented in the staffing plan. The following is one example.

Average RN salary including premiums, overtime	$25.00
% RN on staff	0.60
Average LVN salary including premiums, overtime	$14.00
% LVN on staff	0.20
Average PCA salary including premiums, overtime	$ 8.00
% PCA on staff	0.10
Average registry salary	$30.00
% Registry on staff	0.10

The average wage rate per staffing category is then multiplied by the staffing percentage and then summed to determine the weighted average wage rate for the unit. This is then multiplied by the total hours of care to be delivered to determine the unit's salary costs for the budget year: ($25.00 × 0.60) + ($14.00 × 0.20) + ($8.00 × 0.10) + ($30.00 × 0.10) = $21.60; 64,798.3 total hours × $21.60 = $1,399,643.28.

The number of budgeted nursing hours per patient day is an average based on multiple factors, including patient acuity information. On a daily basis, the individual needs of patients may require the nursing HPPD to be varied. Such variations are managed by the head nurse and staff on each nursing unit based on their professional judgment. Increasing or decreasing acuity or increasing or decreasing number of patients on a given day should result in more or fewer direct nursing staff assigned to the unit that day. The only requirement is that the average nursing care standard be achieved over time (Kirby & Wiczal, 1985). The variable staffing expense component should be designed to enable the manager to staff positions as closely proportional to volume of activity as possible. To determine the number of staff required for a particular shift, the manager needs to multiply the number of beds expected to be filled (30) by the budgeted hours of care per patient day (4.3), then divide by the number of worked hours per day per FTE (30 × 4.3 = 129; 129 hours/8 hours per shift = 16.13 total FTE required for the next day) (Smeltzer & Hyland, 1989).

Finkler (1985) has described another approach to calculating required FTEs, positions, and labor costs. First, as described previously, the nursing care needs for the patient population are predicted, as are those hours of nursing care required to meet the projected needs. The estimates are based on average patient acuity per day. This is used to determine the daily staffing pattern: the number of staff required per 24 hours for the average daily workload of the unit. For example, suppose the average acuity of the patients on a nursing unit is 1.5, and the ADC is 30. The average workload index is thus 45.0 (30 patients × 1.5). If the nursing care standard for the unit is 4.0 hours for each workload unit, including both direct and indirect nursing care time, the total hours of nursing care required for each 24 hour period for the unit is 180, or 22.5 staff for 24 hours, assuming 8 hour shifts (180 hours/8 hours per shift). The unit needs 22.5 staff working one shift each to cover 180 hours of work in a 24 hour period. The unit manager can then design a staffing pattern, distributing the staff according to the desired mix and shift (Table 25–1).

The 22.5 required staff members identified in the daily staffing pattern do not work 7 days a week and do not work all 52 weeks a year. As in the previous examples, staff will take vacations, holidays, and sick time. They will be paid for these hours but not be available for patient care. Therefore, the 22.5 FTEs must be supplemented to maintain the required staffing pattern every day of the week. First, 0.4 FTE is added for weekend coverage (5 shifts = 40 hours = 1 FTE; 2 shifts = 16 hours = 0.4 FTE). For each FTE in a 24 hour staffing pattern, 1.4 FTEs must be hired to maintain the staffing pattern on a 7 day a week cycle. This is obviously not required if the unit is open only 5 days a week. More specifically, staff required per 24 hours × 1.4 weekend adjustment factor = number of FTEs required for a 7 day week: 22.5 × 1.4 = 31.5 FTEs.

To account for nonproductive time, for which coverage must also be provided,

TABLE 25–1 Staffing Pattern

| | SHIFT | | | |
CATEGORY	7–3	3–11	11–7	TOTAL
RN	5	3	2	10
LVN	3	2	2	7
PCA	2	2	1.5	5.5
Total	10	7	5.5	22.5

the manager can use payroll reports or consult with the payroll office to identify nonproductive time as a percentage of productive time. This usually ranges from 9% to 15% (Finkler, 1985). For every required productive FTE, 1.15 (15% nonproductive time) FTEs will be required to maintain the staffing pattern and cover the nonproductive time. The equation (Finkler, 1985) is

FTEs required for 7 day week × 1.15 nonproductive factor = total FTEs, or

$$31.5 \text{ FTEs} \times 1.15 = 36.23 \text{ total FTEs}$$

These conversion factors can be used to determine the required number of FTEs for each nursing unit. Specifically, staff required for 24 hours × factor for days off × factor for nonproductive time = total required FTEs, or in this case

$1 \times 1.4 \times 1.15 = 1.61$, or, alternatively,

$$1 \text{ productive FTE} = 1.61 \text{ total FTEs}$$

This staffing factor can then be used for each unit, multiplying each direct care personnel category on the daily staffing pattern by the conversion factor, so that weekends off and nonproductive time are covered and the required workload standard is met (Finkler, 1985).

Calculations for on-call time also must be included in the FTE budget for units such as the operating room. The total number of projected hours of on-call time must be converted to FTEs and added to total FTEs already identified after calculating nonproductive time.

Fringe benefits are closely related to personnel costs, employee statistics, and personnel policies (Esmond, 1982). Employee benefits usually have not been budgeted by the unit managers. Instead, these items, which include Social Security and Medicare, health insurance, pension plans, tuition reimbursement, worker's compensation, unemployment compensation, life insurance, medical services, and disability insurance, are summed at the organizational level, divided by the total number of FTEs in the organization, and then allocated to individual departments and cost centers based on the number of departmental FTEs relative to the total number of FTEs in the organization (Strasen, 1987). The calculations are as follows.

Total hospital fringe benefit expense/total hospital FTEs =
benefit expense per FTE

Benefit expense per FTE × No. of departmental FTEs =
departmental benefit allocation

Position Control. Because salaries, wages, and fringe benefits represent a substantial percentage of a hospital's total expense budget, it is important that personnel costs be carefully budgeted and controlled. The most important factor in controlling personnel costs is the establishment of a plan that shows what positions should be filled, when, and at what salary level. The position control worksheet is where the required number of FTEs is converted into actual positions, hours, and pay rates. At the beginning of each budget cycle, the manager compares currently authorized positions on the unit's position control worksheet with projected personnel needs and makes any necessary requests for adjustments. FTEs are organized on the departmental or cost center worksheets by job class, grade, work status (FT or PT) and shift. The position control system reflects every approved position, whether filled or vacant. The position control sheet needs to be updated as hospital management approves positions to be added (such as new caregiver categories) and eliminates others (vacant RN positions or eliminated assistant head nurse positions).

In preparing the personnel budget, managers match the previous year's personnel budget to the current payroll file and compare position descriptions, job classification, salary, and number of authorized positions. Discrepancies may result from transferred positions across cost centers or job description changes during the year. Salaries are based on current hourly rates and then adjusted to incorporate planned merit increases, cost-of-living raises, intermittent shift differentials, and on-call premiums. It is necessary to include a vacancy allowance in order to project the dollar impact of filling currently unfilled positions.

Overtime projections are based on projected overtime hours for each department or cost center. Overtime is calculated at a different pay rate. The proportion of work to be allocated to overtime usually is based on the unit's previous overtime experience and is projected for the coming year as a separate line in the budget. Shift differentials also are calculated at a different pay rate. For those employees on a permanent evening or night shift, the differential is part of their average salary rate. For those employees who rotate to an evening or night shift, separate calculations must be done. The number of hours an employee is scheduled to work on an off-shift is multiplied by the hourly differential rate for that shift. For example, a nursing unit needing four RNs on the evening shift and two RNs on the night shift, and which does not have permanent shift assignments, would multiply the differential rate for the evening shift by 8 hours (per shift) and then multiply this by the four nurses scheduled to rotate to the shift. The differential rate for the night shift would be multiplied by 8 hours and then by the two nurses who will rotate to this shift. The incremental amount of salary dollars generated by paying this shift differential is multiplied by 365 days to determine the annual amount of salary dollars that have to be budgeted for shift differentials for the unit.

A matrix worksheet usually allows more accurate and simplified calculations. One worksheet may be the department's overall position control sheet. This is then supplemented with the more specific personnel worksheet (Table 25–2). The department manager would then prepare a monthly worksheet showing base salary, shift differential, on-call pay, holiday pay, and scheduled raises in the applicable months.

Preparation of the personnel budget and position control sheets is the responsibility of the line manager. The manager needs a copy of the hospital's personnel policies, the position control documents for the department or cost center, information on current staffing, and the appropriate budget worksheets.

TABLE 25–2 Example of a Matrix Worksheet

Memorial Hospital
Unit: Renal Medicine 4 South   Date: 1/1/92   Cost Center #085

LABOR GRADE CLASS	CLASSIFICATION	APPROVED FTEs	APPROVED SALARY RANGE
1	RN	15	$15–24/hour
2	LVN	08	10–15/hour
3	PCA	06	4–8/hour
4	Clerk	02	6–10/hour
10	Manager	01	24–32/hour

Memorial Hospital
Unit: Renal Medicine 4 South   Date: 1/1/92   Cost Center #085

JOB CODE	AUTHORIZED POSITION	FTE	CURRENT HOURLY RATE	PROPOSED HOURLY RATE	BASE SALARY
1	Mary Jackson	1.0	$15.50	$16.20	$33,698
1	Reg Sands	1.0	$17.00	$17.77	$36,962

*Shift Differential of $1.50/hour for evenings and $2.00/hour for nights (if not in base pay rate); holiday bonus of 50% on all shifts in applicable months; merit increase to be scheduled in anniversary month.

The policies will cover the methodology for determining wage and salary levels, shift differentials, and vacation and holiday pay. Budgeted payroll expense calculations are based on current actual salaries for filled positions and beginning salary levels for vacant positions.

Once salary increases and differentials are agreed on, the budgeted total for each person should be distributed by month. Budgeted salary for a vacant position should begin in the month the manager realistically thinks it will be filled. Known terminations and retirements should be reflected in the appropriate month. The salaries should reflect step and merit increases in the month they are scheduled to occur, with merit increases usually on the employee's anniversary date. Shift differential is included in the base wage of a staff member on a permanent shift or as a separate line item spread by month if the staff member rotates. Holiday time (usually time-and-a-half or double time) is reflected in the appropriate month. Budgeted amounts for overtime and temporary help are included in separate accounts (Esmond, 1982). A vacancy allowance may be added to the calculations at the end of the process. This is an estimate of the costs that may not be incurred because of unforeseen turnover and vacancies. The manager and budget officer estimate an offset to total salary and wage expenses for the amount that probably will not be paid. It is an educated guess based on past experience and intuition (Esmond, 1982).

Another type of personnel control report is an hourly report. It summarizes paid hours by job category and employee. Hours are broken down into productive (worked) time, including straight time and overtime, and nonproductive time (paid nonworking time, such as sick, holiday, and vacation pay). This can serve as an important management tool (Finkler, 1984) and should be reviewed carefully by the department manager.

Independent contractors, such as agency nurses, are not classified as employees of the health care institution. They are considered outside purchases and are on the nonsalary budget. Since reducing the number of fixed positions reduces the break-even point (volume required to cover the fixed costs of producing services), careful management of these purchased labor services may be a cost-containment strategy for the unit.

Supplies and Services (Nonsalary) Budget

The supplies or commodities budget includes all direct expenses of the unit or cost center other than employment. Supplies are the second most significant budget factor, representing about 10% of the entire nursing budget (Smeltzer & Hyland, 1989; Strasen, 1987). The supply budget includes medical and nonmedical supplies and services not billed directly to the patient, such as linen and dietary. The simplest process for developing the supply budget is to first develop or identify a cost per unit of service ($UOS), such as cost per meal served, based on past experience. Then, to forecast the supply budget, the $UOS is multiplied by the projected number of UOS and then adjusted for price inflation. Although simple, this method does build in past inefficiencies, excessive use, and waste (Strasen, 1987).

Actual medical supply costs 1991/actual UOS 1991 =
medical supply cost per UOS

Medical supply cost per UOS × budgeted UOS 1992 ×
price inflation factor = 1992 medical supply budget

The budgeted units of service are determined by reviewing previous expense reports to determine trends: volume changes, change in patient mix or patient type, and changes in specific procedures or technologies. These will influence the intensity of supply use in particular cost centers. Prices are adjusted to reflect the impact of inflation. One hedge against inflation and midyear price changes is contract purchasing, where the hospital can obtain a quantity discount and guaranteed price for a specified time period.

A more complex process for projecting supply expenses for the next budget cycle requires consideration of three basic factors: the supply price inflation factor, predicted census changes, and predicted changes in intensity of supply usage (Hoffman, 1985). Medical supply price inflation will vary according to whether purchases are direct from the supplier, are part of a contract, or are a portion of shared expenses. Hospital Purchasing Management, a monthly report, provides a complete analysis of health care inflation factors that can be used to project price increases for specific supply categories for the budget year.

Intensity of supply use varies with patient acuity as well as technologic changes. Supply use per patient has increased over time, holding acuity constant (Hoffman, 1985). As the average acuity of patients in the inpatient setting increases, supply use also will increase. Hoffman has described a method for measuring the rate of change in supply use over time to be used in preparing the supply budget for the next budget cycle. First, the percentage change in supply items per patient over the past 5 years (or whatever time span seems reasonable) is calculated. This is the difference between the number of items used per patient over the last few years divided by the number of change periods over the same time frame.

$$1991\text{—supply items per patient} = 20.0$$

$$1986\text{—supply items per patient} = 15.0$$

Change periods = 5
$$(1986–1987, 1987–1988, 1988–1989, 1989–1990, 1990–1991)$$

The difference in use (20 − 15 = 5 more items used per patient) is divided by the number of change periods (5/5 = 1) to determine how many more items are being used per patient per year. This is then converted to a percentage by dividing the incremental amount per year (1) by the number of items used in the first year (15), or 1/15 = 0.066, or 6.6%. This is used to adjust intensity upward for the next budget year.

Census has been declining over the last few years, so this may have to be adjusted downward in the supply budget projections.

$$1991\text{—average patient census} = 29$$

$$1986\text{—average patient census} = 35$$

Change periods = 5 (the trend line; same as in preceding example)

The difference in census (29 − 35 = −6) shows a decrease in average patient census over the 5 years. The annual difference is again determined (−6/5 = −1.2 patients per year). The difference per year is divided by the census for the first year (35) to determine the annual percentage decline, or −1.2/35 = −0.037, or −3.7%. This is the downward adjustment for census changes in the 1992 supply budget.

The manager identifies unusual, one-time expenses that will need to be added to the annual budget estimate. If within-year projections are to be made, they are based on the current year-to-date experience, and expenses are projected for the rest of the year. Fiscal year projections are based on the previous year's expenses and project expenses for a full year into the future (Hoffman, 1985). The previous year's budget must be adjusted downward, however, if it included one-time, nonrecurring expenditures for specific supply items.

The basic equations for the fiscal year projections are as follows (Hoffman, 1985).

A. Base year expense (minus any one-time expenses) ×
    direct purchase inflation factor × intensity factor × census factor ×
                                  % direct purchase

B. Base year expense (minus any one-time expenses) ×
contract purchase inflation factor × intensity factor × census factor ×
% contract purchase

C. A + B + projected one-time purchases = projected supply budget

For example, suppose that last year's supply budget was $70,000, that it included a $5000 one-time expense, that the direct purchase price inflation factor is 7% and the contract price inflation factor is 5%, that 50% of the supply budget is direct purchase, and that a one-time expense of $3500 is planned. The calculations for next year's supply budget are as follows.

A. ($70,000 − $5000) × 1.07 × 1.066 × 0.963 × 0.50 = $35,698.55

B. ($70,000 − $5000) × 1.05 × 1.066 × 0.963 × 0.50 = $35,031.29

C. $35,698.55 + $35,031.29 + $3500 = $74,229.84 1992 supply budget

The unit manager needs to control both the level of supply usage and the cost per item. Strategies employed will vary with the individual unit, depending on such factors as geographic layout, amount of traffic through the unit, type of supplies, and so on. For example, a unit may limit access to supplies by installing locked cupboards. Other units may reduce their inventories, eliminating unused or infrequently used items. Other cost-reducing strategies include substituting less expensive types of supplies and centralizing purchasing to obtain the best prices (Smeltzer & Hyland, 1989).

Capital Budget

The capital budget is a plan that identifies the major asset items that have been assigned high priority for purchase and the expected sources of funds required to make the purchase. The capital budget is built from investment decisions—whether to buy or whether to lease specific capital items. These investment decisions are important because they commit the organization to a pattern of financial demands, production techniques, service selection, and geographic location. To cover all resource requirements completely, the capital budget should include all capitalized expenditures (all items not shown as expenses in the revenue and expense budget) (Esmond, 1982).

Capital equipment budgeting is required if an item costs more than a specified amount (usually $500) and has a useful life of more than 1 year. It is done separately from the operating budget. The capital budget covers a longer time period than the revenue, expense, and cash budgets, which relate to 1 year time periods. However, the capital budget, like the operating budget, is driven by the strategic plan. Well-planned capital decisions are necessary to achieve the long-range objectives of the institution.

Capital is derived from operating income, debt, funded depreciation, unrestricted investments, proceeds from sale of assets, endowment income, grants, and philanthropy. The single largest category is debt, which includes bond offerings, bank loans, and mortgages. The major uses of the capital funds are major construction, renovation, and repair projects, proposed acquisitions of equipment to expand or add new services, and replacement of current equipment. The major capital budget categories are land, buildings, fixed equipment, major moveable equipment, and minor equipment.

Capital expenditure requests originate at the unit or cost-center level. The department manager identifies needs, justifies the specific request, and makes a determination of priority within the department's total capital requests. A centralized capital committee reviews organizationwide requests and prioritizes these requests in accordance with the organization's strategic plan and goals. Evaluation criteria used by the central committee classify the requests as urgent, essential, economically desirable, or generally desirable (Esmond, 1982). Urgent requests usually relate to safety requirements. Essential requests may be associated with accreditation requirements. New equipment, such as MRI scanners, may be economically desirable because of revenue enhancement, and replacing old equipment may be a cost savings for the institution. Building a same-day surgery center may result in a volume increase, whereas renovating the maternity unit may be generally desirable from a patient satisfaction viewpoint. Funding for new capital projects is limited by the facility's ability to generate capital.

Hoffman (1986) has identified seven steps to developing a request for capital funds. These are

- Gather data to document need
- Develop alternative solutions to meet documented needs
- Prioritize the solutions
- Analyze costs and benefits of each solution
- Recommend one best solution
- Develop an implementation plan
- Create an evaluation plan

The need for specific capital items might result from a physician's request or an identified specific patient need. Additional data to support the request might address the projected extent of use of the item, other applications of the item, others' experience with the new equipment, reported effectiveness and liability issues, its potential for revenue generation, any required building changes or additional technical personnel and supply requirements, whether the item replaces or is an addition to other equipment, and specifics about financing options (Hoffman, 1986).

Cash Budget

The cash budget flows from and supports both the operating budget and the capital budget. Cash flows both into and out of the hospital. The statement of cash flows summarizes the effect of organizational activities on the cash accounts.

Cash is generated from the revenue received from patient billings to third party payors, nonoperating revenue sources, such as parking and the cafeteria, and income from investments and other sources. Cash is expended on operations (labor, supplies, equipment), nonoperating activities, such as debt repayment and interest, and reserves (Ward, 1988). The cash budget ensures that the organization will have the necessary cash flow to be able to meet its bills. Usually, the CFO is responsible for the cash budget (Strasen, 1987).

The cash budget is a projection of cash balances at the end of each month throughout the budget year. It compares projected balances to establish standards for desired cash balances. It provides management with a tool to project temporary monetary excesses that can be invested or shortfalls that must be covered through lines of credit or short-term notes. It tests how well the revenue, expense, and capital expenditure budgets have been coordinated (Esmond, 1982) and also assesses the impact of operating, investment, or financing decisions on cash flows.

The lifeblood of the organization is its cash balance. The director of the cash budget or the CFO may spend considerable time developing strategies for increasing cash receipts and reducing cash expenditures. Strategies for increasing the flow of cash into the hospital include quicker internal processing of patient bills, reduced collections float by use of lock boxes in strategic areas, twice-daily bank deposits, requiring deposits before service is rendered, use of credit cards for payment, and identification of new, revenue-generating programs. Strategies to reduce cash expenditures include routine buy/lease analysis, shared purchasing, use of noncash benefits to staff, and increased use of float and on-call personnel (to reduce fixed costs.)

A hospital can experience cash flow problems if it (Strasen, 1987)

1. Experiences an increase in bad debts or uncompensated care
2. Experiences an increase in days in accounts receivable
3. Has an unexpected reduction in census or length of stay
4. Has an unexpected increase in amount of nonproductive time (sick days)
5. Has unplanned capital expenditures (the hospital has a fire or flooding)

VARIANCE ANALYSIS

The unit manager and staff need to concentrate on controllable costs within their budget, which are generally the direct, variable costs. Strategies to reduce direct nursing costs include changing the skill mix to a lesser paid mix, reducing overtime, and omitting or limiting the use of agency nurses. However, in a severely resource-constrained environment, cost-control strategies may involve changes at the organizational level, such as deleting a layer of management, which generally has been considered a fixed cost. Managers need to examine the overhead costs that are allocated to the unit budget. These costs, which include housekeeping, security, building maintenance, hospital administration, and insurance, should be reviewed for accuracy and fairness. More specifically, the assigned square footage, FTEs, patient days, and so on need to be examined to determine whether the allocation statistic is accurate.

Variance analysis is the final phase of the management control process (Cleverley, 1986). Variance analysis involves analyzing the difference between actual and budgeted amounts for any revenue or cost item to determine probable causes of any deviations and possible corrective courses of action. If the amount actually spent on an item is greater than the budgeted amount, it is considered an unfavorable variance. If less was spent than anticipated, it is a favorable variance. Variances are always stated in terms of dollars (Kersey, 1988). Favorable and unfavorable are accounting terms that refer to spending more or less than expected or planned. Higher volumes create an unfavorable variance but mean greater revenue and a wider base for distributing fixed costs, so are favorable from the revenue perspective (Finkler, 1991).

Managers must be able to monitor and control expenses while maintaining high-quality services. Variances help pinpoint specific areas that are over or under budget and point the direction for investigations to determine underlying causes (Finkler, 1984). Differences between actual and budgeted amounts require explanation and justification by the manager who is responsible for the budget (Strasen, 1987). Therefore, managers need to know the amount of any variance, the reason for its occurrence, and the possible corrective actions.

At the simplest level, there are three types of variances.

1. Volume variance—when output level is higher or lower than budgeted. This occurs when the actual census or number of patient days (or other appropriate volume statistic) is higher or lower than planned. If lower, revenue will be lower, and expenses also should be lower. The nurse manager has little control over volume variance, but it is a critical factor when examining the other types of variances.
2. Usage (efficiency, productivity) variance—when the actual quantity of inputs used are different from budgeted levels, such as a difference between planned hours of care and actual hours of care.
3. Price or rate variance—when the prices paid for inputs are different from budgeted prices, for example, the difference between budgeted rate of pay and actual rate of pay (or price for supplies).

Traditional variance analysis is the difference between the actual cost for the actual volume of workload or output and the budgeted cost, which assumes a predicted, fixed volume or workload. This method provides an expected cost for one particular volume of output that is unlikely to be achieved. Flexible budget variance analysis, on the other hand, is a technique derived from cost-accounting principles. The flexible budget is an after-the-fact device that tells what it should have cost for the volume of activity actually attained. It is derived by adjusting the static budget for the actual production volume achieved (Finkler, 1983).

The process of flexible budget variance analysis begins with determining the volume variance. This is the difference between the static budget and the flexible budget. Higher volume means higher cost and going over budget, but revenue also will be over budget. In many cases, nurse managers may be held responsible for the costs but will not receive credit or benefit from the increase in revenue (Finkler, 1985). The flexible budget allows identification of how much of the total variance is due to the changes in workload volume, and the nurse manager can then concentrate on the other, controllable causes of variance (Finkler, 1991). The manager proceeds to flexible budget analysis, or the difference between the actual costs and the flexible budget. The two areas of focus are the quantity variance and the price variance, both of which can be influenced by the nurse manager. The flexible budget variance and the volume variance together equal the total variance. The price, quantity, and volume variance together are equal to the total variance between the actual costs and the original static budget.

Example. The nurse manager has been informed that the unit's budget has an unfavorable variance of $101,350. She knows that the census had been higher than predicted and that as a result she used more overtime and temporary help. The manager needs to determine the exact causes of the unfavorable variance and which of the causes are under her control and require managerial action. The nurse manager has gathered the following information relevant to the unit budget.

Actual price (AP): $20.00/hour   Budgeted price(BP): $18.50
Actual quantity(AQ): 4.5 HPPD   Budgeted quantity(BQ): 4.6 HPPD
Actual volume(AV): 12,000 patient days   Budgeted volume(BV): 11,500 days

The manager first calculates the static budget and actual budget for the unit.

$$BP \times BQ \times BV = \$18.50 \times 4.6 \times 11,500 = \$978,650 \text{ static budget}$$

$$AP \times AQ \times AV = \$20.00 \times 4.5 \times 12,000 = \$1,080,000 \text{ actual budget}$$

The difference between the actual budget and the static budget does indeed equal the total variance of $101,350. However, a lot of the cost overage seems due to the higher volume of care delivered. The manager decides to calculate the volume variance first, which is the difference between the flexible budget and the static budget.

$$BP \times BQ \times AV = \$18.50 \times 4.6 \times 12,000 = \$1,021,200 \text{ flexible budget}$$

This is the amount that should have been budgeted had the correct volume been known. The volume variance is thus the difference between this flexible budget amount and the static budget, or

$$\$1,021,200 - \$978,650 = \$42,550 \text{ unfavorable volume variance}$$

The nurse manager then determines the flexible budget variance, or the difference between the actual budget and the flexible budget, so the manager could proceed to determining the rate and quantity variances.

$$\$1,080,000 - \$1,021,200 = \$58,800 \text{ unfavorable flexible budget variance}$$

The manager notes that the volume variance and the flexible budget variance equal the total variance. She also notes that the volume variance was not a controllable variance. The manager proceeds to calculation of the quantity and price variances, for which responsibility can be assigned. First, the subflexible budget is calculated.

$BP \times AQ \times AV = \$18.50 \times 4.5 \times 12,000 = \$999,000$ subflexible budget

The price variance is equal to the difference between the actual budget and the subflexible budget, or

$\$1,080,000 - \$999,000 = \$81,000$ unfavorable price variance

The quantity variance is equal to the difference between the flexible budget and the subflexible budget, or

$\$1,021,200 - \$999,000 = \$22,200$ favorable quantity variance

The manager notes that price variance is unfavorable because of a higher hourly pay rate than budgeted. Perhaps the additional patient days required extensive use of overtime, at time-and-a-half pay, and the use of registry nurses, who are paid a higher average rate than staff nurses. It is also possible that the negotiated pay increase for nurses was higher than anticipated. The quantity variance is favorable because the actual nursing care standard was lower than budgeted. Perhaps the unit was unable to staff all shifts at the target nursing care standard for the additional days of care delivered. It is also possible that the average acuity level was lower than expected, and the standard was lowered accordingly.

More hospitals are incorporating projections of anticipated acuity levels of patients as well as projections of patient days into their budgeting processes (Finkler, 1985). If the hospital can classify patients into acuity categories, it can calculate nursing time required by projected acuity levels. The same number of patient days can generate substantially different FTE needs depending on the expected average acuity levels (Finkler, 1985). Forecasting of patient days by nursing acuity levels becomes more important as LOS declines but nursing care requirements per patient day increase.

Example:

$$
\begin{array}{lll}
BQ = 4.2 & AQ = 4.6 & \text{Required NHPPD} = 4.5 \\
BP = \$16 & AP = \$18.00 & \\
BV = 9000 & AV = 10,500 &
\end{array}
$$

Static budget $= BQ \times BP \times BV = 4.2 \times \$16 \times 9000 = \$604,800$

Flexible budget $= BQ \times BP \times AQ = 4.2 \times \$16 \times 10,500 = \$705,600$

Actual budget $= AQ \times AP \times AV = 4.6 \times \$18 \times 10,500 = \$869,400$

Subflexible budget $= AQ \times BP \times AV = 4.6 \times \$16 \times 10,500 = \$772,800$

Volume variance $= \$705,600 - \$604,800 = \$100,800$ unfavorable

The difference between the actual amount spent and the flexible budget is due to either price paid for inputs or quantity of inputs used per unit of output.

Price (rate) variance $= \$869,400 - \$772,800 = \$96,600$ unfavorable

Quantity variance $= \$772,800 - \$705,600 = \$67,200$ unfavorable

Part of the quantity variance may be due to a higher average patient acuity level than expected. If the average acuity level changes, a change in the amount of nursing time used per patient day would be expected. The amount of the acuity variance would be contained in the difference between the flexible budget and the subflexible budget, since one contains the actual amount of nursing time and the other contains the budgeted amount of nursing time (Finkler, 1985).

Acuity subflexible budget $=$ BQ (for actual acuity) $\times$ BP $\times$ AV $=$
$$4.5 \times \$16 \times 10,500 = \$756,000$$

Quantity variance (excluding acuity) $=$ acuity subflexible budget $-$
subflexible budget, or $\$756,000 - \$772,800 = \$16,800$ unfavorable

Acuity variance $=$ flexible budget $-$ acuity subflexible budget, or
$$\$705,600 - \$756,000 = \$50,400 \text{ unfavorable}$$

Then, $50,400 plus $16,800 equals the total quantity variance of $67,200. This added to the price variance ($96,600) and the volume variance ($100,800) equals the total variance ($264,600).

METHODS OF BUDGETING
Flexible Budgets

Flexible budgeting is a more sophisticated method of budgeting and is getting adopted more frequently in hospitals. The flexible budget adjusts target levels of costs for changes in volume or activity level. In flexible budgeting, the operating budget for 90% occupancy is different from the operating budget for 75% occupancy. Flexible operating budgets change as the volume of business changes. A flexible budget has the appearance of a series of fixed budgets at various occupancy levels (Esmond, 1982). There are dramatic differences in approved costs resulting from the two methods. Recognizing the underlying cost behavior patterns can change the estimated resource requirements approved in the budgeting process (Cleverley, 1986).

The flexible budget is tied directly to variable costs that increase or decrease as a result of patient days. Direct caregiver salaries, medical supplies, and dietary expenses are expected to change as a direct result of altered volume of services delivered. Therefore, if patient days decline, the manager needs to reduce variable costs in relation to the decrease in volume. If the census goes below the point of minimum staffing levels, fixed cost expenditures will exceed revenues. At this point, management needs to consider consolidating units or closing beds.

Program Budgets

Program budgets are a restructuring of budget information by accumulating revenue and cost information into more meaningful categories (Herkimer, 1978). They are designed to forecast revenues and expenses for one specific project so as to assist management in predicting or monitoring the profitability of the new service. It can be an effective management tool in forecasting and evaluating the cost-benefit ratio of a single project. The program budget is usually a supplement to the institution's master budget plan.

Rolling Budgets

Length of the budget period may be fixed or rolling (continuous). A rolling budget means that the budget is continuously extended 1 more month or one more quarter into the future. The manager always has a full 12-month budget to work with rather than a budget that may have only 1 or 2 months left (Herkimer, 1978). It, therefore, always maintains a yearly planning horizon. It requires more effort to maintain a rolling budget, but it may provide a more realistic forecast for planning and control (Cleverley, 1986). It also relieves the massive problem of doing a whole year's budget in a few short months (Finkler, 1983).

Zero-Base Budgeting

Zero-base budgeting is again gaining popularity. Zero-base review is a way of looking at existing programs and their expenses. The basic premise is that no department or program should last forever (Esmond, 1982) and that no program is entitled to automatic renewal and funding. Because it is very expensive and time consuming, individual programs may be reviewed every few years rather than annually. Whether annually or less frequently, senior management reevaluates all activities to decide whether they should be eliminated or funded. Questions asked during the zero-base review include whether the services are being delivered in an efficient manner and whether the services are being delivered in an effective manner in terms of the organization's goals and objectives (Cleverley, 1986). Appropriate funding levels are determined by organizational priorities. Activities are ranked by top management, and projects are approved or disapproved according to overall availability of funds. There are two basic steps to the review process: (1) development of decision packages, where each package identifies the project, department, or unit and includes the mission, goals, objectives, revenue, expenses, and benefits to the entire organization, and (2) allocation of resources by management according to rankings—the most important programs or departments being first (Herkimer, 1978). The final budget takes all approved decision packages, separates out the revenue and costs, and then develops the total budget.

FORECASTING

Forecasting is a method of determining what may happen in the future based on current driving forces and trends. After potential future scenarios are identified, the process of strategic management is used to bring about the desired future. In budgeting, forecasting is the attempt to predict, in quantitative terms, what a department or institution will produce over a specified period of time. It provides a measure of workload or activity in each department or responsibility center for the coming budget period. Forecasting is a key step in the budget planning and control process. A budget is only as good as its volume or activity forecast.

There are many factors to consider during the forecasting process (Herkimer, 1988).

1. External and internal competition
2. Government and third party policies
3. Department goals and objectives
4. New services and capital expenditures
5. Historical data and trends
6. Other known facts and rumors

If no significant changes have occurred in the environment, the department's historical data and trends provide the most accurate and reliable source for starting volume forecasting.

Methods: Qualitative
Delphi Technique

This technique uses expert opinion and consensus building. Experts individually and then collectively generate opinions about the future and then rank-order them according to importance or probability.

Scenario Building

This is forecasting of potential scenarios and then selecting the desired future based on the organization's mission statement, philosophy, and goals. The process is as follows.

1. Identify the organization's present position
2. Identify the organization's strengths and weaknesses
3. Identify driving forces in the environment that could be threats or opportunities
4. Construct possible alternative future scenarios based on the driving forces and trends in the environment
5. Identify the desired future for the organization

Methods: Quantitative
Graphic Presentation

Graphic presentation is a method of time series analysis. Time is placed on the horizontal axis, and output is placed on the vertical axis. Trends are then determined (upward, downward, steady state, seasonality, random fluctuation). Graphic representation requires an adequate number of data points.

Weighted Moving Average

Weighted moving average is a time series method of forecasting future activity or volume. Each projected number in the moving average sequence is the weighted average of a number of past consecutive months.

$$\text{Forecast} = 3M^1 + 2M^2 + 1M^3/6$$

where M_1 = latest month's data, M_2 = data from 2 months ago, and M_3 = data from 3 months ago. The most recent month's data are weighted more heavily than the data of the month before, which in turn is weighted more heavily than the data from 3 months ago. This technique allows the manager to forecast short-term future volume measures that are more sensitive to current trends than are annual budget projections.

Linear Model (Least Squares Method)

The purpose of linear modeling is to fit a straight line to time series data to determine the trend line and to project next year's volume. This technique has been used most frequently to determine trends in days of patient care. The equation for fitting a straight line for days or hours is

$$Y^\wedge = a + bX$$

where $Y^\wedge$ is projected days, a is the intercept, b is the slope of the line or rate of change in days, and X is time (years or months). The midpoint method of the least squares approach (Herkimer, 1978) is as follows.

X (year)	Y (patient days)	X DEV (from midyear)	X² (squared deviation)	XY
1986	120,000	−2	4	−240,000
1987	124,000	−1	1	−124,000
1988	132,000	0	0	0
1989	136,000	+1	1	+130,000
1990	140,000	+2	4	+280,000
1991(?)				

$\Sigma Y = 652,000 \qquad \Sigma X = 0 \qquad \Sigma X^2 = 10 \qquad \Sigma XY = 52,000$

Mean = 130,400 $\qquad\qquad \Sigma XY/X^2 = 52,000/10 = 5200 = b$

(652,000/5) $\qquad\qquad\qquad\qquad$ (Rate of change)

CALCULATIONS:

1986:	130,400 + (−2 × 5200)	= 120,000
1987:	130,400 + (−1 × 5200)	= 125,200
1988:	130,400 + (0)	= 130,400
1989:	130,400 + (1 × 5200)	= 135,600
1990:	130,400 + (2 × 5200)	= 140,800
1991:	130,400 + (3 × 5200)	= 146,000

This represents the line that best fits the data; 146,000 days of care are predicted for 1991. The number of predicted days must next be distributed across the annual budget by month. The following techniques are in order of increasing accuracy.

Monthly Volume Distribution

1. Even month distribution process

   Total patient days/total calendar months =
   $$\text{monthly patient days per calendar month}$$

   $146,000/12 = 12,166.67$ days for January 1991

2. Calendar month distribution process

   Total patient days/total calendar days = daily patient days

   $146,000/365 = 400$; 31 days $\times$ 400 = 12,400 for January 1991

3. Percentage distribution process: use last year's actual monthly distribution and calculate the monthly percentage of the total annual volume.

   1990 January = 12,321 days

   1990 total days = 140,000

   $12,321/140,000 = .088$

   $146,000 \times 0.088 = 12,848$ for January 1991

4. Two year percentage distribution process
   Add the last 2 years total of patient days for the month, and then divide by the 2 year patient day total.

   1990 January = 12,321   1990 total = 140,000

   1989 January = 11,950   1989 total = 136,000

   2 year total = 24,271 days 2 year total = 276,000 days

   $24,271/276,000 = 0.08794$

   $146,000 \times 0.08794 = 12,839.2$ for January 1991

CONCLUSION

Koontz, O'Donnell, and Weihrich (1986) have identified several dangers in the budgeting process. There is the danger of overbudgeting, where the budgeting process itself becomes cumbersome, meaningless, and expensive. The budget may spell out minor details, which results in lack of managerial freedom and low morale. There is a danger that the organization's goals may be overridden by budgetary goals. The overriding mission may be lost when budget goals become more important than institutional goals and objectives. The budget may hide inefficiencies in operations. The managers need to review constantly the standards and conversion factors on which the budget is built. Finally, the budget may lead to inflexibility in the organization. This inability to change and lack of creativity may nullify the usefulness of any budget.

The key to effective departmental management and leadership is information (Kersey, 1988). The more information managers have about the financial operation of the department or unit, the more likely they are to make informed decisions and be in control. This can only work to the advantage of the parent institution.

References

Cleverley, W.O. (1986). *Essentials of health care finance*. Rockville, MD: Aspen.

Esmond, T.H. (1982). *Budgeting procedures for hospitals*. Chicago: American Hospital Association.

Finkler, S.A. (1983). *The complete guide to finance and accounting for nonfinancial managers*. Englewood Cliffs, NJ: Prentice-Hall.

Finkler, S.A. (1984). *Budgeting concepts for nurse managers*. Orlando, FL: Grune & Stratton.

Finkler, S.A. (1985). Flexible budget analysis extended to patient acuity and DRGs. *Health Care Management Review, 10*(4), 21–34.

Finkler, S.A. (1991). Variance analysis: Part I. Extending flexible budget variance analysis to acuity. *Journal of Nursing Administration, 21*(7/8), 19-25.

Finkler, S. A. (1992). *Budgeting Concepts for Nurse Managers*. (2nd ed). Philadelphia: W.B. Saunders Company.

Herkimer, A.G. (1978). *Understanding hospital financial management*. Germantown, MD: Aspen.

Herkimer, A.G. (1988). *Understanding health care budgeting*. Rockville, MD: Aspen.

Hoffman, F.M. (1985). Projecting supply expenses. *Journal of Nursing Administration, 15*(6), 21–24.

Hoffman, F.M. (1986). The capital budget: Developing a capital expenditure proposal. *AORN Journal, 44*(4), 604–610.

Kersey, J.H. (1988). Increasing the manager's fiscal responsibility. *Nursing Management, 19*(1), 30–32.

Kirby, K.K., & Wiczal, L.J. (1985). Budgeting for variable staffing. *Nursing Economic$, 3*(3), 160–166.

Koontz, H., O'Donnell, C., & Weihrich, H. (1986). *Essentials of management*. New York: McGraw-Hill.

Lusk, E., & Lusk, J. (1979). *Financial and managerial control: A health care perspective*. Rockville, MD: Aspen.

Mark, B.A., & Smith, H.L. (1987). *Essentials of finance in nursing*. Rockville, MD: Aspen.

Scodro, J. (1988). Basic concepts in financial management and budgeting. In D.R. Blaney & C.J. Hobson (Eds.). *Cost-effective nursing practice: Guidelines for nurse managers*. Philadelphia: J.B. Lippincott Company.

Smeltzer, C.H., & Hyland, J. (1989). A working plan to understand and control financial pressures. *Nursing Economic$, 7*(4), 208–214.

Strasen, L. (1987). *Key business skills for nurse managers*. Philadelphia: J.B. Lippincott Company.

Ward, W.J. (1988). *An introduction to health care financial management*. Owings Mills, MD: Rynd Communications.

CHAPTER 26

COST: CONCEPTS AND MEASUREMENT

PAUL L. GRIMALDI
MICHAEL L. MOORE

EXECUTIVE SUMMARY

Knowing where the money goes is an important job in the efficient operation of any organization. We must know how much is spent on labor, materials, and overhead so that we can control costs, establish prices, and calculate profit margins. This chapter provides an overview of how costs are tracked and evaluated in the health care setting.

The first section of the chapter reviews the different ways that costs are classified. The areas of incurred vs paid costs, cost relative to output, and historical vs replacement costs are covered in an easy to understand manner. The rest of the chapter is devoted to costing methods, in particular the two methods used for determining Medicare costs: stepdown cost finding and the use of the resource-based relative value scale (RBRVS). These costing methods are discussed at length, and practical examples of both methods are provided.

This chapter provides an in-a-nutshell look at these complex areas and serves as a valuable resource for the nurse manager.

A ll businesses must analyze their costs to understand relationships among costs, output, prices, and profit margins. Imprecise information may lead to poor production decisions, unrealistic prices, large losses, and eventual bankruptcy.

This chapter begins by explaining different ways to classify and examine an organization's costs. It then provides an overview of certain methods that accountants frequently use to estimate the cost of specific products and services. The chapter concludes by describing two costing methods that Medicare applies to hospital care and physician services.

COST CONCEPTS

Accountants, economists, and other professionals employ a variety of cost concepts to measure costs, control costs, establish prices, and calculate profit margins (Suver & Neuman, 1981). In so doing, costs may be classified by their nature, their relation to and variability with the volume of output, the accounting period to which costs apply, and the analytic purposes at hand (American Hospital Association, 1980).

Natural Categories

An organization's total costs (before income taxes) can be sorted into three major categories: labor, materials, and overhead. The first two of these categories usually include direct and indirect costs. Direct costs are clearly attributable to specific products or services, such as the compensation paid to nurses and technical support staff rendering care in a coronary care or intensive care unit. Indirect (or overhead) costs are not directly attributable to specific products or services but instead are incurred for many services combined or for an organization as a whole. For example, a portion of the total cost a hospital incurs for housekeeping, medical records, accounting and finance, and general administration is attributable to the intensive care units. Other portions are attributable to outpatient services, routine inpatient care, and so on. In practice, various methods are used to allocate a proper share of a hospital's indirect total costs to each type of output a hospital produces.

Cost Relative to Output

Direct or indirect costs may be fixed, variable or semi-variable. Total fixed cost (TFC) does not vary with output; examples include rent, insurance, mortgage interest, and compensation paid to salaried personnel. Total variable cost (TVC) varies directly, although not necessarily proportionally, with output, such as the total wages of hourly employees, materials, and supplies. Semivariable cost consists of partly fixed and partly variable costs.

Fixed costs occur only during the short run, which is a flexible time period that depends on the circumstances. During this period, a fixed cost is the same regardless of the level of output. In the long run, no costs are fixed. Instead, all costs are variable. Leases can be renegotiated or canceled, mortgages are paid or refinanced, and salaries are changed, or personnel find employment elsewhere.

Given TFC, average fixed cost (AFC) must decline as output increases as the same total cost is spread over an increasingly larger output. In contrast, average variable cost (AVC) may increase, decrease, or remain unchanged as output increases. AVC will decrease if output increases faster than total variable costs. AVC will increase if the opposite situation prevails. AVC will remain unchanged if total variable cost and output increase at the same rate.

Average total cost (ATC) equals the sum of AFC and AVC. As output increases, ATC will decrease if AFC and AVC decrease or if AFC decreases more than AVC increases. Conversely, ATC will increase as output expands if AVC increases by a greater amount than AFC decreases.

Marginal cost (MC) represents the cost of producing an additional unit of output. MC depends on variable cost, since fixed costs are constant. MC may rise, fall, or remain constant as output increases. MC may be a large or small proportion of ATC, depending on the types of products or services an organization provides.

TABLE 26–1   Relationships Between Cost and Output

Unit of Output (Q)	Total Fixed Cost (TFC)	Total Variable Cost (TVC)	Total Cost	Average Fixed Cost[a] (AFC)	Average Variable Cost[b] (AVC)	Average Total Cost[c] (ATC)	Marginal Cost (MC)
0	$1000	$ 0	$1000	—	—	—	
1	1000	500	1500	$1000	$500	$1500	$500
2	1000	900	1900	500	450	950	400
3	1000	1200	2200	333	400	733	300
4	1000	1400	2400	250	350	600	200
5	1000	1550	2550	200	310	510	150
6	1000	1650	2650	167	275	442	100
7	1000	1900	2900	143	271	415	250
8	1000	2200	3200	125	275	400	300
9	1000	2700	3700	111	300	411	500
10	1000	3400	4400	100	340	440	700

[a]TFC/Q = AFC.
[b]TVC/Q = AVC.
[c]AFC + AVC = ATC.
[d]$TVC_2 - TVC_1$ = MC (marginal cost).

Table 26–1 illustrates the calculation of different types of cost. TFC and TVC are given. Average and marginal costs are derived from these givens. The figures show that

- TFC remains unchanged at $1000 as output expands.
- AFC declines continuously from $1000 to $100.
- AVC declines over the first seven units and then rises as TVC increases faster than total output increases.
- ATC declines until the eighth unit of output and then increases thereafter.
- For eight units, AFC decreases along with AVC, causing ATC to fall as output expands.
- MC decreases for six units and then rises rapidly thereafter.

Explicit and Implicit Costs

We have so far addressed explicit costs—that is, costs for which cash outlays have been or will be made. Explicit costs are recorded in a company's accounting records. Almost always, however, explicit costs do not equal total costs. The difference between total costs and explicit costs equals implicit costs.

Implicit costs are costs that do not involve any cash outlay. One example relates to the funds investors use to operate a business. These funds could have been put into treasury bills, certificates of deposit, or savings accounts, earning interest with little or no risk of nonpayment. By foregoing such opportunities, an implicit cost is incurred equal to the lost interest. Similarly, an implicit cost occurs whenever an individual foregoes a salary in order to operate a business.

Implicit costs are as important as explicit costs in setting prices. If implicit costs are not recovered, an individual can do better financially by taking advantage of other opportunities, such as investing elsewhere or shutting down to take a salaried position.

Incurred vs Paid Costs

A cost or expense may be incurred in one accounting period but reported in a different accounting period. The total cost reported for a given period, therefore, depends on whether costs are counted on an incurred or paid basis. Most large businesses report costs on an incurred (or accrued) basis in an attempt to match revenue with the cost incurred to generate the revenue.

Recently, the issue of reporting costs on an incurred vs paid basis has been debated extensively for retiree health benefits. Virtually every company that provides these benefits records the cost on a cash or pay-as-you-go basis. However, the cost is incurred during an employee's working life. Since retiree health benefits are a relatively new fringe benefit, a company's paid cost generally is significantly lower than its incurred cost, which understates today's reported costs and thus overstates net income. To minimize the possibility of misleading financial statements, the Financial Accounting Standards Board requires companies to report retiree health benefits on an incurred rather than paid basis, generally beginning January 1, 1993.

Historical vs Replacement Cost

The cost of a building or major equipment is not expensed when a cash outlay is made, as is done for most other explicit costs. Instead, the capital asset's cost is amortized as it depreciates over time. Depreciation expense depends on the asset's expected useful life and salvage value. Various methods are used to depreciate a capital asset (Table 26–2). For a given year, these methods ordinarily yield different depreciation expenses for the same asset.

Capital assets eventually become obsolete and are subject to wear and tear. The account depreciation expense is designed to recover the original cost of capital assets consumed during production processes.

Generally accepted accounting principles allow firms considerable latitude in calculating depreciation. The two most widely used approaches—the straight-line and accelerated methods—may yield different results at any point. In addition, accounting depreciation for a given year may differ from economic depreciation—that is, accounting principles may permit a depreciation write-off that differs from the amount of capital actually consumed during the production period. Furthermore, unforeseen technologic developments may terminate an asset's useful life long before the currently planned retirement date.

Table 26–2 shows the annual depreciation expenses for a $20,000 asset with an assumed zero salvage value and an estimated useful life of 10 years. Accelerated depreciation methods—double-declining balance and sum-of-the-years digits—generate more depreciation during the early part of an asset's useful life than does the straight-line method. Consequently, accelerated methods allow a

TABLE 26–2 Comparisons of Various Depreciation Methods on a
$20,000 Asset with Zero Salvage Value and Estimated Useful Life of
Ten Years

		ACCELERATED METHODS	
YEAR	STRAIGHT-LINE METHOD[a]	DOUBLE-DECLINING BALANCE[b]	SUM-OF-YEAR DIGITS[c]
1	$ 2,000	$ 4,000	$ 3,636
2	2,000	3,200	3,273
3	2,000	2,560	2,909
4	2,000	2,048	2,545
5	2,000	1,638	2,182
6	2,000	1,311	1,818
7	2,000	1,049	1,455
8	2,000	839	1,091
9	2,000	671	727
10	2,000	537	364
Total	$20,000	$17,853[d]	$20,000

[a](Historical cost-salvage value)/estimated useful life.
[b](Historical cost-accumulated depreciation) × double the straight line annual rate of depreciation.
[c]Historical cost times the ratio of the number of years of useful life remaining to the sum of the years comprising the useful life, i.e., 10/55 in the first year, 9/55 the second, 8/55 in the third, and so on.
[d]Special accounting rules apply to the balance of $2147.

quicker recovery of an asset's costs. At the end of the fourth year, double-declining depreciation totals $11,808, as compared to $8000 for straight-line depreciation.

Accountants dispute the value to be placed on a depreciating asset. One approach is to value the asset at its historical cost, which is the amount paid for the asset at acquisition. This amount would be the basis for depreciation, regardless of the length of the asset's useful life. The competing approach is to value the asset at replacement cost, which is the cost of replacing it today. Given inflation and the passage of a decade or more, historical cost and replacement cost may diverge significantly. Historical cost is the conventional basis for valuing an asset, partly because of the highly subjective nature of determining an asset's replacement cost.

COSTING METHODS

Every business needs a rational, objective, and systematic way to measure the cost of the services and products sold. Flawed methods may lead to poor production decisions, low prices, and large losses. The cost of producing a particular product or service may be determined on an actual or standard basis. An actual cost system typically accumulates direct costs as they occur and apportions indirect costs to specific products at predetermined rates. Based on historical experience, for example, direct costs might be increased 50% to recognize the associated indirect costs.

A standard cost system uses predetermined unit costs and predetermined production rates to estimate the standard cost of producing a specific number of units of output. Actual production costs are tallied as they occur. Differences between actual and standard costs, also known as variances, are recorded in separate accounts and are used to revise predetermined unit cost and production rates.

Cost Accumulation

The cost of producing a particular product or service may be accumulated by the job order cost method or the process cost method. Under the job order method, the focus of concern is the cost of specific jobs, contracts, or engagements for which varying amounts of labor and other resources are required. Several jobs may be ongoing concurrently. Each job is assigned a job sheet that is used to accumulate the hours spent working on the job as well as the materials and supplies used. The hours are costed based on the hourly compensation rates (wages and fringe benefits) of the persons performing the tasks. Materials are costed based on invoices and other financial records. To these direct costs are added a share of all the indirect costs incurred during the production period. Certain indirect costs may be assigned entirely to a few jobs. Other indirect costs may be spread equally among all jobs.

Table 26–3 shows a hypothetical job order cost sheet. The top part reports the hours devoted to the job along with the corresponding hourly wage rates. The middle part shows the cost of materials and supplies. The bottom part shows the amount of total overhead or indirect cost allocated to this job.

A process costing system frequently is used when homogeneous products are produced under mass production or by a continuous process. Because the products are indistinguishable from each other, process costing assumes that the same amount of labor, material, and overhead is required to produce each unit of output. Each unit is, therefore, assigned the same average amount of total costs. No distinction is made between direct and indirect costs.

MEDICARE COST FINDING

Medicare applies two costing methods to hospitals and physicians. The first method—stepdown cost finding—has been used by Medicare for over two decades to calculate its share of a hospital's total inpatient and outpatient costs. This method, with or without modifications, is or has been used also by various state Medicaid programs, Blue Cross plans, and other insurers to determine their respective share of a hospital's total costs. Medicare's stepdown method is generally consistent with standard cost accounting principles, as applied in other industries.

The second method—resource-based relative value scale (RBRVS)—applies to physician services as of January 1992. Medicare, Medicaid, and several other

TABLE 26–3 Job Order Cost Sheet

		LABOR		
DATE	EMPLOYEE	HOURS	RATE/ HOUR	TOTAL COST
9/1/90	Jones	2	$ 8.00	$16.00
9/3/90	Smith	3	10.00	30.00
9/5/90	Moore	4	12.50	50.00
Total		9		$96.00

		MATERIALS			
DATE	REPORT NO.	DESCRIPTION	UNITS	UNIT COST	TOTAL COST
9/1/90	10-1	Paint	2 gallons	$12.25	$24.50
9/3/90	10-2	Plywood	2 pieces	25.75	51.50
Total					$76.00

OVERHEAD

Allocated indirect cost: 50 cents of overhead for every dollar of direct
costs = 0.50 ($96 + $76) = $86.00

TOTAL COST	
1. Labor	$ 96.00
2. Materials	76.00
3. Overhead	86.00
Total	$258.00

insurers are using all or some part of RBRVS. The RBRVS costing method is not a formal cost accounting method but, instead, applies statistical principles to information from various sources to estimate the cost of, or payment for, individual physician services.

Hospital Care

Hospitals (as well as nursing facilities and home health agencies) that participate in Medicare must complete a complex report that estimates the cost of the services that Medicare patients receive. Currently, Medicare's cost report exceeds 175 pages, and the companion instructions total approximately 280 pages. A hospital must complete the sections of the report that apply to the services for which Medicare reimbursement is sought. Typically, the larger the hospital, the greater the time and expense of capturing the requisite information and completing the report. Medicare cost reports must be submitted annually and are audited for accuracy and completeness. Fraud and abuse are punishable by fines, imprisonment, and termination from the program.

The Medicare cost report begins with an account-by-account listing of a hospital's total costs. An intricate cost-finding method is employed subsequently to determine Medicare's share of total inpatient cost, total outpatient cost, and other costs for which Medicare reimbursement is sought. Detailed manuals explain the computational methods and procedures that must be used for cost-finding purposes. This includes definitions of the types of costs that Medicare reimburses and any limits Medicare imposes on the amount of allowable costs that are deemed reasonable for reimbursement purposes.

The essential features of Medicare's stepdown method are explained below, along with two competing approaches. The explanation is necessarily limited and greatly understates the method's complexity (Braganza, 1988). Second, most hospitals are generally not reimbursed today on a cost basis for services rendered to Medicare inpatients. Nevertheless, a participating hospital must still submit a completed cost report because Medicare reimburses certain inpatient costs and the cost of most outpatient services on a cost basis. Nursing facilities and home health agencies must submit completed cost reports in order to receive Medicare reimbursement.

Cost Centers

A cost center is an organizational unit or department over which a manager is responsible for the costs incurred. The cost center may be a revenue-producing department or a nonrevenue-producing department. As the nomenclature suggests, the crucial distinction between these departments is whether patients are charged directly for their services. Examples of revenue-producing departments include radiology, laboratory, pharmacy, anesthesiology, physical therapy, occupational therapy, and the emergency room. Nonrevenue-producing departments include nursing, laundry and linen, medical records, accounting and finance, housekeeping, social services, dietary, administration, and maintenance and repairs.

Cost Allocation Bases

The total cost of operating a revenue-producing department includes an appropriate share of the costs of the nonrevenue-producing departments, which are indirect patient care costs or overhead costs. The estimation of each revenue-producing department's appropriate share lies at the heart of Medicare's cost-finding method.

Table 26–4 lists many of the statistical bases that Medicare requires hospitals to use to allocate costs among departments. A hospital may use different bases if Medicare approves. Requests for alternative bases are scrutinized because Medicare reimbursement may change measurably as the allocation bases change. In general, there are four types of allocation bases: (1) volume of services used, (2) dollar value of services used, (3) departmental size (e.g., as indicated by square footage or costs), and (4) special studies. Different bases are used to allocate the cost of different nonrevenue-producing departments. The guiding principle in selecting a base is the achievement of an equitable cost allocation

TABLE 26–4 Selected Statistical Bases to Allocate Overhead Costs for Medicare Reporting Purposes, 1992

Cost Center	Allocation Basis
Depreciation (buildings)	Square feet
Depreciation (movable equipment)	Cost of equipment in each department; specific expenses of each cost center per fixed asset records
Employee health and welfare	Specific expense of each cost center per the payroll records; gross salaries and wages; number of full-time equivalent employees
Administration and general	Accumulated cost
Admitting	Number of admissions; inpatient charges by department
Data processing	Machine hours
Purchasing	Cost of supplies purchased
Repairs and maintenance	Costed work orders
Laundry and linen	Weight or pieces of laundry processed
Housekeeping	Hours of service and square feet
Dietary	Number of meals prepared
Nursing administration	Time spent
Central supply	Costed requisitions
Pharmacy	Costed requisitions
Medical records	Number of patient days and weighted outpatient visits
Social services	Time spent
Interns and residents	Assigned time spent

at a reasonable cost. One base may be more accurate than another base, but the gain in computational precision may not justify the incremental data collection costs.

To clarify, assume that the housekeeping department costs $50,000 to operate and that it provides services to two revenue-producing departments. Department A contains 3000 square feet and Department B contains 7000 square feet. Under these assumptions, $15,000 (= $50,000 × 3000/10,000) of housekeeping costs would be allocated to Department A and $35,000 (= $50,000 × 7000/10,000) to Department B. Housekeeping costs also could be apportioned by square footage, but the expense involved might far exceed the expected benefits.

Cost Allocation Methods

Allocation bases may be applied in several ways to allocate the costs of nonrevenue-producing departments to revenue-producing departments. The most common approaches are direct allocation, stepdown, and double apportionment.

TABLE 26–5 Example of Statistical Bases to Allocate Costs Among Departments[a]

Cost Center	Employee Benefits (Gross Salaries)	Repairs (Costed Orders)	Laundry and Linen (Pieces)	Housekeeping (Square Feet)
Nonrevenue-producing				
Employee benefits	100%			
Repairs	5	100%		
Laundry	10	15	100%	
Housekeeping	5	20	10	100%
Revenue-producing				
Routine care	35	30	60	60
Pharmacy	20	20	15	20
Radiology	25	15	15	20

[a]Each nonrevenue-producing department is assumed to provide services to other departments only and no services to itself.

A fourth approach employs simultaneous equations to apportion the costs of nonrevenue-producing departments to revenue-producing departments. The functional relationships tend to vary by hospital because of organizational or operational differences. Simultaneous equations pay closer attention to interdepartmental cost relationships than do the other methods. A nonrevenue-producing department is not closed until it has received all of the costs of the nonrevenue-producing departments from which it receives services. Unlike other allocation methods, the order of the cost allocation is unimportant because of the simultaneous nature of the allocation process. These methods employ different assumptions about interdepartmental cost relationships. The assumptions affect the hierarchical order in which nonrevenue-producing departments are closed into revenue-producing departments.

Table 26–5 exemplifies the percentages used to allocate the costs of four nonrevenue-producing departments to three revenue-producing departments. It is noteworthy that each nonrevenue-producing department is assumed to provide services to other departments only and no services to itself. In any event, when the process is complete, the $200,000 spent to operate the nonrevenue-producing departments will be closed into, or transferred to, the revenue-producing departments.

Direct Allocation Method

The direct allocation method assumes that the nonrevenue-producing departments furnish services solely to revenue-producing departments. In other words, no nonrevenue-producing department provides service to any other nonrevenue-producing department. The costs of nonrevenue-producing departments are, therefore, allocated directly to the revenue-producing departments.

As Table 26–6 illustrates, housekeeping cost of $20,000 is distributed to the three revenue-producing departments based on square footage. Since Pharmacy has 20% of the square footage of the revenue-producing departments, it receives

TABLE 26–6 Direct Apportionment Method

Cost Center	Direct Cost	Employee Benefits (Gross Salaries)	Repairs (Costed Orders)	Laundry (Pieces)	Housekeeping (Square Feet)	Total Cost
Nonrevenue-producing						
Employee benefits	$ 80,000					
Repairs	40,000					
Laundry	60,000					
Housekeeping	20,000					
Revenue-producing						
Routine care	$250,000	$35,000[a]	$18,462[b]	$40,000[c]	$12,000[d]	$355,462
Pharmacy	150,000	20,000	12,308	10,000	4,000	196,308
Radiology	100,000	25,000	9,230	10,000	4,000	148,230
Total	$700,000	$80,000	$40,000	$60,000	$20,000	$700,000

[a] $35,000 = $80,000 × 35/80. The denominator (80) is the sum of the percentages for employee benefits applicable to the revenue-producing departments. These percentages are in Table 26–5. The numerator (35) is the percentage applicable to routine care in Table 26–5.
[b] $18,462 = $40,000 × 30/65.
[c] $40,000 = $60,000 × 60/90.
[d] $12,000 = $20,000 × 60/100.

20% of the housekeeping costs, or $4000. Similarly, Pharmacy receives 30.8% of repairs and maintenance because it has 30.8% of the costed work orders.

The direct allocation method is relatively simple to employ and minimizes data collection requirements. However, the assumption that nonrevenue-producing departments do not produce services for other nonrevenue-producing departments is usually false and may lead to highly inaccurate allocations.

Stepdown Method

Medicare requires hospitals to use the stepdown method to calculate the cost of diagnosing and treating Medicare patients. The stepdown method recognizes that certain nonrevenue-producing departments render services to both revenue-producing and other nonrevenue-producing departments. A critical issue is the order or sequence in which the costs of the nonrevenue-producing departments are allocated. Sequencing is important because a department is closed after its costs are allocated and, therefore, cannot receive costs from other nonrevenue-producing departments that remain open.

Medicare has issued guidelines governing the sequence in which costs are allocated and nonrevenue-producing departments are closed. In principle, costs are allocated first for the nonrevenue-producing department that furnishes the largest volume of service for the greatest number of other nonrevenue-producing departments and receives the smallest amount of service from the fewest nonrevenue-producing departments. The second nonrevenue-producing department that is closed ranks second in terms of these criteria, and so on. In practice, application of these criteria is far from clear-cut and requires assumptions and judgment.

Table 26–7 illustrates the stepdown method. Employee (health and welfare) benefit costs are distributed first to the remaining nonrevenue-producing departments and to the revenue-producing departments based on each department's proportionate share of the allocation statistic. Thus, $16,000 of total fringe benefits is allocated to Pharmacy because it accounts for 20% of the allocation statistic (gross salaries). The employee benefit cost center is closed after the $80,000 is distributed to the other cost centers, and it cannot receive costs from other nonrevenue-producing departments, even if it actually received services from them.

The second nonrevenue-producing department to be closed is repairs and maintenance. Total costs of $44,000 ($40,000 of direct costs plus $4000 of allocated fringe benefits) are apportioned to the remaining departments. A similar procedure is used for the two remaining nonrevenue-producing cost centers. In each case, costs are distributed based on the percent of a department's costs allocable to the remaining open departments.

Double Apportionment Method

The double apportionment method pays greater attention to interdepartmental cost relationships than does the stepdown method. Specifically, this method

TABLE 26-7 Stepdown Method

Cost Center	Direct Cost	Employee Benefits (Gross Salaries)	Repairs (Costed Orders)	Laundry (Pieces)	Housekeeping (Square Feet)	Total Cost
Nonrevenue-producing						
Employee benefits	$ 80,000					
Repairs	40,000	$ 4,000[a]				
Laundry	60,000	8,000	$ 6,600[b]			
Housekeeping	20,000	4,000	8,800	$ 7,460[c]		
Revenue-producing						
Routine care	$250,000	$28,000	$13,200	$44,760	$24,156[d]	$360,116
Pharmacy	150,000	16,000	8,800	11,190	8,052	194,042
Radiology	100,000	20,000	6,600	11,190	8,052	145,842
Total	$700,000	$80,000	$44,000	$74,600	$40,260	$700,000

[a]$4,000 = $80,000 × 0.05.
[b]$6,600 = $44,000 × 0.15.
[c]$7,460 = $74,600 × 0.10.
[d]$24,156 = $40,260 × 0.60.

involves two allocations of the costs of nonrevenue-producing departments to revenue-producing departments.

Like the stepdown method, the sequencing of the first round of cost allocations depends on the number of nonrevenue-producing departments served and the number of departments from which services are received. (The percentages in Table 26–5 would have to change to accommodate the fact that the nonrevenue-producing departments are still open after the first round is completed. These percentages are available from the authors on request.) Unlike the stepdown method, a nonrevenue-producing department is not closed after its costs are allocated initially. Instead, the department remains open and receives costs from the nonrevenue-producing departments that served it. The second round of cost allocations is the same as the stepdown method, and each nonrevenue producing department is closed after its costs are allocated.

Table 26–8 shows how to apply the double apportionment method. The first round of cost allocations is conceptually the same as the stepdown method, except that no nonrevenue-producing department is closed after its costs are allocated. This means that the initial percentages showing the distribution of the costs of nonrevenue-producing departments are used to apportion costs rather than the percentages used in the stepdown process. In the second round of allocations, the stepdown percentages are used to apportion the costs of non-revenue-producing departments.

Cost Comparison

Table 26–9 shows the fully allocated cost of the revenue-producing departments under the direct, stepdown, and double apportionment methods. The high and low values differ by 1% to 2%. The higher a department's fully allocated cost, the greater the amount of cost reimbursement, all other things being equal.

Medicare's Cost Share

Medicare needs to know its share of each department's fully allocated costs to determine its financial liability under Part A (inpatient care) and Part B

TABLE 26–9 Comparison of Three Cost Allocation Methods

Cost Center	Direct Apportionment	Stepdown	Double Apportionment	Percent Difference (High to Low)
Routine care	$355,462	$360,116	$358,752	1.3
Pharmacy	196,308	194,042	194,544	1.2
Radiology	148,230	145,842	146,704	1.6

TABLE 26–8 Double Apportionment Method

ROUND/CENTER	EMPLOYEE BENEFITS	REPAIRS	LAUNDRY	HOUSEKEEPING	ROUTINE CARE	PHARMACY	RADIOLOGY	TOTAL
Direct costs	$80,000	$40,000	$60,000	$20,000	$250,000	$150,000	$100,000	$700,000
Round 1								
Employee benefits	−80,000	+4,000	+8,000	+4,000	+28,000	+16,000	+20,000	0
	0	$44,000	$68,000	$24,000	$278,000	$166,000	$120,000	$700,000
Repairs	+4,000	−44,000	+6,000	+8,000	+12,000	+8,000	+6,000	0
	$4,000	0	$74,000	$32,000	$290,000	$174,000	$126,000	$700,000
Laundry	+3,364	+3,364	−74,000	+6,727	+40,364	+10,091	+10,090	0
	$7,364	$3,364	0	$38,727	$330,364	$184,091	$136,090	$700,000
Housekeeping	+704	+1,056	+1,761	−38,727	+21,124	+7,041	+7,041	0
	$8,068	$4,420	$1,761	0	$351,488	$191,132	$143,131	$700,000
Round 2								
Employee benefits	−8,068	+403	+807	+403	+2,824	+1,614	+2,017	0
	0	$4,823	$2,568	$403	$354,312	$192,746	$145,148	$700,000
Repairs		−4,823	+723	+965	+1,447	+965	+723	0
		0	$3,291	$1,368	$355,759	$193,711	$145,871	$700,000
Laundry			−3,291	+329	+1,974	+494	+494	0
			0	$1,697	$357,733	$194,205	$146,365	$700,000
Housekeeping				−1,697	+1,019	+339	+339	0
				0	$358,752	$194,544	$146,704	$700,000

(outpatient care). This discussion focuses on how Medicare determines its share of routine and ancillary inpatient costs. On average, Medicare costs based on settled (with or without audit) cost reports are somewhat lower than Medicare costs based on submitted cost reports (Cowles,1991).

Medicare's share of fully allocated routine inpatient costs (e.g., nursing services, room and board, dietary, and minor supplies) is calculated by multiplying total routine costs by the ratio of Medicare inpatient days to total inpatient days. If Medicare patients account for 35% of the days, 35% of routine inpatient costs would be assigned to Medicare patients. Thus, if total routine inpatient costs equal $1.5 million, Medicare's share would be $1,500,000 × 0.35 = $525,000.

Medicare's share of the fully allocated cost of an ancillary service (e.g., radiology or pharmacy) can be calculated in the following two equivalent ways.

$$\text{Department total cost} \times \frac{\text{department charges to Medicare inpatients}}{\text{department total charges}} \tag{1}$$

$$\frac{\text{Department charges to Medicare inpatients}}{} \times \frac{\text{department total costs}}{\text{department total charges}} \tag{2}$$

According to Equation 1, if Medicare inpatients account for 15% of a department's total charges, 15% of the department's total costs would be assigned to Medicare inpatients. Similarly, Equation 2 states that if a department's ratio of total cost/total charges was 0.15, 15% of the department's total charges to Medicare inpatients would be assumed to equal the cost of treating these patients.

Specific Services

If the services an ancillary department renders are relatively homogeneous, the cost of a particular service can be approximated by dividing total departmental cost by the units of service. If, however, the services are heterogeneous, the resultant average cost may differ significantly from the actual cost of a particular service, test, procedure, or patient.

When services are heterogeneous, formal cost accounting techniques or statistical methods could be employed to estimate the cost of certain services. One approach involves the construction of a scale that assigns a relative value to each service. The cost of the average service would be multiplied by a given service's relative value to estimate its cost. Thus, if the typical service cost $20 and the service's relative value was 1.35, the service's cost would be $27.00 ($20 × 1.35 = $27.00).

In 1983, Medicare researchers used stepdown principles to estimate the cost of about 470 diagnosis-related groups (*Note:* DRG costing is analogous to job order costing) (for additional information, see Grimaldi & Micheletti, 1985). Specifically, the cost of treating a Medicare patient assigned to a DRG was calculated by summing the following three items.

- The cost of routine care, found by multiplying the number of days the patient spent in a regular room by the hospital's fully allocated routine cost per day

TABLE 26–10   Cost of Treating a Medicare Patient Assigned to a DRG

SERVICE	CALCULATION	COST
Routine care	$200 × 8	$1600
Special care	$350 × 2	700
Ancillary services		
Radiology	$300 × 0.70	210
Pharmacy	120 × 0.75	90
Laboratory	230 × 1.10	253
Inhalation therapy	100 × 1.40	140
Total		$2993

- The cost of special care (e.g., intensive care), found by multiplying the number of days spent in a special care unit by the hospital's fully allocated special care cost per day
- The cost of ancillary care, found by multiplying the charge for a service by its cost/charge ratio

To illustrate, assume that a patient discharged from Hospital A is assigned to DRG 1. This patient spent 8 days in a regular room (allowable per diem cost of $200) and 2 days in a special care unit (allowable per diem cost of $350) and received four ancillary services with cost/charge ratios ranging from 0.70 to 1.40. (A ratio less than 1 indicates that charges exceed costs; a ratio greater than 1 indicates the opposite.) The cost of treating this patient is $2993, as is shown in Table 26–10. A similar calculation is made for every Medicare patient. If five patients discharged from Hospital A are in this DRG and the estimated costs are $2993, $2248, $3950, $4200, and $3109, the cost per Medicare discharge for DRG 1 would be $3300.

Resource-Based Relative Value Scale (RBRVS)

Starting January 1, 1992, Medicare began to phase in a new payment system for physician services. The core of the new system is a nationally applicable RBRVS developed largely by Harvard researchers. The total resources needed to produce a physician's service are divided into three components: physician work, practice expenses, and malpractice insurance (Grimaldi, 1992; Physician Payment Review Commission).

A relative value has been established for each component of each physician service. Specialty-specific physician panels established a relative value for the physician services within their purview. Specialty by specialty, the work required to render a service was measured in terms of a reference (or standard) service for different specialties. Some work values were established through direct measurement. The rest (most) were established through extrapolation techniques. Statistical methods were employed subsequently to link the relative values of different specialties into a single uniform scale that essentially applies to all physician services. The scale allows the value of one physician service to be expressed in terms of the value of any other physician service.

Physician Work

The RBRVS divides physician work into preservice, intraservice, and postservice components, each of which was measured along the following dimensions.

- Time required to provide a service
- Technical skill and physical effort
- Mental effort and judgment
- Physician stress due to possible iatrogenic risk or complications or both
- Total work

The time dimension is self-explanatory. The next three dimensions capture the complexity and specialty training required for a physician to render a service. Total work is a composite measure of the time and complexity variable. Total work divided by time is the rate of work per unit of time (e.g., minute or hour) or, alternately, the intensity with which a service is rendered. Intensity may increase, decrease, or remain constant as physician work time increases. The direction and rate of change may vary by service or procedure.

Practice Expense

Expenses other than malpractice insurance (e.g., nurse compensation, rent and utilities) that physicians incur in providing patient care form the practice expense component of the RBRVS. Practice expense varies as a proportion of a physician's gross revenue, ranging in 1989 from 23.2% for anesthesiologists to 52.2% for family/general practitioners (Federal Register, 1991).

In general, the relative value of the practice expense for a service (or class of services) was obtained by multiplying the service's 1991 national average prevailing charge by its weighted practice expense percentage. An average charge for 1991 was estimated by updating the 1989 charge for changes in payment rules between 1989 and 1991. The corresponding weighted practice expense percentage was calculated in two steps. First, the proportion of the service rendered by each specialty was determined using Medicare Part B claims data for 1989. Second, the proportion for a specialty was multiplied by the specialty's practice expense percentage, and the products were summed.

To clarify, assume that 25% of a service is furnished by general practitioners, 45% by cardiologists, and 30% by orthopedic surgeons. Further assume that the corresponding practice expense percentages are 43.9, 61.2, and 47.4, respectively. The weighted practice expense percentage would be $52.7 = (25 \times 0.439) + (45 \times 0.612) + (30 \times 0.474)$. If the average charge were $150, the relative value would therefore equal $150 \times 0.527 = $79.05.

Malpractice Insurance

For two reasons, this expense is separated from other practice expenses. First, malpractice insurance varies considerably across specialties, including about 2.7% for internal medicine and 7.4% for orthopedic surgeons (Federal Register, 1991). Second, malpractice insurance may increase significantly in a short time, depending partly on the dollar value of settled claims.

The relative values for malpractice insurance were derived in the same manner as were the values for practice expenses. In other words, 1991 average charges were multiplied by specialty-specific malpractice insurance percentages.

Actual RBRVS

Relative values have been established for roughly 7000 HCPCS/CPT codes. Table 26–11 shows the relative values for selected services and procedures, including a value of 71.78 for a coronary arteries bypass (code 33512). This service, therefore, has a relative value that is almost 72 times higher than the value of the average (or reference) service, which is a level 3 office visit by an established patient (code 99213, relative value = 1.00).

TABLE 26–11 Relative Value Units for Selected Physician Services, 1992

HCPCS CODE[a]	DESCRIPTION	PHYSICIAN WORK	PRACTICE EXPENSE	MALPRACTICE INSURANCE	TOTAL UNITS
General surgery					
44145	Colectomy, partial; with anastomosis, with coloproctostomy (low pelvis anastomosis)	19.11	14.28	3.00	36.39
47600	Cholecystectomy without cholangiography	9.73	7.93	1.67	19.33
49505	Repair inguinal hernia, age 5 years or over	5.08	4.75	0.99	10.82
Cardiology					
33207	Insertion of heart pacemaker	7.67	9.49	1.40	18.56
33405	Replacement of aortic valve	25.84	32.12	5.62	63.58
33512	Coronary arteries bypass	26.41	38.61	6.76	71.78
Radiology					
73120	X-ray examination of hand (global)	0.16	0.57	0.04	0.77
73120	X-ray examination of hand (professional)	0.16	0.07	0.01	0.24
73120	X-ray examination of hand (technical)	0.00	0.50	0.03	0.53
Office or other outpatient, established patient					
99211	Level 1	0.21	0.20	0.02	0.43
99212	Level 2	0.40	0.30	0.02	0.72
99213	Level 3	0.58	0.39	0.03	1.00
99214	Level 4	0.93	0.55	0.04	1.52
99215	Level 5	1.46	0.81	0.07	2.34

[a]CPT HCPCS codes copyright American Medical Association.

TABLE 26–12 RBRVS Fee for Office Visit, Established Patient (Level 4, Code 99214, 1992)

ITEM	CHICAGO		DALLAS		LOS ANGELES	
Relative value units						
Physician work	0.93		0.93		0.93	
Geographic adjustment	× 1.044		× 0.996		× 1.060	
Adjusted value		0.971		0.926		0.986
Practice expense	0.55		0.55		0.55	
Geographic adjustment	× 1.114		× 0.971		× 1.196	
Adjusted value		0.613		0.534		0.658
Malpractice insurance	0.04		0.04		0.04	
Geographic adjustment	× 1.773		× 0.504		× 1.370	
Adjusted value		+0.071		+0.020		+0.055
Total adjusted value		1.655		1.480		1.699
Conversion factor		× $31.001		× $31.001		× $31.001
RBRVS fee[a]		$51.31		$45.88		$52.67

[a]Full fee before any other adjustment, including the 5% reduction for nonparticipating physicians. The example assumes that the full RBRVS fee applies in 1992 rather than the transition fee. In general, the latter is paid when the old and RBRVS fee differ by more than 15%. A blend (or weighted average) of the old and RBRVS fee will be paid until 1996, when the RBRVS fee will take effect.

Geographic Adjustment

The resource-based relative values for physician work, practice expense, and malpractice expense are adjusted for geographic differences between regional and national resource unit costs. Geographic practice costs indexes (GPCIs) have been developed for 240 areas. An index of 1.028 indicates an area that is 2.8% more costly than average; an index of 0.95 indicates an area that is 5% less costly than average.

RBRVS Fee

The relative cost of, or fee for, a service can be found by multiplying the service's relative value by a conversion factor. This factor essentially equals the dollar value of one relative value unit. Medicare's conversion factor for 1992 is $31.001. Table 26–12 shows how to calculate the RBRVS fee for a level 4 office visit by an established patient (code 99214). For the areas shown, the fee ranges from $45.88 to $52.67.

CONCLUSION

An organization's costs can be categorized and analyzed in a variety of ways, depending on the purposes at hand. Ideally, costs are measured accurately and completely. In practice, estimation techniques are inescapable because of the expansiveness of the information and the cost of collecting and sorting it. For these reasons, primary analytic attention is paid to the large proportion of the costs (e.g., 80%) that typically account for a small proportion of total output (e.g., 20%). If the 80% figures are reliable, costs related to 100% of output also are likely to be reliable.

References

American Hospital Association. (1980). *Managerial Cost Accounting*. Chicago: American Hospital Association.

Braganza, K. E. (1988). Cost Finding. In W. O. Cleverly (Ed.), *Handbook of health care accounting and finance* (Chap. 11 and instructions to the latest cost report, HCFA Form 2552-92). Rockville, MD: Aspen.

Cowles, C. M. (1991). Review effect on cost reports: Impact smaller than anticipated. *Health Care Financing Review, 12,* 21–25.

Federal Register. (1991, November 25). *6,* 59568.

Grimaldi, P. L. (1992). *RBRVS: Untangling the web* (Chap. 3). Westchester, IL: Healthcare Financial Management Association.

Grimaldi, P. L., & Micheletti, J. A. (1985). *Prospective payment: The definitive guide to reimbursement* (Chap. 5). Chicago: Pluribus Press.

Physician Payment Review Commission. *Annual Reports 1989, 1990, 1991.* Washington, DC: Author.

Suver, J. D., & Neuman, B. R. (1981). *Management accounting for health care organizations* (Chaps. 2, 6, 7). Oak Brook, IL: Hospital Financial Management Association.

CHAPTER 27

RESOURCE ALLOCATION AND MATERIALS MANAGEMENT: PURCHASE OF SUPPLIES AND MINOR EQUIPMENT AND CAPITAL ACQUISITION PROCESS

KATHRYN J. MCDONAGH

EXECUTIVE SUMMARY

One of the greatest challenges to the nurse manager is to couple clinical knowledge and business acumen to provide the highest possible level of nursing care. This means that the manager must know what dollars are available and what processes are used for equipment purchase and materials management activities. This chapter provides a look at these important areas and provides excellent examples to guide the nurse manager through the processes.

The chapter starts with a glossary of materials management terms, followed by a discussion of the purchasing process. We also see how the relationship between the nurse manager and manager of the materials management department must be carefully cultivated to maintain well-stocked supplies and an efficient replacement system.

The chapter contains samples, such as purchase requisitions, new product evaluation forms, and capital requisition forms, as well as brief, easy to read policies relating to purchasing, capital equipment approval and acquisition, and how to deal with vendors. A review of cost–benefit analysis and some examples of how this is done are provided.

This chapter, along with many others in the handbook, emphasizes the diverse roles required of today's nurse manager. Clearly, one of those roles is understanding how capital expenditures are evaluated and made in an attempt to provide quality nursing care.

T he nurse manager plays a critical role in hospital resource allocation through informed decision making regarding the purchase of supplies and equipment. The increasing financial pressures on hospitals as a result of shrinking reimbursements make the purchase of equipment even more important and worthy of a higher degree of scrutiny than in the past. Prior to the onset of prospective payment under Medicare in 1983, hospitals spent money liberally on new equipment and technologies. The attraction of new technologies and new services proliferated in communities across the country, often resulting in duplication of costly services and a poor return on investment for many hospitals. Regulations resulted, such as state certificate of need laws, that required certain criteria to be fulfilled before purchase of major technologies or construction of new facilities. Today, although new medical discoveries and technologies proliferate, more care is taken by hospitals to conserve scarce resources and purchase equipment in a more prudent and systematic manner. The ideal method for equipment purchasing is to develop a financial strategic plan that is congruent with the hospital's strategic plan and make purchase decisions using a set of criteria reflecting the overall strategic direction of the organization. To avoid haphazard purchasing based simply on physician demands or sales pressure, the development of a strategic plan assists managers in making the most appropriate decisions. Nurse managers should play a key role in the development of that plan and, most importantly, assuring compliance with it.

Other ways to promote systematic and objective purchasing decisions include having policies and processes in place to ensure this. Examples of these types of policies include capital equipment approval and acquisition, contracts, purchases, and agreements, product evaluation, stock supplies, and purchase requisitioning. The materials management department manager typically ensures compliance with these policies so that equitable decisions are made throughout the organization. Nurse managers need to educate themselves on all of these policies and practices, since they may differ from one organization to the next. Nurse managers who are knowledgeable about materials management will be able to provide their patients and staff with the most appropriate clinical and office equipment. The competition for resources that exists internally in hospitals makes it important for the nurse manager to understand acquisition processes and the financial data necessary to support requests.

Major medical equipment companies or vendors are realizing more than ever before the important role that nursing plays in the selection, implementation, and evaluation of new equipment. In fact, these companies are hiring nurses to sell equipment, since they can relate so well to the nurses using the technologies in the clinical setting. These companies often exhibit their wares at nursing conferences, knowing that nurses will have a strong vote in purchase selections. Focus groups are routinely conducted with nurses so that companies can get feedback on existing and new products. As customers, nurses should take advantage of these opportunities to learn more about various products. An important role of any manager is that of steward or guardian of an organization's resources. As consumers or representatives of the hospital consumer, nursing managers should keep in mind the caveat emptor, or let the buyer beware caution. That means it is essential to do your homework before making purchases and not be influenced unduly by strong sales pitches. Taking the responsibility as purchaser and evaluator of equipment for an organization is a serious one that a prudent nurse manager should be well educated and prepared for.

Nurse managers act as patient and nurse advocates and, therefore, need to ensure that patient care can be conducted in a clinical setting that is well equipped and maintained. Having the right equipment and supplies and being able to manage the availability of these items are what materials management is all about. Expertise in this field will enable the nurse manager to provide an environment conducive to excellence in patient care.

DEFINITIONS

This glossary is provided so that nurse managers can become accustomed to terminology commonly used in relation to materials management.

Capital Budget: A plan, expressed in dollars, that contains approved projects expected to provide economic returns and goal accomplishment for an organization. The capital budgeting process includes a series of steps that identify, analyze, and select appropriate capital expenditures (Helfert, 1987).

Capital Expenditure: A commitment of resources that is expected to provide benefits over a reasonably long period of time, at least 2 or more years. There are various ways to classify capital expenditures, such as

- Time period over which the investment occurs
- Types of resources invested
- Dollar amount of capital expenditure
- Type of benefits received (Cleverley, 1986).

Cost–Benefit Analysis: A process of evaluating the attractiveness of an investment that includes examination of the amount invested, the potential benefits (both financial and other), the economic life of the investment, and the risks associated with the investment decision.

Depreciation: An accounting allowance made in recognition of the decrease or loss in value of property or capital expenditures over time due to wear, age, or technologic obsolescence.

Inventory Management/Control: The process of having the necessary equipment and supplies available at the appropriate time. This requires knowledge of demand cycles and peaks in order to minimize costs of storage or stock out costs. Developing a par level system for items commonly used and in need of replenishment is one way to manage inventory.

Minor Equipment: Items that are relatively small in size and cost, available in large quantities, and usually have a maximum useful life of 3 years. Minor equipment items are requested and used by various departments in the organization.

Product Evaluation Committee: A multidisciplinary group of staff (including clinical, engineering, financial) working collaboratively to identify, implement, and evaluate current and new products in the hospital. This group's written analyses and recommendations are used for purchasing decisions.

Purchase Requisition: A systematic process for ordering equipment and items, which includes a standardized form that requires appropriate signatures for approval of a purchase. A purchase order number for each request is used as a means of tracking the requests, prices, item descriptions, and other necessary information.

PURCHASE OF SUPPLIES AND MINOR EQUIPMENT

Hospitals typically have a written policy describing the internal process required for ordering supplies and equipment. A sample purchasing policy is shown in Appendix 27–A. Standardized forms, called requisitions, are used to ensure control over the process. Financial and managerial control is important, since the materials management department acts as a central clearinghouse for large quantities of equipment and inventory in the hospital. This can represent substantial dollars for the hospital. In fact, internal auditing processes often are established related to purchasing because of the significant financial impact to an organization. These audits help prevent loss from lack of controls or possible fraudulent behaviors.

Purchase requisitions require authorized signatures from the requesting manager and an appropriate administrator. This check and balance is an example of managerial control of the system. The authorizing signatures are validating that funds have been allocated in the budget for this purchase and that the item is being evaluated and ordered appropriately. Further substantiation of the order then occurs in materials management to prevent any inappropriate purchasing.

A purchase order number is originated in the materials management department as a means of tracking each requisition. Most requisition systems are computerized now, so that tracking of such essential information as item description, price, and cost center allocation is relatively simple. A sample purchase requisition is shown in Figure 27–1.

STOCK SUPPLIES

Nursing departments usually have supplies that are used frequently and in large quantities. This includes many paper and office supplies, forms for medical records, and bandages, catheters, bedpans, needles, and other commonly used items. These routine items are stocked in the department and are replaced on a periodic basis.

A unit clerk or secretary is usually responsible for monitoring stock levels and ordering items as needed to prevent depletion of stock items, which is known as stock out. Stock out can be costly, since it may result in emergency orders and extra trips to the materials management area and may compromise patient care or result in hoarding of stock supplies by staff. If staff members fear depletion of certain critical items, they may begin hoarding stock, which can result in high inventory or storage costs.

PAR LEVEL SYSTEMS

One method to prevent erratic inventory levels for commonly used items is to develop a par level system for stock supplies in each department. This process begins with a meeting between the nurse manager and the materials management manager. They negotiate the quantity needed for each item in that department. Quantities may vary from department to department based on the patient population and needs of the department. The types of stock items also varies between departments. For instance, a surgical unit will need more suture removal kits than a cardiology unit, which needs various telemetry supplies.

Purchase Order No._____

SAMPLE PURCHASE REQUISITION

Department_____ Depart.Deliver To_____ Cost Center_____ Date_____ 19____

USE THIS REQUISITION TO ORDER ITEMS NOT LISTED IN STOCK

Quantity	Unit	Catalog Number		Unit Price	Total
Requested by:	Approved by:		Order Placed With:	Total:	
	Administrator				
Approved by:	Ordered From:		Delivery Time:		
Dept. Head	To be filled in by Materials Management Department				

Figure 27–1 Sample purchase requisition. (Courtesy of St. Joseph's Hospital, Atlanta, GA.)

Once the par levels are agreed on, the materials management department replenishes the stock supplies on a daily or weekly basis. The items used are replenished back up to the par level to maintain a consistent inventory level. Records are maintained on use of all items so that the par levels can be changed if necessary. This prevents aging of underused stock items or stock out of frequently used items. In addition to monitoring the par level records, the nurse manager should periodically discuss stock items with the staff nurses so their concerns about stock levels or ideas about new stock items can be considered.

COMPANY REPRESENTATIVES

Most hospitals have guidelines for the activities of company representatives or vendor salespersons in order to promote fairness and ethical standards in the purchasing process. If vendor sales representatives were allowed to talk to and show products to hospital staff at any time, this could result in excessive sales pressure and circumvention of established approval channels, such as product evaluation committees. When company representatives are in contact with personnel other than materials management and key staff members, negotiation of prices also may be difficult. Usually, price negotiation for products is handled by materials management staff, who are knowledgeable about competitive pricing, warranty contracts, and negotiation strategies. A sample hospital policy delineating guidelines for company representatives is shown in Appendix 27–A.

COLLABORATING WITH MATERIALS MANAGEMENT

It is imperative for nurse managers to develop effective working relationships with the materials management manager and staff to maximize the benefits that result from good purchase decisions and efficient inventory control. Too often in hospitals, the relationship between materials management staff and nursing staff are adversarial, primarily due to a lack of structure or opportunity to collaborate. A nurse manager should invite the manager of materials management to the clinical area to help educate the manager about clinical operations and the need for appropriate equipment to facilitate good patient care. Then, the nurse manager should ask to be invited to the storeroom or warehouse so that he or she can understand the operations of materials management and the pressures that can result from so many hospital departments requesting items all at once and often Stat. Working together with materials management can promote collaboration and improved nursing input on the purchasing process.

ROLE OF THE NURSE MANAGER ON PRODUCT EVALUATION COMMITTEE

A product evaluation committee is a multidisciplinary group in the hospital responsible for evaluating and selecting new products for use. Members usually include representatives from materials management, nursing, medicine, biomedical engineering, engineering, and education. Departments that use high volumes of equipment, such as surgery, IV therapy, cardiac catheterization laboratories, and central supplies, should have representatives as well. This diversity of membership provides the necessary perspectives that pull together the technology and tools of the trade with the human caregiving provided in hospitals (McConnell, 1991).

The product evaluation committee solicits input from staff throughout the hospital on the need for certain products and equipment. Research is done into the various vendors for products, and presentations or demonstrations may be done for the committee. Once several brands of equipment are selected for review, the committee decides what departments or areas should act as pilot demonstration units for the purpose of conducting trials and evaluating new equipment. Pilot units may be selected because the staff have expressed an interest in conducting a specific product review or because it is the most appropriate department for the application of a new product. Care should be given to the rotation of nursing areas for product evaluation so that all nurses feel that they have a voice in the selection of the equipment they are asked to use.

A time period for an evaluation is established by the committee, and a written evaluation process is undertaken. Figure 27–2 is an example of a new product evaluation form to be completed by staff members who try the new products. The nurse manager may need to encourage staff nurses to take the time to

NEW PRODUCT EVALUATION FORM

Date_____

Reason for Evaluation

(1) New Product ◯
(2) Improved Product ◯
(3) Re-evaluation of Product in use ◯
(4) Replacement of existing product ◯
(5) Special Request ◯

Criteria for Evaluation

(1) Does this product have a sterility guarantee?   Yes___ No___ N/A____ (not applicable)
(2) Does this product have a warranty period?   Yes___ No___
   If yes, how long? _____
(3) Can this product be used in other departments?   Yes___ No___
(4) Is product and/or service available locally?   Yes___ No___
(5) Audiovisual and/or inservice equipment available?   Yes___ No___

Product Identification

Brand _____   Name of Product _____

Approximate Cost _____ (+/-)

Instructions

Please complete this form after using the listed product having had an opportunity to evaluate thoroughly and become familiar with its use.

(1) Does product offer
   (a) Easier Procedure   Yes___ No___ N/A___ Same___
   (b) Safer Procedure   Yes___ No___ N/A___ Same___
   (c) Better Patient Care   Yes___ No___ N/A___

(2) Do you like the packaging?   Yes___ No___ N/A___

(3) Is this product easy to open?   Yes___ No___ N/A___

(4) Does product store easily? (i.e., on supply carts)   Yes___ No___ N/A___

(5) Is equipment designed or arranged in an easy-to-use fashion?   Yes___ No___ N/A___

(6) Are directions for use clear and understandable?   Yes___ No___

(7) Does the product perform as indicated in the directions?   Yes___ No___

(8) Is it easier to use than the product we are now using?   Yes___ No___

Why?_____

(9) Would you like to use this product in the future?   Yes___ No___

Why?_____

(10) Is there a similar product you would like the hospital to evaluate?_____

_____

(11) Comments_____

_____

Thank you for your cooperation in evaluation of this product.

_____   _____

Signature   Department

Please return this form to your department head by_____

Figure 27–2 New product evaluation form. (Courtesy of St. Joseph's Hospital, Atlanta, GA.)

complete the form so that the best decisions can be made. The product evaluation committee then compiles and analyzes the data from the study period and makes a decision. The committee coordinates educational programs so that the staff can learn about new equipment and its use. This committee structure provides an effective liaison with materials management and provides ample opportunity for input on purchase selections from nurses, physicians, clinical managers, and others using the products or equipment. This exemplifies the strength and effectiveness of shared governance in the complex health care arena and how shared decision making can result in the most cost-effective and beneficial decisions for patient care and user satisfaction (McDonagh, 1990). It is essential that nurse managers take an active role in the product evaluation committee. If such a committee does not exist in the organization, it would be advantageous to initiate the development of this collaborative effort (Satwicz, Treston-Aurand, & Zangara, 1991).

To ensure appropriate levels of nursing input into the product evaluation process, another alternative is to have a nurse assume the role of the products nurse specialist (Stahler-Wilson & Worman, 1991). This products nurse specialist is responsible for coordinating all evaluation, education, and problem resolution with products in the clinical setting. She or he works closely with the hospital product evaluation committee. Whatever strategies are undertaken, it is essential to link the use and purchase of health care technology with the nursing practitioners providing the patient care.

CAPITAL ACQUISITION PROCESS

A major challenge facing health care organizations is a rapidly escalating demand for services combined with increasing public scrutiny of the costs associated with health care. This increasing demand, brought on by an aging population with chronic illnesses and an increasing indigent population and societal trends, coupled with shrinking capital funds creates the need for a thorough, objective, and systematic process for acquiring capital items.

Hospitals, in particular, since they are large purchasers of capital items, will need to make more efficient use of available capital (Sadock, 1990). This includes assessing future capital needs based on the strategic plan of the organization. Capital investments represent long-term commitments that are congruent with the organizational strategy and make the provision of goods and services to customers possible (Helfert, 1987). Capital expenditures are differentiated in the budget from operational spending because of the long-term time frame associated with them.

Capital acquisitions may include land, buildings, facilities, or equipment that result in future economic gain for the organization. Like other major investments, there is a need for management to evaluate the effectiveness of capital purchases continually in light of economic conditions, financial status, and the competitive position of the organization.

Capital acquisition budgets usually are projected 3 years into the future. The type and quantity of capital allocation planning depends on the nature of the services provided, past purchase practices, and the necessary cash flow to allow capital acquisitions.

The capital acquisition process is a part of the organization's overall financial strategy and is complex in hospitals because of the many regulations controlling health care expenditures, such as Medicare capital reimbursement regulations, and because of the many individuals and groups involved in the process.

Hospital Policy and the Nurse Manager

Nurse managers, as one of the interested constituencies in the hospital capital acquisition process, should become educated about what capital expenditure planning is and, specifically, how the hospital undertakes this process. When making capital requests, nurse managers need to thoroughly analyze and justify the necessity for expenditure. They should provide detailed explanations of

- Benefits of the purchase
- Cost of the implementation or change
- Long-term effects of the project

Appendix 27–A contains a sample hospital policy on capital equipment approval and acquisition. This policy describes the multidisciplinary process that is used in capital acquisition planning in most hospitals. Figures 27–3 and 27–4 are samples of capital requisition forms commonly used by department managers.

The TEAM Method

Another way of analyzing capital purchases is the use of the TEAM method. This stands for technology, evaluation, and acquisition methods for hospitals (American Hospital Association, 1979). This approach includes a comprehensive and systematic set of procedures and guidelines to assist hospitals in the task of assessing technology. Assessing and evaluating capital items and technology in health care is complex and multifaceted. Therefore, this process includes clinical, financial, engineering, and maintenance considerations. Study of this process has been helpful in developing the multidisciplinary framework for capital decision making that would work best in each organization.

Just as the multidisciplinary approach to the product evaluation committee was so fundamental to its success, the same is true for capital acquisition planning. Capital planning represents a major financial process, and if left to the financial staff only, it would exclude the critical input of nurses, physicians, engineers, and others. Therefore, a systematic process needs to be established so that appropriate input for the long-term financial success of the organization is obtained.

COST–BENEFIT ANALYSIS

An important component of any purchase decision, whether it be major capital items or supplies and equipment, is the translation of the value of that purchase into economic or financial terms. Cost–benefit analysis provides a means of

CAPITAL REQUEST FORM (CRF-1)

Category of Request

___ 1. Medical Equipment   ___ 3. Information Systems & Telecommunications

___ 2. Construction/Renovation   ___ 4. All Other   Furniture

==

Department Information

Dept Name _____ Cost Center _____ Date _____ Req By _____

Phone # _____ Dept Dir/Mgr Approval _____ Amt Budgeted _____ if unbudgeted, list

funding _____

Justification _____

_____

_____ Date needed_____

Alternative approaches considered _____

_____

_____

Attach program evaluation (if required).

==

All Capital Equipment Requests

Equipment description/supplier _____

Quantity _____ Estimated Cost _____

Equipment description/supplier _____

Quantity _____ Estimated Cost _____

Annual supply cost _____ Annual maintenance cost _____

Cost savings/revenue enhancement: give explanation/estimate _____

_____

Materials Management review/date _____

==

All Software/Computer/Telecommunication Requests

Expectations of system/equip (ie, financial, operation, etc._____

_____

_____

Data processing review/date _____ Estimated cost _____

CAPITAL REQUEST FORM (CRF-1)

Figure 27–3 Capital request form (under $100,000). (Courtesy of St. Joseph's Hospital, Atlanta, GA.)

Capital Request Form (CRF 1)
Page 2

Facility Improvement/Capital Equipment Requests

Description of work _____

_____

_____

_____

Plant oper review/date _____ Est By _____ Est Cost _____

Actual $_____ Completed _____ Date _____

(required)

===

Purchasing Use Only

Director _____ Date _____ Buyer_____

Vice Pres _____ Date _____ Date Ordered _____

C.F.O. _____ Date _____ P.O.# _____

Capital asset# _____
Project # _____

Figure 27–3 Continued

describing the cost and benefits of an item in relation to cash inflows and outflows. "In essence, capital is invested for one basic reason: to obtain sufficient future economic returns to warrant the original outlay, that is sufficient cash receipts over the life of the project to justify the cash spent. Analytical methods should take into account in one way or another, this basic trade-off of current cash outflow against future cash inflow" (Helfert, 1987, p. 201). Nurse managers should be prepared to understand, discuss, and develop reports that include cost–benefit analysis for purchase decisions.

There are several ways to analyze an investment. However, three essential elements should be included in the analysis (Helfert, 1987).

- Net investment, or the amount expended
- Operating cash flows, or the potential benefits
- Economic life, or the time period over which the investment will provide benefits

Some of the methods of analyses that the nurse manager needs to be cognizant of include

- The payback method

Capital Request Form Over $100,000 (CRF-2)

Cost Center:_____ Department Name:_____

1. Name of new or expanded program: _____
2. Hospital strategy or goal: _____
3. Description of the new or expanded program:_____
   _____
   _____

==

I. Costs

A. Estimate cost of equipment including shipping $_____

B. Estimated cost of installation, building modification (attach details) $_____
   Source/Approval _____

C. Depreciable life of project (years) _____

D. Equipment to be replaced:
   1. Description _____
      _____
      _____
   2. Fixed asset number_____
   3. Assigned useful life _____
   4. Present age _____
   5. Current book value $ _____
   6. Current market value $ _____

E. Associated Increase/Decrease in Expense

	Yr 1	Yr 2	Yr 3	Yr 4	Yr 5
Training					
Labor					
Utilities					
Supplies					
Other					
Totals					

==

Additional review and input from the Finance Division may be appropriate, ie. Medical reimbursement, impatient and outpatient mix, etc.

Figure 27–4 Capital request form (over $100,000). (Courtesy of St. Joseph's Hospital, Atlanta, GA.)

Capital Request Form Over $100,000 (CRF-2)
Page 2

Other review criteria to be incorporated and considered may be:
-Support of EMHS contracts
-Service Contracts
-Trade in allowances
-Mercy Philosophy Support
-Fixed asset control
-Scheduled receipt dates

	New Clinical	**Replacement Clinical**	**New Nonclinical**	**Replacement Nonclinical**
II.	☐	☐	☐	☐

III.   New Revenue _____

New Payroll Expenses _____

New Supply Expenses _____

IV.   Check List: Signatures Required

A. Engineering Review _____

B. Biomedical Engineering Review _____

C. Purchasing Review _____

D. Assistant Vice President Signature _____

E. Vice President Signature _____

Figure 27–4   Continued

- Net present value
- Minimum required revenue per procedure
- Internal rate of return or yield

Consideration needs to be given to financing alternatives as well. This may include a comparison of the benefits of a cash purchase, loan, or leasing options.

Since capital expenditures have an impact over a number of years, risk analysis and projections about future considerations need to be made as well in the cost–benefit analysis. A variety of financial methods of sensitivity or risk analysis can assist in these projections for the future. It is a function of management to periodically evaluate decisions made based on certain assumptions that were made at the time of purchase, so the supporting documentation needs to be saved to compare what actually happened to what was projected. This is a way of measuring the quality of management investment decision making.

CASE STUDIES

Two examples of multidisciplinary cost–benefit analysis for major capital expenditures were recently completed at Saint Joseph's Hospital of Atlanta. One project was the study and evaluation of a needleless system to reduce needlestick injuries of staff (Dugger, 1992). The other was the comparative analysis of intravenous infusion pumps for purchase (Saint Joseph's Hospital of Atlanta Report, 1992). Common characteristics of both of these case study projects include

- Problem identified
- Multidisciplinary group assembled
- Strong nursing and clinical input
- Cost–benefit analysis completed
- Pilot unit/product trials conducted
- Written documentation of analysis and trials compiled
- Research conducted (data collection, interviews, literature review)
- Decision made by the multidisciplinary group

This process proved to be successful in both of these case studies. The purchase of the needleless system resulted in a dramatic reduction of staff needlesticks. The purchase of the new intravenous infusion pumps proved to be the most cost-effective choice, and early indications show that staff satisfaction and quality improvement are positive. Since so much staff involvement occurred in the process, both decisions have been well accepted in the hospital. This team approach has been a true success story as a responsible method of making prudent investment decisions for the hospital.

CONCLUSION

The nurse manager is in a pivotal role in the hospital to combine clinical expertise with financial and business skills to make effective decisions related to resource allocation and materials management. Since nursing has such a central coordinative function for patient care in hospitals, it is appropriate for nursing managers to promote high-quality patient care through the provision of safe, effective equipment and technology.

References

American Hospital Association. (1979). Technology evaluation and acquisition methods for hospitals. Chicago: Author.

Cleverley, W. O. (1986). *Essentials of healthcare finance* (2nd ed.). Rockville, MD: Aspen.

Dugger, B. (1992). Saint Joseph's Hospital of Atlanta study on use of needleless system to reduce needlestick injuries of staff (unpublished).

Helfert, E. A. (1987). *Techniques of financial analysis* (3rd ed.). Homewood, IL: Richard D. Irwin.

Herkimer, A. G., Jr. (1988). *Understanding healthcare budgeting*. Rockville, MD: Aspen.

Hibbs, C. W. (1987, November–December). Taking charge of high tech equipment purchases. *Journal of Healthcare Materiel Management*, pp. 42–46.

McConnell, E. A. (1991, November). Key issues in device use in nursing practice. *Nursing Management, 22*(11), 32–33.

McDonagh, K. J. (Ed.). (1990). *Nursing shared governance: Restructuring for the future*. Atlanta: K J McDonagh & Associates.

Sadock, J. M. (1990, November). Capital equipment acquisition: Coping with the present and planning for the future. *Hospital Materiel Management Quarterly, 12*(2), 37–40.

Saint Joseph's Hospital of Atlanta Report. (1992, February). Infusion pump proposal (unpublished).

Satwicz, M. J., Treston-Aurand, J., & Zangara, A. (1991). Nursing and product selection = quality care. *Nursing Management, 22*(11), 30–31.

Stahler-Wilson, J. E., & Worman, F. E. (1991). Products nurse specialist: The compleat clinical shopper. *Nursing Management, 22*(11), 36–38.

Sample Hospital Purchasing Policy

PURCHASING REQUISITIONING

Every hospital purchase requires a completed purchase requisition prior to issue of a purchase order.

Procedure

1. Purchase requisitions will be processed on a daily basis with emergency requisitions receiving priority.
2. Requisitions will be processed in the following manner.
    a. Authorized signature: All requisitions will be approved by department managers who have been authorized in writing to purchase by the appropriate administrator.
    b. Requisitions are to be typed or printed and completely filled out before submission to the purchasing department or other specified department. One copy of each requisition will be returned to the requesting department with the addition of the following information: purchase order number, anticipated delivery date, revised price information, if applicable.
    c. The director of purchasing is responsible for procuring the requested items.
    d. Upon receiving the ordered items, the receipt will be signed by the authorized purchasing department representative.
3. A purchase requisition must be cosigned by the appropriate administrator before its submission to the purchasing department when it contains a single unit cost greater than $500 or an aggregate cost exceeding $2000. Amounts greater than $2000, but less than $15,000 must be approved by the appropriate vice president. Amounts greater than $50,000 require authorization by the president/CEO.
4. Purchase requisitions for capital equipment must be clearly marked as such, specify the month for which the purchase was approved by the capital equipment committee, and be signed by the appropriate administrator.
5. All equipment (regardless of cost) that needs installation must be coordinated with the engineering department prior to submission of the purchase request, which should also contain an estimate of the installation cost.

COMPANY REPRESENTATIVES

It is the responsibility of the purchasing department to direct the search for sources of supplies and equipment.

Procedure

To achieve equal opportunity in the hospital for every potential company (vendor) representative, the following regulations must be followed by all vendor representatives and hospital personnel.

1. The purchasing department has the following hours set up for vendor representative calls and interviews on a first-come, first-served basis.
   Tuesday–Thursday: 9:00 AM–Noon
   1:00 PM–3:00 PM
2. All vendors are required to report first to the purchasing department, sign in on the vendor log, and be issued an identification tag, which is to be worn at all times while in the hospital. If the vendor needs to call on a department head, he or she is to be cleared through the purchasing department, at which time the department head will be contacted for the interview.
   Anyone found violating this policy will have all privileges for interviews cancelled, and the company represented will be contacted. This applies to all vendors, excluding pharmaceutical salesmen and food representatives only.
3. Any vendor going directly to a department without clearing through the purchasing department should be directed to do so before seeing hospital personnel. Purchasing should be informed that an unauthorized vendor is in the department. This person can be identified by the absence of an identification badge or an incorrect date on a badge.
4. All orders for merchandise and equipment must have a purchase order number assigned to them before shipment. All purchase orders must be filled out completely, showing quantity, description, and price.
   Any price changes that occur before shipment is made must be forwarded to the purchasing department so these changes can be recorded on the purchase order before the invoice is received. All merchandise and equipment received must have the purchase order number clearly displayed on the outside packaging.
5. Emergency orders needed when the purchasing department is closed will require a purchase order number from this office on the next working day after the item is ordered.
6. Vendor representatives may not show and detail any new product to hospital employees without the proper approval of the appropriate department head or purchasing department. At the request of the department head, these products may be referred to the product evaluation and standardization committee for review and evaluation.
7. Vendor representatives will not contact the physician on the hospital staff in the name of the hospital unless previously approved by the purchasing department.
8. Vendor representatives are asked not to make a sales call on the physicians within the hospital unless at the personal request of that physician. Sales calls should be made at the physician's office.

Any vendor representative who refuses to operate under these approved guidelines will forfeit any visiting privileges and potential sales resulting from these efforts.

CAPITAL EQUIPMENT APPROVAL AND ACQUISITION

Policy: To provide a process for the approval and acquisition of capital equipment.

Procedure

1. **General:** Capital items consist of renovations or equipment valued at $500 or more. Equipment is classified as follows. Categories of request
   a. Medical equipment and patient care items
   b. Information systems and telecommunications
   c. Renovations/construction projects; furniture
   d. All other
      Note: In all cases, capital requests will delineate if the equipment is for an existing program or if it is intended to support a new clinical program or business venture. Program evaluation for new programs will be conducted in accordance with hospital criteria.
   On an annual basis, four working groups will be assigned to assist in prioritizing and making recommendations to administration on all capital equipment items. Each working group will be assigned to review equipment in one of the four categories of request as indicated above.
2. **Capital budget requests:** All capital items, included in the annual budget process, are reviewed by the hospital staff and the medical director, or the appropriate department chairman or section chief. The president/CEO approves all items for inclusion in the capital budget. In addition to this approval process, the finance committee reviews and approves all capital expenditures in excess of $500,000, and the board of directors will be asked to approve line items in the capital budget in excess of the following dollar amounts.
   a. New equipment in excess of $250,000
   b. Replacement equipment in excess of $500,000
   c. Renovations in excess of $500,000
3. **Capital budget requests under $100,000:** All requests for capital expenditure will require a completed and approved capital request form (CRF).
   a. When initiating a capital request (medical equipment, information systems/telecommunications, construction/renovation/furniture, or other), the requesting department will be required to complete the appropriate section(s) of the capital request form. If additional space is needed for explanation or justification, additional pages should be attached to the CRF.
   b. On completion of the department section, the initiating department should forward the CRF to the director of materials management. If additional reviews are required (i.e., capital request that requires a plant modification), the director of materials management will be responsible for for-

warding the CRF to the subsequent review area and tracking the status of the request.

c. On completion of review for costs estimates, the completed capital request form will be reviewed by the appropriate work group. Notification of approval or disapproval will be provided once the budget process is complete.

4. **Capital budget requests over $100,000:** In addition to requirements outlined in paragraphs 2 and 3 above, capital requests in excess of $100,000 will require a completed value analysis. The requesting department will be responsible for completing the value analysis.

5. **Acquisition of capital equipment:** Once the capital budget is approved for the fiscal year, a hospital capital committee will be convened on a quarterly basis in order to approve acquisition of capital equipment and monitor progress of ongoing renovations. The committee will prioritize requests and approve the timing of equipment acquisition. The capital committee will consist of the president/CEO, vice president for patient services, chief financial officer, chief of medical staff, as well as other medical staff representation.

6. **Request for nonbudgeted or emergency capital items:** A capital contingency fund is established for equipment needs that are unforeseen during the budget preparation process or that represent opportunities for new business ventures. Assistant vice presidents have discretionary authority up to $5000 to approve emergency replacement capital items. Emergency requests beyond $5000 require the approval of the appropriate vice president as well as the president/CEO. Nonbudgeted expenditures for capital equipment or renovation in excess of $100,000 require the approval of the board of directors.

7. **Reporting:** The president/CEO will provide the board of directors with a report on capital expenditures on a quarterly basis.

CHAPTER 28

CONTROLLING DRUG DISTRIBUTION AND ABUSE

JANE ENGLEBRIGHT POLLOCK

EXECUTIVE SUMMARY

The control and distribution of medication are functions shared by nurses, physicians, and pharmacists. As a part of this function, nurse managers are called on to help design, monitor, and improve distribution systems and to be alert for signs of abuse among the nursing staff. This chapter provides an excellent review of drug distribution systems, discusses techniques for monitoring medication distribution and substance abuse, and looks at the harrowing issue of drug abuse by nurses.

There is an initial review of four types of medication distribution systems: routine, used for inpatient settings, floor stock for procedural areas, such as emergency rooms, and emergency and narcotic systems, variations of the floor stock method. The chapter then moves into a discussion of substance abuse. This discussion ranges from ignoring the problem to prevention and early detection, are discussed as methods of dealing with this critical situation.

Excellent, step-by-step guidelines are provided for stress reduction as a means of reducing substance abuse, how to monitor narcotic use, and how to do a substance abuse investigation.

This chapter offers information that can lead to a well-designed and well-monitored medication distribution system. Such a system can provide patients with the timely and accurate delivery of needed medication. The same system can also limit the devastating problem of substance abuse in the nursing profession.

T he nurse manager is accountable for the quality of care delivered to patients within his or her assigned area of responsibility, including the accurate and timely administration of medication. Designing or redesigning distribution systems, monitoring the effectiveness of distribution systems, recognizing the need for improvement, and dealing with abuse of the system are responsibilities the nurse manager shares with the pharmacy manager and physicians. Medication distribution and administration are interdisciplinary and highly integrated functions that cannot be undertaken in isolation.

Several regulatory agencies set standards for medication distribution, including Medicare, the Joint Commission on Accreditation of Healthcare Organizations, and state laws regarding controlled substances. Abuse of medications involves state licensing bodies, professional standards of ethics, and human resource policies.

EVALUATING MEDICATION DISTRIBUTION SYSTEMS

Medication distribution systems are established early in the life of an organization. They tend to be replicated in new areas as the organization grows. In many work redesign strategies, medication distribution systems are being analyzed and reorganized to create more efficient and more patient-focused care delivery.

Medication distribution systems are highly integrated functions. Improvements in the process must be undertaken within a multidisciplinary work group. Although nursing and pharmacy are the primary departments involved, physicians are also vitally interested in the effectiveness and responsiveness of the medication distribution system.

Ancillary departments also may be affected. Information systems may be intimately involved in computer program changes and charting form changes. Respiratory therapy, physical therapy, anesthesia, and other departments that order medications from the pharmacy may be affected by changes made for the benefit of the inpatient unit. Long-term success of the changes made depends on identifying the people affected by the change and including them in the change process.

The primary function of all medication distribution systems is to deliver medications to patients accurately, rapidly, and with minimal consumption of resources. Patients are the ultimate consumer of the medication distribution system. Physicians and nurses are intermediate consumers, and pharmacists are the suppliers.

Patients require a medication system that is free from errors and timely. Patients would like a system that allows for customization in response to individual preferences. For example, some patients may want bedtime medications at 8 PM, whereas others consider 10 PM bedtime. Patients also would like a medication system that prepares them or their caregiver for self-medication after discharge.

Physicians are concerned with accuracy and timeliness. Some medications are administered by a physician, usually during a procedure. Physicians do not want to wait for anesthetics or other agents to be delivered. They have a duty to monitor the effects of the medications they prescribe. To do this, they need to be able to review the medication administration schedule of their patients, compare the information to other data, such as laboratory results and vital sign records, and make treatment decisions. Easy access to this information is important to physicians seeking to monitor their patient's progress in a timely manner.

Nurses require a system that meets the needs of the patient efficiently. Nurses desire a system that prevents errors, facilitates patient education, and makes efficient use of the time and talents of the nursing staff.

Pharmacists require a system that complies with regulatory requirements, allows for tight inventory control, and prevents lost revenue. Pharmacists also are concerned with using the time and talents of the pharmacy staff in an efficient manner.

TYPES OF MEDICATION DISTRIBUTION SYSTEMS

Medications are generally distributed through four different types of systems: routine, floor stock, emergency, and narcotic. Most nursing departments use all four types of medication distribution systems. The predominant system, however, varies with the type of patient care delivered in the department. Inpatient units deliver most of the patient medications through the routine system. Procedural areas, such as the emergency department, deliver most of their medications through the floor stock system.

Problems with medication distribution systems usually include problems with communication, timing (Stevens, 1985), or resource consumption. Frequently, nursing, pharmacy, and medicine spend a great deal of time blaming each other for the failure of a system. Flow diagrams are a useful technique for refocussing attention on analysis of the system and identification of opportunities to improve the system (Stevens, 1985). Figure 28–1 is an example of the process of refilling nonnarcotic p.r.n. medications at one institution.

Automation is gradually entering medication distribution systems. Total parenteral nutrition (TPN) admixture machines, automated stock drug and narcotic lockers, and computerized medication administration records are a few examples. Introduction of these technologies presents a wonderful opportunity to evaluate the system and improve both quality and cost. The introduction of technology must be considered within the framework of the entire medication distribution system. Isolated changes in a highly integrated system can create havoc for other users.

Routine Distribution System

The routine distribution system is usually established by the pharmacy. Nursing input revolves around order entry processes, documentation systems, refill and reorder procedures, and standard administration times.

Self-medication programs are an emerging form of medication administration. Self-medication programs usually are designed and administered by the nursing staff. Patient selection, patient/family education, and training and monitoring of medication administration are key components of a self-medication system (Platts, 1989). The distribution system is shifted from the central nurses' station to the patient room. Self-medication programs present a challenge to most distribution systems, but the clinical advantages for the patient make them worth the struggle.

Floor Stock Distribution System

Floor stock systems provide ready access to urgently needed medications. They are crucial to the functioning of many departments. They also pose a logistical challenge for upkeep and financial control.

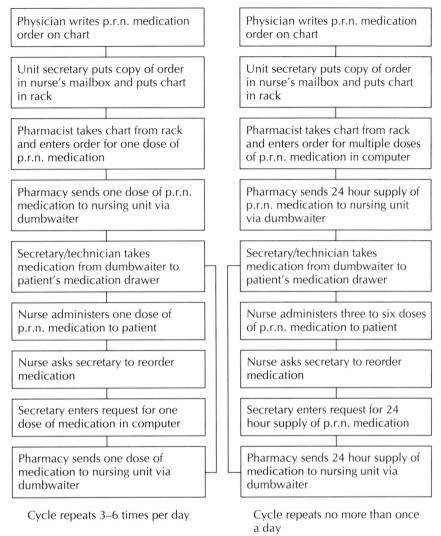

Cycle repeats 3–6 times per day   Cycle repeats no more than once a day

Figure 28–1   Example of flow chart analysis of medication distribution.

The types of medications and numbers of medications included in a floor stock system should be established by physicians, nurses, and pharmacists working in the department. The medications included in the floor stock system should be unique to each nursing department. When developing the contents list, the group should consider the historical use of specific medications by the department, the timeliness of delivery from the main pharmacy on the night shift, and the cost of the medications. Infrequently used medications would not be included on the list if pharmacy delivery times for emergency medications are acceptable on the night shift. Very expensive medications would not be included unless charging mechanisms ensure that each medication will be charged properly.

Floor stock should be labeled or tagged in such a way that charging the medication generates a refill request for the pharmacy. In addition to the automatic refill system, floor stock systems need to be counted or inventoried on a regular basis—daily in high use areas. Missing medications are replaced at this time, and uncharged items usually are charged to the nursing department. The inventory can be conducted by nursing or pharmacy personnel. Expiration dates are checked during the inventory process, and expired medications are replaced. The nurse manager should review the list of medications replaced due to expiration annually. The manager should consider reducing the inventory of medications that are expiring in the floor stock system.

Charging systems are critical to the financial viability of the floor stock system. Tags, stickers, and bar codes are all systems that can work. The key is to make the system convenient to the nurse users and to ensure that the nurses understand their responsibility for charging for the medications. Automated floor stock systems provide an exciting alternative. These machines provide accurate inventory and timely patient billing and reduce nursing and pharmacy staff time spent in inventory control, billing, and tracking lost charges.

Floor stock also should contain medications for staff use. Pain medications, decongestants/antihistamines, and antacids frequently are stocked for employee use. Convenient access to such medications removes the temptation to borrow from patient supplies.

Emergency Distribution System

Emergency distribution systems are a specific type of floor stock system. The contents of the emergency medication system are determined by physicians, nurses, and pharmacists. The group should consider the historical use of medications in emergency situations and the medications used in emergency treatment protocols for the institution. The contents of the emergency medication system should be standard for each department to allow staff to participate in emergency treatment in any area of the institution.

Emergency medication systems should include premixed, ready to administer medications whenever possible. The emergency medication supply should be sealed and dated with the first expiration date of the medications inside. The emergency medication supply should be used only in a patient emergency. The integrity of the system should not be broken for special procedures or nonemergency care. If this is occurring, consider revising the floor stock system to include the items that are being used from the emergency medication supply.

The integrity of the emergency medication supply should be checked each shift and documented. Each new nurse should be oriented to the emergency medication system for the department. In departments where the emergency medication system is rarely used, periodic review of the system in staff meetings or inservices is desirable.

Narcotic Supply System

Narcotic supply systems are another variation of floor stock systems. The contents of the narcotic supply system should be determined by physicians, nurses, and pharmacists. The group should consider the historical use of narcotics within the department when compiling the contents list. The amount of medication stocked will depend on the frequency of restocking by the pharmacy department.

Narcotic inventories should be different for different types of departments. Critical care areas will stock primarily injectable narcotics, whereas rehabilitation and outpatient areas will stock primarily oral narcotics. Postoperative areas will have more pain medications, and medical areas will have more sedative medications. The narcotic inventory should reflect the needs of the primary patient population and the prescribing patterns of the primary physician users of the unit.

The narcotic supply system provides very tight inventory control for medications. This degree of control increases the cost of providing these medications to patients. When nonnarcotic alternatives are available, they offer a more cost-effective approach to patient treatment (Kitz et al., 1989). At the same time, the narcotic supply system can provide a mechanism for establishing tighter inventory control for nonnarcotic medications that have a tendency for misuse or abuse. For example, furosemide is a medication frequently stolen by dieters and drug abusers facing a urine drug screen. Furosemide can be added to the narcotic drug supply. Each dose will then be signed out by the administering nurse, wastages will be cosigned, and inventory will be counted on each shift.

TECHNIQUES FOR MONITORING MEDICATION DISTRIBUTION

Incident reports should be used to improve system problems and problems with individual performance. The staff should view incident reports as confidential communications from them to the organization to point out problems and to begin problem resolution. If incident reports are used in a punitive manner, the staff will underreport problems. For instance, if the number of incident reports the nurse is named in shows up on his or her annual evaluation, the nurse will be less likely to self-report incidents.

TECHNIQUES FOR MONITORING SUBSTANCE ABUSE

Substance abuse among nurses is a major problem in our society and in the nursing profession. Early studies indicated higher rates of substance abuse among nurses as compared to the general population. More recent studies indicate that substance abuse among nurses corresponds to the rate of abuse in the nonnursing population (Trinkoff, Eaton, & Anthony, 1991). The American Nurses Association estimates that 6% to 8% of the 1.5 million registered nurses working in nursing have a substance abuse problem (Gelfand et al., 1990).

Substance abuse accounts for the majority of disciplinary actions taken by state boards of nursing *(News)*. Managers are concerned not only with disciplinary actions but also with the effects on quality of patient care and the cost of maintaining or returning the nurse to work (Mazzoni, 1988).

There are four basic approaches to dealing with substance abuse that the nurse manager can adopt: ignore the problem, punish the nurse, work cooperatively with the nurse in a treatment and return to work process, and proactively strive to prevent, identify, and seek treatment for nurses with a substance abuse problem (Kemp, 1989).

Ignoring the problem is not an option in many states. Mandatory reporting of impaired nursing practice has been enacted in several states. Codes of ethics also require managers to take action to protect the safety of patients.

Punishing the nurse usually involves focusing on the behavior rather than the cause of the behavior. The nurse may be disciplined and even terminated for attendance problems but not reported to the state board or required to seek treatment. Although this approach relieves the nurse manager of the problem, it does not relieve the profession or protect the public from an unsafe practitioner.

The cooperative approach involves both notifying the board of nursing of the nurse's impaired practice and supporting the nurse through a treatment process and return to work. This is a time-consuming and energy-consuming process that more nurse managers were willing to undertake during the nursing shortage of the 1980s. The best possible outcome from this approach is a nurse retained within the profession and returned to safe practice.

The proactive approach includes all the attributes of the cooperative approach plus an emphasis on prevention and early detection. The proactive approach requires institutionwide policies and programs for all hospital employees. The human resource department is a key component in this approach. Policies within the institution should describe drug screening programs, reporting requirements and procedures, confidentiality and anonymity, and return to work guidelines. Drug screening programs can include preemployment, incident-related, probable cause, random, or a combination of any of these testing regimens (Baldwin, 1989). Employees should be made aware of the institution's policy during the employment process and sign a statement indicating that they are aware of the policy.

Drug awareness and prevention programs within the institution should inform employees of reporting requirements and procedures. The information should include how to identify an employee who is abusing alcohol or drugs. The institution's philosophy of helping the employee to seek treatment, retain licensure, and return to work needs to be emphasized in presentations to employees. Employees also need reassurance of protection and anonymity for the reporter (Baldwin, 1989).

Employee assistance programs provide confidential counseling and referral programs for employees. The employee assistance counselor can be a valuable resource for the manager in confronting and counseling employees.

Strategies To Prevent Substance Abuse

Substance abuse among nurses is attributed to high stress levels, variable work patterns, a knowledge of drugs, the caregiver role, peer protection, and easy access to drugs. One effective strategy to prevent substance abuse is to reduce

TABLE 28–1 Some of the Stressful Situations Facing Nurses

- Rotating shifts
- Evening and night hours
- Weekend and holiday shifts
- Physician-dominated health care system
- Involvement with death, dying, and illness
- 24-hour responsibility for patient care
- Downsizing and redesign efforts in many organizations
- Inability to control or predict pace of work
- Frequent inability to take breaks
- First-line response to complaints from physicians, patients, and families

Data from Mazzoni (1988) and Baldwin (1989).

or eliminate the stressors nurses experience. The list of stressful situations nurses deal with is long (Table 28–1).

Some techniques for reducing stress include

1. Support groups to deal with specific incidents or ongoing groups to facilitate team development
2. Ready access to the manager or the problem-solving process
3. Elimination of confrontations with abusive physicians
4. Access to employee assistance programs
5. Education on policies and procedures related to substance abuse by employees and reporting requirements of the institution and of the state
6. Prompt resolution of conflicts within the work group
7. In-depth discussion of the reasons for poor performance during routine evaluations and after specific incidents

Another effective strategy to prevent substance abuse is to establish and maintain optimal work schedules. This includes eliminating rotating shifts and implementing flexible scheduling options. Instituting a self-scheduling policy is an innovative solution to a long-standing problem.

A management strategy for dealing with nurses' knowledge of drugs involves giving them additional knowledge. Nurses may believe that their knowledge gives them control. They need additional information on the lack of control that comes with substance abuse. They need information on substance abuse within nursing, incidence, risks, signs and symptoms, and consequences for patients and for the nurse.

Management strategies directed toward the caregiver role are intimately related to stress reduction strategies. Nurses are expert caregivers, but they often are very poor care receivers. Encourage the staff to care for themselves. An example is 5 minute massages for tired staff provided by other staff or managers. Provide a relaxation room with tapes and visual aids available to the staff. Group exercise, weight reduction, or stop smoking initiatives are all examples of the staff caring for themselves and for each other.

Management strategies to decrease peer protection also involve education. The staff need to know their legal and ethical requirements to report impaired nursing practice. They also need assurance of the manager's and the institution's practice of supporting the nurse thorough treatment and reentry into practice. Staff may exhibit enabling behavior toward the nurse, excusing the nurse from full responsibility for errors, omissions, and inappropriate behavior (Cannon & Brown, 1988). The manager must be alert to the development of enabling behaviors and confront the enabler and the impaired nurse promptly.

Management strategies to decrease access to medications are necessary but not sufficient to prevent substance abuse. One key to effective control is to change the processes periodically. Elements of narcotics use monitoring include

1. Intershift narcotic counts include a review for cosignatures on all wasted narcotics.
2. Narcotic signout sheets are monitored on a routine basis in the pharmacy and periodically by the nurse manager. The manager should look for pages with the same drug signed out by the same nurse more than other nurses.
3. All nonroutine narcotic refill requests are logged and reviewed for trends. The manager should look for the same nurse requesting refills of the same medication.
4. All instances of narcotic count irregularities are investigated. Incident reports should include the names of everyone working in the department at the time of the irregularity. A statement from each employee should be attached. The nurse manager should compare all incidents of narcotic count irregularity with previous trends, and look for the same name on multiple reports.

Detecting Substance Abuse Among Nurses

The typical nurse who abuses drugs does not fit the profile of a drug addict that most nurses look for in their patients. The nurse addict is usually a hard worker, often volunteering for overtime or extra duties. The nurse is generally well liked. Mood swings and irritability often are attributed to the amount of overtime the nurse is working or to problems at home.

The nurse is usually several years into the disease process before the effects begin to show at work. When a good nurse begins to have changes in behavior and changes in quality of work, substance abuse is a possible cause. There is not a specific behavior that indicates substance abuse (Table 28–2). Rather it is the change from overachieving behaviors to underachieving behaviors that is a clue to substance abuse. Many nurse managers want to rule out all other possible causes before considering substance abuse, but statistics clearly point to substance abuse as a problem for nurses. Family problems and financial problems are also symptoms of substance abuse, and they usually precede problems at work (Patrick, 1984).

Detection often begins with an unusual incident. A narcotic count irregularity, a syringe found in the staff bathroom, empty vials in the narcotic drawer, or an

TABLE 28–2 Changes that Often Indicate Impaired Nursing Practice

- Increasing absences, often associated with days off or paydays
- Tardiness at beginning of shift or returning from breaks
- Increased isolation from peers
- Often initiates orders or changes in orders for p.r.n. medications
- Excessive early arrival
- Does not have drug wastages cosigned
- Makes frequent trips out of the unit
- Waits until alone to open narcotics cabinet
- Often confused about work schedule
- Consistently signs out more controlled drugs than others
- Consistently signs out more controlled drugs for others
- Gives elaborate excuses for behavior
- Consistently volunteers to count narcotics
- Documentation is illogical, incomplete, or sloppy
- Has periods of low and high activity
- Often has runny nose or dry sniffles, diaphoresis, or unusual body odor
- Often looks tired
- Inattention to details
- Sudden weight gain or loss
- Physical appearance becomes sloppy
- Difficulty recalling past events
- Frequent incidents, such as needlesticks, back strains, or breaking equipment
- Simple mathematical errors
- Questionable judgment in patient care decisions
- Complaints from co-workers, patients, and families
- Frequently complains about policies, peers, and patients, often without a specific reason
- Avoids contact with the manager
- Blame others for errors or misunderstandings
- Denies having any problems
- Displays wide swings in mood
- Borrows money from co-workers
- Overreacts to criticism
- Increased irritability, often argumentative and defensive, with unexpected blowups

Data from Mazzoni (1988), Baldwin (1989), and Caroselli-Karinja & Zboray (1986).

emotional outburst in the unit. Once suspicion is aroused, careful investigation must follow. The investigation should be thorough, and the pharmacist responsible for narcotics within the institution should be included as an objective reviewer. The investigation may include

- A review of narcotic signout sheets

- A review of nonroutine requests for narcotic refills
- An audit of patient charts, comparing medication signed out to medication given. (The nurse manager should look for differences in p.r.n. medication administration patterns among nurses caring for the same patient.)
- An interview with patients to evaluate their perception of pain relief from medications administered by the nurse
- An interview with co-workers to determine if they have any concerns about the nurse's job performance or behavior

On completion of the investigation, the nurse manager discusses the findings with the immediate supervisor or a colleague. The nurse manager should ask for feedback on the thoroughness of the investigation and the validity of the conclusions. The manager should review the reporting requirements of the state board of nursing and the human resources policies of the institution.

The next step is to confront the nurse with the evidence and with the concerns about substance abuse. The purposes of the confrontation are to initiate the treatment process, to initiate the disciplinary process, and to fulfill reporting requirements. A time for the confrontation should be scheduled when the nurse manager and an advocate for the nurse can meet with the nurse without interruption. The advocate can be a representative from the human resources department or the employee assistance program, a substance abuse counselor, or a recovering nurse.

The nurse manager should meet with the advocate before the confrontation and role play some of the potential responses the nurse may present. Denial is a common characteristic of substance abuse, and the manager should be prepared for denial, anger, indignation, relief, and confession. By knowing the resources in the area, the nurse manager is prepared to escort the nurse to a treatment program at the end of the confrontation. Many states have peer assistance programs that are very willing to send representatives to participate in the confrontation. The American Nurses Association publishes *Addictions and Psychological Dysfunctions in Nursing,* a guide to state programs and contact persons, annually.

A written summary should be prepared describing the questionable behavior in as specific and concrete a manner as possible. Disciplinary forms, leave of absence forms, and an action plan outlining expectations should be prepared before the confrontation.

The manager should start the confrontation by presenting the facts and then expressing concern that the nurse is using drugs. The nurse manager then demonstrates willingness to help if that is the problem. The rest of the meeting will be dictated by the nurse's response. The nurse should be allowed to talk, and the nurse manager should listen carefully to her response until she is finished.

During this conference, it is important for the nurse manager to remember that he or she is responsible for providing quality nursing care to the patients in the department. A caring and helpful manner toward the employee must be maintained, avoiding the role of nurse to the employee. The advocate will assume the caregiving role for the employee. The manager must be an advocate for the patient and the profession in this confrontation.

At the end of the meeting, the nurse must be told of any reporting requirements, and the nurse manager must document the meeting as would be done with any performance problem. The nurse must review and sign the documentation. Future performance expectations, monitoring and reevaluation requirements, and the consequences of noncompliance with the expectations are outlined for the nurse.

Dealing with Co-Workers

The amount of information given to the staff on the unit is limited. The nurse is entitled to confidentiality about disciplinary processes and health problems. The staff will know, however, and they will feel betrayed. This is a nurse they trusted, and she has betrayed their trust.

Self-recrimination is common among nurses who may have signed for narcotic wastages that they did not witness or helped cover some of the lapses in care the nurse may have had. Guilt and fear are common among nurses who may have participated in recreational drug use with the nurse.

The staff need to discuss their feelings with each other. Inservices on substance abuse among nurses often are helpful mechanisms for giving information and reassurance. It is often helpful for the manager to review the narcotic administration procedure and discuss the current process for handling narcotics within the unit. Are partial doses of unused narcotics passed from nurse to nurse or taped to the patient's headboard? Are narcotics returned to the pharmacy in an open bin? Many nurses will want to return to strict adherence to the narcotic supply administration policy. The nurse manager should request that the staff adhere strictly to the policy.

Returning the Impaired Nurse to the Workplace

Substance abuse is a chronic, incurable disease. The recovery phase of substance abuse usually lasts 1 to 2 years (Mazzoni, 1988). Once the nurse has completed the acute phase of treatment, he or she will contact the manager and request return to work. Many states have very specific guidelines under which nurses can return to work after treatment for substance abuse. Each nurse will require an individualized contract that specifies performance and behavioral expectations. The contract should include the following:

1. The nurse should be assigned to work straight shifts, preferably days or evenings.
2. A supportive supervisor should be working the same unit and the same shift as the nurse at least 80% of the time. The supervisor will be responsible for assessing the nurse to determine if he or she appears to be impaired by any substance at the beginning of each shift and for monitoring behavior throughout the shift. The supervisor will modify the work environment to reduce stress and limit access to narcotics as much as possible.
3. The nurse should agree to submit to a urine drug screen whenever the supervisor suspects drug use or whenever patient care errors occur. The nurse also should agree to a specified number of random urine drug screens

during the first 1 to 2 years after returning to work. The nurse should have the right to request a urine drug screen whenever he or she feels a need to clear himself or herself of the suspicion of drug use by the supervisor or by co-workers.

4. The nurse should have limited access to narcotics. Often the nurse can partner with another nurse by agreeing to give all the baths for the partner if the partner will administer all the narcotics. If total access cannot be denied, the nurse should be restricted from carrying the narcotic keys. The supervisor should observe her signing out, administering, and wasting narcotics as much as possible.

5. In instances where the nurse must give narcotics independently, for instance, the anesthetist role, stronger measures to assure sobriety are needed. One option is to have the nurse report to the supervisor at the beginning of the shift, take an Antabuse tablet in the presence of the supervisor, and then assume patient care responsibilities. Antabuse results in severe nausea and vomiting when taken with alcohol.

6. The nurse agrees to continue to receive treatment and participate in peer assistance programs or support groups.

7. The employee assistance or peer counselor should be a part of the contract negotiation process.

8. The contract should specify who will pay for the costs of laboratory tests. In most cases, the institution absorbs the cost of testing.

The first challenge the manager and the returning nurse will have is informing the staff of the planned return and the limitations on practice. This is particularly difficult when the nurse is returning to the same unit where the substance abuse occurred. The nurse should be encouraged to meet with the staff before the first day back. Discussing the substance abuse problem with colleagues on staff is an important step in recovery.

Substance abuse is a chronic disease prone to relapses, and the nurse manager must be prepared for relapses. The nurse should know that the nurse manager is aware of how difficult the return to work is going to be. She or he should be encouraged to come to the nurse manager if there is a relapse or a feeling that a relapse is about to occur. After supporting the nurse through a treatment process and return to work, it is worth the additional investment by the nurse manager to support the nurse through a relapse. Usually, stricter monitoring and additional limitations on practice are instituted after a relapse. The nurse manager should continue to document the behaviors associated with the relapse through the disciplinary processes of the institution. With a second relapse, termination is usually the result.

Substance abuse is a significant problem in our society and our profession. Well-designed and well-managed medication distribution and administration systems limit substance abuse, but management of substance abuse by a staff member requires strong interpersonal skills and a strong sense of caring for the staff member.

References

Baldwin, D. (1989). Drug screening in the workplace. *Occupational Health Nursing Journal, 37*(9), 379–381.

Cannon, B.L., & Brown, J.S. (1988). Nurses: Attitudes toward impaired colleagues. *Image: Journal of Nursing Scholarship, 20*(2), 96–101.

Caroselli-Karinja, M.F., & Zboray, S.D. (1986). The impaired nurse. *Journal of Psychosocial Nursing, 24*(6), 14–19.

Gelfand, G., et al. (1990). Prevention of chemically impaired nursing practice. *Nursing Management, 1*(7), 76–78.

Kemp, D. (1989). Evaluating chemical dependency in critical care nurses. In S. Cardin & C.R. Ward (Eds.). *Personnel management in critical care nursing* (pp. 176–188). Baltimore: Williams & Wilkins.

Kitz, D.S., et al. (1989). Examining nursing personnel costs: Controlled versus noncontrolled oral analgesic agents. *Journal of Nursing Administration, 19*(1), 10–14.

Mazzoni, J. (1988). Management of drug abuse in the hospital environment. *Topics in Health Record Management, 9*(1), 54–61.

News. Washington, DC: American Nurses' Association.

Patrick, P.K.S. (1984). Self-preservation: Confronting the issue of nurse impairment. *Journal of Substance Abuse Treatment, 1*, 99–105.

Platts, S. (1989, November). A self-medication pilot program. *Dimensions, XX,* XX–XX.

Stevens, B.J. (1985). *The nurse as executive* (3rd ed.), Rockville, MD: Aspen.

Trinkoff, A.M., Eaton, W.W., & Anthony, J.C. (1991). The prevalence of substance abuse among registered nurses. *Nursing Research, 40*(3), 172–175.

Part C. Managing Quality

CHAPTER 29   •   •   •   •   •   •

QUALITY MANAGEMENT

HARRY J. SCHULER

EXECUTIVE SUMMARY

In this chapter, the concepts and methods of total quality management (TQM) have been highlighted. As the Joint Commission continues its work on TQM development, it is essential that health organizations respond by demonstrating their commitment to total quality. Research efforts clearly indicate that total quality is a potential management solution to many organizational problems.

However, if there is one thing that is certain, it is that organizations are facing some common barriers to full implementation of the TQM process. First, the management literature on change suggests that the change process can be threatening at all levels of employment. Therefore, TQM must be introduced very slowly and with great caution. Senior management must be fully committed to TQM, take a leading role, and be involved in continuous quality improvement throughout the implementation process.

Second, organizational culture changes very slowly. Even under the best of circumstances, cultural change can take many years. Education and training are the keys here. It is critical to embark early on the development of a comprehensive, in-house training progam that is ongoing and updated to respond to changing organizational needs. TQM will flourish when education is a cornerstone of all service production and quality control activities.

Third, special attention must be paid to quality problem-solving techniques for corrective action in TQM. Research findings suggest that system failure and not the providers themselves is responsible for nonconformance and reduced quality functioning. The use of statistical quality control points to root causes of problems and appropriate corrective actions. The approach is a step-by-step model that aids in arriving at preferred solutions to improve quality performance. Remember that quality problem solving is the key to effective decision making in quality functioning.

TQM holds enormous promise for organizations willing to make the commitment to improve total quality. The next challenge is to ensure that commitment to the quality improvement process succeeds.

In the decade of the 1990s, the dimensions of quality in patient care activities are more difficult to manage, as the concept itself is growing in complexity. To illustrate that point, we need only look at the shift in professional interest from the more fundamental areas of definition and measurement of patient care quality to the more complex issue of patient care total quality management (TQM). The proliferation of articles, seminars, and scholarly research on quality management is recognition of the fact that total quality is much more than inspecting patient care outcomes.

The quality management concept is best described as knowing how everyone in the organization views and understands what patient care quality is and what their individual role is in making continuous quality improvement a reality. Widespread adoption of this concept has led to an evolution of quality thinking in the health industry from reliance on outcome assessment and inspection-based quality programs to full integration of the TQM concept. The latter is based primarily on organizational commitment to total quality in service production through process-oriented control.

A process is a set of interrelated activities requiring resources (inputs) that, when combined, produce units of patient care service (output). The term, process control, attempts to discover, through analysis, cause and effect relations that dampen the quality functioning of patient care service delivery.

This chapter focues on TQM in order to better understand the concepts, issues, and evolving nature of quality assurance programming. To keep the discussions within reasonable bounds, emphasis is placed on three types of interrelated quality activities

1. Quality measurement
2. Quality planning
3. Quality improvement

PRINCIPLES AND METHODS IN QUALITY ASSURANCE

Quality assurance is best described as a process-oriented, clinical function performed by a wide range of health care professionals. This process orientation recently has been expanded to include patients' needs and expectations as part of the process analysis. The range of patient care activities carried out by the nurse manager is very broad in scope, encompassing several functions, including drug use and handling, infection control, discharge planning, and utilization management. Improvement of patient care services is the primary objective of quality assurance programming.

In practice, quality assurance takes the form of ongoing and systematic monitoring and evaluation of patient care quality based on a multistep, quality assurance model. The model evaluates patient outcomes in terms of the definition and measurement of patient care quality. With regard to process, it is recognized that quality assurance activities are dependent on the changing nature of quality standards, federal and state regulation and law, the provider–patient relationship, and the health care organization. Each activity is dynamic and has a direct impact on quality assurance programming.

A quality assurance program is mandated by the Joint Commission on Accreditation of Healthcare Organizations (JCAHO) to oversee adherence to preestablished standards on the quality of patient care. In December 1988, the Joint Commission adopted a process-oriented definition of patient care quality as follows.

> . . . the degree to which patient care services increase the probability of desired patient outcomes and reduce the probability of undesired outcomes, given the current state of knowledge.

This definition rivets our attention on both the structures and processes of patient care. Emphasis is placed on understanding the process and the importance of dedicated workers in the workplace and their role in patient care service delivery.

A note of caution is presented here. The management literature clearly states that structure must follow process in the design of effective health care organizations. A simple translation of the foregoing suggests that first-work activities must be defined, understood, and implemented in health care facilities. Subsequently, a suitable organizational structure must be established to support the workers, the work environment, and the productivity systems.

Unfortunately, in the health industry, the organizational design process described is not widely practiced. In reality, process more typically must adapt to existing (or modified) structure. This simple observation has profound implications in the provision of patient care services.

PROCESS OF TOTAL QUALITY MANAGEMENT IN PATIENT CARE

TQM in patient care is emerging as the dominant management theme in health care policy and patient care practice. The total quality concept subsumes

- The technical question of quality measurements (i.e., the measure of health care practitioners' performance in patient care delivery)
- Organizational measures of quality that focus on structure and process variables

The former includes the dimension of total patient satisfaction (as defined by the patient), and the latter details such elements as quality planning, quality strategy, and organizational commitment to quality. The total quality concept emphasizes the system in developing integrated quality programming in a price-competitive, customer-centered organization.

A related theme addresses the question of participation. The total quality concept requires the participation of all units (e.g., divisions, departments) and all employees (e.g., CEO, management team, rank-and-file) of the organization. The intent of organizationwide participation is straightforward. It means that everyone in every unit of the organization must actively participate in the quality control process. In short, quality is everyone's job! In practice, this is accomplished through education and training of everyone in every unit so that each individual can actively promote total patient care quality.

A TQM system for patient care delivery includes three interdependent and essential ingredients.

1. A focus on the patient
2. A comprehensive plan
3. A change in the organization's culture

The first element is introduced to focus our attention on the patient's basic needs, wants, and expectations in regard to medical care. In the 1990s, patients are exercising much more control over medical treatment decisions. There simply is no avoiding it. A straightforward example of the foregoing is the increased use of advance directives by patients. The advance directive is a document (e.g., Durable Power of Attorney, the Living Will) through which the patient can dictate instructions about medical care before a medical emergency prevents the patient from doing so. Historically, this was not the case. Too often, the physician's reaction to a medical condition was a treatment plan independent of the patient's (or patient's family's) wants or needs. A focus on patients means to listen to their opinions and to act in a way that will take their views into account.

Planning for total quality is the second basic element. The need for a comprehensive, total quality management plan recognizes the enormous task and complexity of transforming an organization and building a total organizationwide quality program. The planning process must involve all workers and carefully integrate purposeful work that will lead to the development of innovative ways to achieve continuous quality improvement.

The third element introduces the concept of organization culture. In its simplest form, organization culture is described as the integrated pattern of work behavior, which includes language, actions, and artifacts, that is learned by and transmitted to employees. Since the elements of organization are fundamental beliefs and learned behaviors that are held in common by employees, they cannot be changed quickly. That fact is consistent with the literature on habit-forming behavior.

Culture is thought to endure for a long period of time and change very, very slowly. A cultural change must permeate the entire organization and be instilled in every employee to be successful. In large complex organizations, the process of cultural transformation can take up to 10 years. Therefore, the health care facility undergoing cultural transformation and its leadership team must be forward looking and think long term. Organizational communication must be increased substantially and sustained at a higher level over longer durations to be effective. Management must encourage ongoing and active participation among employees at all organizational levels to better understand and manage the change process. These considerations are of paramount importance if organization culture is to be transformed successfully.

Quality Methods

Health care providers have looked to the manufacturers of products (e.g., AT & T, Ford Motor Co., IBM) for guidance on total methods to produce higher quality patient care services. The rationale for turning to the producers of consumer products was simple—leaders in the manufacturing sector are credited with the successful implementation of total quality programming, under the rubric of TQM.

TQM and the quality improvement techniques that are used worldwide are based on the extensive writings of three Americans—W. Edwards Deming (1986), Philip B. Crosby (1979, 1984), and Joseph M. Juran (1986, 1989).

- Deming's principles and work on statistical quality control guided the quality turnaround in Japan's post-World War II economy.
- Crosby defines quality as conformance to requirements and advocates zero defects in a quality program that focuses on prevention.
- Juran has developed a quality trilogy—planning, control, and improvement—as a universal way of total quality thinking.

Their philosophies on total quality control are summarized eloquently in a recently published article (Sahney & Warden, 1991) and are not repeated here. Instead, the concepts common to their quality philosophies are applied to this discussion of quality methods and patient care considerations. Patient care quality is the health industry's watchword phrase in the 1990s.

There is an ongoing quality movement in the U.S. health care system. The movement is an inclusive label that encompasses all efforts to define, measure, and improve service quality and overall patient satisfaction. Many health care professionals attribute the quality movement primarily to three sources: JCAHO, employees, and the insurance industry. The Joint Commission has concentrated its efforts primarily on developing quality standards for health care organizations. The quality standards are made operational through quality programming approaches.

Alternatively, employers and insurance carriers have emphasized the collection and use of both quality and cost data. The two considerations are intertwined, but in today's reimbursement environment, cost considerations are predominant in managed care contracting agreements.

In the health care organization, the total quality methods applied generally are based on four key principles.

1. The team concept
2. Benchmarking
3. Quality problem solving
4. Employee education and training

The Team Concept

The team concept is the first of the major techniques used by managers in TQM practice. Team members include both clinical and nonclinical persons who are organized into both patient care and management teams. The team members are commonly referred to as principal stakeholders because they are directly responsible for work flow and production.

Their primary function is twofold: to define problem areas in work flow and production that interfere with quality functioning—the problem recognition stage, to recommend possible courses of action—the solution stage. To be successful, the team must focus its attention on the first stage and make every effort to fully understand the problem(s). That task is best accomplished when team members have quality authority and actively participate in brainstorming sessions.

No team member is forced to take sides—that is, there is no politicking and no perception of winners and losers. During the problem recognition stage, all relevant issues are debated until there is agreement on the essence of the problem. The aim here is at achieving consensus on defining the problem(s). Team members are reminded that during this stage, there is no mention of possible solutions. Alternative courses of action are discussed only after consensus is achieved.

The problem recognition stage rivets management attention to essentials and leads to the logical conclusion that commitment follows understanding. This makes for effective decisions and is time well spent.

The approach just described is very different from a management process that emphasizes the decision or the right solution to the problem(s). In the health industry, there is much more emphasis on the solution stage of the process. Too often, the tradeoff is a cursory examination of the problem. Managers are required to develop systematic approaches to arrive at the right solution to the problem quickly. This observation is analogous to placing the solution before the problem.

This observation points up two related considerations. First, the decision process is heavily biased toward senior management in health care. Junior managers and rank-and-file workers are practically excluded from the decision process. This lack of involvement dampens the enthusiasm of those stakeholders who are directly responsible for decision implementation and quality improvement. Second, the quest for decision is fraught with political bias and frequently lacks the commitment of senior management. As a consequence, the political issue rarely yields real changes in work attitudes and behavior that improve quality functioning.

Adaptations of the team concept provide the basis for the quality movement in the U.S. health care system. The rationale is simple—quality problems are best addressed by a team of people. However, like many good ideas, the teams do not always work well together, and an external party, a consultant, is sometimes used to aid team members at each stage in the process.

Benchmarking

The term, benchmarking, is used as an analog for the process of measuring baseline performance of quality functioning in patient care services. The benchmark is comparable to an average measure of clinical performance in quality monitoring. Although the concept is appealing in health care, benchmarking can have some negative side effects. For example, it seems obvious that when clinical performance is high, quality monitoring may seem unnecessary and unwanted by practitioners. Many clinical persons resent the task and ask the obvious question: Why waste valuable resources to reaffirm that the organization is doing a good job clinically? Moreover, when the task of quality monitoring is undertaken, a real concern becomes perfunctory performance.

Alternatively, when clinical performance is low, quality monitoring efforts are likely to be interpreted as a threat to the organization's status quo. Herein lies the basic dilemma. The organization must address the possibility that not all clinical practitioners are capable of providing high-quality patient care services. In this case, the organization may be required to replace personnel, improve recruitment strategies, and provide inservice training. Many organizations may not be willing to accept the fact that low-quality patient care is systemic of deep-rooted organizational problems.

An organization can act most effectively when benchmarking is one element of a larger quality programming effort. The benchmark becomes the basis for a relative comparison in a self-improvement mode as the organization engages in both process evaluation (i.e., task performance) and program evaluation (i.e., outcome assessment). Moreover, improvements in the benchmark can be linked directly to incremental cost increases to answer the fundamental question: Quality improvement, but at what cost?

Quality Problem Solving

Problem solving is an integral part of the quality management process. Indirectly, the problem-solving concept was alluded to during the discussion of problem definition and solution in the team concept section. However, because the topic is complex, it is introduced at this time to more fully explain its technical requirements.

In its simplest form, the problem-solving process consists of a set of activities that take the team members through five basic steps:

1. **Problem definition**—Identification and articulation of the quality problem (What is it?)
2. **Data gathering**—Assembling of relevant information about the quality problem (What data are needed?)
3. **Problem solving**—Analyzing work flow and service production (What is the cause-and-effect relationship?)
4. **Solution formulation**—Implementing the preferred alternative (What is the preferred course of action?)
5. **Follow-up activities**—Evaluating the selected alternative and initiating follow-up action (What feedback information is needed?)

Needless to say, the technical aspects of problem solving are the most cumbersome. If the five steps are carefully assessed, the following is a reasonable set of corresponding observations.

1. A well-defined problem is essential. Team members must be in total agreement before proceeding further.
2. Analysis of the quality problem requires good information. The information must lend itself readily to quantification (i.e., numerical form) and measurement. Information generally is coded, stored, and maintained on computer files for easy access and retrieval.
3. The information is analyzed, with a range of statistical probabilities, to understand the cause-and-effect relationships in statistical quality control. Possible causes are tested to determine their ability to explain the problem.
4. An appropriate solution is designed and implemented on the basis of the cause-and-effect analysis. The analysis points up a cause that warrants further investigation.
5. It must be verified that the solution has eliminated the problem, permanently. If the problem is not eliminated, follow-up, corrective action must be taken.

More detailed remarks on the technical problem just described go beyond the scope of this discussion. Persons with technical expertise can lead the organization's efforts in this area. Alternatively, it is perhaps more important to ask the fundamental question: Why are these five steps undertaken?

To answer that question, consider the following example. If an incident report is used to determine a corrective action in clinical performance, the organization's quality assurance committee could be in a position of changing the patient care system based on the random occurrence of an event. If the cycle is repeated, the organization might very well make another system level, corrective action that is inappropriate. This pattern could repeat itself again and again and prove to be very destructive in terms of quality management.

The random occurrence of an event is a chance happening that must be dealt with as a special circumstance. The random occurrence event is infrequent, has special causes, and requires an individual corrective action. To do otherwise could put the organization in a constant state of making inappropriate adjustments in patient care systems.

Alternatively, if an event occurs more frequently and has common causes, it lends itself rapidly to statistical analysis and systemwide management action that is appropriate. In statistical quality control, if systematic variability of events in a patient care system is understood, the researcher can move rapidly toward explaining root cause(s) to fundamental quality problems. This can lead to problem elimination and a permanent solution.

Employee Education and Training

Employee education and training is an organized process by which the employee acquires knowledge, skills, and attitudes that are needed to be successful in the workplace. That definition is straightforward and, in operational terms, is quite simple to implement. However, with few exceptions, the education and training component within health organizations rarely lives up to expectations.

Why so? In general, the answer lies in the organization's modest level of commitment to the concept.

For example, employee education is considered to be the individual's responsibility in most health facilities. The individual is expected to be trained or licensed or have a degree before being hired. If continuing education is required for relicensure, employees usually secure the training outside the organization.

If the organization does train new employees, the training is considered minimal and restricted to selective managerial and professional employment categories. In most health facilities, quality assurance education lasts only a few days or weeks at most. In short, in-house education and training are insufficient.

In Japan, employee quality education as an organized process takes place over several months. Education is a cornerstone of all production and quality control activities. Further, there is no other nation that promotes and supports employee education as vigorously. In discussing employee education, Ishikawa (1985, p. 37), one of the world's foremost authorities on total quality control, states that

> Quality control is a thought revolution in management, therefore, the thought processes of all employees must be changed. To accomplish this, education must be repeated over and over again.

The intent of employee education and training is to support directly the organization's commitment to continuous quality improvement. In health care, quality education does not mean copying the Japanese, but the industry can emulate their success. Very detailed education and training programs are called for when

- Behavior modification is essential
- New knowledge is required to be successful
- A modified skill mix or level is mandatory

Employees faced with these challenges in quality assurance can rely on education and training programs as an opportunity to perform the job correctly, to improve job performance, and to contribute to quality problem solving. Ishikawa (1985) concludes that "Quality control begins with education and ends with education."

Senior management must understand and be taught to apply TQM philosophy. Equally important, the organization's leadership must develop an education and training plan and ensure that all quality education programs are continuous.

The activities described are always conducted by professionals trained in continuous learning techniques. The education component involves training in TQM methods and principles that are common to all employees, including senior management. This means that education is made available for each job level and category, including board members, the CEO and medical staff director, the executive management team and all physicians, registered nurses and allied health professional employees, and workers in other hourly or staff positions. In addition, education programs must be updated because new employees enter the organization each year and the needs of the organization change over time.

Up to this point, employee involvement in education and training has been discussed only in terms of job level or category. This involvement is much more inclusive and requires both consultant-led and self-directed team training. Not only are the team members or stakeholders trained in TQM problem solving and decision approaches, but they also are required to instruct others. Educators have long asserted that to instruct others is the best way to learn.

Incentives often are used to encourage nonperfunctory participation. The incentives typically focus on team accomplishments, and rewards are based on specific achievements in quality problem solving and decision making. The rewards should be progressive and relate specifically to improvement in quality functioning. At the individual level, quality performance can be recognized in promotion and compensation criteria.

DEVELOPMENT OF TOTAL QUALITY MANAGEMENT MONITORS AND TOOLS

The use of TQM monitors and tools is consistent with JCAHO's quality-oriented accreditation objectives. The history of the Joint Commission's approach to quality is one of progressive development toward TQM. Early in the 1980s, JCAHO introduced a requirement for ongoing monitoring of quality functioning. This monitoring involved systematic data collection on a continuous basis as well as emphasis on quality indicators to evaluate important aspects of patient care.

The monitoring and evaluation process was a forerunner to the Joint Commission's Agenda for Change project (1986). The demonstration project led to new research on quality indicators and introduced outcome-oriented monitoring and evaluation. The approach is designed to assist health facilities in improving the quality of care they provide (Carroll, 1991).

The new directions being pursued by the Joint Commission build on the foregoing. First, clinical evaluations are based on quality-driven processes that focus on organizational measures of structure and process. Second, the more technical question of quality measurement is analyzed using statistical procedures to understand cause-and-effect relationships. The search for root causes seeks to eliminate quality problems permanently.

Standards to represent TQM are scheduled for field testing and adoption by JCAHO in 1992. Shortly thereafter, health facilities will need to collect, code, store, and maintain the standardized quality indicator data on computer files for easy access, retrieval, and management reporting.

WORK PROCESS FOCUS

Quality-driven processes in patient care seek to bring about systemwide improvements (e.g., increased patient satisfaction, increased cost savings) through definition and analysis of patient care processes. A quality driven process is defined, as a set of interrelated quality activities—a quality process sequence, that requires resource use (inputs) to produce units of patient care service (output). More simply stated, the process sequence identifies the work steps undertaken by practitioners and the resources that are used in this overall effort. In short, the quality process sequence details work flow in patient care activities.

In the problem recognition stage, principal stakeholders emphasize the analysis of patient care processes. This action is accomplished by carefully undertaking work process (or work flow) analysis. (In the TQM literature, the terms are used interchangeably.)

The inventory of work process activities is recorded and described in terms of process inputs (e.g., practitioners, equipment) and expectations and process outputs (e.g., patient satisfaction, outcome assessment) and expectations. The analysis of process inputs addresses the question, What is it that we do? The analysis of process outputs addresses the question, What is it that we provide? The label, expectations, is a surrogate for desired results in service production.

It is important to note that work process analysis takes place at all levels of the organization and in all departments, not just the clinical units. Direct patient care activities are important to quality functioning, but so are materials management, human resource management, and financial management. Patient care is intertwined with all of these organizational functions.

DATABASE SYSTEMS

Historically, computerized databases in health facilities were used primarily to manage patient care financial information. Recent technologic changes in microcomputers, such as networking and advanced software applications, have opened possibilities to develop clinical database systems for the monitoring of quality functioning and patient care outcomes. Today, the primary focus of data managers is to develop and implement more integrated databases that link organizational information directly to quality indicator information.

The organizational information is representative of the organization's culture, leadership, planning, philosophy, mission statement, and quality improvement processes. The quality indicator information is collected from many sources, including clinical, management, and other organizational support systems. Using a common database system to manage and integrate these functions is consistent with the Joint Commission's new direction in accreditation standards development.

TQM requires database systems that are both valid and reliable.

- Quality reports result in a time and cost savings in information gathering and processing. Sources of information are designated, and duplication of effort is minimized.
- Quality reports are used to develop quality improvement plans for each

department or division in the organization. Processes are analyzed, and quality problems are eliminated.

- Quality reports are used to better understand patient wants and needs. Patient satisfaction is increased.
- Quality reports are the basis for communicating organizational commitment to quality, results achieved in problem solving, team recognition, and all other quality matters.

Although the reports themselves can be very different in design, content, and intent, the data requirements for each are not significantly different.

FEEDBACK AND CORRECTIVE ACTION

Feedback and corrective action in TQM require a two-step process. First, the corrective action is designed and implemented on the basis of cause-and-effect analysis. In quality problem solving, patient care processes are analyzed using a range of statistical procedures to understand cause-and-effect relationships in statistical quality control. Possible root causes are tested to determine their ability to explain quality functioning. After the quality problem's root cause has been identified, an appropriate solution—corrective action—is undertaken. Second, feedback and follow-up activities occur when the corrective action is evaluated following its implementation. During this step, quality teams are assessing the corrective action to determine whether the problem has been eliminated permanently. If the problem is not eliminated, appropriate follow-up action is required.

In practice, corrective action is always applied by the appropriate level of management. For example, if the quality problem is departmental (e.g., waits or delays), the corrective action is implemented by the department manager. The department's quality team may require a change in work method to improve quality functioning. If, however, the quality problem is organizational (e.g., duplication of effort across departments), the corrective action is moved up to the appropriate level of senior management (e.g., division manager). The division's quality team must analyze the work flow process and then select an appropriate corrective action. Stakeholders may require the elimination of activities in one or more departments to improve quality functioning. The division manager is responsible for implementation of the corrective action.

The situations described here are different from other problem-solving scenarios because team members are empowered to both select and implement the corrective action. The implications of empowering employees in decision making are important in TQM.

First, the problem solving process allows stakeholders to solve their own quality problems. As a consequence, stakeholders are part of the quality solution and not part of the quality problem. Second, stakeholders are taught to focus on what the problem is all about and not what the right decision should be. This enables stakeholders to openly debate all viewpoints and bring out minority as well as majority opinions. Open debate of problem issues is a healthy activity in organizations. Third, stakeholders build up to effective decision making through consensus. The problem-solving activities lead to total organizational commitment with regard to decision making.

COST CONTAINMENT AND QUALITY IMPROVEMENT

Successful TQM models are being developed, tested, and implemented in health organizations. A major purpose is to improve operations and assist organizations in becoming more competitive. However, the cost-containment issue in TQM is not well documented.

In general, the cost of quality is made up of two components.

1. The price of conformance
2. The price of nonconformance

The price of conformance includes such factors as education/training, testing, audits, and quality functioning process documentation. The cost of nonconformance includes all failure costs or error costs in patient care systems—reject, redo, rework service activities. Although the formula for cost of quality is highly simplistic, there are enormous difficulties associated with developing an operational format.

It is essential, first, to identify and cost-out the elements of patient care service quality. This step includes a detailed analysis of process input, process sequence, and process output factors. Next, the organization must identify sources of information to do the actual cost of quality estimates. Possible sources of information include reports, audits, tests, inspections, and other available documentation.

The third step is to calculate the cost of quality. This task is accomplished following the integration of patient care process information and financial data. Calculating the cost of quality highlights the need to develop a common database system for use in TQM.

Insurance carriers and other fiscal intermediaries have long emphasized the collection and use of both quality and cost data. The two considerations are often intertwined in the business literature and lead to the logical conclusion that higher patient care quality will attract the best health care professionals and lead to increased patient satisfaction and higher overall profits. Unfortunately, this view contradicts the more traditional thinking among health care providers that high-quality patient care increases costs and leads to lower overall profits. Not enough information is available to prove that high quality costs less in health care. It is an issue that must be studied further.

If there is one argument that has been resolved, it is that physicians and health organizations alike are rewarded by insurance carriers and other third party payors for reducing cost. What is not clear is whether providers of patient care are rewarded for increased quality functioning. There are indications in today's managed care environment that purchasers of medical care are not willing to direct increased patient volume to providers solely on the basis of quality care.

PATIENT SATISFACTION

Too often we forget that quality of service is defined by patients. That statement is independent of the fact that patients' judgments on the technical aspects of care are likely to be invalid. Patients simply lack the technical knowledge to understand fully the complexity of patient care service delivery. Despite these limitations, patients' attitudes, perceptions, and opinions are essential to quality monitoring.

A monitoring system that incorporates a comprehensive measure of patient satisfaction can assist the organization in quality improvement efforts. Its potential is enormous. For example, an understanding of patient satisfaction helps to break down barriers between patients and practitioners. The system can aid in building cohesiveness in patient care systems and improving the morale of patients. These efforts are enhanced only when patient satisfaction is broadly understood.

In the health industry, an increased effort must be applied to identify those attributes of service quality that are valued by patients or their families. Undoubtedly, this is a research topic worthy of investigation. In TQM, there are a number of information sources and techniques that are used for this purpose.

First, patient questionnaires are analyzed by applying survey-based consulting tools. The intent of the survey research is twofold.

1. To develop outcome measures
2. To design profiles

The outcome measures for patients relate to the technical question of practitioners' performance in patient care delivery. The measures make it easier for patients to provide feedback on specific service delivery issues. The patient profiles attempt to quantify patient satisfaction on the basis of patient perceptions and expectations. Both sets of information seek to identify patient requirements in addressing the fundamental question, Do we really understand what the patient wants and needs in patient care service? Monitoring performance and the organization's efforts to increase patient satisfaction must be an ongoing process.

Second, patients and patients' families frequently are interviewed by applying direct interview or focus group techniques. In a direct interview situation, the interviewer collects information from the patient in a face-to-face meeting. Alternatively, a focus group uses a moderator to lead a group session in which patients are asked to comment on patient care service delivery issues. The intent is to integrate the information provided by patients directly into quality programming efforts.

Finally, the measures of patient satisfaction should be used to develop standards of quality in patient care that are performance based. One approach would be to develop standards that describe the level of service that patients can expect. Practitioner's performance can then be evaluated in terms of the predetermined quality standards.

References

Carroll, J.G. (1991, March). Continuous quality improvement and its implications for accreditation standards. *Topics in Health Record Management, 11,* 27–37.

Crosby, P.B. (1979). *Quality is free.* New York: McGraw-Hill.

Crosby, P.B. (1984). *Quality without tears.* New York: McGraw-Hill.

Deming, W.E. (1986). *Out of crisis.* Cambridge, MA: MIT Press.

Ishikawara, K. (1985). *What is total quality control?* (D. Lu, Trans.) (p. 37). Englewood Cliffs, NJ: Prentice-Hall.

Juran, J.M. (1986, August). The quality trilogy. *Quality Process, 19,* 19–24.

Juran, J.M. (1989). *Juran on planning for quality.* New York: The Free Press.

Sahney, V.K., & Warden, G.L. (1991, summer). The quest for quality and productivity in health services. *Frontiers of Health Services Management, 7,* 2–40.

CHAPTER 30

QUALITY MANAGEMENT IN THE HOSPITAL SETTING: NEW HORIZONS

NANCY E. ROYAL
MARYANN F. FRALIC

EXECUTIVE SUMMARY

Quality management in today's health care environment reflects a complex and evolving process. Traditional quality assurance activities are being integrated with hospitalwide quality improvement initiatives to produce more viable and productive quality management programs. Although quality management may vary from institution to institution, there are several intrinsic characteristics of effective programs.

- Maintaining basic elements of traditional quality programs while simultaneously implementing hospitalwide quality improvement initiatives to produce a new quality paradigm
- Identifying customers
- Focusing on process improvement
- Measuring variation
- Maintaining leadership commitment
- Encouraging employees to own the change process
- Crossing organizational boundaries in the improvement process
- Celebrating success

Because nurses are involved in all aspects of patient management, it is often nurses who are pivotal in identifying opportunities to improve care. Nurse managers play a key role in supporting staff participation in the quality improvement process. Not only must they coach and train employees, but they also must provide consistent feedback and recognition of success. Staff ownership of quality activity is critical to the success of quality management programs. Nursing leaders recognize that true quality improvement is based on truly empowering the caregiver to effect positive change.

QUALITY IN TRANSITION

Traditional hospital quality assurance is in transition to an innovative quality model, incorporating the best elements of quality monitoring with the new paradigm based on continuous quality improvement (CQI) and total quality management (TQM).

Multiple forces are driving the changes in health care quality.

- Health care costs continue to escalate.
- Payors, both private and governmental, are demanding better value for their health care dollars.
- Patients are expecting improved technology, services, and outcomes.
- Regulatory agencies are requiring more exacting compliance with increasingly proscriptive standards.
- Health care workers question the value of current quality monitoring programs.
- Health care executives are becoming more aware of industrial quality management models that reduce and control cost while simultaneously improving the quality of goods and services.

These forces, in conjunction with the general failure of inspection-based quality monitoring programs to significantly improve quality, have clearly mandated the need for a new and innovative approach. Although current regulatory standards still mandate many of the inspection-based elements of quality assurance, innovative organizations are now integrating traditional quality assurance programs with organizationwide CQI or TQM (or both) initiatives. The blending of elements of conventional quality assurance with the hospitalwide quality improvement process (whether it is called continuous quality improvement, total quality management, or any of a number of analogous terms) is the foundation of quality management.

Evolution of Traditional Quality Assurance: A Retrospective

Health care has a long history of addressing quality issues. As Williamson noted, "Health professionals have always striven for excellence and attempted to maintain and improve their knowledge and skills as a major responsibility of being a professional" (1991, p. 52). During the Crimean War, Florence Nightingale cited mortality statistics of soldiers in an effort to empirically document unacceptable standards (Nielsen, 1992, p. 66). In 1917, the American College of Surgeons formulated a Hospital Standardization Program to specify the elements required by a hospital to provide good care: qualified physicians, credentialled staff, proper facilities, and resources (Spath, 1991, p. 1). A requirement to review the care of surgical patients was added by the College in the 1940s. In 1951, the hospital accreditation program was assumed by the Joint Commission on Accreditation of Hospitals. The first Joint Commission standards published in 1953 mandated review but did not recommend specific mechanisms for the review process. Generally, hospitals implemented, as a minimum, a morbidity and mortality review process. The Medicare Act also established utilization review and medical necessity determination in 1965. By 1972, additional legislation required physician review of the care provided to patients whose care is federally funded. Current peer review organizations (PROs) are a direct result of that legislation. The complex federal regulatory structure that has evolved is designed to control health care costs and evaluate quality.

During the 1970s and 1980s, hospitals were attempting to comply with the evolving Joint Commission on Accreditation of Healthcare Organizations (JCAHO) standards related to quality. Initially, compliance involved retrospective audits to monitor patient care. Later standards emphasized the need for hospitalwide problem resolution to improve outcomes. By 1985, the standards had evolved to a quality review process based on the systematic monitoring and evaluation of important aspects of care (JCAHO, 1991, p. 8). A traditional inspection-oriented quality review process was firmly entrenched in hospitals accredited by the Joint Commission and monitored by the PROs.

Strongly influenced by external requirements, most hospitals have organized quality programs with three primary elements: assessing and measuring performance, monitoring conformance to standards, and improving performance when standards are not met (Laffel & Blumenthal, 1989). The traditional method does assure the public of a certain level of safety and competence based on compliance with standards and regulations. Additionally, some improvements in the quality of patient care have resulted from a combination of compliance with these externally imposed requirements and with the innate desire of health care workers to improve patient care.

Weaknesses in Traditional Quality Assurance

There are numerous weaknesses in the conventional inspection-based system. Williamson notes that "Perhaps the most serious is the fact that traditional methods often use externalized, negative incentives. Consequently, professionals often feel resentment and resist QM [Quality Management] participation whenever possible" (Williamson, 1991, p. 53). Berwick graphically describes the inspection-oriented approach to health care quality as the Theory of Bad Apples (Berwick, 1989). The Bad Apple approach leads to defensiveness and an attempt by professionals to justify themselves and their institutions as satisfactory (Berwick, 1989, p. 54). A focus on self-justification frequently subverts the search for ways to improve quality.

Another inherent problem with traditional quality programs is that they are based on conformance to standards. Although compliance does assure a minimum level of performance, conforming to standards rarely fosters creativity. Instead, it is a "static approach" (Laffel & Blumenthal, 1989, p. 2869), which may lead to conformity, complacency, and mediocrity.

Yet another weakness in traditional quality assurance is the tendency to focus on departmentalized monitoring and evaluation in which pertinent information may not be shared with the appropriate individuals or departments. For example, both the orthopedic service QA committee and the nursing service QA committee may be concerned about a sudden increase in the occurrence of postoperative wound infections in total knee replacement patients. Working independently to resolve the problem, members of each committee may identify possible causes and corrective actions related to their practice areas. The physicians may identify timeliness of preoperative antibiotics as a potential problem, whereas the nurses determine that postoperative dressing change techniques are problematic. Working independently, neither group recognizes the areas of patient management shared by both disciplines. Although corrective actions may be implemented by both physicians and nurses, failure to share information with the other discipline may hinder timely and optimal resolution of the problem. Thus, the departmentalized quality assurance activity leads to fragmentation of monitoring and follow-up corrective actions and evaluation. Long term, this lack of system integration may delay or impede patient care improvement.

As traditional quality assurance evolved during the 1980s, some American manufacturing and service industries were simultaneously beginning to implement and apply quality improvement philosophies and programs that had proved so successful in post-World War II Japan. Concepts, such as customer identification and satisfaction, measurement and reduction of variation, continuous process improvement, and active employee participation, were keystones of the new approach. The names of Deming, Juran, and Crosby were becoming well known in American companies. Based on the positive experience with quality improvement in industry, some health care organizations began implementing similar initiatives.

Continuous Quality Improvement

The Joint Commission also identified a need for continuous quality improvement. O'Leary addressed this issue (1991, p. 74).

> I speak of quality improvement with a small q, small i, and no abbreviations or acronyms. We are all well aware of the variety of labels and constructs, and their welter of initials, within which total quality management and continuous quality improvement have been set forth. . . . When we use any initials within the Joint Commission, we tend to use CQI, for continuous quality improvement, because to us the term means the way of life in an organization, whether that's inside the Joint Commission, your organization, or any organization. We might contrast that with, for instance, total quality management (TQM), which might imply that there is a simple management style that is necessary for all of this change to happen within an organization. That may or may not be true—time and experience will tell.

In 1987, The JCAHO launched "the Agenda for Change—multi-year initiatives designed to make future accreditation an effective stimulus for continuous improvement in the performance of health care organizations" (JCAHO, 1991, p. 9). In the 1992 *Accreditation Manual for Hospitals,* the previous Quality Assurance chapter was replaced with a Quality Assessment and Improvement chapter, which mandates the initiation of continuous quality improvement activities within hospitals (JCAHO, 1992, p. 139).

The Joint Commission will continue to revise standards to reflect an increasing emphasis on continuous quality improvement. Modifications launched by the Joint Commission will include the following areas (JCAHO, 1992, p. xiii).

- Increased emphasis on the role of leadership in improving quality
- Expansion of the scope of assessment and improvement activities beyond the strictly

clinical to the interrelated governance, managerial, support, and clinical processes that affect patient outcomes

- Emphasis on continuous improvement rather than only on solving identified problems
- Use of other sources of feedback (in addition to ongoing monitoring) to trigger evaluation and improvement of care and services
- Organization of assessment and improvement activities around the flow of patient care and services, with special attention to how the "customer and supplier" relationships between hospital departments (as well as within departments) can be improved, rather than compartmentalizing activities within departments and services
- Emphasis on the processes of care and service rather than only on the performance of individuals
- Increased emphasis on maintaining improvement over time

The 1994 *Accreditation Manual for Hospitals* has many standards chapters organized by key activities (JCAHO, 1994). This change promotes cross-departmental attention to quality and reiterates the concept that quality is an organizationwide responsibility. The Joint Commission has opened the door to change. The challenge for hospitals will be to comply with the traditional inspection-oriented standards that remain while embarking on the implementation of a hospitalwide CQI process. The opportunity to integrate both elements creates tremendous challenge and opportunity in quality management.

COMPONENTS OF QUALITY IMPROVEMENT

Although quality improvement in hospitals is going through an evolutionary phase, key elements of the paradigm can be identified. CQI will be a permanent component of quality programs. If quality is not adopted for economic or philosophical reasons, mandates by the Joint Commission will ensure its ongoing place in hospital quality programs.

Walton described six companies that have attempted to implement Deming's ideas about quality (Walton, 1990, p. 14).

> The companies share a common approach. They are pledged to Dr. Deming's notion of continual improvement. The top management of each organization is committed to quality transformation. The people in these organizations understand who their customers are. They recognize the need to base decisions on data. And they are beginning to understand that there is variation in every process. The quality journey never ends, and people are at different points along the way.

All of the quality improvement elements identified by Walton also apply to successful hospital quality programs. They include

- Commitment by hospital leadership
- Customer satisfaction
- Process focus
- Display and measurement of variation

Commitment by Hospital Administrative Leadership

Members of the hospital's administrative leadership must be committed to quality improvement. The institutional commitment and organizational culture must be established by the chief executive officer, senior management, and key administrative leaders. There must be "constancy of purpose" (Deming, 1986, p. 24) in which both short-term and long-term quality goals are identified. Quality must be defined and incorporated into the vision and strategic plan of the hospital, and the board of directors should be involved in the overall planning and evaluating of quality activity. Sufficient resources should be allocated for quality training and education. Information systems need to be mobilized to support quality improvement activity. It is helpful to designate key leaders who will be responsible for assessing and prioritizing targeted projects and initiatives. Ultimately, successful hospitalwide quality improvement programs will be led by administrative leaders who personify a total commitment to continuously enhancing quality within the institution.

Role of the Nurse Manager

Nurse managers play a key role in facilitating quality improvement activity. They must provide ongoing coaching and training to employees. Because quality improvement concepts may be unfamiliar, consistent positive reinforcement from nurse managers is critical to successful employee involvement. Educational and communication tools, such as videos, newsletters, books, and articles, may provide additional means for the nurse manager to utilize in training activities.

Timely and appropriate feedback from nurse managers is important. Nonjudgmental feedback will encourage employee creativity and enthusiasm. Managers may need to assist employees in identifying additional sources of information or in assessing the impact of improvement projects on other areas of the hospital. Feedback may be as simple as encouraging employees to put their ideas on paper or to participate in group quality activities. Employees need to feel free to offer suggestions, to participate in process change and evaluation, and to cross organizational boundaries in order to address interdepartmental and multidisciplinary issues.

Recognition of employee success is yet another important management role. Commonly used mechanisms for recognizing success include newsletters, storyboards, posters, pictures, and awards ceremonies. The effective nurse manager will seek to recognize employees in ways that are most meaningful to the employee. Public recognition of success enhances pride in achievements and encourages further involvement.

Staff ownership of quality improvement activity is critical to success. When provided with legitimate support from administrative leadership and nurse managers, clinical nurses are fully capable of effecting positive change through quality improvement projects. Streamlining documentation forms, reducing the occurrence of skin breakdown in rehabilitation patients, developing new strategies for family and patient education, reducing the level of noise on nursing units— all are examples of intradepartmental quality improvement projects in which clinical nurses can implement changes that have a positive impact on patient care.

Because many departments and disciplines contribute to the patient care delivery process, clinical nurses may participate actively in multidisciplinary and interdepartmental quality improvement teams. These teams might undertake such diverse projects as simplifying the admission process for same-day surgery patients, minimizing delays in completion of x-rays and diagnostic examinations, reducing the length of stay for coronary artery bypass patients, or eliminating errors in the charging of patient care supplies and equipment. Vesting accountability with the nurses who provide patient care results in improved care and enhanced self-esteem and professional satisfaction for the nurses involved in quality improvement activities.

Customer Satisfaction

Another element of the new era quality management program is a hospitalwide commitment to meet and exceed customer needs. Because all processes in hospitals are based on customer–supplier relationships, identification of customer needs and expectations is a key element in the improvement process. The patient is, of course, the ultimate customer in the hospital setting. However, linked customer–supplier processes throughout the organization are the basis of the care delivery system. The examples in Table 30–1 identify their relationship.

Identifying and implementing improvements in the customer–supplier process ultimately lead to more efficient care delivery for the patient.

Clinical competence and appropriateness have always been a basic tenet of patient care. However, the patient who has a prolonged wait in the admitting office may still remember this negative experience after his or her discharge, despite an excellent clinical outcome. Therefore, a quality improvement program may include assessing and improving waiting time in the admitting office as well as monitoring clinical aspects of care through more traditional inspection-oriented quality assurance.

Process Focus

Another key concept related to quality improvement is that processes, not individuals, are analyzed. Quality improvement focuses on improving process or work flow. Deming's 85–15 rule postulates that 85% of what goes wrong is

TABLE 30–1   Customer–Supplier Relationship

SUPPLIER	INTERNAL CUSTOMER
Radiology department	Physician waiting for a stat chest film
Central service	Nurse waiting for sterile supplies before doing a dressing change
Nurse	Physician receiving report on status of postoperative patient
Information systems	Admitting clerk waiting for data on previous patient admission

with the system and only 15% is with individuals or things (Walton, 1990, p. 20). The focus on process improvement instead of on individual bad apples is an important distinction from traditional quality assurance.

In many traditional inspection-oriented quality assurance programs, there is a tendency to address individual problems without resolving the underlying causative process issues within the system. For example, patients on a medical unit who have intravenous antibiotics ordered every 6 hours frequently receive their 6:00 AM doses 1 to 2 hours late. Several night nurses who are responsible for administering the late 6:00 AM doses have been counseled by the nurse manager about the need for timely medication administration. The nurses have explained that the antibiotics are administered late because medications are frequently not available on the unit for 6:00 AM doses. The nurse manager could respond by recommending that the nurses should plan ahead and check medication bins early in the shift, thereby identifying and obtaining missing doses before 6:00 AM.

However, a nurse manager who understands the concepts of quality improvement will recognize that the delayed medication administration times reflect an underlying problem in the medication delivery process. Inefficient processes within the system result in problems with medication availability. Improving processes involved in medication delivery systems will ultimately prove more effective than trying to correct isolated problems with individual practitioners. Improved processes will allow nurses to focus on providing better patient care rather than on resolving recurring problems in the system.

Tools and Techniques: Display and Measurement of Variation

Analysis of process variation is a key concept in quality improvement. This analysis is based, in part, on the use of graphic tools and techniques that visually display process variation. Using display and measurement of variation, process problems can be more easily identified, analyzed, and modified. The quality improvement and management literature contains many detailed explanations of quality improvement tools and techniques. A particularly helpful resource is *The Memory Jogger Plus +* (Brassard, 1989).

Application of some of the tools and techniques is described in the following example. The nursing leadership of a large metropolitan hospital noted an increasing problem with bed availability for admissions and transfers to both critical care and medical–surgical units. With the support of the hospital administration, they established a multidisciplinary quality improvement team with the goal of increasing bed availability within the institution. Team members represented nursing, environmental services, admitting, social services/discharge planning, laboratory, and administration.

The team initially brainstormed ideas about the possible causes of bed unavailability and then displayed this information on a cause and effect diagram (Fig. 30–1). Development of the cause and effect (fishbone) diagram encourages group participation and provides a useful mechanism for displaying complex issues.

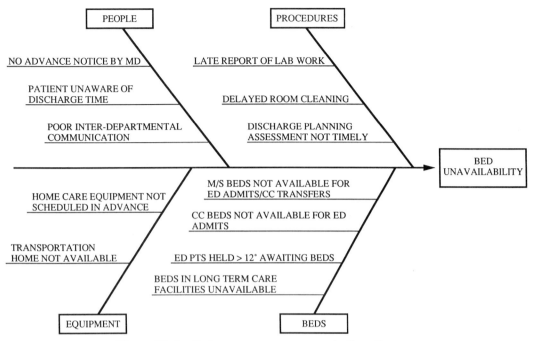

Figure 30–1   Bed management cause and effect diagram.

The team members believed that all of the causes identified contributed to bed unavailability. Some issues, such as faulty communication between nursing and admitting, were addressed immediately by establishing a daily multidisciplinary bed management meeting to prioritize and coordinate transfers and admissions. All routinely admitted patients are now provided with information about hospital discharge times. The environmental services department rescheduled administrative office cleaning for evening and nights to allow for cleaning of patient rooms during peak patient discharge periods.

With the help of the social service/discharge planning department, a data collection tool was developed to objectively identify the primary reason for delays (over 3 hours) in discharge and the frequency of these delays. Based on their findings, the team developed a Pareto chart to aid in prioritizing discharge issues and to measure the frequency of the delays (Fig. 30–2). Corrective actions to expedite the discharge planning process were implemented. At the request of the quality improvement team, the chief of staff sent a letter to all house staff and attending physicians requesting 24 to 48 hours advance notice of discharge planning or of home care needs. One additional FTE was added to the social service/discharge planning department to allow for more timely screening of discharge planning needs. The process changes implemented by the team significantly reduced the discharge delays within the facility and created the opportunity for increased admissions and additional revenue. A follow-up analysis

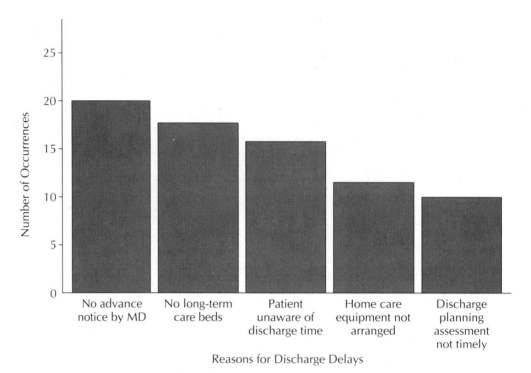

Figure 30–2 Discharge delays, January 1, 1991, to January 31, 1991.

conducted 9 months after the initial assessment documents the improvement (Fig. 30–3).

Because it is primarily due to problems in the external health care system, availability of long-term care beds remains an unresolved issue. The quality improvement team is continuing to work on methods to alleviate this problem. Additionally, the team is proceeding to resolve remaining bed management issues.

THE ORGANIZATIONAL QUALITY TEMPLATE

Hospital-based quality management programs are entering a period of transition. Current quality programs generally are based on identification of problems and opportunities for improvement, implementation of corrective actions, and remonitoring to ensure that the corrective actions have been effective. Clinical indicators and outcome measures selected by the various departments and committees are the primary methodology by which problems and opportunities to improve care are identified. Information from departmentalized quality improvement activity in the medical staff, nursing, and ancillary and support areas is generally reported through a central hospitalwide quality committee to the governing board. Although the traditional program has significant flaws, it does support the hospital's efforts to comply with externally mandated regulations

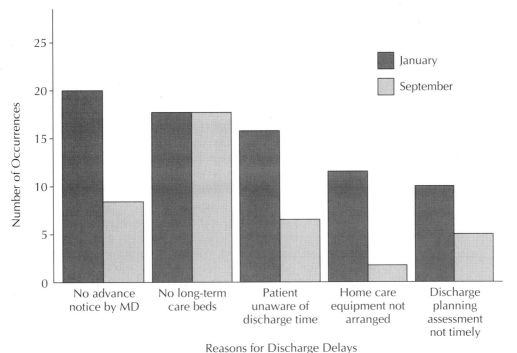

Figure 30–3 Comparative discharge delay analysis.

and standards and provides the primary internal mechanism for improving the quality of care delivered in the institution. However, better systems are possible.

Continuous Quality Improvement Trigger Points

Hospitals are struggling with ways to integrate the inspection-oriented traditional quality programs with the philosophy of CQI. They are not mutually exclusive. Traditional quality assurance can, in fact, serve as one of several mechanisms to trigger the CQI process. Additional trigger points may include

- Ineffective processes
- Customer satisfaction
- Third party payor demands for better value for health care dollars

For example, a clinical quality indicator in the SICU may be unplanned extubations. Through the traditional quality assurance monitoring process, a sudden increase in the frequency of unplanned extubations is identified. Rather than addressing the issue by looking for faulty practitioners, the SICU quality team employs quality improvement tools to analyze possible process variations within the care management system. Based on their findings, they implement changes in the processes involved in managing intubated patients and, over time, demonstrate an improvement in the clinical management of the intubated patient.

A much more complex example of trigger points leading to quality improvement is the implementation of practice guidelines or clinical protocols. For instance, a hospital that has an active open heart surgery program may be competing for patients with another hospital in the same city. If the quality of care (as defined by adjusted mortality and length of stay data) at both hospitals is within national norms, there may not be a clinical incentive to improve care. However, a powerful health care coalition in the city offers to shift a large number of patients to the hospital that can provide the best quality at the best price. Consumer and cost issues may become the trigger points for implementing quality improvement initiatives. These initiatives may take the form of implementation of clinical practice protocols (guidelines) that reduce variation within the care delivery process. Reduced variation generally leads to improvement in clinical management and may reduce the cost of providing care. Thus, there is an incentive for hospital management and clinical leaders to work cooperatively on quality improvement projects to achieve desired outcomes.

Operationalizing the integration of traditional quality programs with continuous organizationwide quality initiatives is a major challenge. The degree of integration between the two must be determined by the leaders within the organization. However, whether there is a close integration or a loose communication network between the two systems, hospital leaders must begin the implementation of at least limited quality improvement initiatives.

Schaffer and Thompson (1992, p. 82) suggest implementing "results driven improvement processes that focus on achieving specific, measurable operational improvements within a few months." They contend that when short-term incremental projects are substituted for large-scale amorphous improvement goals, managers and employees can more quickly identify tangible results. Over time, many small success stories can contribute to significant positive organizational change.

Fully implementing a hospital quality improvement program is a long-term process that may, even with strong management support, require years to fully integrate within the system. However, many hospitals can share success stories about effective short-term and long-term clinical and organizational quality improvement projects. The total integration of the old and the new approaches to quality management is, for the most part, still an evolving process and an emerging paradigm.

Implementation: The 14 Points for Success

Because quality improvement initiatives require a prolonged implementation period, hospitals cannot afford to wait to evaluate "how everyone else is doing it." Based on the preliminary experience of hospitals that are integrating traditional quality programs with organizational quality initiatives, certain key implementation principles seem to be emerging.

1. Involve the governing board from the inception of the integration process.
2. Establish a senior management council to coordinate and to participate in the organizationwide quality improvement program.

3. Identify the organizational vision and define the meaning of quality within the organizational culture.
4. Allocate sufficient resources to support the necessary organizational changes.
5. Maintain established mechanisms for quality monitoring during the initial stages of integration to ensure compliance with regulatory agencies and to maintain current levels of quality.
6. Develop mechanisms and structures to facilitate communication and to minimize duplication.
7. Promulgate the vision that everyone in the organization shares responsibility for quality.
8. Provide sufficient education and training related to conducting meetings, group process, conflict resolution and quality improvement principles, tools, and techniques.
9. Establish a quality assessment and improvement library that is accessible to all interested staff.
10. Use preexisitng quality assurance linkages, such as committees and reporting functions, to facilitate information flow.
11. Establish mechanisms to link current quality functions with both clinical and nonclinical project teams.
12. Form quality improvement project teams composed of individuals who have a vested interest in the success of the project.
13. Support active multidisciplinary participation on project teams.
14. Recognize, celebrate, and share successes and accomplishments.

QUALITY MANAGEMENT IN THE NURSING DIVISION

Just as there is an institutional template for a quality management program, the nursing division also must have such a plan. Just as a hospital organizes and structures for quality monitoring, so must nursing. Yet they are not totally separate and distinct endeavors but rather must be interactive and interdependent. The nursing quality management program should be a functional program (i.e., for nursing) as well as cross-functional and cross-disciplinary. Nursing, a major clinical discipline within the organization, bears serious responsibility for the continuous improvement of patient care services. This can be accomplished only through a well-planned and systematically executed program that will ensure a consistently high level of quality.

Today's Systems: One Hospital's Example

The continuous improvement of quality takes many forms. It is not a single activity but a continuum of multiple and diverse actions, all focused on enhancing the patient care product. These activities must coalesce into a comprehensive framework for a responsibly designed and executed quality program.

Many mandates are driving the actions of hospital nursing divisions. The JCAHO's Nursing Standards now contain a strong and clear emphasis on quality. There are stringent requirements for ensuring that these standards are met. The new requirement for development of The Hospital Plan for Nursing Care is further evidence of the firm commitment to ensuring that the entire organization is mobilized to provide the resources, structure, and leadership for the provision of high-quality patient care.

Therefore, one can conclude the following about the design of effective programs.

- The chief nursing officer and senior nursing management staff must provide unequivocal endorsement of the program.
- Structures, processes, and systems must be thoughtfully developed.
- Resource requirements, including dollars, people, system support (such as data analysis, materials), must be identified and provided.
- There must be a clearly articulated vision that is operationalized to support the constant assessment and improvement of patient care services.

To improve quality, one must vest authority and accountability with the clinical nurse who is close to the patient and actually delivering care. Instilling the feeling of the staff's ownership of quality is the goal. Clinical nurses are anxious to continually improve the quality of their care. Given the appropriate authority and resources, they will do so, and practice will improve continuously.

Practical Application

An illustration of this premise is the Professional Practice Analyst Program developed at Robert Wood Johnson University Hospital (Fralic, Kowalski, & Llewellyn, 1991). This is a unit-based quality monitoring system that has proven to be extremely effective. The philosophy that drives the system is that the nurse who provides the care is best positioned to evaluate and improve that care. Clinical nurses are best able to influence their peers regarding practice issues.

The Professional Practice Analysts are registered nurses, one from each nursing unit, elected by their peers to serve as their unit's agent for quality. Nurses who are elected are considered to be top clinicians in their area of practice. They willingly assume responsibility for quality on their unit for a 1 or 2 year term. They spend 1 day per month in business clothes on their unit—without patient care responsibilities—as they monitor quality. They review charts, interview patients and families, consult with staff, and monitor specifically selected quality indicators. They then meet monthly with their peers from throughout the hospital to discuss divisionwide and unit-specific quality issues. They receive support from the nursing systems department relative to data organization, collation, and analysis. They develop clinical quality indicators, identify areas for improvement, formulate action plans, communicate results to staff, and serve as the catalyst for CQI.

Before the inception of this program, quality was monitored in very traditional ways. Moreover, the nurses who delivered care were not involved with quality management in any substantive way, nor were they directly accountable for the process. They could not influence policy or systems effectively and predictably to enhance quality. The Professional Practice Analyst Program addressed all of these deficits.

The success of the program is clearly related to a firm management commitment to the program and its support. Time is made available for nurses to engage exclusively in quality monitoring activities, and a support structure was established to help them meet these responsibilities. Staffing hours on each unit that are not devoted to direct patient care are certainly an additional cost. However, effectively monitoring the quality of patient care, consistently enhancing practice, and critically analyzing the outcomes of nursing practice were deemed to be well worth the institution's investment (Fralic et al., 1991).

Quality escalates with a unit-based program operated by the staff nurses themselves. Centralized programs directed by QA nurses often do not have that major advantage. Hospitalwide resources can be mobilized when quality issues are systematically identified. Because of the staff nurses' contributions, significant clinical and systemwide improvements have been made. Such programs provide a highly effective and powerful stimulus for clinical nurses, they respond to their innate desire to continually enhance their practice, and they make major contributions to the overall clinical and financial integrity of the institution.

THE FUTURE PROMISE

New ways will be found to involve staff nurses consistently in the evaluation and improvement of clinical care. They will have significant institutional impact, since their contribution is critical. There will be a mobilization of the entire organization toward quality, and nursing will be an integral part of that effort. Ad hoc groups, matrix relationships, and multidisciplinary teams will characterize future systems for quality. These teams will not be satisfied with merely meeting standards. Rather, they will be driven by the mandate for continuously enhancing the quality of the patient care product. The process is never complete. Once processes are improved, the cycle of assessment and improvement continues.

Exceeding the standard will be the endorsed expectation. The nursing division's systems for quality management will be characterized by fluid boundaries, moving easily throughout the entire organization, and influencing broad changes in patient care systems. There will be more participation and self-determination by the grass roots caregivers.

As more health care organizations redesign their practice systems, new opportunities will continue to emerge. Patient care will be delivered increasingly by multidisciplinary and multifunctional groups, with nurses in pivotal positions. This will present the opportunity for the emergence of high performance teams dedicated to exceptional patient care quality. As the team delivers care and constantly evaluates that care, the CQI process will be molded and strengthened. Nursing will exert strong leadership in the design of enhanced systems that are committed to patient-centered care delivery.

The emergence of the nurse case manager also presents great opportunity for quality improvement. Nurse case managers epitomize the potential for nursing to be prominent in managing the cost–quality equation in health care. Effective nurse case managers in hospital situations go far beyond simply managing the stay. They manage both the cost and the quality of the care that patients receive. They track this care through clinical protocols, which are, in effect, practice guidelines. These protocols increasingly will be developed with multiprofessional groups, incorporating all key caregivers. Nurse case managers follow these guidelines, identifying both positive and negative variances as they occur. They analyze these variances with other disciplines, thus creating a true quality improvement team. Their analysis of the patient care process provides useful information for the entire organization. Through such processes, quality can only improve.

For example, the nurse case managers on the orthopedic unit at Robert Wood Johnson University Hospital in New Brunswick, New Jersey, noted that patients undergoing major joint replacement surgery had a prolonged length of stay. Data related to length of stay and treatment variances were collected. A targeted analysis resulted in identification of the need to increase availability and use of weekend physical therapy services. With the expansion of physical therapy support, patients were ready for earlier discharges, having met all quality targets. A follow-up analysis of the length of stay of joint replacement patients demonstrated significant improvement directly attributable to the intervention resulting from the quality improvement project. This process change resulted in measurable dollar savings to the institution and more appropriate clinical management for the patient.

These examples illustrate the quality cycle, that is, the contant assessment and improvement of quality (Fig. 30–4). Quality is a moving target in which assessment and improvement are a never ending cycle. Indeed, the quality assessment and quality improvement cycle is a continuous process without end.

Thus tomorrow's paradigm is quite exhilarating. Nursing's quality management activities will be far less compartmentalized, much more comprehensive,

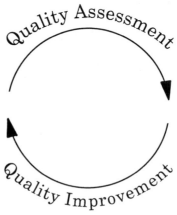

Figure 30–4   The quality cycle.

much less restrictive, and certainly more challenging. It is clear that the future health care system will be driven equally by both cost and quality. Nursing is extremely well positioned to make significant contributions by balancing these elements skillfully and simultaneously. As Dobyns and Crawford-Mason (1991) convey in the title of their provocative book, it will indeed be "quality or else."

CONCLUSION

The patient is the customer and the focus of health care. Hospitals must design and synchronize all systems to maximize attainment of this goal. Internally, barriers must be removed and collaborative practices supported. O'Leary (1991, p. 75) makes the following observations.

> But the successful organizations today are the organizations that have erased the lines between those boxes. They have figured out that in order to be successful, people must work together. Cooperation, coordination, and most difficult of all, communication are the keys to success. The organization must pull as one team in order to succeed . . . units in an organization exist in order to make the organization successful and not the other way around.

Organizations with a true passion for quality have the greatest chance of success in the challenging years ahead. That passion for quality must pervade the organization at every level and in every endeavor. Despite the increasing costs and regulatory constraints in all health care environments, the dedication to quality ultimately will translate to survival for organizations. All else being equal, customers—both individual patients and third party payors—will always opt for quality. It is up to us to deliver.

References

Berwick, D. M. (1989). Sounding board: Continuous improvement as an ideal in health care. *The New England Journal of Medicine, 320*(1), 53–56.

Brassard, M. (1989). *The memory jogger plus + .* Massachusetts: GOAL/QPC.

Deming, W. E. (1986). *Out of the crisis.* Boston: Massachusetts Institute of Technology, Center for Advanced Engineering Study.

Dobyns, L., & Crawford-Mason, C. (1991). *Quality or else: The revolution in world business.* Boston: Houghton Mifflin.

Fralic, M. F., Kowalski, P.M., & Llewellyn, F.A. (1991). The staff nurse as quality monitor. *American Journal of Nursing, 91*(4), 40–42.

Joint Commission on Accreditation of Healthcare Organizations. (1991). *An introduction to quality improvement in health care.* Chicago: Author.

Joint Commission on Accreditation of Health-

care Organizations. (1992). *Accreditation manual for hospitals.* Chicago: Author.

Joint Commission on Accreditation of Healthcare Organizations. (1994). *Accreditation Manual for Hospitals.* Chicago: Author.

Laffel, G., & Blumenthal, D. (1989). The case for using industrial quality management science in health care organizations. *Journal of the American Medical Association, 262*(20), 2869–2873.

Nielsen, P. A. (1992). Quality of care: Discovering a modified practice theory. *Journal of Nursing Care Quality, 6*(2), 63–76.

O'Leary, D. S. (1991). Accreditation in the quality improvement mold—a vision for tomorrow. *Quality Review Bulletin, 17*(3), 72–77.

Schafer, R.H., & Thomson, H.A. (1992, January–February). Successful change programs begin with results. *Harvard Business Review,* pp. 80–89.

Spath, P. L. (1991). *Health care quality: A prac-*

tical guide to continuous improvement. Oregon: Brown-Spath & Associates.

Walton, M. (1990). *Deming management at work.* New York: Putnam Publishing.

Williamson, J.W. (1991). Medical quality man-agement systems in perspective. In J.B. Couch (Ed.), *Health care quality management for the 21st century* (pp. 23–67). Tampa, FL: American College of Physician Executives.

Suggested Readings

Batalden, P.B. (1991). Building knowledge for quality improvement in healtcare: An intoductory glossary. *Journal of Quality Assurance, 13*(5), 8–12.

Crosby, P.B. (1979). *Quality is free: The art of making quality certain.* New York: McGraw-Hill.

Jeffer, E.K. (1992). Quality assurance and quality improvement: The 1990s and beyond. *Journal of Healthcare Quality, 14*(3), 36–40.

Kriegel, R.J., & Patler, L. (1991). *If it ain't broke . . . break it!* New York: Warner Books.

Longo, D.R., & Bohr, D.B. (Eds.). (1991). *Quantitative methods in quality management: A guide for practitioners.* Chicago: American Hospital Publishing.

The memory jogger: A pocket guide of tools for continuous improvement. (1988). Massachusetts: GOAL/QPC.

Peters, T., & Austin, N. (1985). *A Passion For Excellence.* New York: Random House.

Walton, M. (1986). *The Deming Management Method.* New York: Putnam Publishing.

CHAPTER 31

ETHICAL ISSUES IN NURSING PRACTICE

BARBARA J. YOUNGBERG

EXECUTIVE SUMMARY

The practice of nursing continues to evolve with nurses now finding that they are an integral part of a collaborative approach encompassing all elements of patient care. Where in the past the physical aspects of patient care received the most significant attention and nursing education focused on the science of caring for the physical manifestations of illness there is now an emerging importance placed on a holistic approach to patient care which takes into consideration not only the physical aspects of illness but the legal, ethical and psychological components as well. Understanding the nature of the ethical conflict and successfully addressing it through an appropriate and collaborative framework will be a continued challenge for the nurse and all other members of the health care team.

The health care system finds itself in a challenging position as the rapid advancements in health care technology compete with the rise in individual patient rights and the ability of the health care practitioner to significantly prolong life with the introduction of new drugs and procedures clashes with the rights of patients and their families to refuse such care. Ethical issues and the problems associated with those issues seem to have arisen because technology has developed faster than the ethical guidelines that would have enabled people to deal with the effects of that technology. In addition, the process of providing medical and nursing care historically has centered on making patients well, prolonging life and curing illness rather than assisting in the decision-making process that could shorten life or limit treatment.

This issue is further complicated because theology, medicine, and the law have all converged on the conflicts between the right to individuality and the prohibition against ending life or limiting or controlling it. Added to those theories postulated by lawyers, theologians, and physicians is the additional expectation created by the media, which suggests an often unrealistic expectation of what our current health care system is capable of providing.

In one of the sentinel cases to address ethical decision making, the New Jersey

Supreme Court *In re Quinlan, 70 NJ 10, 355 A.2d 647, 70 ALR 3d 205, cert den 429 US 922, 50 L Ed 2d 289, 97 S Ct 319 (1976)* stated

> Medicine with its combination of advanced technology and professional ethics is both able and inclined to prolong biological life. Law with its felt obligation to protect the life and freedom of the individual seeks to assure each person's right to live out his human life until its natural and inevitable conclusion. Theology with its acknowledgement of man's dissatisfaction with biological life as the ultimate source of joy . . . defends the sacredness of human life and defends it from all attack.

United States Supreme Court Justice Warren Burger admitted that in the triad of theology, medicine, and law, law was the last to evolve. He said, "The law always lags behind the most advanced thinking in every area. It must wait until the theologians and the moral leaders have created some common ground, some consensus."

In a more recent and well-publicized court decision *(Nancy Cruzan v. Missouri Department of Health),* the United States Supreme Court attempted to look to the wishes of patients as evidenced by written statements or verbalizations these patients had with others relating to decision making about health care, specifically the withholding or withdrawing of medical treatment. Although the Court did not allow for the termination of life support in this case, it recognized that competent individuals have a constitutionally protected right to refuse unwanted life-saving or life-prolonging treatment but must clearly express such wishes verbally or in writing.

THE ROLE OF THE NURSE

Although ethical decision making seems to receive its greatest attention when addressing end-of-life decisions, many other ethical issues complicate and compound the problems associated with the delivery of health care. These issues can relate to a varied population of patients with many different problems.

All of these convergent issues have added to the challenge of nursing, for it is the nurse who often is placed in the position of not only having to identify when an ethical issue is evolving but also to assist with its resolution. It is often the nurse who speaks with patients or their families and finds issues in conflict or questions about the appropriateness of care. The discussion of ethics and ethical decision making is fairly new to the practice of nursing. As with the profession of medicine, nurses are trained to be healers, supporters of life, professionals who have considerable skill at maintaining life and preventing death. Now, nurses are being asked to recognize that they have an equally important role in supporting patients in their death and assisting them in a decision making process that could actually hasten death or greatly influence the treatment provided. In addition to supporting patients and their families in this critical decision-making process, nurses are being asked to become educators, assisting patients and families in understanding all of the legal and ethical issues associated with making ethical decisions. Because there are many types of ethical issues that can arise, it is important to develop a process for handling ethical dilemmas in general rather than addressing a specific and isolated set of circumstances.

Ethical decision making as it relates to end-of-life choices spans a wide range of options. At one extreme are the well-publicized activities of Dr. Jack Kevorkian (referred to by the press as "Dr. Death"), who invented the "suicide machine," which enables terminally or chronically ill persons to self-administer lethal doses of drugs when they decide they no longer wish to live. At the other end of the spectrum is the recently enacted Patient Self-Determination Act, which promotes the belief that patients deserve to be advised of their right to make end-of-life decisions and should be given ample and appropriate information to assist them in this process. The responsibilities of the nurse as they relate to assisting the patient to make choices about treatment or refusal of that treatment fit somewhere between these two extremes. Often, the nurse's role as patient advocate makes discussion of these ethical dilemmas even more complicated. As the caregiver who has the most direct and sustained contact with the patient and the patient's family or significant others, the nurse may find that she or he is in the best position to address the issues related to ethical decision making and life support. However, the nurse may find that these discussions may be in conflict with the treatment plan that the physician has developed for the patient. Resolving these issues in a multidisciplinary manner so that the patient has a voice is a significant challenge for nurses and other members of the health care team.

Defining the many other ethical issues that arise within the hospital setting is part of the challenge to the health care professionals within the hospital.

IDENTIFYING OTHER ETHICAL ISSUES IN HEALTH CARE

Although most persons think of ethical decision making as related primarily to the refusal or withdrawal of life support, many other issues related to health care also give rise to ethical conflicts. A broad list of ethical dilemmas in the health care setting might include the following.

- The decision made by a competent patient to limit life-sustaining treatment or to not be resuscitated in the event of a cardiac or respiratory arrest
- The decision made by a family member or significant other to limit or terminate treatment in an incompetent patient or minor and the determination that this decision is representative of what the patient would have decided
- The decision to terminate a pregnancy and abort a fetus conceived through an act of violence, found to be genetically or physically impaired, or endangering the life of the mother
- The decision to aggressively treat and administer costly therapy to a preterm, low-birth-weight infant who may survive but be faced with multiple lifelong physical problems
- The decision to support the care of a preterm infant born with multiple anomalies attributed to drug abuse by the mother when there is an indication that the child will require lifelong care
- The decision to sterilize or castrate a patient—even when consent is obtained—or the decision to conceive a child so that its bone marrow or organs can be used to treat another sibling
- The decision to disseminate to patients information that may be in conflict

with the hospital's mission or philosophy or the beliefs or values of the nurse (such as, affording birth control or termination of pregnancy information to patients in a Catholic hospital)

- Decisions related to providing costly treatment, with limited proven efficacy, to patients with no means to pay for such treatment
- Issues related to access to care, rationing of care, and patient selection for procedures (such as organ transplant) where demand may exceed supply or where costs may be prohibitive
- Ethical conflicts among professional staff who may disagree on the treatment plan appropriate for a particular patient
- The appropriateness or duty of releasing information about a patient when withholding such information could jeopardize another's life or health
- The decision made by a health care facility to notify patients of the HIV-positive status of a caregiver with whom the patient had contact
- The decision to refuse to give consent on behalf of a minor for blood or surgery because of religious or cultural beliefs held by the parent or guardian when such refusal could result in the death of the child

All of these issues affect not only the person seeking or refusing treatment but also the caregivers involved in the decision-making process. Reaching a consensus that is consistent with the patient's wishes as well as with the mission of the hospital and the values of the caregivers and the community is a great challenge for the health care professional. It is a challenge that the nurse should be involved in from the outset.

ESTABLISHMENT OF AN ETHICS COMMITTEE

If not already involved in the hospitalwide ethics committee, nursing should begin to become represented in this forum. In the 1992 standards of the JCAHO *Accreditation Manual for Healthcare Organizations,* nursing participation on ethics committees is mandated. Ethics committees within hospitals should meet regularly to discuss actual ethical issues as well as to plan for potential ethical conflicts. The committee, if it is to provide the most value to the organization, should not be an ad hoc forum that meets only to resolve crises but should become a regular forum for establishing guidelines for staff specific to hospital policy. It should educate staff about state and federal laws that may affect ethical decision making and recognize in a proactive way instances or circumstances during which ethical conflicts may arise. Hospital ethics committees should have a broad cross-section of representatives from the organization. The multidisciplinary team should consist of members of all of the groups in the hospital who will be affected by the decisions reached and who can present a variety of views and opinions. Some hospitals have added to their ethics committees members of the community, so that the values of the community also can be considered in the decision-making process. Suggested members of a hospital ethics committee include the following.

- Members of the nursing staff—both staff and administration

- Members of the medical staff
- Hospital administration
- A health care attorney or hospital lawyer
- A hospital chaplain, ethicist, or community church leader
- Representative from the hospital marketing department, who may have to deal with the public's response to a decision made or to issues that receive media attention
- Laypersons who can represent the values of the community
- Other ad hoc members who may bring particular expertise if the ethical problem is a particularly complex or unusual one

Nurses play an important role in assisting the other members of the committee in identifying the many ethical issues that arise in the inpatient and outpatient settings. Many of these issues can arise from questions asked by patients and their families that relate to if and how care will be provided.

DEVELOPING A FRAMEWORK IN THE HOSPITAL TO ADDRESS ETHICAL DECISION MAKING

The nature of the business occuring within the hospital guarantees that a number of ethical challenges will arise. Though most persons equate ethical decision making with life and death decisions, a number of other circumstances may give rise to an ethical dilemma. Examples of other ethical conflicts that have received attention recently are listed in the preceding section. Although each conflict is different and once resolved will have different ramifications, the process used to evaluate the issue can be similar. Steps in the process might include the following.

1. What precisely is the ethical conflict? Is the conflict internal to the patient, or are the patient and the caregivers in conflict? Will the decision made affect the patient's prognosis, treatment, and outcome? Are potential additional conflicts likely to arise if a particular course of action is chosen? How does the law view the resolution of the conflict or the varying positions of the persons in conflict?
2. Who is involved in the ethical conflict? Are the appropriate people discussing the ethical conflict and its potential outcome? This question should include analysis of the patient and his or her family as well as the staff caring for the patient.
3. What are the possible alternatives that should be considered, and what is the likely outcome if a particular alternative is chosen over another? Have these alternatives been fully explained to the patient or surrogate decision maker?
4. Which (if any) of the alternatives fit most closely with the underlying philosophy of the organization and its staff?
5. Does the alternative chosen by the patient or family comply with state law or, if the law is silent, with the values and mores of the community?
6. What type of educational program can be developed to address issues

wherein ethical conflicts may arise? How can this information best reach the hospital staff? Does the hospital have the responsibility for also providing information to the community on these ethical issues?

Educational Initiatives

The nurse involved in education for staff should begin to develop resources for nursing staff that address the following issues. Becoming proactive in this area will enhance the likelihood that when ethical dilemmas or questions of choice arise, appropriate decisions will be made. Coincidentally, one of the components of the Patient Self-Determination Act is the education of persons within the staff and community relative to the Act.

The Patient Self-Determination Act

The Patient Self-Determination Act became effective December 1, 1991. The Act requires that all hospitals, nursing homes, home health agencies, hospices, and other institutions that receive Medicare or Medicaid funding (or both) provide patients, at the time of their admission, written information about their rights under state law to accept or refuse medical care and to formulate advanced directives. Specific provisions of the Act require that documentation be placed in the medical record indicating whether or not an advanced directive has been signed. The Act further requires that care not be conditional on whether or not a patient has executed an advanced directive. Hospitals are to have in place a policy that indicates how the Act will be operationalized within the hospital and how issues already settled by a companion state legislature will be addressed. The need to educate others about this Act is the final provision.

Advanced Directives

Advanced directives can take a number of forms. Basically, advanced directives are documents that provide a means to allow for self-determination even if the patient loses the capacity to make important end-of-life decisions. Advanced directives can take the form of the living will or the durable power of attorney.

Living Wills

Living wills are intended to provide documentation, in advance of illness, of a patient's preferences regarding administration of mechanical or artificial means of life support in the event of a terminal illness or condition. Although state statutes vary in their specificity, most allow for a living will to become effective when it has been determined that the patient has no reasonable hope of recovery and, because of the illness or condition, is unable to make decisions about continuation or termination of care. The living will can be modified or revoked by the person executing the document at any time during the person's life. If the document is executed in accordance with the relevant state statute, it is considered binding on all health care providers.

Although these documents can be very valuable in assisting family members and health care providers in making decisions for patients who are unable to make such decisions for themselves, problems often arise when the documents fail to provide with specificity the exact type of treatments or procedures being refused. An additional shortcoming of the living will is that the document can be executed using a standard form document and often is completed with dialogue occurring between the patient and the health care provider. This part of the process is essential to ensure that there is a clear understanding of the ramifications of the decisions made.

Durable Power of Attorney

The durable power of attorney is the legal empowerment of a designated person other than the patient to make decisions for the patient when the patient becomes incompetent. The word "durable" is important and can be contrasted with the simple power of attorney, which becomes ineffective immediately on the patient's incapacity. A durable power of attorney allows for the designation of a legally recognized surrogate decision maker for the incompetent patient. The responsibility of the person holding the durable power of attorney is to consider the medical choices available to the incompetent patient and to choose that course of treatment consistent with the type of care the patient would have chosen had he or she been in the position to make that decision. If no living will has been executed, the durable power of attorney allows for the transfer of decision making to the designated surrogate or agent.

This method of health care decision making obviously will work best if the person executing the durable power of attorney and the surrogate have a clear understanding of the decisions to be made in the event of incapacity of the patient. If no such discussions take place, such an instrument can place a significant burden on the designated surrogate or agent.

Surrogate Laws

A number of states recently have enacted laws that enable surrogates to make treatment decisions for incapacitated patients or patients otherwise unable to communicate their wishes (Table 31–1). Although these laws vary in their language, the important thing to recognize is that in most cases they allow for decisions to be made by someone other than an immediate family member,

TABLE 31–1 States with Surrogate Acts in Place

Oregon	Texas	Iowa
Montana	Hawaii	Illinois
Nevada	Ohio	North Carolina
Utah	Florida	Connecticut
New Mexico	Virginia	Maine
Arkansas	Louisiana	

provided that person has been named in the appropriate legal documents.

Having these issues worked out in advance and having a copy of the document itself in the hospital record can greatly minimize the likelihood that inappropriate treatment decisions are made or that a conflict arises between the provider and the family members of the incompetent patient.

The Role of the Nurse as Articulated by the American Nurses Association

The American Nurses Association (ANA) has articulated a position relative to the role of the nurse in the Patient Self-Determination Act. Although each hospital will establish its own policies on how they will comply with the Act, nurses generally have the following responsibilities.

- Be knowledgeable of state laws regarding advanced directives and be familiar with the various types of advanced directives
- Assist in providing patients with basic information about their right to consent or to refuse medical treatment as well as their right to execute advanced directives
- As part of the initial nursing assessment, determine whether the patient has executed an advanced directive, and if so, ensure that a copy of the document is placed with the patient's record and that all appropriate individuals are notified
- Help to ensure that advanced directives are current and reflect any changes in treatment decisions
- Ensure proper documentation of the medical record to indicate facility compliance with information provided and received from patients regarding advanced directives

Considering the breadth of ethical issues that the nurse may face in the course of providing care, it is advisable to develop similar methods for addressing other common ethical issues.

SPECIFIC ETHICAL ISSUES AFFECTING NURSING
Refusal of Surgery or Blood

Issues related to the refusal of blood or treatment often arise in critical or emergency situations. Many treatment decisions are influenced by religious beliefs or values that are protected under the Constitution. In most cases, the courts have decided that a competent adult can refuse blood or surgery even if such refusal could result in death. Courts are less willing to allow such refusal in the case of minors or incompetent persons, who may not understand the implications of such a decision.

Nurses should be aware of the steps the hospital has developed to address such concerns. In many cases, hospitals have specific forms denoting a patient's refusal of consent that must be completed and placed in the patient's permanent record. Emergency nurses, critical care nurses, or operating room nurses should know the process by which court orders can be obtained and who in the hospital must obtain them if such a refusal of treatment by a patient or family member seems inappropriate.

Issues Related to Children: Appropriateness of Consent for Treatment

A very difficult ethical dilemma can arise for the health care professional when the parents or legal guardians of a hospitalized child refuse consent for treatment that could improve the child's condition. When these issues arise, the nurse should feel comfortable in addressing the problem with the ethics committee. Using the framework established earlier in this chapter could assist the nursing staff and members of the ethics committee to better understand the dynamics behind this problem. In some cases, hospital staff may find that refusal is based on an unclear appreciation of either the gravity of the child's illness or of the consequences of refusing treatment. In other instances, the parent or guardian may fear that the treatments proposed will be too painful or dangerous, and it is that fear that results in the decision—not a desire to do the child harm. Although some states have addressed these issues through state child protective statutes or precedent-setting court decisions, most have not. It is, therefore, important that the hospital address how these treatment issues are handled.

Child Abuse

The incidence of child abuse continues to rise and has become a well-recognized cause of morbidity and mortality among children. Many stories reach the media illustrating what can happen when suspected abuse goes unreported for fear that the person suspecting the abuse is in error about how the injury actually occurred.

The role of the nurse (and any other health care providers) in reporting actual or suspected child abuse is clear. Many states require physicians and nurses to report all actual or suspected cases of child abuse—even if the parents vehemently deny such allegations. Health care providers should be aware that a majority of the mandatory reporting laws allow for immunity from civil suits filed by the parents provided the report was made in good faith and was based on a reasonable belief that the injuries were a result of negligence or an intent to harm.

Nurses working in pediatrics or the emergency department should seek to work with physicians, social workers, and legal counsel to define what state laws govern their practice. They should attempt to develop patient profiles (or obtain profiles already developed) that correlate certain types of injuries, presenting complaints, and behaviors as consistent with child abuse. This information should be included in the educational process of all nurses working in the area.

Abortion/Sterilization

A woman's right to terminate an unwanted pregnancy has been recognized by the U.S. Supreme Court since the landmark case of *Roe v. Wade*. In this case, the Court acknowledged a woman's right to privacy and her right to be responsible for decisions concerning her own body. Many recent cases have challenged this right, insisting that there is a countervailing right of the unborn fetus to be protected. Although the rights of women to make procreative decisions are being eroded continually, current law affords women the ultimate authority in the first trimester of pregnancy, with consideration of other factors as the pregnancy continues.

Nurses may find that such decisions are difficult for them to support or that they work in a setting that refuses to perform such procedures or to discuss them with patients. Although it may be difficult to put one's own beliefs or values aside, the nurse often will be expected to do so. The nurse should recognize that it is not appropriate to attempt to influence a patient in one way or another but rather to provide appropriate and complete information to a patient so that she can make an informed decision.

It is recommended that nurses look at the policies of hospitals with strong positions against birth control or abortion before accepting a position where basic values and beliefs will be in conflict. Following the ever changing legal developments in this area is critical so that hospital policies undergo frequent review and revision, and the nurse and the health care facility can maintain full compliance with the law.

The nurse also may find that ethical issues arise in cases related to sterilization. In general, legal decisions on this subject have dealt with two main issues. One, which is grounded in negligence rather than ethics, addresses failed sterilization. The other involves the appropriateness of sterilizing incompetent persons or persons who have been deemed by society as unfit to have children. In general, the courts have been reluctant to support the sterilization of incompetent persons. In a recent case, a man convicted of rape agreed to undergo castration as part of his punishment for the conviction. There was an uproar from the community at this prospect, which could have been related to the fact that the person agreed to be castrated but had minimal understanding of the ramifications of the procedure. The procedure was never performed.

Hospitals generally have very specific procedures related to sterilization. In some instances, these policies require that if the patient is married, consent of both partners is required. Understanding of these policies and procedures and adherence to them often after dialogue with the patient is part of the nurse's responsibility.

Clinical Research and Human Experimentation

Many new technologies and drugs are being developed that promise to bring about miraculous results and cures. As can be expected, patients with terminal illnesses with little hope of survival often fall prey to this new technology, willingly accepting any amount of pain or discomfort in exchange for the possibility that their lives will be prolonged. Abuse of a patient in the pursuit of medical research has been well documented and in most cases has been addressed appropriately by hospital research committees or institutional review boards (IRBs).

Nurses who work in settings where clinical research is conducted should familiarize themselves with the conditions for research described in the hospitals IRB documents. They should be familiar also with research protocols that govern current research and should, through their conversations with patients, verify their ongoing understanding of the positive and negative aspects of the research.

Bibliography

Annas, G. R. (1989). *The rights of patients: The basic ACLU guide to patients' rights.* Carbondale, IL: Southern Illinois University Press.

Beauchamp, T. L., & Childress, J. F. (1989). *Principles of biomedical ethics* (3rd ed.). New York: Oxford University Press.

Benjamin, M., & Curtis, J. (1986). *Ethics in nursing* (2nd ed.). New York: Oxford University Press.

Buchanan, A. E., & Brock, D. W. (1989). *Deciding for others: The ethics of surrogate decision making.* New York: Cambridge University Press.

Cohen, C. B. (1988). *Casebook on the termination of life-sustaining treatment and the care of the dying.* Bloomington, IN: Indiana University Press.

Culver, C. M., & Hanover, N. H. (Eds.). (1990). *Ethics at the bedside.* Dartmouth, NH: University Press of New England.

Forman, E. N., & Ladd, R. (1991). *Ethical dilemmas in pediatrics: A case study approach.* New York: Springer-Verlag.

Fowler, M. D. M., & Levine-Ariff, J. (1987). *Ethics at the bedside: A sourcebook for critical care nurses.* Philadelphia: J. B. Lippincott.

Gorovitz, S. (1991). *Drawing the line: Life, death and ethical choices in an American hospital.* New York: Oxford Universtiy Press.

Hosford, B. (1986). *Bioethics committees and health care decision making.* Rockville, MD: Aspen.

Jonsen, A. R., Siegler, M., & Winslade, W. J. (1986). *Clinical ethics: A practical approach to ethical decisions in clinical medicine* (2nd ed.). New York: Macmillan.

Kane, R. A., & Caplan, A. L. (Eds.). (1990). *Everyday ethics: Resolving dilemmas in nursing home life.* New York: Springer.

Kapp, M. B., Pies, H. E., & Doudera, A. E. (Eds.). (1986). *Legal and ethical aspects of health care for the elderly.* Ann Arbor, MI: Health Administration Press.

Kopelman, L. M., & Moskop, J. C. (Eds.). (1989). *Children and health care: Moral and social issues.* Boston: Kluwer Academic Press.

Lyon, J. (1985). *Playing God in the nursery.* New York: W. W. Norton.

Monagle, J., & Thomasma, D. C. (Eds.). (1988). *Medical ethics: A guide for health professionals.* Rockville, MD: Aspen.

Ross, J. W., et al. (1986). *Handbook for hospital ethics committees.* Chicago: American Hospital Publishing Co.

Society for the Right to Die. (1991). *Refusal of treatment legislation.* New York: Society for the Right to Die.

Thompson, J. B., & Thompson, H. O. (Eds.). (1990). *Professional ethics in nursing.* Malabar, FL: R. E. Krieger.

Weir, R. F. (Eds.). (1986). *Ethical issues in death and dying* (2nd ed.). New York: Columbia University Press.

Weir, R. F. (1989). *Abating treatment with critically ill patients: Ethical and legal limits to the medical prolongation of life.* New York: Oxford University Press.

Youngberg, B. J. (Ed.). (1991). *Quality and risk management in health care: An information service.* Gaithersburg, MD: Aspen Publishers.

CHAPTER 32 • • • • • • •

PATIENT CARE DELIVERY SYSTEMS

KAREN KOHRT RINGL

EXECUTIVE SUMMARY

Patient care delivery systems design, individualize, and delegate patient care activities in hospitals and other environments to nursing staff in order to meet the unique needs of patients. They provide the framework for registered nurses to assure that each patient's nursing care needs are met by an appropriate caregiver.

This chapter provides the reader with an in-depth overview of the traditional delivery systems used by nurses to deliver patient care and a review of the most common alternative delivery systems that have been developed in response to the changing health care environment. The key elements of each system are explained, including the origin and specific features of the system, the role and responsibilities of the staff nurse in the system, patient and physician satisfaction, quality and cost issues, and the role of the nurse manager.

First, the traditional systems are explained in detail. These are

- Case method or total patient care
- Functioning nursing
- Team or modular nursing
- Primary nursing

The reader is then challenged to rethink the way patient care is delivered and consider alternative delivery systems.

- Case management and managed care
- ProACT
- Partners in practice
- Health care technicians

Fiscal and clinical accountability of nurse managers is emphasized as they are challenged to evaluate each system to determine which one is best for their institution. Issues to consider and questions to ask are presented to assist the reader.

OVERVIEW OF DELIVERY SYSTEMS

A patient care delivery system is a method by which nursing care is delivered to patients. It is an assignment system that designs, individualizes, and delegates patient care activities in hospitals and in other environments to nursing staff in order to meet the unique needs of patients. Delivery systems provide the framework for registered nurses to assure that each patient's nursing care needs are met by an appropriate caregiver.

The best way to deliver patient care has been debated for over 50 years. During this time, no one system has been determined to be better than others because of the many variables in each institution. However, four traditional systems have evolved as professional nursing has continually attempted to improve the quality and decrease the cost of patient care.

1. Case method or total patient care
2. Functional nursing
3. Team or modular nursing
4. Primary nursing

The rapid changes in the health care environment initiated by implementation of the prospective payment system (PPS) have challenged professional nursing to rethink the way patient care is delivered and develop alternative models. Many models have been introduced that focus on restructuring the delivery of patient care. The most widely used alternative models are discussed.

1. Case management and managed care
2. ProACT nursing
3. Partners in practice
4. Health care technicians

The alternative models have used the best of the traditional systems and redesigned them to focus on clinically excellent, cost-effective care. They emphasize that registered nurses must proactively manage the delivery of patient care. In the face of a rapidly changing health care environment, a decreasing pool of nurses, and continually declining hospital revenues, nursing leaders must assure that patient care is delivered at the highest quality and the lowest cost possible.

DETERMINING THE BEST SYSTEM

Different systems are needed in different settings. For nurse managers to determine which system is best for their institutions, they need to consider the many variables that influence the health care system. The philosophy and policies of the health care organization and the nursing department are especially important. The effectiveness of any system will depend also on such variables as organizational climate, abilities of the nurses, needs of the patients, preferences of the medical staff, and requirements of the board of trustees. The availability of registered nurses, access to education and training, cultural diversity, and support for change also are variables the nurse manager should consider.

To make an intelligent decision about the best system for their area, nurse managers must understand the various components of patient care delivery systems. The key elements to consider in making a decision are

- The origin and features of the system
- The role and job satisfaction of the staff nurses
- Patient and physician satisfaction
- Quality and cost issues
- Role of the nurse manager

TYPES OF DELIVERY SYSTEMS
Traditional Delivery Systems
Case Method or Total Patient Care

Case method or total patient care is the oldest patient care delivery system (Marquis and Huston, 1992a). The case method has been used to deliver care since the beginning of the nineteenth century, when it was practiced in both hospitals and homes. In this system, one nurse assumes total responsibility for the complete care of the patient while she or he is on duty. Thus, it is essential that the nurse be competent to provide all of the care the patient needs. This method is used frequently in intensive care units to provide care to the most critically ill patients. It also is used as a method for teaching student nurses and assisting them to gain experience. A form of the case method is widely used in home health agencies.

Advantages and Disadvantages. Some staff nurses like this method of patient care because they can focus their complete attention on their patient(s) without having to worry about supervising other caregivers. Other nurses, however, do not like this method for that same reason. They believe their skills and time are wasted doing some of the patient care activities that could be done by less skilled workers. Thus, nurse satisfaction is greatly dependent on the skills and attitudes of the nurses.

Patient satisfaction is high with this method as long as continuity of care and communication are maintained between nurses. Patients and families feel a sense of security knowing one nurse will be with them throughout the shift but become concerned at change of shift when a different nurse appears. Physicians also are satisfied with case or total patient care, especially because they only have to find and communicate with one nurse. The key issue, as mentioned previously, is the competence of each nurse and her or his ability to establish a relationship with the patient quickly.

The quality of patient care under this system is high because registered nurses deliver all the care. However, quality of care can be compromised significantly when the nurse assigned to deliver total care to a patient is inadequately prepared to provide that care. Care planning with a strong focus on continuity of care and clinical expertise is a key area to address to assure that high-quality care is delivered to patients.

The cost of care in the case method or total patient care is probably the most detrimental factor. Because of the high percentage of registered nurses used to deliver direct patient care, this method is probably the most expensive to implement. Additionally, turnover or a shortage of nurses can make this system dependent on agency personnel or other temporary nurses. These nurses frequently are associated with high costs, low quality, and limited continuity of care.

The major role of the nurse manager when the case method or total patient care is used is to hire and maintain highly competent staff. The nurse manager needs an in-depth knowledge of her staff because the total needs of the patient will be met by one person during each shift. Thus, it is very important that the nurse assigned to each patient is competent to meet those needs. The nurse manager also must assure that each patient's continuity of care is maintained between nurses. Because only one nurse cares for a patient during a shift, there is no problem coordinating care during a shift. However, because each nurse has accountability during her tour of duty, there can be significant inconsistencies between nurses, and fragmented care can result.

Functional Nursing

Functional nursing was introduced during World War II because registered nurses were needed overseas and there were not enough nurses to meet the demands caused by the war (Marquis and Huston, 1992b). In the functional method, work assignments are divided into tasks and assigned to nursing and ancillary personnel. Each staff member has a fixed task that he or she is responsible for completing. One staff member will be assigned to pass medications, another to administer treatments, others to provide hygiene and assist with activities of daily living. An experienced staff nurse (or the nurse manager) usually is placed in charge of the other caregivers and frequently is responsible for assuring that nonlicensed personnel complete their tasks. Additionally, the registered nurse is responsible for all documentation in the medical record. Less experienced nurses are assigned tasks like other team members.

Advantages and Disadvantages. This method of care delivery was borrowed from industry, where this assembly line approach had proven to be very successful. It requires a lower level of commitment by the nurse or other caregiver to the patient because each caregiver is responsible for completing a task, not caring for a patient. The job satisfaction of nurses who desire a closer involvement with their patients is usually low. However, although research documents low satisfaction in nurses working in a functional setting, some nurses are more secure in a repetitive, task-oriented job. This is especially although not exclusively true in nonprofessional staff.

Regardless of the job satisfaction of the nursing staff, physicians and patients almost exclusively do not like functional nursing. Both are concerned about the fragmentation of care and the inability to find anyone who feels accountable for the total patient. Patients especially complain that there is a continual parade of staff coming into their rooms with a single purpose. None of the staff have the time to stop and talk with the patients because they have to go to the next patient and complete the task again.

The quality of patient care in this system has been highly criticized. Because of the task assignment mode, patient problems or needs frequently are overlooked because they do not fit into a defined assignment. Despite its problems, functional nursing is an excellent delivery system in a disaster or in periods of severe staffing shortages.

The cost efficiencies in functional nursing are very good. It has the greatest administrative efficiency because the division of labor is clearly stated, and there is little confusion regarding who does what. Functional nursing can be done with the smallest amount of staff, which makes it the most economical and the method of choice in a disaster. This method also best uses different skill levels. It requires minimal management time to coordinate activities of the staff because each level has clear task assignments.

The role of the nurse manager in functional nursing is usually that of an organizer and supervisor to assure that all tasks are completed. In this system, the nurse manager is a manager in the purest sense because only she has an overview of all of the patients on the unit and only she is responsible for assuring that all aspects of the patients' care have been met. Additionally, the nurse manager may be the only experienced registered nurse on the unit or one of only a few RNs.

Team or Modular Nursing

Team or modular nursing was introduced in the 1950s to address the problems associated with functional nursing (Marquis and Huston, 1992). By modifying the depersonalized and task focus of functional nursing, team nursing attempted to increase both nurse and patient satisfaction. Team or modular nursing uses a group of health care workers with varied skills, training, and licensure. They are directed by a leader to provide total services for a defined patient population. It is based on the premise of cooperation among team members.

Teams usually refer to larger groups of patients, whereas modules refer to smaller groups of patients. Other than this somewhat arbitrary definition, team and modular nursing are the same. The team or module should be led by a professional nurse with leadership skills and training. This nurse directs health care workers who, as a group, have agreed to work collaboratively and cooperatively to provide care to patients. The team shares the assessment, planning, implementation, and evaluation of care.

The role of the staff nurse in this method frequently is that of team leader. The team leader's primary responsibility is to assure that each patient assigned to the team is cared for by the mutual sharing of work by the team. She is responsible for coordinating and supervising the work of the team and assuring that all team members fully participate in the successful functioning of the team. Through the team process, the team leader plans, coordinates, supervises, evaluates, and participates in the delivery of care to patients. Because assignments are less routinized than in functional nursing, more time must be spent checking on the work of team members.

Advantages and Disadvantages. This system works well if the staff nurse has the training and experience necessary to lead a team. Frequently, however, insecure or inexperienced nurses are assigned the team-leading function. These nurses often do the work assigned to other team members because they are uncomfortable supervising and delegating to others. This problem definitely decreases the efficiency of team nursing. It also causes the team leader to be overworked and frustrated. This problem is one of the leading causes of turnover among nurses functioning in team-leading roles.

Despite the frustrations associated with team nursing, esprit de corps is usually high among the team because of the close interaction among the staff. When this occurs, nurse satisfaction is higher. Also, because the team assignment is associated with a group of patients instead of specific tasks, team members feel a greater sense of accomplishment and satisfaction because of closer nurse–patient relationships.

Patient and physician satisfaction is higher in team nursing than functional nursing because the patient has a greater sense that his or her needs are being identified and met. This satisfaction is even greater in modular nursing because the group of patients assigned to a module is less than the number assigned to a team. Thus, each patient feels a greater sense of personalized care.

A major problem with team or modular nursing that affects patient and physician satisfaction is the amount of time needed by the team to meet and share ideas and coordinate efforts. A frequent complaint is that patient lights are not answered or physicians cannot find anyone to answer their questions because everyone is in a team conference or at team report. Despite this problem, physicians generally are satisfied with this method because there are more nurses who are aware of their patients' needs and available to work with them. In some team situations, the physician will become part of the team and actively contribute in team conferences and rounds. This is easier to implement when physicians are assigned to a unit or service, as is done with medical school students or when a unit or team is assigned to one physician or physician group.

Quality of care in team or modular nursing is higher because the nurse has responsibility and accountability for less patients. Thus, she can know more about each of them. The team leader will be better able to match the needs of the patients with the skills of the staff and provide more direction, coordination, and supervision. This is important because having nurses doing many complex tasks increases the risk of errors. The team leader must know the skills of the team and evaluate the care closely to assure that errors are detected.

The increase in quality, job satisfaction, and patient satisfaction that resulted from team nursing came at a very high cost. There is significant loss of efficiency in team nursing. Good staff are restricted to a limited group of patients. This is especially true when large teams are broken into small modules. Most important, however, is the inefficiency caused by the loss of productive work time. The time spent in conferences and in coordinating, delegating, and supervising care makes team or modular nursing one of the most expensive models of patient care delivery.

In team or modular nursing, the nurse manager is responsible for assuring that the system is implemented properly and functions appropriately. Team nursing can become functional nursing without the proper guidance. The nurse manager must assure that the team leaders are qualified to lead. Inadequately trained team leaders and improper implementation are major reasons why team nursing does not work. The role of the nurse manager becomes one of educator, facilitator, supporter, and developer of the team leaders. As team leaders become experienced, the nurse manager can delegate many of the day to day management functions to the team leaders and expand her own managerial functions. Responsibilities for budget development and management and personnel functions, such as hiring, firing, counseling, and evaluating staff, are assumed by the nurse manager instead of by an area supervisor when team nursing is implemented appropriately.

Primary Nursing

Primary nursing was introduced by Manthey in the early 1970s as an entirely different method of patient care delivery (Manthey et al., 1970). It is a system for delivering nursing service that consists of the allocation and acceptance of 24 hour responsibility for patient care decision making by one nurse. It involves individualized, patient-centered care and direct communication with the patients, their families, physicians, and other nursing and support staff to assure continuity of care.

The principles of responsibility, authority, and accountability are essential to the successful implementation of primary nursing. Each primary nurse has a case load of patients for whose care she is responsible and accountable 24 hours a day. The primary nurse is responsible and has the authority to act in planning, organizing, and evaluating the effectiveness of the patient's nursing care in the same manner as the primary physician is responsible and has the authority to direct the patient's medical care. The primary nurse is responsible for introducing herself to the patient and explaining her responsibilities so the patient understands the role of the primary nurse.

It is important to note that the responsibility for planning and coordinating care does not mean that the primary nurse must deliver all the care any more than the primary physician delivers all the care he orders. However, many institutions implemented primary nursing with an all RN staff. When financial problems arose, many administrators associated primary nursing with an all RN staff and determined that they could not afford primary nursing. What they could not afford was the all RN staff. Primary nursing is a design concept that emphasizes professional practice in the delivery of patient care. It does not require an all RN staff.

The role of the staff nurse changes radically when adapting primary nursing from functional or team nursing. Primary nursing states that the staff nurses have full accountability for the care of their patients. The primary nurse must form therapeutic relationships with her or his patients and make decisions regarding their care. The primary nurse must be able to assess patients and obtain data and communicate this effectively to physicians and other health care colleagues.

Associate nurses may be assigned to deliver care to the patient under the primary nurse's direction or care for the patient following the primary nurse's care plan when the primary nurse is off duty. Associate nurses are usually RNs who work part time or evening or night shifts when it is difficult, although not impossible, to function as a primary nurse. New graduate nurses or other nurses who do not feel competent or compelled to carry out the responsibilities of a primary nurse may choose to function as associate nurses. LPNs and nurses' aides assist primary and associate nurses in the delivery of direct patient care.

Advantages and Disadvantages.   Nurses in primary nursing experience high job satisfaction. They are able to practice nursing the way they were taught and establish strong nurse–patient relationships. The patient outcomes are the direct result of the primary nurse's work and are not shared with a team of people. Thus, the nurse's job and career satisfaction is higher. Primary nursing allows the nurse to function in a highly professional capacity and allows for great professional autonomy.

Because nurses function highly autonomously, they sometimes feel isolated. This is especially true with nurses who enjoyed the highly social team nursing. This can be a problem that affects job satisfaction if other means of socialization are not created.

Despite the high satisfaction usually experienced by nurses delivering primary nursing, satisfaction is greatly dependent on the preparation of the nurse for the role of a primary nurse. A nurse who is not secure in her practice will feel threatened by the increased responsibilities of primary nursing. Patient care may be affected by a primary nurse not competent to fulfill her or his responsibilities. Despite this problem, primary nursing has very high patient satisfaction. Patients truly feel that they have one special nurse who is responsible for them. Many primary nurses have business cards that they give to their patients. The patients proudly show this to relatives and friends and talk about the wonderful things their nurse did for them.

Physicians have been very positive about primary nursing mainly because their patients like it so much and because they can go to their primary nurse for information on subtle changes in their patient's condition.

The quality of care is very high in primary nursing because the primary nurse can define and resolve the patient's problems. Better and faster patient outcomes result. The higher retention rate documented in primary nursing also creates higher quality.

Primary nursing has been demonstrated to be very cost effective when not implemented with an all RN staff. The best way to monitor cost is to review and carefully evaluate the cost per patient day of the staff. Mix of staff, regardless of the delivery system, is one of the key indicators of cost. Also, turnover costs and the resulting expense of hiring and training staff can be very expensive.

The role of the nurse manager in primary nursing is very different from that in the other delivery systems. In order for primary nursing to be successful, the nurse manager must empower the primary nurses. The role of the nurse manager becomes one of facilitator and supporter of staff. Since the primary nurses are the patient advocates, the nurse manager does not need to support the patients but does need to assure that the staff are empowered to fulfill this role. The nurse manager functions as a teacher and staff developer. Primary nurses must be competent to function in their roles, and the nurse manager must assure this competency. Monitoring and evaluation are very important to assure quality of care because no other nurses are doublechecking the primary nurse.

However, the manager must trust her staff to function in the independent role that primary nursing requires. The nurse manager must have the clinical skills to ensure development of standards of care that will achieve the desired patient outcomes and the managerial skills to monitor and evaluate the quality of care and the cost of care. The nurse manager also must incorporate an effective leadership style that allows the primary nurses to grow and develop professionally.

RESTRUCTURING CARE

The change from retrospective to prospective payment mandated the fiscal management of patient care. These changes have put the traditional nursing care delivery systems at risk of being outdated. Additionally, the changes limited the ability of hospitals to finance increasing nursing labor costs. Nursing shortage concerns in some parts of the country put pressure on institutions to offer competitive salaries and sometimes even bonuses. These factors indicate that nurses must be used more judiciously than ever before and delivery systems must be redesigned to enable fewer nurses to work more effectively. Thus, professional nursing has had to reexamine traditional patient care delivery systems and revise, adapt, or restructure them to achieve fiscal and clinical accountability.

Alternative practice models were designed to reduce the demand for registered nurses by better using their skills and supporting them with ancillary personnel. The new models frequently created two different RN roles, recognizing that some nurses desired to function in an expanded capacity and assume a managerial role in patient care, whereas other nurses wanted to deliver care during their tour of duty and did not want the added responsibility of planning and managing care. The alternative models recognized different nurses' experience and career goals.

Alternative models generally adopt one of the traditional systems as the core of the model. Thus, it is important to understand the key components of both the alternative model and the traditional model on which it was based. The design of these new systems is based on a clarification and refocus of professional practice that maximizes the role of registered nurses and holds them accountable for the outcomes of care. The models support clinical practice with appropriate ancillary services and focus on high quality at reasonable cost. The new models are structured to support clinical standards and continuous quality improvement (CQI).

Alternative Delivery Systems
Case Management and Managed Care

Case management and managed care are probably the most frequently used new systems (Zander, 1990). Managed care is a planned approach to the efficient use of economic, technologic, and human resources. In hospitals, it is a process of delivering care on a unit organized by specific case types. Accountability for the outcomes of care remains with the nurse manager.

Case management is a systematic approach to identifying the high-volume, high-cost, high-risk patients and coordinating and managing their care. Case managers are accountable for the outcomes of care of their patients wherever they are located. Both methods require a change from nurses planning care to nurses managing care. The patient care delivery system is adapted to focus on low-cost and high-quality outcomes.

Managed care and case management can be implemented with any traditional patient care delivery system but usually build on primary nursing. The primary nurse continues to maintain accountability for the clinical care of her patients and also continues to delegate nonnursing functions to support staff.

Case management may allocate the responsibility and authority to manage cases to case managers instead of line managers. Case managers manage patients in specific diagnostic categories throughout the patient's illness. Case managers usually are clinical specialists or experienced staff nurses who work in a collaborative practice with physicians. Case management attempts to connect the previously unconnected parts of the health system into a continuum of care.

Critical paths are a tool of managed care and case management. They are a framework for the care of the patient with a specific diagnosis. They define the specific aspects of care needed each day from admission through discharge for patients to assure that the patient's stay is as short as possible. Critical paths assure that the desired outcomes are achieved within the desired time frame. The critical path is a multidisciplinary plan, negotiated by physicians, nurses, other health care team members, and the patients and their families.

Nurses direct patients' care according to the critical path and evaluate variances from the path. Variances can then be used to identify quality concerns and improve care. Case managers or nurse managers evaluate their patients' progress according to the critical path, review variances from the path, determine if there is a problem to be fixed or an opportunity to improve care, and plan what they need to do to get their patients back on their path.

Advantages and Disadvantages.   Nurse satisfaction is high in managed care and case management especially because of the increased opportunities for nurses in expanded roles. Patient and physician satisfaction is usually high, although the pressure to follow the critical path and leave the hospital has created complaints from both doctors and patients.

Managed care and case management control costs by managing patient care to ensure optimum outcomes. In managed care, the nurse manager is responsible for assuring that the staff nurses follow the critical paths. The nurse manager is frequently the person accountable for the aggregate data, evaluating care and identifying opportunities to improve care. In case management, the case manager assumes these functions, and the nurse manager can play a more direct managerial and leadership role.

ProACT Nursing

ProACT model or professional advanced care team was developed by Tonges in the late 1980s (Tonges, 1989a,b). The ProACT model has two distinct roles for RNs: clinical care manager and primary nurse. ProACT maintains primary nursing as the patient care delivery system and expands it by creating an expanded role of clinical care manager that focuses on patient outcomes and variance analysis. The clinical care manager also trends data, determines potential problems, and develops solutions. Although the two positions are different in scope, they are equally important to the success of the model.

The responsibility of the clinical care manager is to coordinate patient care services, with an emphasis on fiscal accountability or the business of nursing. The clinical care manager is responsible for assuring that patients reach desired outcomes according to developed clinical protocols. The primary nurse is responsible for all nursing care on a 24 hours basis. She assesses, plans, and evaluates care and directs implementation through the use of LPNs and nurses' aides, who assist with care delivery.

ProACT creates more efficient use of clinical and nonclinical support services. Clinical and nonclinical support services are expanded to accomplish the non-nursing activities. In ProACT, expanded support services include creating support-service hosts to do housekeeping and other unit hotel-type tasks that free the nurse from these responsibilities.

ProACT initiated the role of clinical care manager so the management of patient care could be accomplished while focusing on the role of the primary nurse in care delivery. This allows nurses who do not want to assume responsibility in managing care to function as primary nurses.

The objectives of ProACT are to reduce the hospital stay and provide optimal clinical outcomes at minimal cost while assuring maximum reimbursement. Changes in the mix of staff, especially at the support level, have increased job satisfaction while cutting costs.

Advantages and Disadvantages. In ProACT, patient satisfaction is high. Nursing satisfaction is also high because nurses are able to choose the role of primary nursing or clinical case managers based on their individual career desires and talents. Physicians also have responded positively to the model.

In the ProACT model, the role of the nurse manager is much more administrative than in traditional systems because the clinical care manager manages patient care. The nurse manager also functions as teacher and supporter of the primary nurses.

Partners in Practice

Partners in practice is a nurse extender program developed by Manthey in the mid-1980s (Manthey, 1988). This is an alternative model that can be implemented with any delivery system, although it is most frequently implemented with primary nursing. It is based on the premise of an experienced nurse working in partnership with a practice partner. The practice partner is a technical assistant to the nurse. She is someone who can provide direct patient care and perform tasks under the supervision of the nurse. The difference between this system and other nurse extender systems is that the experienced nurse has the authority to hire her practice partner and determine work allocations. Thus, the practice partner functions only in a relationship with one RN. This RN, the senior partner, makes the final decision on the selection of her partner, and the two work the same schedule.

Partners in practice empowers the RN to make decisions about the care of the patients and allows her or him to work collaboratively with someone that she or he has hired and who has made a commitment to work in partnership with the RN. The previous problems RNs had of finding a nurse assistant when the nurse really needed help or trying to supervise aides who actually reported to and were evaluated by the nurse manager are eliminated by this system.

One of the most important aspects of this program is to train senior partners appropriately. Delegation skills, as well as hiring, firing, coaching, counseling, and teaching skills, need to be taught to the senior partners.

Determining the appropriate number of partnerships for each clinical area is very important. Not all RNs need to be senior partners, nor should they be assigned this role. Senior partners should be experienced nurses who want to work directly with a partner and who have the collaborative skills to do so. Senior partners should be promoted to the position after interview by the nurse manager. It is important to include the senior partners in assessment of the workload on their unit to determine what needs to be done by an RN and what can be delegated to the practice partner. In almost all cases, the RNs determine that much of the work they have been doing could be delegated to a practice partner they trust and who reports to them. State and federal licensing agencies need to be consulted to assure compliance with legal requirements, but careful discussion about the actual work nurses are doing reveals that much could be done by unlicensed personnel. In determining the workload and number of partnerships needed, it is important to ask what the nurse needs to know compared with what the nurse needs to do.

Advantages and Disadvantages.   Job satisfaction of the senior partner and the practice partner increases because work assignments are fair and nurses are not delegating work to a few assistants who do not know what to do first.

Patients and physician satisfaction is very high in this system because, like primary nursing, the patients feel that their nurse and the partner are accountable for their care. They know if their nurse is busy, her or his partner can help them or get their nurse.

The greatest savings come from the changes in the skill mix and the decrease in the numbers of registered nurses. However, decreased orientation costs and decreased turnover because of job satisfaction of both RNs and partners also provide significant savings.

The role of the nurse manager in partners in practice is complex because she or he has to assure that the partnerships are functioning appropriately and also maintain the delivery system that is being used. Scheduling the partners (on the same schedule) is usually a difficult task when combined with the usual problems of scheduling. However, the satisfaction of the nurses and their partners outweighs the problems in most situations.

Health Care Technicians

Health care technicians are not specifically an alternate delivery system but are used in almost all of them. As health care changes, the reexamination of delivery systems and skill mix requires that they be addressed seriously. Health care technicians frequently are renamed and retrained nurses' aides and other ancillary support staff used in expanded roles.

Advantages and Disadvantages.   Many innovative ways of using health care technicians are being tried. The most successful are those that use technicians to support patient care while freeing the registered nurse to do what only an RN can do. They incorporate the technicians into the unit under the direction of the nurse manager and eliminate unnecessary support service supervisors and traditional interdepartmental problems. By using health care technicians, hospitals can provide the patient care, housekeeping, clerical, transportation, and ancillary support that patients and nurses need without using the expensive resource of RNs.

Health care technicians are called by a variety of titles in many institutions. The major task in alternative delivery systems is to define clearly those functions and activities that can be performed by staff other than registered nurses and assure that the health care technicians, instead of nurses, perform those tasks. These decisions need to consider the skill and training of the technicians, state licensure laws, board of registered nursing regulations, and Joint Commission on Accreditation of Healthcare Organizations requirements.

Once these decisions are made, criterion-based job descriptions and written standards of care need to support the expectations. Among the most innovative uses of health care technicians are those being spearheaded by the ServiceMaster Company. They are incorporating traditional housekeeping tasks with those of passing dietary trays, transportation, and other hotel-type services into a role called "patient services representative." This technician role has job enrichment because of expanded functions and more patient involvement while incorporating employees into the health care team at the unit level who previously were not part of the team or concerned about the quality of patient care.

STRATEGIES FOR CHANGE

Change is hard work and very stressful. Many human elements have significant effects on successful change. Changing the delivery system can be unsuccessful if the change is not planned carefully or if the necessary resources and support necessary to make the change are not available. The nurse manager should carefully consider the following questions before beginning any change in delivery systems.

- What is the mission of the organization?
- Would a change in the patient care delivery system continue to support the mission?
- What is the philosophy of nursing?
- Does the proposed change continue to support the philosophy?
- Does the change support or hinder the goals of the organization and the department of nursing?
- Is the proposed system cost effective?
- Will the quality of patient care improve?
- Does the new system enhance patient and family satisfaction?
- Will the medical staff support a change to a new system?
- Will the job satisfaction of the nursing staff and other support staff improve?
- Can this job satisfaction be measured by increased productivity and decreased turnover?
- Does the new system enhance communication between all members of the health care team?
- Does the nurse manager have the necessary RNs to implement the system?
- Do they have the skills needed to meet the challenges of the new system?
- Does the nurse manager have the training support necessary to implement the change?
- Does the nurse manager have the support of top nursing administration to make change?
- Will the majority of the staff support changes in their roles and job descriptions?
- Will the changes negatively affect the communication patterns of the unit?
- Will the changes adversely effect the social relationships of the unit?
- Does the nurse manager have the desire and will to lead the change process from beginning to end?

Nurse managers are challenged more than ever before to provide the highest quality care at a very low cost. As Drucker frequently has emphasized, efficiency is doing things right; effectiveness is doing the right things. Doing the wrong things, regardless of how inexpensively they are done, is not what health care needs. Nurse managers have a tremendous opportunity to do the right things right. The resulting change will be the effectiveness of patient care.

References

Bennett, M. K., & Hylton, J. P. (1990). Modular nursing: Partners in professional practice. *Nursing Mangement, 21*(3), 20–24.

Brett, J. L., & Tonges, M. C. (1990). Restructured patient care delivery: Evaluation of the ProACT℠ model. *Nursing Economic$, 8*(1), 36–44.

Cronin, C. J., & Maklebust, J. (1989). Case-managed care: Capitalizing on the CNS. *Nursing Management, 20*(3), 38–47.

Ethridge, P., & Lamb, G. S. (1989). Professional nursing case management improves quality, access and costs. *Nursing Management, 20*(3), 30–35.

Ethridge, P., & Rusch, S. C. (1989). The professional nurse/case manager in changing organizational structures. *Series on Nursing Administration, 7*(2), 146–164.

Gardner, K. G. (1989). *The effects of primary versus team nursing on quality of patient care and impact on nursing staff and cost*. Rochester, NY: Rochester General Hospital.

Loveridge, C. E., et al. (1988). Developing case management in a primary nursing system. *Journal of Nursing Administration, 18*(10), 36–39.

Manthey, M., et al. (1970). Primary nursing: A return to the concept of "my nurse" and "my patient." *Nursing Forum, 9*(1) 65–83.

Manthey, M. (1988). Primary practice partners (a nurse extender system). *Nursing Mangement, 19*(3), 58–59.

Manthey, M. (1989). Practice partnerships: The newest concept in care delivery. *Journal of Nursing Administration, 19*(2), 33–35.

Manthey, M., & Kramer, M. (1970). A dialogue of primary nursing. *Nursing Forum, 9*(4) 356–379.

Marram, G., et al. (1976). *Cost effectiveness of primary & team nursing*. Wakefield, MA: Contemporary Publishing.

Marquis, B. L., & Huston, C. J. (1992a). *Leadership roles and management functions in nursing*. Philadelphia: J. B. Lippincott.

Marquis, B. L., & Huston, C. J. (1992b). *Organizing groups for patient care and committee work*. Philadelphia: J. B. Lippincott.

Melia, K. (1990). A decade of change. *Nursing Times, 86*(26), 33–34.

O'Malley, J., & Llorente, B. (1990). Back to the future: Redesigning the workplace. *Nursing Management, 21*(10), 46–48.

Pearson, M. A., & Schwartz, P. (1991). Primary practice partners: Analysis of cost and staff satisfaction. *Nursing Economic$, 9*(3), 201–204.

Spitzer, R. (1986). *Nursing productivity: The hospital's key to survival and productivity*. Chicago: S-N Publications.

Stevens, B. (1985). *The nurse as executive*. Rockville, MD: Aspen.

Tonges, M. C. (1989a). Redesigning hospital nursing practice: The professionally advanced Ca team (ProACT™) model, Part 1. *Journal of Nursing Administration, 19*(7), 31–38.

Tonges, M. C. (1989b). Redesigning hospital nursing practice: The professionally advanced Ca team (ProACT™) model, Part 2. *Journal of Nursing Administration, 19*(9), 19–22.

Wood, J., et al. (1990). An effort to indentify the optimum method of patient care delivery. *Critical Care Nursing Quarterly, 12*(4), 5–9.

Zander, K. (1990). Differentiating managed care and case management. *DEFINITION: The Center for Nursing Case Management, Inc. Newsletter, 5*(2), 1–2.

CHAPTER 33 • • • • • •

MANAGEMENT OF PATIENT EDUCATION

BARBARA KLUG REDMAN

EXECUTIVE SUMMARY

There is ample literature describing the benefits of patient education, arguably more than for many other technologies. Perhaps in part because this service has largely remained outside the reimbursement system, the delivery and documentation of patient education constitute a managerial challenge. In addition, there is not a strong and consistent group of professionals in this field who follow research findings and incorporate them into new programs. In other words, there is a weak technology development and dissemination system.

Especially in hospitals, organizational forms that especially support education have been reported. In most ordinary care situations, structure in the form of protocols, documentation forms, and training of staff to fulfill clear patient education responsibilities are useful. Where there has been careful development of a coherent program to treat a group of patients with a common clinical problem, education often is appropriately delivered, and these conditions of structure are met.

Philosophical and political forces advocating for patient autonomy and better involvement in health care decision making will likely continue. Education could play a significant role in better patient outcomes, including quality of life for the large population coping with chronic disease and in patient and family satisfaction with health care. There is considerable opportunity to further develop this service so that it is delivered with reliably high quality, costs are covered, and benefits are obtained for our patients as well as for the health care system.

P atient education is not only a very old element of nursing practice, it is also central to the profession's sense of purpose. Notions of nursing as an educational instrument, as a prime means by which patients develop self-care abilities, as an interpreter of the situation for the patient, and as a coach that helps shape the illness experience for the patient are spread liberally throughout the profession's theory base.

Whether any information was shared with the patient was for a long time thought to be a private matter decided by the physician. In recent years, however, nurse practice acts have become explicit about education being a function of nursing practice. Nurses, therefore, are responsible for inclusion of competent patient education in their practice. During the 1970s, the American Hospital Association endorsed a patient's bill of rights, and gradually, case law has found institutions liable if an untoward event occurred because they had not ensured adequate education of patients. Hospitals began to organize patient education services into programs so as not to depend solely on the interest or practice style of a particular professional.

The most recent survey of patient education programs, completed in 1987, showed that 87% of responding hospitals offered inpatient education programs, and 73% offered community health promotion programs. The nursing department or an education department was most commonly the mechanism for administering the education program. Twenty-one percent of responding hospitals, especially larger ones, reported having a consumer health library (AHA, 1987). Although there are no statistics that describe the amount of patient education currently delivered in any setting, it seems that the cost and reimbursement environment in which health care is now provided has decreased support for programs of patient education.

Management of the patient education function provides an opportunity and a challenge for nursing. As the largest health profession and the one whose practice is most centrally concerned with patient education, nursing has an opportunity to establish itself firmly as competent in delivering and managing these services. This is especially important because self-care, prevention of disease, and promotion of health, all of which require teaching, will inevitably be emphasized in the coming reform of the health care system, precipitated by issues of cost and lack of access. Nursing's Agenda for Health Care Reform (1991) describes a community-based, consumer-driven health care system that takes full advantage of educational services.

The challenge comes from the fact that patient education is an invisible service, supposedly provided by everyone but for which no one is held accountable, with few financial incentives and modest legal threats for practitioners but with an enormous potential for patient welfare. The literature on management of patient education is small compared with the immense literature dealing with the clinical functions of patient education. Yet there are good ideas about organizational forms that enhance delivery of these services, necessary staff development and motivation, and examination of the quality of care and outcomes to which education contributes.

For most managers of nursing services, ensuring an adequate flow of quality patient education services will require conscious and constant effort. This chapter focuses on ideas and tools necessary to attain this goal.

INCORPORATION OF PATIENT EDUCATION INTO HEALTH SERVICES

Incorporation of particular services into health care requires a legal and ethical base as well as the philosophic and regulatory base noted previously. Informed consent is the legal doctrine under which most patient education falls, yet it is widely understood that this doctrine is unevenly applied in clinical situations— usually applied in surgery and other invasive procedures but infrequently applied with drug therapy and in rehabilitation settings. Actual patient understanding about the decision he or she is to make is not the criterion against which practice is judged in many jurisdictions. Instead, practice is judged against the criterion of what patients are commonly told in that community of practitioners. Some physicians still believe that informed consent is an invasion of the physician–patient relationship. Many informed consent forms are written in such a complicated fashion that it is predictable that patients have little recall of what they signed (Redman, 1992). Fiesta (1991) notes that a nurse who obtains consent for a physician may become part of informed consent litigation, and if the hospital, by policy, involves its nurses this way, the hospital must understand that it is picking up liability exposure. The ethical base supporting patient education is even less well developed than is the legal base. I have defined it as encompassing access to these services if they are necessary when one is receiving care, and competent practice in attaining goals and avoiding negative side effects including indoctrination, to the level described in research-based practice standards. Perhaps one of the most difficult aspects for nurses is that they frequently find themselves in work situations where they must implement moral decisions in which they do not participate. This situation contributes to occupational stress and ethical anguish.

Patient education is delivered in all sites in which direct care is given. As hospital stays are shorter and chronic disease common, increasingly technology assists the continuation of education across care environments. Telephone programs have become important as a means to provide support and teaching as well as transmission of electrocardiograms. Education is given to caregivers for frail elderly or those with Alzheimer's disease and to families who are dealing with various stages of cancer in a loved one. In the past decade, education has been used with patients who are schizophrenic and with their families who must cope positively with their illness. In 1988, 8000 home care agencies were making 2 million home visits per week, many involving teaching. High-tech home care is now common and includes antibiotic therapy and chemotherapy, ventilation, cardiac monitoring and defibrillation, dialysis, and total parenteral nutrition (deLissovoy & Feustle, 1991).

Evidence of Efficacy of Patient Education

Although health care professions are gradually moving to research-based practice standards and guidelines, many standards and guidelines that now exist are based on professional consensus. There is a relatively large body of research about the outcomes of patient education, and it has been well summarized in some 35 review articles and meta-analyses. The latter are preferred, since they use a more statistically rigorous method of combining the results of individual research studies. Table 33–1 provides a brief summary of the most recent and relevant studies. A complete listing can be found in Redman (1992). An effect size (ES) of 0.5 means that the study group did 0.5 standard deviation better than did control or comparison group on the outcomes. An effect size of 0.3 standard deviation is small, 0.3 to 0.5 is moderately large, and over 0.5 is large.

TABLE 33-1 Sampling of the Literature on Outcomes of Patient Education

AUTHOR, DATE	FINDINGS
Broome, Lillis, & Smith, 1989	Analysis of 27 studies, 40% of which used cognitive and affective pain management interventions, usually immediately before the painful event. The pain management programs resulted in at least 30% reduction in children's distress responses.
Brown, 1990	Summarizes findings from 82 studies. Results indicate that patients who receive diabetes patient education experience improved knowledge, self-care behaviors, metabolic outcomes, and psychologic outcomes.
Devine & Cook, 1986	Summarizes findings from 102 studies of adult surgical patients. There were statistically reliable and positive effects on recovery, pain, psychologic well-being, and satisfaction. Average duration of treatment was 42 minutes.
Jones, 1986	Summarizes 27 studies completed from 1960 to 1981, finding an average effect size of 0.38. Compared with parents who did not take childbirth education, parents participating in it were more attentive and responsive to their infants, were more satisfied with the behavior of the infants, reported fewer feeding problems, had more positive feelings and attitudes toward their infants, and spent more time playing with and cuddling their infants.
Padgett et al., 1988	Diet instruction showed an effect size of 0.68, and social learning/behavior modification interventions an effect size of 0.57, with positive effects retained but decreased at 6 and 12 months.
Suls & Wan 1989	Combined sensory-procedural preparation for coping with stressful medical procedures yielded the strongest and most consistent benefits in terms of reducing negative affect, pain reports, and other rated distress. Procedural details provide a map of specific events, and sensory information facilitates their interpretation as nonthreatening.

The research base is perhaps strongest in the area of preparation for surgical and other procedures. In general, it is clear from the variety of reviews that a combination of information and psychosocial support and skill teaching is more effective than is any of these elements alone.

Contributions to the Business of Health Care

Reimbursement for patient education has been obtained as a part of skilled care for Medicare, for freestanding programs when the education and the caregivers meet stringent standards, and for programs integrated with other care. Education can be used as a marketing tool, to compete with other health care institutions offering similar services. One institution that found itself in intense price competition for mammography services used education for breast self-examination, a breast awareness promotional campaign with a hotline for a week, and information centers set up at shopping malls. Although the campaign cost $12,000, it brought in $17,000 of revenue. Had direct advertising been used, it would have been much more expensive (Marketing, 1989). Revenue can be obtained through program fees, contracts for services with businesses and other groups, sales of educational materials, and grants.

Increasingly, patient education managers in hospitals must be able to articulate the role of patient education in decreasing costs and nonprofitable DRGs and increasing appropriate admissions of profitable DRGs. Education before admission and after discharge generates increased revenue and can decrease inpatient hospital costs (Weinraub, 1985).

ORGANIZATIONAL FORMS FOR DELIVERY OF PATIENT EDUCATION

In the early 1970s, conscious attention to management of patient education in hospitals began to appear. Such management occurs on three levels.

1. Management of the educational process for individual patients
2. Management of educational programs for target groups of patients, such as those with diabetes
3. Management of patient education activities and programs throughout the institution

A series of surveys by the American Hospital Association, beginning in 1975 and extending through 1987, showed that in 1987 about two thirds of hospitals reported offering patient education services "with written goals and objectives for the patient and/or family related to therapeutic regimens, medical procedures and self-care" (Giloth, 1990). Many hospitals had multiple programs, most frequently coordinated by nursing or by an education department.

To coordinate and make patient education services efficient, several management structures were thought to be important.

1. Formal statement of a policy supporting patient education, usually issued by the CEO or board of trustees
2. A person to coordinate patient education services in the institution
3. A budget
4. An interdisciplinary committee with authority to
   - Identify, specify, and prioritize patient education needs in the institution
   - Develop and implement patient education policies and procedures
   - Oversee development and implementation of education programs, including their coordination and review
   - Train and develop staff
   - Identify and allocate resources to patient education programs, including purchase of teaching materials
   - Establish standards of quality and documentation of patient education

Perhaps the Department of Veterans Affairs most thoroughly developed the blueprint for this set of management structures (VA, 1987).

In institutions that retain some centralized management of patient education, there is much variation. These programs are administratively housed within different organizational units, may operate as separate departments or be subsumed within larger divisions, may have direct patient teaching responsibilities or function purely in a management capacity, may generate revenue or be non-revenue generating, and may maintain staff development or community education functions as well as a patient education focus. Rykwalder (1987) describes the department she heads at the University of Virginia Medical Center as responsible for the management of patient, family, and community health education services, organizationally placed in the division of clinical services headed by an associate hospital director, and having no direct patient education responsibility, since this is assumed by each care provider.

Some innovative care delivery models have used patient education as a central service. Perhaps most notable is the cooperative care unit pioneered at New York University Hospital in 1979. It emphasizes a structured health education program of general and specific education relating directly to the patient's illness for patient and care partner, usually a family member. The setting is homelike, and patients are brought to the centralized hospital service for clinical nursing and medical care and for educational sessions. Its development reflects at least two goals: that the traditional inpatient acute hospital setting is organized primarily for intensive management of disease but not well suited for patient education, leading to subsequent independent home self-management, and second, that significant costs can be saved by placing selected patients in a less care-intensive setting.

Six thousand patients have entered the program each year since 1981, most frequently with a diagnosis of infectious disease, neoplasms, or cardiovascular disorders. The length of stay averaged 4.5 to 5 days (Greico et al., 1990). There are perhaps 10 other facilities that have established cooperative care units based on the NYU model. The program recently underwent an evaluation (Chwalow et al., 1990). The study found that the less expensive cooperative care did not result in poorer health or functional status or increased use of services. There was, on the other hand, evidence of the positive effect of the unit on patient understanding, adherence to treatment, satisfaction, and self-management. NYU's cooperative care unit charged one third of the room rate for the hospital's acute care beds (Berg, 1991).

A similar model developed by Planetree focuses on a philosophy of teaching patients and caregivers as partners in care as well as improving their own wellness. Patients have access to their medical records and to a health information library and a self-medication program. There are five Planetree sites nationwide (Berg, 1991).

Other institutions have responded to changes in reimbursement and length of stay by developing outpatient education programs. Through its community nursing center, the Medical Center of Long Beach provided access to such programs as

1. A lactation service, which educates and supports breastfeeding mothers
2. A preoperative/preadmission education program
3. An enterostomal outpatient service

4. Living with Lung Disease, focusing on self-care skills training to patients with lung disease

Patients pay directly or by third party (Pappas & Van Scoy-Mosher, 1988).

Personnel Delivery Systems

There are several nursing roles in which patient education is firmly integrated and in which new roles are being developed. Ethridge (1991) describes the professional nurse case manager in a nursing HMO. Nurses provide care to patients who are physiologically imbalanced, emotionally challenged, have no caregivers or caregivers with a knowledge deficit, need more home care than qualified for, or consistently use the emergency room or the hospital for immediate health care needs. Clients consistently say that the nurse case managers have helped them recognize and manage early warning signs of acute exacerbation of their chronic illnesses. The nursing HMOs cut by one third the number of inpatient days for these enrollees, and those who were admitted had lower acuity.

Lind (1991) describes expansion of the RN role in a pediatric outpatient department from that of an assistant to that of an income-producing provider. This department served primarily patients covered by Medicaid and also used nurse practitioners. In the expanded role, the RNs independently provided care to children and families in need of education visits, many for lead poisoning, nutritional anemia, and complex prescriptive needs. They also provided direct services to children who needed vision or hearing screening, dressing changes, suture removal, immunizations, medication administration, or follow-up cultures. Standards of care and protocols were written, and RNs were provided with education about teaching. Revenue generated from RN visits rose 150% in 1 year.

Although these innovative models are to be applauded, there is still the widespread perception that the health care environment is full of obstacles to adequate delivery of patient education. Woodrow (1979) outlined those obstacles more than a decade ago, and the efforts of the 1980s in building systems of patient education were meant to address these concerns.

- Materials are not available for staff to use in patient education, and there is no system to keep materials current.
- Patients are too sick during hospitalization to learn, and there is no follow-up system.
- Hospital staff must reinvent the wheel because they are not aware of what has already been done in the area both inside and outside the hospital.
- The acuity/staffing system does not adequately reflect the patient's educational needs.
- There is no mechanism or system established whereby staff can charge time spent in patient education activities.
- There is lack of third party reimbursement for outpatient education.
- Space for patient education is extremely scarce.
- The cost of implementing a widescale program is high.

- Some professional staff members are not comfortable with the principles of teaching patients.

Webber (1990) further described the situation as clustering around problems of territorial imperatives between the professions about who is in charge of patient education, around lack of education of health professionals, especially physicians, for teaching responsibilities, and the low priority given by administrators to this function. Perhaps contributing to this set of problems is the near absence in the patient education literature of discussion of costs. Webber's recommendations include providing flexibility of present structures in health care, holding professionals responsible for outcomes they achieve—patient satisfaction—and indicators of health.

What little research literature there is on management of patient education programs suggests that more than just loosening structures is necessary. Several studies completed by Redman, Levine, and Howard (1987) found that the degree of structure for implementation (chart forms, procedures), provider perception of reinforcement for doing patient education, and perceived payoff from the program were significantly related to reported receipt of instruction by patients and reported delivery of instruction by providers. Age of the program, administrator support for social change, and staff support for the program did not show significant relationships with delivery of education. The study also found that in moderately developed institutional programs it was rare for there to be a single hospitalwide coordinator for patient education. Instead, coordinative functions were carried out by a variety of personnel.

In the diabetes education programs studied in community hospitals, according to patients an overall average of 43% of the topics commonly taught in such programs were taught to them, with between a third and three fourths of patients in the various study hospitals indicating that they had received no instruction. Staff reported that they lacked basic materials and incentives for carrying out instruction. A second study of the same research questions, carried out in a teaching hospital, found wide variability in the amount of structure available to support the education programs. Providers from the postpartum teaching program in this hospital indicated that these elements were present and adequate or excellent: program manual or guidelines, sample teaching plans, materials available for teaching, staff training materials, and chart forms for recording education. Audits including patient education, with feedback to staff, were reported to be in place about half the time. Materials to evaluate patients' learning were not well developed for any of the programs studied.

Reinforcements perceived by the providers were less a part of the formal reward structure by the employer (chance for promotion or raise in which excellence in patient education played a significant part, recognition from superior or colleagues for doing good patient education) and more likely to come from patients and from providers' own expectations of their professional role (Redman et al., 1987).

The other major study of management of patient education asks a narrower question about whether staff nurses are able to deliver efficacious educational services (O'Connor et al., 1990). The authors note that nearly all studies of the effectiveness of education with surgical patients, summarized in the review articles cited previously, used researchers to deliver the intervention. They ask whether staff nurses can deliver education with reliable patient benefits as part of their normal workload. Workshops were used to prepare these nurses for teaching surgical patients, which included learning by doing and observing models doing good teaching to generate the social energy and self-confidence necessary to carry out a new behavior. Nurses were familiarized with the teaching protocol, focusing on those elements that had been received by fewer than three fourths of the patients. Impediments to teaching were shared with administrators, and they were asked to make supportive environmental adjustments. Staff nurses indicated that patient education was barely mentioned in their annual evaluations and that their head nurses rarely discussed it with them. Much information and support were delivered, resulting in shorter lengths of stay, less use of sedatives, antiemetics, and hypnotics, and there was no adverse effect on other work activities. What seems clear is that teaching was accomplished concurrent with physical care, and probably the reason that teaching of skills related to postoperative care did not increase is that it frequently requires a separate block of time.

A number of surveys report that nurses place a very high value on patient education and see it as an important component of their jobs. There is spotty evidence, however, to show that nurses frequently believe that patients are not adequately taught before discharge (Redman, 1992).

The studies by O'Connor et al. (1990) and by Redman, Levine, and Howard (1987) attempt to identify elements in the system of caregiving and staff development that will better support consistent delivery of good quality patient education. There are also ways to hire or develop staff with special skills in this area of care. There are certified diabetes education specialists available, and childbirth education has for some time been a specialty. Institutions may use these specially trained persons to provide direct care or to serve as consultants to regular staff who may do the routine teaching, leaving complex educational cases to the specialists. Sometimes, institutions train their own nurses to increase their expertise in a particular area of patient education so that several individuals trained in different areas serve as resources for peers, patients, and families. One hospital used an expert patient education consultant to work with head nurses and staff nurses to develop and improve patient education, with the consultant withdrawing when the staff's skills had been developed. There is virtually no research addressing which of these strategies yields the best educational services.

This discussion has focused on development of personnel to serve the needs of individuals or target groups of patients. Individuals who manage complex programs of patient education for an institution need additional skills, which have been described by Young and Johnson (1984) (Table 33–2). It is worth noting that educators in these kinds of positions have organized themselves into local regional councils to share resources and to network.

Innovations in Organizational Management of Patient Education

There are reports in the literature of innovation in the management of patient education services. One example, described by Harvey and Hanchek (1991), was undertaken in response to early discharge. It included the need to reflect

TABLE 33–2 Competency Statements for Patient Education Director

I. Policy development
   A. Develop goals and philosophy statements for the patient education service
   B. Establish appropriate policies and procedures that support recognized standards of legal, cost, and quality accountability for institutionwide patient education services
   C. Maintain current knowledge regarding local, state, and federal legislation policy and trends related to patient education
II. Management
   A. Manage institutionwide patient education services
   B. Provide sound fiscal direction of patient education service-related resources
   C. Use current media and technology to ensure optimum quality of patient education services
III. Coordination of institutionwide patient education services
IV. Consultation
   A. Provide consultation to individuals, groups, and organizations institutionwide and seek consultation with outside experts to achieve patient education goals
V. Training and continuing education
   A. Assess training needs of those responsible for patient education

   B. Develop specific program goals, objectives, content, and implementation strategies for each program
VI. Program development for target populations
   A. Identify patient education needs through data collection and analysis
   B. Develop specific program goals, objectives, content, and implementation strategies for each program
   C. Organize and develop multidisciplinary task forces for patient education programs for specific target populations
   D. Analyze behavioral theory and empirical evidence from research and make interpretations to the practice of patient education
   E. Direct the implementation of patient education services
VII. Evaluation of patient education services
   A. Design and manage the evaluation and revision of patient education programs and activities
   B. Advocate the development of greater accountability for and quality of patient education services
VIII. Generic knowledge and skills (verbal and written communication, group meetings, liaisons, and cooperation)

From Young, B., & Johnson, L. (1984). The development of hospitalwide patient-education director competencies. *Patient Education and Counseling, 6,* 19–24, 1984. Used with permission.

standards of practice for their specialty and to meet JCAHO requirements and the need to adapt to a computerized information system for communication and documentation. The authors operated within their institution's interdisciplinary patient education committee, which appointed a task force to work on the transition. This group identified that they would use computer-generated teaching plans that could meet three essential needs.

1. A teaching/education guide
2. An informational handout for reference by patients
3. A documentation tool

These plans from Harvey and Hanchek (1991) were called interdisciplinary, to encourage their use by many disciplines. They contained common components and were written in patient objective format.

1. Disease process/risk factors
   Identifies . . .
2. Diagnostics/treatments
   Verbalizes rationale for . . .
3. Nutrition
   Describes the importance of . . .
4. Activity
   Identifies appropriate activity level . . .
5. Medications (purpose, dose, schedule, precautions, side effects)
   Verbalizes understanding of . . .
6. Additional self-care management
   Demonstrates . . .
7. Follow-up
   Identifies resources . . .
   Identifies warning signs in need of follow-up . . .
8. Special precautions/comments
   Identifies . . .*

The teaching plans became computer-generated forms, selected from an index of such forms. Instructions for use of the teaching plans came up on the computer when the teaching plan was selected. Before a patient's discharge, the nurse reviewed the plan, updated the status of the outcomes, noted any final patient instructions, and completed the documentation of the patient's responses. The copy of the plan that had been used for documentation was placed in the patient's chart, and the second copy was given to the patient for reference postdischarge. The authors reported that chart audits showed teaching plan usage and documentation to be improving slowly. They expected to develop a quality assurance monitoring tool that would evaluate whether the patient teaching system had influenced expected outcomes and documentation of patient progress (Harvey & Hanchek, 1991).

*Copyright by University of California, Irvine. Used by permission.

EDUCATION IN MANAGEMENT OF COMPLEX CLINICAL PROBLEMS

In addition to systems for the assignment of personnel to deliver educational services, sometimes complex care problems are addressed by interdisciplinary teams, establishing innovative protocols. The examples cited represent a program addressing serious degrees of noncompliance accompanied by social problems, a program to support safe self-care that would have cost considerably more if provided by professionals, and a home care program that relieved the hospital of considerable loss of money.

Glasgow et al. (1991) describe a program that identified a certain subset of adolescents with diabetes mellitus, who were repeatedly readmitted for ketoacidosis. They were generally poor, with limited community and social support, from one parent families, and lacking private insurance. The one major cause for this pattern was the failure to take insulin. An interdisciplinary team developed a focused program that addressed the problem through sequential steps. The first step was to explain that the readmissions were due to missed insulin injections and to fill patient and family knowledge gaps. If this did not solve the problem, the team confronted the patient and worked with him or her to take responsibility for the situation. Subsequent interventions were more directive and included having the parents assume administration of insulin, sending in a home care nurse to do so until the family could be reintegrated, and if all else failed, obtaining a court order. Readmissions were decreased by 47%.

Bradshaw, Sloane, and Chamberlain (1989) describe a college self-care cold clinic designed to help students decide

- If their symptoms were cold related
- How to reduce discomfort associated with symptoms
- When to see a health care provider
- When to use self-treatment strategies

The cold clinic provided mirrors, flashlights, tongue depressors for self-examination of throats, and thermometers, with photos of normal and abnormal throats. Over-the-counter medications were provided and accessible 24 hours a day. Before the course, many students with minor cold symptoms were occupying large amounts of clinicians' time, and others should have been seen early because of serious or advanced complications.

Goldberg et al. (1987) describe considerable economic losses to a hospital due to prospective payment policies that allowed insufficient reimbursement in an acute care setting for ventilator-assisted children. This hospital established a program to discharge a growing number of these children, including standards for reeducation and training of parents, family members, and home caregivers. Parents were first encouraged to assist in their child's basic care of feeding, dressing, and bathing, then taught tracheostomy care, suctioning, and bronchial drainage, and use of the ventilator and related equipment. If providers had concerns about the parents' preparedness, a contract was established with the family to perform their child's care in the hospital for a specified length of time, during which their capabilities were observed. The transition to home included

24 hours a day nursing care. The predischarge quality assurance checklist for this program is shown in Table 33–3.

There are many more examples that incorporate patient education more or less centrally to the resolution of important clinical problems. There is also much new knowledge about patient learning that could be incorporated into clinical care to improve outcomes. Unlike most of scientific medicine, there generally is a very weak system by which new knowledge about patient education is picked up and translated into improved care. Some involves new technology, such as the wallet-sized learning memory decision support system that helps patients with IDDM adjust their insulin dosages based on blood glucose, food intake, and exercise (Peters et al., 1991). This device serves as a catalyst of the learning process, as opposed to a technical controller of blood glucose.

Perhaps even more basic is the work that finds patients' cognitive models of their illnesses as highly predictive of their returning to work and their general adaptive functioning (LaCroix et al., 1991). These models or schemas include

- A belief in the relatedness of a variety of physiologic and psychologic functions
- A cluster of sensations, symptoms, emotions, and physical limitations in keeping with that belief
- A naive theory about the mechanisms that underlie these elements
- Implicit or explicit prescriptions for corrective action

The schemas not only organize the symptoms and emotions and beliefs but also serve as a guide to direct the patient to carry out active searches for symptoms and for causes. This finding may partially explain why there is often considerable discrepancy between the symptoms and the underlying pathologic conditions and why symptoms may vary widely in patients with similar underlying pathologic conditions. Patients who understood their symptoms and the relationship between them and their medical condition functioned at a higher level in their daily lives than did less well informed patients. The clinical implications are straightforward. It is important for patients to both understand and believe in correct schemas, and it is equally important to disentangle any previous misconceptions that patients or families may have developed.

TOOLS FOR PLANNING CARE AND JUDGING QUALITY

Quality can be defined as the degree of conformity with accepted practice standards, degree of fitness for the patient's needs, and degree of attainment of achievable outcomes (Slee, 1991).

Of the limited surveys that have been done, most report that nurses place a very high value on patient education and see it as an important part of their jobs but frequently believe that patients are not adequately taught in their institutions (Redman, 1992). Documentation is inevitably a problem, although a study by Sinclair (1991) showed that a nursing information system increased discharge teaching documentation and patient recall by 14%. A study of malpractice claims in four medical specialties in New Jersey found that 4% in obstetrics and gy-

TABLE 33–3 Children's Memorial Hospital Ventilator-Dependent Discharge Program Predischarge Quality Assurance Checklist*

Patient's name: _____ Date: _____

Parent's name: _____

	Satisfactory	Unsatisfactory	Does not apply
1. Each parent has a copy of the education program/orientation manual.			
2. Parents have copies of correspondence with community services and know who to contact if need arises.			
3. Parents understand who to call for emergency care.			
4. Parents understand who to call for medical advice.			
5. Parents understand who to call for equipment troubleshooting/repair.			
6. Parents have copies of all DME warranties, repurchase agreements, and service and preventive maintenance contracts as applicable.			
7. Parents understand how and when to order disposable supplies, as well as the mechanism for payment.			
8. Parents understand the mechanism of scheduling and payment for caretakers.			
9. Parents understand the medical conditions for their child that warrant a. contacting a physician and b. immediate rehospitalization.			
10. The VDDP coordinator has documentation of parent/caretaker knowledge and demonstrated skills for the child's medical home care.			

*A checklist helps to assure that parents have had the training that they need in order to care for their ventilator-dependent child at home.
From Goldberg, A.I., et al. (1987). Quality of care for life-supported children who require prolonged mechanical ventilation at home. *Quality Review Bulletin, 13* (March), 81–88.

TABLE 33–3 Children's Memorial Hospital Ventilator-Dependent Discharge Program Predischarge Quality Assurance Checklist* *Continued*

	Satisfactory	Unsatisfactory	Does not apply
11. Parents feel capable and are willing to provide for their child's			
• oxygen therapy;			
• artificial ventilation (includes manual resuscitators and phrenic pacers when applicable);			
• artificial airway management/tracheostomy care;			
• emergency care;			
• bronchial drainage;			
• portability;			
• medications; and			
• cardiopulmonary resuscitation (CPR).			
12. Parents feel comfortable enough with their child's medical home care protocol and equipment to take their child home.			

Parent's signature: _____ Presented by: _____

necology and 3.5% in general surgery were due to problems in communicating with the patient (Kravitz, Rolph, & McGuigan, 1991). Frequently, standards of patient education are process oriented; an example may be found in Wyness (1989). From the limited available evidence and from observations where health care is delivered, it seems clear that there is much that can be done to improve the quality of education.

A number of tools are available to measure quality and to improve the process of care. It is well known that patient education affects patient and family satisfaction with care. Reeder and Chen (1990) have developed a client satisfaction survey for home care, combining previously separate tools (Table 33–4). Hays et al. (1991) have developed a short-form patient judgment questionnaire that collects data about ease of getting information, clarity and completeness of discharge instructions, and explanations about costs.

Discharge represents a time during which patients move to the next phase of care, and institutions have a legal duty to protect patients from reasonably forseeable harm postdischarge, including a plan of care that patients understand. Garrard et al. (1987) have developed a patient discharge status checklist of inpatient behaviors, problems, or conditions that might warrant home health services (Table 33–5).

TABLE 33–4 Client Satisfaction Survey

Please circle the answer that best describes the nurse(s) caring for you.

	STRONGLY AGREE	AGREE	UNCERTAIN	DISAGREE	STRONGLY DISAGREE
1. The nurse listened well to what I had to say today.	1	2	3	4	5
2. When I need to talk to someone, I can go to the nurse with my problems.	1	2	3	4	5
3. The nurse should be more attentive to my needs.	1	2	3	4	5
4. The nurse asks a lot of questions; but once he or she finds the answers, he or she does not seem to do anything about them.	1	2	3	4	5
5. Just talking to the nurse makes me feel better.	1	2	3	4	5
6. I feel free to ask the nurse questions.	1	2	3	4	5
7. The nurse understood what my main health problem was today.	1	2	3	4	5
8. I feel the nurse talks down to me.	1	2	3	4	5
9. The nurse was understanding when she listened to my problems.	1	2	3	4	5
10. The nurse did not involve me as much as I wanted in deciding what I am expected to do for my health before my next visit.	1	2	3	4	5
11. The nurse gives directions at just the right speed for me.	1	2	3	4	5
12. The nurse involves my family or friend in supporting my health care.	1	2	3	4	5
13. The nurse makes it a point to show me how to carry out the doctor's orders.	1	2	3	4	5
14. The nurse and I decided together what needs to be done in order for me to stay as healthy as possible.	1	2	3	4	5
15. The nurse gives good advice about my health.	1	2	3	4	5
16. The nurse is just not patient enough with me.	1	2	3	4	5
17. I do not understand what I need to do in order to stay as well as possible.	1	2	3	4	5

Reprinted from Reeder, P.J., and Chen, S.C. (1990). A client satisfaction survey in home health care. *Journal of Nursing Quality Assurance, 5*(1), 20–21, with permission of Aspen Publishers, Inc., © 1990.

TABLE 33–4   Client Satisfaction Survey *Continued*

	Strongly Agree	Agree	Uncertain	Disagree	Strongly Disagree
18. The nurse explains things in language that I can understand.	1	2	3	4	5
19. The nurse seems too busy to spend time talking with me.	1	2	3	4	5
20. The nurse is often too disorganized to appear calm.	1	2	3	4	5
21. The nurse really knows what he or she is talking about.	1	2	3	4	5
22. The nurse is too slow to do things for me.	1	2	3	4	5
23. The nurse is not efficient in doing his or her work.	1	2	3	4	5
24. The nurse always gives complete enough explanations of why tests or certain procedures are ordered.	1	2	3	4	5
25. It is always easy to understand what the nurse is talking about.	1	2	3	4	5
26. The nurse is skillful in carrying out procedures.	1	2	3	4	5
27. The nurse spends as much time as necessary with me.	1	2	3	4	5
28. Too often the nurse thinks you can not understand the medical explanation of your illness, or he or she just does not bother to explain.	1	2	3	4	5
29. I have some complaints about my nursing care.	1	2	3	4	5
30. The nurse is pleasant to be around.	1	2	3	4	5
31. I wish the nurse would tell me more about the results of my tests or procedures.	1	2	3	4	5
32. The nurse should be more friendly.	1	2	3	4	5
33. The nurse is a person who can understand how I feel.	1	2	3	4	5
34. The nurse discussed whether or not there were changes in my health since his or her last visit.	1	2	3	4	5
35. I'm very satisfied with the nursing I receive.	1	2	3	4	5

TABLE 33–5 Patient Discharge Status Checklist

Instructions: √ all items that apply.

	√	HEALTH/MEDICAL PROBLEMS
1		End-stage disease with poor prognosis (cancer, COPD, end-stage renal, CHF, etc.)
2		Enteral or parenteral nutrition
3		IV therapy
4		Right atrial catheter (Broviac, Hickman, Leonard)
5		Open wound(s) and/or draining/non-draining tubes
6		Unresolved pain control
7		Needs frequent post-hospitalization monitoring of lab values/vital signs/health status/or self-medications
8		Recent dependency in activities of daily living (hemiplegic, paraplegic, quadraplegic, total body case, amputee, etc.)
9		Recent body image change (ostomy, trach, disfiguring surgery, etc.)
10		Health status significantly impacts on normal growth and development
11		Other (please specify)
12		Status reviewed, no service needs observed
		PSYCHOSOCIAL/BEHAVIORAL PROBLEMS
13		Patient and/or family non-acceptance of disease/prognosis
14		Patient and/or family making inappropriate or inadequate plans for post-hospitalization care
15		Emotional, behavioral or mental health problems substantially impairing daily functioning
16		Evidence or suspicion of lack of compliance with or understanding of care plan
17		Other (please specify)
18		Status reviewed, no service needs observed
		EDUCATION/COORDINATION OF CARE NEEDS
19		Additional patient and/or family education is needed to provide self-care after discharge
20		Care needs to be coordinated with other services (e.g., P.T., O.T., home health aide, etc.) or other agencies
21		Lack of competent care provider in the home if patient is dependent on self-care
22		Home needs physical modifications for care of patient
23		Patient and/or family needs help with obtaining medical equipment
24		Other (please specify)
25		Status reviewed, no service needs observed
	COMMENTS:	

From Garrard, J., et al. (1987). A checklist to assess the need for home health care: Instrument development and validation. *Public Health Nursing, 4,* 212–218. Reprinted by permission of Blackwell Scientific Publications, Inc.

There are a number of case examples of quality assurance studies in which patient education is central. One is reported by nurses in the medical critical care unit (MCCU) at a VA medical center, targeting patients admitted with a preliminary diagnosis of rule out myocardial infarction. The initial monitor of quality measured the immediate improvement in patient knowledge. The long-

TABLE 33–6 Palo Alto VAMC Nursing Service Ward QA Report

for ward: MCCU   for: April 1990

CLINICAL INDICATOR: 90% of patients will verbalize knowledge of symptoms of angina and appropriate responses to symptoms after receiving MCCU Patient Education Program. 75% of returning patients will demonstrate compliance with taking appropriate actions when angina is recognized.

FINDINGS	CONCLUSION	RECOMMENDED ACTIONS	ACTIONS TAKEN	EVALUATION OF ACTIONS TAKEN
1. 14 of 19 pts. (75%) admitted in April for R/O MI rec'd education.	1. Sevenfold increase in teaching.	1. Continue reinforcing need to teach all admissions. Inservice staff as needed. Include completed sample monitor as a model in Patient Education binder.	1. First revision of tool completed.	1. Tool simpler to use; clearly documents pts. understanding.
2. Only 2 of 14 pts. (14%) responded appropriately to chest pain preadmission.	2. Pts. continue to show need for teaching.		2. QA monitor report presented to both nursing/multidisciplinary staff in April.	2. All staff feedback very positive.
3. All pts. post-education verbalized knowledge.	3. Teaching successful in the short-range.	2. Patient Education Committee to critique forms at May meeting.	3. Rough draft of pamphlet approved by Cardiology.	3. Solid foundation for future expansion of project.
4. No patients previously taught returned to MCCU.	4. Long-range result unknown.			

Staff: Joan Keenan, RN; Joan McAuliffe, RN, CCRN; Marina Pabinguit, RN; Laurel Schott, RN, CCRN; Carol Yamane, RN, (MCCU QA Coordinator); Head Nurse Kim Coppin, RN, CCRN
Original: August 1987
Revised: November 1989

From Arnoldussen, B., Coppin, K., and Schott, L. (1991). Patient education as a quality indicator in critical care: Ischemic heart disease—recognition and response. *AACN: Clinical Issues in Critical Care Nursing, 2,* 56–62.

range monitor was the assessment of improvement in patients' compliance as some returned to the MCCU on rehospitalization. At this time, the nurses compared patients' most recent behavioral response to angina with their original behavior (Arnoldussen, Cappin, & Schott, 1991). Their quality assurance report is reproduced in Table 33–6.

WILL PATIENT EDUCATION REMAIN PERIPHERAL?

Since it is likely that health care will face significant reforms in the next few years, it is not entirely possible to predict whether patient education will occupy a more central role than it does now. Most parties calling for reform are addressing primarily the financing of the system. Fewer groups, nursing included, call for reform of the delivery system and of the balance of services between primary and preventive care and acute care.

Patient Self-Determination Act

There are several trends in health care that affect patient education and that seem likely to continue. One is public demand that patients have authority to make a broad range of choices. Perhaps the most recent indication of this trend is the Patient Self-Determination Act, which went into effect December 1, 1991. It requires that Medicare- and Medicaid-reimbursed agencies have in place written policies and procedures regarding use of advanced directives and provide written information to patients at admission about their right to an advanced directive. Agencies could comply with the act by giving patients complicated written information, or they could assist patients to understand and make true self-determinations (Flarey, 1991). The American Nurses Association (1991) recommends that questions about advanced directives be part of the nursing admission assessment.

A goal of the statute is to encourage but not require adults to fill out advanced directives. The quality of patient decisions depends a good deal on the quality of the counseling they receive. So, also, must providers work with proxies, helping them to identify their own matters of concern, to separate those from the patient's, and to focus on the patient's wishes and interests in making decisions about treatment.

Educating Chronically Ill Patients

A second trend should be recognized. Since the initial work in diabetes education occurred after the discovery of insulin, those working with various disease entities have, almost in turn, discovered the benefits and necessity of patient education. The two most recent areas to do so include psychiatry and epilepsy. Within the last decade, instruction has become available for patients who are schizophrenic or depressed and for their families who must assist them with daily living. It is believed that the lag in development of these interventions occurred partly because of the assumptions that these patients might be unable to comprehend and were unmotivated to learn. Instruction may focus on screening and prevention of those who may be depressed, on community adjustment and medication adherence skills, and on simply understanding the disease.

Until recently, pharmacologic and surgical approaches dominated treatment of epilepsy. Now, behavioral approaches to seizure control and patient self-management have been developed. Patients are taught how to monitor and self-regulate behaviors affecting seizure susceptibility, such as stress, sleep, photic stimulation, and excessive use of recreational drugs and alcohol (Legion, 1991). These techniques, as well as appropriate use of antiepileptic medications, can yield a better quality of life for patients and family. Clearly, this is a single example of the tremendous challenges before us to help patients and families deal with chronic illness and one that our acute care-oriented system has not addressed sufficiently.

Educating Patients on Proper Medication Use

A revolution in accountability is occurring in health care and clearly will be part of health care reform, which seems imminent. One example of the part that patient education can play in this reform has been pointed out by the Commissioner of the Food and Drug Administration. He notes that evidence suggests that inadequate communication about drugs is one of the principal reasons why 30% to 55% of patients deviate from their regimens, and patients' misunderstanding of the proper use of medications also is an underlying cause of many adverse drug reactions. In the mid-1980s, a nationwide poll found that one third of patients did not receive counseling at either the physician's office or the pharmacy unless they asked for information. Just over 30% were warned at their doctors' offices about the potential risks of prescribed medication. At the pharmacy, similar counseling was half as frequent. The FDA has plans to assume a supportive role in fostering the development of computer-based patient information materials (Kessler, 1991). Nursing's Agenda for Health Care Reform (1991) emphasizes consumer responsibility for personal health, self-care, and informed decision making in selecting health care services.

References

American Hospital Association. (1987). Census of hospital-based health promotion and patient education programs. Chicago: Author.

American Nurses Association. (1991). Nursing and the Patient Self-Determination Act. Kansas City, MO: Author.

Arnoldussen, B., Coppin, K., & Schott, L. (1991). Patient education as a quality indicator in critical care: Ischemic heart disease—recognition and response. *AACN: Clinical Issues in Critical Care Nursing, 2,* 56–62.

Berg, E. (1991). Teaming up to improve quality of patient care. *Modern Healthcare, 21*(31), 27–32.

Bradshaw, J.F., Sloane, B.C., & Chamberlain, M.D. (1989). Implementing a college self-care cold clinic: Administrative, educational and program planning issues. *Patient Education and Counseling, 14,* 147–158.

Broome, M.E., Lillis, P.P., & Smith, M.C. (1990). Pain interventions with children: A meta-analysis of research. *Nursing Research, 38,* 154–158.

Brown, S.A. (1990). Studies of educational interventions and outcomes in diabetic adults: A meta-analysis revisited. *Patient Education and Counseling, 16,* 189–215.

Chwalow, A.J., et al. (1990). Effectiveness of a hospital-based cooperative care model on patients' functional status and utilization. *Pa-tient Education and Counseling, 15,* 17–28.

deLissovoy, G., & Feustle, J.A. (1991). Advanced home health care. *Health Policy, 17,* 227–242.

Devine, E.C., & Cook, T.D. (1986). Clinical and cost-saving effects of psychoeducational interventions with surgical patients: A meta-analysis. *Research in Nursing and Health, 9,* 89–105.

Ethridge, P. (1991). A nursing HMO: Carondelet St. Mary's experience. *Nursing Management, 22*(7), 22–27.

Fiesta, J. (1991). Informed consent process—whose legal duty? *Nursing Management, 22,* 17–18.

Flarey, D.L. (1991). Advanced directives: In search of self-determination. *Journal of Nursing Administration, 21*(11), 16–22.

Garrard, J., et al. (1987). A checklist to assess the need for home health care: Instrument development and validation. *Public Health Nursing, 4,* 212–218.

Giloth, B.E. (1990). Management of patient education in US hospitals: Evolution of a concept. *Patient Education and Counseling, 15,* 101–111.

Glasgow, A.M., et al. (1991). Readmissions of children with diabetes mellitus to a children's hospital. *Pediatrics, 88,* 98–104.

Goldberg, A.I., et al. (1987). Quality of care for

life-supported children who require prolonged mechanical ventilation at home. *Quality Review Bulletin, 13,* 81–87.

Greico, A.J., et al. (1990). New York University Medical Center's cooperative care unit: Patient education and family participation during hospitalization—The first ten years. *Patient Education and Counseling, 15,* 3–15.

Harvey, C.V., & Hanchek, K. (1991). Interdisciplinary patient teaching plans: Design and implementation. *Orthopaedic Nursing, 10,* 55–62.

Hays, R.D., et al. (1991). Hospital quality trends: A short-form patient-based measure. *Medical Care, 29,* 661–668.

Jones, L.C. (1986). A meta-analytic study of the effects of childbirth education on the parent–infant relationship. *Health Care Women International, 7,* 357–370.

Kessler, D.A. (1991). Communicating with patients about their medications. *New England Journal of Medicine, 325,* 1650–1652.

Kravitz, R.L., Rolph, J.E., & McGuigan, K. (1991). Malpractice claims data as a quality improvement tool. *Journal of the American Medical Association, 266,* 2087–2092.

LaCroix, J.M., et al. (1991). Symptom schemata in chronic respiratory patients. *Health Psychology, 10,* 268–273.

Legion, V. (1991). Health education for self-management by people with epilepsy. *Journal of Neuroscience Nursing, 23,* 300–305.

Lind, P.H. (1991). Making the most of the R.N. in a pediatric outpatient setting. *Maternal Child Nursing, 16,* 267–271.

Marketing mammography: Education key. (1989). *Hospitals, 63*(4), 44.

Nursing's Agenda for Health Care Reform. (1991). Kansas City, MO: American Nurses Association.

O'Connor, F.W., et al. (1990). Enhancing surgical nurses' patient education: Development and evaluation of an intervention. *Patient Education and Counseling, 16,* 7–20.

Padgett, D., et al. (1988). Meta-analysis of the effects of educational and psychosocial interventions on management of diabetes mellitus. *Journal of Clinical Epidemiology, 41,* 1007–1030.

Pappas, C.A., & VanScoy-Mosher, C. (1988). Establishing a profitable outpatient community nursing center. *Journal of Nursing Administration, 18*(5), 31–33.

Peters, A., et al. (1991). Clinical evaluation of decision support system for insulin-dose adjustment in IDDM. *Diabetes Care, 14,* 875–879.

Redman, B.K. (1992). *The process of patient education* (7th ed.). St. Louis: C.V. Mosby Co.

Redman, B.K., Levine, D., & Howard, D. (1987). Organizational resources in support of patient education programs: Relationship to reported delivery of instruction. *Patient Education and Counseling, 9,* 177–197.

Reeder, P.J., & Chen, S.C. (1990). A client satisfaction survey in home health care. *Journal of Nursing Quality Assurance, 5,* 16–24.

Rykwalder, A. (1987). Achieving fiscal fitness: Budgeting basics for patient education managers. *Patient Education and Counseling, 9,* 73–79.

Sinclair, V.G. (1991). The impact of information systems on nursing performance and productivity. *Journal of Nursing Administration, 21,* 46–50.

Slee, V.N. (1991). Quality management nee quality assurance. *Journal of Nursing Administration, 21*(5), 9–12.

Suls, J., & Wan, C.K. (1989). Effects of sensory and procedural information on coping with stressful medical procedures and pain: A meta-analysis. *Journal of Consulting and Clinical Psychology, 57,* 372–379.

Veterans Administration. (1987). *Patient health education profile in VA medical centers.* Washington, DC: Author.

Webber, G.C. (1990). Patient education: A review of the issues. *Medical Care, 28,* 1089–1103.

Weinraub, H. (1985). The impact of prospective pricing on hospital health education: The New Jersey experience. *Patient Education and Counseling, 7,* 337–343.

Woodrow, M. (1979). Cost consciousness prompts three-phase education service. *Hospitals, 53*(9), 98–102.

Wyness, M.A. (1989). Devising standards for patient education in a teaching hospital. *Quality Review Bulletin, 15,* 279–285.

Young, B., & Johnson, L. (1984). The development of hospitalwide patient-education director competencies. *Patient Education and Counseling, 6,* 19–24.

CHAPTER 34 • • • • • •

DISCHARGE PLANNING AND CASE MANAGEMENT

LINDA J. PIEROG

EXECUTIVE SUMMARY

Case management is an overall term for resource management and patient outcome determination. Discharge planning is an integral initiating step in the case management process. All caregivers who come in contact with the patient are contributors and controllers of the patient's case management plan. It is essential to a hospital's well-being and quality patient care delivery that a case management program be identified and orchestrated, using discharge planning as the primary initiator of outcomes.

T he health care management objectives that optimize the value of health care delivery led to the development of a case management program. Achieving a more cost-effective practice and quality outcomes in individual patient care and aggregate patterns of care is the premise for such a program. Professional nurses have seized this opportunity to integrate clinical care and management data into empowered decision making. Absolute decentralization is promoted, with integrated cost savings, efficiency, and quality patient care accomplishing the case management objectives.

Discharge planning is the initial strategic step in this case management process, where the empowered decision making begins. It is one of the many multidisciplinary collaborative practices that promote the clinical path and accomplishment of care outcomes. The clinical path is the tool of professional collaboration and achievement of patient care outcomes while encouraging cost effectiveness and efficiency. Before admission, through registration notification, a patient can receive education, length of stay information, and clinical outcome information, thus encouraging patient satisfaction through the clinical path.

Nursing has been doing case management since the early 1900s in the public health field. Encouraging this scope of coordinated services from preadmission to discharge is an incorporation and translation of the service provided in the early part of the century. The same service intake activities of assessment, case plan development, implementation of plan, follow-up, ongoing assessment of adherence to plan, variances of plan, case recording, supervision of ancillary caregivers, collaboration with physicians, and quality assurance are essential. This service of resource management within the means of the patient and the care available was and is the kind of case management needed. Following are the acute care–case management components.

- Intake assessment
- Case management plan development
- Plan implementation
- Plan follow-up
- Ongoing assessment of plan adherence
- Case recording
- Supervision of ancillary caregivers
- Collaboration with physicians
- Quality assurance

CASE MANAGEMENT COLLABORATION

An effective patient care system aligns resource use, quality assurance, clinical decision making, and discharge planning into a collaborative force. The seven essential elements of this collaboration are listed in Table 34-1. Using all seven element of an effective clinical case management program develops well-informed clinicians and managers who design, implement, and monitor effective cost-contained patient care with the least amount of delay in obtaining care outcomes. Typically, clinicians and managers use hospital services with little

TABLE 34–1 Case Management Elements

ELEMENT	DESCRIPTION
1. Informative	Information exists for all caregivers through open communication
2. Longitudinal	Planned treatment desired outcomes continue despite changes in staff delivery site
3. Flexible	Clinical path plans allow for changes in a patient's condition
4. Individualized	Each clinical path is orchestrated for the best quality outcome for that patient
5. Comprehensive	All services are made available to all patients 24 hours a day, 7 days a week
6. Personal	The relationships established with a patient are honored, and interest in each patient as an individual is essential
7. Accessible	Services and resources are delivered in an appropriate setting and in a timely, efficient manner using the most appropriate process

understanding of the impact this resource consumption has on the hospital, ancillary services, and budget. Case management plans achieve real savings and shortened lengths of stay through bringing the clinicians and managers into the process and production of care. All this is initiated before the hospitalization, with an understanding of the true cost efficiency plus average and marginal costs associated with the management control issues of care delivery.

CASE MANAGEMENT PLANS

Clinicians and managers using a case management system use time and process to focus on providing quality care outcomes. Protocols are developed across service lines, called clinical pathways or case management plans. These plans define the length of stay, resource use, patient care goals, and ancillary staff involvement for an entire hospital stay. Variances, cost-containment strategies, and resource strategies are realized in real-time and process-directed outcomes. Clear pictures of care delivery are presented for the bedside nurse, nurse associates, laboratory personnel, respiratory therapists, and others in sequenced fashion. These plans become the enforcer, communicator, and monitor of patient care delivery.

The decentralized empowered decision making and integration of care delivery are provided through the case management plan. Production processes associated with patient care delivery are articulated clearly to protect against lapses in quality and service consistency 24 hours a day and 7 days a week among all clinicians and managers. Individual practice patterns align through case management plans by generating mechanisms to encourage capacity building with maintained and enhanced quality.

Specific case management plans must be developed by a task force of experts within the facility. These plans are one-page abbreviated overviews of a patient's expected hospitalization for every discipline to use (see Appendix 34-A). The task force, composed of clinicians, ancillary staff, and managers, is required to determine the needed daily treatments, consultations, medications, diagnostic testing, timing, and processing of ordered resources (Table 34-2). Secondarily, consideration is given to management strategies and cost-containment interventions necessary to achieve specified clinical and financial outcomes of the case

TABLE 34-2 Case Management Plan Task Force

TASK FORCE MEMBERS	WORK PRODUCT
Nursing	Care plan
Physician	Treatment interventions
Discharge planning	Pre- and posthospitalization needs identified
Laboratory	Timing of tests
Radiology	Timing of tests
	Length of stay
Utilization	Payor demands

management plan. Anticipated lengths of stay, intermediate goals, and the subsequent quality outcomes will empower the caregiver to generate the desired patient and team satisfaction.

Of particular import is the longitudinal view of care delivery given by a case management plan, permitting analysis of process and timing. Cases that adversely affect use can be identified at the point of service. The ability to define the point of service issues, especially in complex cases, such as AIDS and cancer, allows even the multiply linked concerns to be analyzed and corrected. This type of information can lead to improved quality and effective case management within the total facility. Continuous monitoring of the case management plan reveals potential clinical problems, problems in the process, or the statistics-generated revised plans. Plans can then meet the ever changing internal, external, and professional demands placed on caregivers and their facilities. Regular, timely reviews and continued enhancement further bring clinicians and managers into alignment regarding the care given and the outcome goals.

Case management plans contribute to new staff, part-time staff, and registry staff orientation. A case management plan gives the caregiver a quick overview of the care direction, easily bringing the novice to a level of physician collaboration and awareness of desired outcomes. The visible reminder of process and timing is essential and cannot be interrupted because of staffing changes. Case management plans alleviate the problems of changes in the care provider by further promoting the goal of continued and constant quality.

CASE MANAGEMENT STAFF/ADVISORS

Overall responsibility for supporting the case management program falls to all involved caregivers and the case management department. Maintenance of physician confidentiality and cooperation is necessary and should be kept by the case management department, with meeting minutes under the auspices of medical staff quality assurance. Numerous physicians, nursing, and ancillary staff participate in this collaborative process, reviewing historical patient care information. One aspect of case management is the service delivery analysis portion, which relates directly to the need for continuous quality improvement and assists the hospital in meeting the challenge of JCAHO regulations. The essential key to health care facility survival is how well departments interrelate to achieve outcomes. A cooperative effort by case management and quality assurance personnel facilitates the highest quality of care in the most cost-effective manner while meeting external requirements. Through the commitment of the medical staff, nursing staff, and administrative staff to the concept of case management, all can accomplish individual and facility goals.

Who then is the case manager, case management advisor, gatekeeper, controller of the case management plan? Anyone who comes into contact with the patient is a case management plan controller. However, there must be one assigned individual for collecting the concurrent data and fulfilling the role responsibilities for the case management department. The responsibilities of this individual, the case management advisor, are

- Assessment
- Planning
- Monitoring
- Reassessing
- Case finding
- Gatekeeping

- Intake assessment review
- Cost containment monitoring
- Capacity building
- Termination of the plan
- Evaluation/analysis

Providers of the case management function should be akin to utilization review nurses, with an excellent clinical skills base. A clinical specialist with utilization review knowledge would be the perfect person for the position. The continuum of care monitoring is maintained through collaboration with patient care personnel and then brought together with prospective planning, concurrent review, and retrospective analysis.

The skills of the clinical nurse specialist and the utilization review nurse become combined into a case management advisor role, allowing those with direct patient care contact to assume the responsibility of patient case manager 24 hours a day 7 days a week with the assistance they need to be empowered in their decision making. Everyone who is in contact with the patient should be a case manager, and the role of the case management advisor becomes one of developing the case management plans, reassessing the plans, and determining compliance and variance rates for future reassessment of the plan.

In summary, the survival of any health care facility is dependent on two main factors.

1. How well resources are used
2. How well the facility can meet the quality expectations of the physician, patient, third party payor, and regulatory agencies

Therefore, it is essential that through the commitment of the hospital and its medical staff, case management and all its objectives be adopted.

DISCHARGE PLANNING

Discharge planning looks beyond the walls of the hospital and is the first and last step in developing the case management plan. Whatever is necessary to achieve a continued recovery after hospitalization is effected through coordination of the case management plan from the beginning until the patient's total recovery. It is true that discharge planning has never been more important than it is today, since acute care stays are compressed and the use of resources outside the hospital has expanded dramatically. Discharge planning sets the case management plan into action by alerting and communicating to the health care team the expectations and needs of an individualized assessment.

The discharge plan is prepared during the initial patient intake by any member of the team coming in contact with the patient. The case management plan is well on its way to achieving outcome goals when the discharge planning is properly initiated on preadmission or admission. Mutually agreed on timing, processing, and outcomes become the property and responsibility of all caregivers. Case management plans accommodate assessment of individual patient discharge needs when identifying

- Recovery stage
- Knowledge deficits
- Support systems
- Dietary needs

- Medication needs
- Durable medical equipment needs
- Follow-up needs/timing/extent

These are then processed through the acute care continuum. Total team accountability in achieving the discharge outcome motivates positive team activities toward outcome attainment. Individual members of the health care team are not isolated in their roles of promoting family and patient responsibility for the transition to home or another care facility.

The entire caregiving team becomes involved in realizing that the acute care stage is a small part of the total patient care necessary for a return to wellness or function. Promotion of continuity and fragmentation of resource involvement is eliminated. Control of the health care continuum is then put in its rightful place, with the patient and case management team. It is unifying, connecting the multidisciplinary team with outcome-driven decision making while remaining patient centered and focused at all times.

Discharge planning, using a case management system, blends prospective assessment, planning efficiency, and quality as mutually supportive concepts. The patient's discharge needs are determined on admission with scheduled, written time frames for delivery of home health aids, visits of home health nurses, or transition to lesser levels of care. Shared goals with the family, patient, and health care team on admission promote highly decentralized functioning in a highly integrated manner. Harmony of roles, with a consistent decision framework, can facilitate achieving the goal of optimizing the health care resources expended.

Bibliography

Blendon, R.J. (1988). The public's view of the future of health care. *Journal of the American Medical Association, 259,* 3587–3593.

Enthoven, A. (1988). Managed competition: An agenda for action. *Health Affairs, 7,* 25–47.

Iglehart, J.K. (1987). Health policy report: Problems facing the nursing professional. *New England Journal of Medicine, 317,* 646–651.

Nelson, A.R. (1989). Humanism and the art of medicine. *Journal of the American Medical Association, 262,* 1228–1230.

Roper, W.L., Winkenwerder, W., Hackbarth G.M., et al. (1988). Effectiveness in health care: An initiative to evaluate and improve medical practice. *New England Journal of Medicine, 319,* 1197–1202.

Wilensky, G. (1989, June). An economic analysis of the nursing shortage. Paper presented at the Sixth Annual Meeting of the Association for Health Services Research and the Foundation for Health Sciences Research.

Case Management Plans*

Patient Name:_____
M.D.:_____
D.O.S.:_____
L.O.S. 6 DAY

CORONARY ARTERY BYBASS
OPTIMAL RECOVERY GUIDELINES

Expected D/C:_____
Risk Assessment:_____

	DAY 1	DAY 2	DAY 3	DAY 4	DAY 5	DAY 6
SURGERY/ RECOVERY		ICU	4W	TCU	TCU	TCU
TESTS Pre-Adm Testing Chest X-Ray EKG CBC Panel 7		H&H Plat CT Panel 7 Chest X-Ray ABG's			CBC Panel 7 Chest X-Ray As Needed	
TREATMENT		FOLEY VENT (EXTUBATE) Pulse Ox CHEST TUBE ART. LINE SWAN	DC

DC | | | |
| MEDICATION | | IV PAIN PRN MANAGEMENT IV ANTIBIOTICS | CARDIAC Meds DC ORAL PAIN

IV ANTIBIOTICS | CARDIAC MEDS

ORAL PAIN

ORAL ANTIBIOTICS | | DISCHARGE |
DIET		NPO REGULAR WHEN EXTUBATED	REGULAR DIET	REGULAR DIET	REGULAR DIET	DISCHARGE
INTRAVEN.		IV's Saline Lock	Saline Lock	Saline Lock	Saline Lock	DISCHARGE
ACTIVITY		BR	BRP, room, chair	AMB.	AMB.	DISCHARGE
ALTERATION IN COMFORT POST-OP	PAIN CONTROL IV MEDS		PAIN CONTROL PO MEDS	CAN PARTICIPATE PATIENT IN CARE		DISCHARGE/PO MEDS
ANXIETY HOSPITALIZATION			Verbalizes decrease anxiety--able to cooperate post-op			VERBALIZES UNDERSTANDING OF WOUND CARE
DISCHARGE PLAN			DISCHARGE PLANNING	SOCIAL SERVICES as needed	CARDIAC REHAB	HOME HEALTH FOLLOW-UP
TEACHING			DIET INST.	Understands importance of activity	DIET VERBALIZES UNDERSTAND ING OF MENU	DISCHARGE Booklet, notified of follow-up call

R.N.

IF PATIENT IS AN MEDICARE - PATIENT MAY GO TO TCU DAY 4 IF STABLE
EACH YES EQUALS TWO (2) AND REFLECTS THE NUMBER OF HOME VISITS

PHYSIOLOGICAL INDICATORS FOR HOME CARE: WOUND INFECTION YES NO	FUNCTIONAL MEASURES OF INDEPENDENCE: DOES THE PATIENT EXHIBIT A NEED FOR CONTINUAL SUPPORT YES NO

EACH PATIENT IS AN INDIVIDUAL AND THE RESPONSES MAY VARY. THE OPTIMAL RECOVERY PATH IS TO BE USED AS A GUIDELINE.

*Developed by Tania Bridgeman, RN, MPA, William E. Ostermiller, MD, Linda J. Pierog, RN, MBA, CCRN, and Joetta Tjaden, RN, BS.

CORONARY ARTERY BYBASS
PERSONAL RECOVERY PATH

PATIENT NAME: _____
MD: _____
PHONE NUMBER: _____

WHAT I NEED TO REMEMBER: TAKE MEDICATIONS WEIGH DAILY PACE MY ACTIVITY WATCH MY DIET REST 1 HOUR AFTER EACH MEAL	DO I HAVE QUESTIONS? WHAT ARE THEY??????	YES	NO

	DAILY	WEEKLY	MONTHLY	SOCIAL ENVIRONMENT
DIET	WATCH SALT INTAKE DAILY DON'T ADD SALT IRON RICH DIET VITAMIN C	EAT 3-4 MEALS A DAY REMEMBER TO EAT SLOWLY REMEMBER TO REST	REVIEW YOUR DIET RECORD SALT CONTENT ASK IS MY DIET IRON RICH?	READ MENU CAREFULLY LOOK FOR HEALTHY HEART SECTIONS OR LIGHT MENU
ACTIVITY	PACE ACTIVITY YOU MAY CLIMB STAIRS ARM & LEG EXERCISE AS PRESCRIBED SHOWER-MILD SOAP	PACE & GRADUALLY INCREASE ACTIVITY ARM & LEG EXERCISE AS PRESCRIBED SHOWER-MILD SOAP	AM I TAKING ADEQUATE REST PERIODS? LOG ACTIVITIES THAT CAUSE STRESS	DON'T HURRY DON'T WORRY VISITORS FOR SHORT PERIODS OF TIME AVOID IRRITATING SITUATIONS
SPECIAL TREATMENTS	WEIGHT YOURSELF SAME SCALE SAME TIME OBSERVE INCISIONS -TENDERNESS -SWELLING -DIFFERENT DRAINAGE	REVIEW ALL DAILY WEIGHTS (IF A GAIN ALWAYS REVIEW DIET & FLUIDS INTAKE)	LOG WEIGHT (HOW AM I DOING?) CONTINUE ASSESSING WOUND ON A REGULAR BASIS	IF AWAY FROM HOME TAKE PORTABLE SCALE WITH YOU. NO NEED TO PAINT YOUR INCISIONS WITH BETAINE CREAM - OINTMENT
MEDICATIONS	-READ YOUR SCHEDULE -DON'T SKIP A PILL -CHECK FOR UNFAVORABLE REACTION	REVIEW THE PAST WEEK: -QUESTIONS? -UNTOWARD REACTIONS?	REVIEW YOUR SCHEDULE -ARE THERE QUESTIONS FOR YOUR M.D. -WRITE THEM DOWN	TAKE YOUR SCHEDULE AND MEDICATIONS WITH YOU.
SIGN & SYMPTOMS TO REPORT TO M.D.	-HOW DO I FEEL -IS MY WEIGHT OKAY -IS MY INCISION -REDDENED -TENDER -SWOLLEN -CHECK FOR UNFAVORABLE REACTIONS	-DO I HAVE STERNAL ROCKING OR EXCESSIVE MOVEMENT -HAVE I A FEVER OF 100 OR MORE THAT CONTINUES 24 HRS OR MORE AND DOESN'T RESPOND TO TYLENOL OR BUFFERIN	LOG ALL QUESTIONS TO ASK -SURGEON -CARDIOLOGIST -OFFICE NURSE	TAKE M.D. PHONE NUMBER WITH YOU

EACH PATIENT IS AN INDIVIDUAL AND THE RESPONSES MAY VARY. THE OPTIMAL RECOVERY PATH IS TO BE USED AS A GUIDELINE.

CARDIOLOGIST - CALL:	STERNAL MOVEMENT:	MOOD SWINGS:
-CHEST PAIN/PRESSURE ANGINA LIKE PAIN THAT INCREASES WHEN LYING DOWN OR TAKE A DEEP BREATH -AT REST, A GREATER THAN 120 MIN HEART RATE -IF YOU FEEL YOUR HEART SKIP OR FLUTTER -CHANGE IN STOOLS (IRON MAKES STOOL BLACK) - WEIGHT GAIN 2LBS IN 24 HOURS	IS EXPECTED THE FIRST ONE TO THREE MONTHS. A CLICKING, POPPING, OR SHIFTING FEELING IS NOTED AND SHOULD OCCUR INFREQUENTLY DO NOT LIFT OBJECTS HEAVIER THAN 10 LBS.	ALONG WITH THE HEALING PROCESS OCCURRING IN YOUR BODY, YOU MAY EXPERIENCE MOOD SWINGS DURING THE FIRST FOUR TO SIX WEEKS AFTER SURGERY. THIS IS EXPECTED AND CONSIDERED NORMAL.

CLINICAL PATH WITH HOME VISIT

	WEEK 1 V1	WEEK 2 V2	WEEK 3 V3	WEEK 4 V4
KNOWLEDGE DEFICIT	INSTRUCT ON DISEASE PROCESS / ANATOMY & PHYSIOLOGY	SYMPTOM MANAGEMENT FOR: – CHEST PAIN – MEDICATION INTERACTION	SYMPTOM MANAGEMENT FOR: – FLUID BALANCE – SHORTNESS OF BREATH	REINFORCE SYMPTOM MANAGEMENT
TREATMENTS	ASSESS WOUND OBSERVE PT TRANSFER	OBSERVE WOUND OBSERVE ADL	QUESTION BOWEL FUNCTION	HOME PT FINAL EVALUATION
DIETARY	REINFORCE DIET AVOID SALT IRON RICH	QUESTION APPETITE REVIEW DIET	REVIEW DIET CONTENT NA	
MEDICATIONS	REVIEW MEDICATIONS LEAVE SCHEDULE	ASSESS COMPLIANCE REVIEW	QUERY KNOWLEDGE OF MEDICATIONS AND INTERACTIONS	
SAFETY/ACTIVITY	EMERGENCY PHONE NUMBERS M.D. NUMBER	INSTRUCTION ON ACTIVITY PACING NO SMOKING	REINFORCE PACING ACTIVITY NO DRIVING	QUERY RESPONSE TO PACING ACTIVITY
SOCIAL SERVICES	OBSERVE FAMILY ENVIRONMENT ASSESS SOCIAL NEEDS	ASSESS CARE GIVER SKILLS	QUERY CARE GIVER ON PT's PROGRESS	RE-ASSESS SOCIAL SERVICE NEEDS
PATIENT OUTCOMES				
GENERAL ASSESS	VITAL SIGNS STABLE HEART & LUNG SOUNDS STABLE	VITAL SIGNS STABLE NO EXCESSIVE PAIN	DIET BALANCE INTAKE & OUTPUT BALANCED	PACING AMBULATION NO SHORTNESS OF BREATH
COMPLICATION POTENTIAL	PT KNOWLEDGEABLE IN WOUND CARE NO SIGNS OF INFECTION	PT WITHOUT EVIDENCE OF INFECTION OR WOUND LESS REDDENED	PT IS WITHOUT EVIDENCE OF INFECTION AND EXCESSIVE PAIN	NO EVIDENCE OF PENDING COMPLICATION
KNOWLEDGE DEFICIT	PT. ORIENTED TO PLAN OF CARE UNDERSTANDING WOUND CARE, AMBULATION, DIET AND PT IF ORDERED	PT VERBALIZES RISK FACTORS AND SIDE EFFECTS UNDERSTANDS MEDICATION REACTIONS	PT CAN DISCUSS ACTIVITY ISSUES WOUND ISSUES	DEMONSTRATES UNDERSTANDING OF EXERCISE, MEDICATIONS, AND WHEN TO CALL M.D.

**Assess the presence of support and reassurance for the patient at each visit.

CARDIOLOGIST APPOINTMENT (MAKE AFTER HOME 1 DAY) DATE:_____TIME:_____	CARDIAC SURGEON APPOINTMENT (MAKE AFTER HOME 1 DAY) LET NURSE KNOW WHETHER YOU HAVE STAPLES IN YOUR CHEST OR LEG DATE:_____ TIME:_____

CHAPTER 35 • • • • • •

RISK MANAGEMENT

SUE E. PARKS

EXECUTIVE SUMMARY

Today's nurse manager has more responsibility than ever before in the history of modern nursing. Learning to identify and manage risk within the health care team is a challenge, but an achievable goal. Becoming educated about basic risk management principles and implementing a proactive approach are the keys to avoiding litigation. If a claim is filed or an unintended outcome occurs, the nurse manager should develop an action plan to identify and implement the necessary changes to minimize the potential for further exposure.

An awareness must be maintained of the common areas of potential nursing liability exposure, which include the following.

- Failure to manage the patient's health care experience
- Failure to observe the patient and take appropriate action
- Failure to document or communicate appropriately
- Failure to follow a physician's order in an accurate and timely manner
- Failure to administer medications appropriately
- Failure to follow appropriate protocols
- Failure to function within the scope of training and experience
- Failure to provide for a safe patient environment
- Failure to use equipment properly

Risk management requires changes that are not always comfortable. Staff will need to be encouraged to work through the discomfort. The business of nursing is service to our patients. A machine can be recalibrated. A computer can be reprogrammed. A process can be refined. But staff cannot be controlled, cajoled, or coerced into managing risk or improving quality. They can be offered the tools, but managing risk and quality is a dynamic process made possible only because the nurse manager is committed, receives satisfaction from it, and works to achieve it (Peterson, 1990).

The current health care environment has placed the burden of responsibility on the nurse manager to function in a variety of new roles that historically have not been within the scope and depth of basic nursing curriculum. Risk management and the law are gaining greater attention as nurses and hospital administrators are recognizing the significance of their shared risk within the health care environment and the financial and emotional consequences of litigation.

There is a movement by payors to advance patients through the health care environment more quickly in order to manage an ever increasing national health care budget, which is nearing $800,000,000.00 per year and consuming approximately 12% of our gross national product. Consequently, the risks involved with providing care are increasing at dramatic rates. According to a 12-year study conducted by the Risk Management Foundation of the Harvard Medical Institutions, the number of medical malpractice claims involving all nurse specialties increased nearly 100% from 1982 to 1987 (Risk Management Foundation, 1989).

Nurse managers are being mandated to control costs, manage risk, and improve the quality of care being provided in an atmosphere of managed care, liability concerns, nursing shortages, and hospitals struggling to maintain their financial viability. Nurses are suffering from information overload and scarcity of time.

Nurses are the vital link in providing reasonable care at a reasonable cost to those in need. The management of these challenges will dictate nursing's viability in the future as a significant contributor to the solution of accessibility and quality. Managing liability risk as responsibilities increase presents a unique challenge and an opportunity for growth to affect a system in need of change.

As the trend for more care and treatment to be delivered in the ambulatory care setting increases, patients are being admitted with more acute needs and are receiving discharge planning on admission. Gone are the days when nurses really knew their patients and families and professional nurses could provide health education, and preoperative and postoperative teaching. The patient back rub and handholding have become relics of the past. The system can no longer afford to justify those nonquantifiable benefits.

Nurse managers in the home health care setting have a growing need to understand the principles of risk management, as their accountability has increasing demands and skill levels that place them at higher risk as well.

There is an emerging need for all nurse managers to develop a greater understanding of the legal process and risk management strategies to minimize liability exposure within their management areas. This will provide the basis for an optimal patient outcome.

YESTERDAY'S AND TODAY'S MALPRACTICE ENVIRONMENT

The early 1970s gave rise to what has been referred to as the "medical malpractice crisis." In 1965, predating the crisis, an important case turned the table of malpractice as it related to hospital nurses. The *Darling v. Charleston Community Hospital* case is significant to help gain an understanding of the temporal effect of nursing and malpractice and often is referred to in basic legal curriculum and hospital risk management presentations (Creighton, 1986).

The case involved a young football player who broke his leg during a game.

He was taken to the Charleston Community Hospital emergency department, where the leg was placed in a cast. Two days later, the patient allegedly complained of pain, and his toes were swollen and became cyanotic. After 2 weeks, he was transferred to another medical center, where the leg eventually was amputated. Mr. Darling filed a lawsuit against the hospital and won. The hospital and nurses providing the care were held liable under the legal doctrine of respondeat superior because they allegedly did not appropriately observe the patient and failed to report the worsening condition to the physician. The physician settled out of court.

The significance of this case established that the hospital had an independent duty separate from the physician to respond appropriately to a given set of circumstances. Because attorneys do not sue buildings or hospitals, the Darling case has provided an avenue for nurses to be sued. As a result, hospitals and nurses have experienced an increase in the filing of lawsuits that culminated in the malpractice crisis of the mid-1970s.

Jury Verdict's Research, an organization based in Ohio that reviews and tracks data as it relates to medical malpractice cases, recently reported that 1991 was a record year for verdicts greater than a million dollars. Although the courts experienced a mild slowing in the frequency with which lawsuits were filed, greater sums of money were awarded to plaintiffs who allegedly suffered from iatrogenic disease.

A number of environmental factors have contributed to the patient's interest in filing a lawsuit. One cannot read a paper or watch television without being made aware of some recent litigation. The large awards are published on the front pages of newspapers, and society has consequently developed a lottery mentality. Attorneys are advertising with offers to potential plaintiffs of no payment until the final settlement or judgment has been entered. Our children are being raised to believe that the only means to problem solving is through litigation. Count the number of television programs and movies that focus on the courtroom as the site for problem resolution. There is even a book for young adults *Can You Sue Your Parents for Malpractice?* (Danziger, 1983).

An increase in technology has tended to remove the human component from care, causing depersonalization and a breakdown in the nurse–physician–patient relationship. Specialized equipment has its inherent problems as medical devices and the users present additional opportunities for exposure.

The age of nursing and medical specialization has increased the propensity of persons to file lawsuits because of the lack of continuity of care, which is addressed later in this chapter. Managed care and the new reimbursement schedules have dictated where and by whom an individual may seek care and have contributed to the breakdown in the nurse–physician–patient relationship.

As a result of decreasing reimbursement, some physicians are increasing the volume of patients to maintain current income levels. Because of increases in medical office overhead, other physicians are hiring unskilled personnel to handle office triage and patient care management, which increases the chances of an error occurring.

The malpractice problem is multifactorial, and the areas identified as contributory variables are certainly not exhaustive but should provide some rationale in gaining a better understanding of the magnitude of the problem in our society. Huber (1988) has referred to the cost of liability as the safety tax, one of the most ubiquitous Americans pay. It has been estimated that $300 has been assessed to every family per pregnancy in New York to pay for the $85,000 annual malpractice insurance premium of an obstetrician.

RISK MANAGEMENT AND QUALITY IMPROVEMENT RELATIONSHIPS

Journals, workshops, and conventions have reached epidemic proportions in their efforts to convert health care providers to total quality management (TQC) or continuous quality improvement (CQI). Just as Juran, Demming, and Berwick are addressing process and outcome, nurse managers need to integrate the concepts of proactive risk management and CQI. Every risk management issue is a quality issue. All quality issues, however, do not necessarily become risk management issues. The potential for improvement efforts is endless.

Delivering quality care has been assumed by most health care providers as their mission. The important distinction is whether the quality perspective has been clinically driven or patient driven. Both are essential risk management components and are necessary to prevent claims. However, patient-driven quality, if managed properly, has the ability to minimize the chances of a lawsuit being filed after an unintended outcome or complication (Cunningham, 1991). Traditionally, clinical quality has been measured and rewarded or punished by the Joint Commission on Accreditation of Healthcare Organizations, professional review organizations (PROs), state nursing and medical licensing boards, and hospital quality assurance programs. When nurses or physicians are asked if they provide quality care, their responses are generally from a clinical perspective rather than based on whether they have satisfied and delighted patients. The patient's perception of quality is often quite different from that of the providers.

The majority of patients have come to expect that they will receive clinical quality as a given in the health care delivery process. A patient's ability to discern clinical quality from lack of clinical quality can be difficult, although many patients are becoming more educated through the medical media and are desiring a more active role in planning their medical regimens.

Patient-driven quality is typically focused on the service component of quality care. This is what the patient remembers about the care that was rendered: "Was I treated with respect and dignity? Did the health care providers follow through with their commitments? Was I kept informed? Were the health care providers responsive to my needs and did they sometimes anticipate them? Were my questions and concerns addressed to my satisfaction? Was my time valued?" Answers to these questions are the pieces of information that a patient synthesizes to determine whether or not the system has provided patient-driven quality.

A favorite example is the practicing nurse or physician in the rural area who has maintained a meaningful nurse–physician–patient relationship. Assume that a patient had a medical condition that warranted emergent attention as a result of either a misdiagnosis or a delay in diagnosis. The patient was transported to a big city hospital and received the best available clinical care, but a poor outcome resulted. A lawsuit was filed against the city hospital. The patient did not have an opportunity to establish the same meaningful relationship with the big city health care providers because of the crisis situation. Therefore, the patient's perception of quality was negative. The rural practitioners are not named parties because the patient refused to believe that they could have done anything wrong.

The application and integration of risk and quality principles in managing the patient's experience is a critical connection. Patient satisfaction is often referred to as a quality indicator. It may also be an indicator of lack of quality, which can lead to the ultimate step on the patient satisfaction continuum—the filing of a lawsuit (Table 35-1).

PROFESSIONAL LIABILITY INSURANCE

Nurses working in hospitals generally are not named individually in lawsuits. The hospital has the deep pocket, and plaintiff's attorneys are in the market to secure the greatest dollar recovery possible for their clients. Because most hospitals carry millions of dollars worth of professional liability insurance and because the focus of civil litigation is to recover as much as possible in money damages—as opposed to criminal litigation, where those violating the law may be put in jail—an independent nurse's policy usually is not the primary target.

Nurses often ask whether they should carry their own individual professional liability policy. This is a judgment decision. Basically, if a professional nurse is functioning within her role as an employee of an organization that carries adequate amounts of coverage, the need diminishes. In most cases, the organization will provide its employees with coverage in the event of a claim. Some nurses' comfort level increases with their own policy. As a nurse manager, investigating the coverage issue with the organization's risk manager or corporate legal counsel is recommended.

The majority of plaintiff's attorneys are not aware of nurses carrying their own individual policies. This is one of the best kept secrets, and nurses should keep it that way for as long as possible. When the plaintiff's attorneys learn that there may be another million dollars or more, the chance is that nurses will become named parties with greater frequency, and liability premiums for nurses will skyrocket.

The professional liability insurance market has received a respite during the past few years as some states have attempted to reduce the flood of lawsuits through a variety of approaches to tort reform. However, the consensus in the industry predicts that within the next few years, the insurance market will begin to harden. History has demonstrated the cyclic process. This means that it is likely that insurance premiums will soon begin to climb, and the rates will increase as more lawsuits are filed. Even if significant tort reform were to take place, an individual's constitutional right to litigation will remain. It is time for nurse managers to prepare and be armed with the strategies to manage liability risk in the future.

TABLE 35-1 Managing the Patient's Experience

- If you **meet** the patient's expectations, you will decrease your potential for liability.
- If you **exceed** the patient expectations, you will increase your potential for viability.

PATIENT SATISFACTION CONTINUUM				
Awful >	Bad >	Good >	Very good >	Excellent
PATIENT ACTION CONTINUUM				
Sue	< Report to credentialing body	< End relationship	<Question value	<Satisfied

COMMON REASONS WHY PATIENTS MAY FILE A LAWSUIT AGAINST A NURSE

There are a number of reasons why patients file lawsuits, and it is critical to understand the problem before the solutions can be implemented. There is an important distinction in the preceding statement that deserves mentioning. Nurse managers need to understand that attorneys manage the litigation process, but it is the patient, or whomever may have a cause of action for the patient, who files the lawsuit in the first place. Therefore, gaining a clear understanding of how the patient's experience is managed throughout the health care system may be the most significant determinant of whether or not litigation is pursued.

The following is a list of potential areas that may cause a patient to file a lawsuit. They are not listed in an order of magnitude but are prioritized in terms of the author's experience and expertise.

- Patients sue, not necessarily because of a bad outcome, but because of the manner in which they have been treated within the health care system.
- Patients sue because of a nurse's failure to observe and take appropriate action.
- Patients sue nurses and physicians because of a lack of continuity of care.
- Patients sue nurses and physicians because of inadequate medical record documentation.
- Patients sue nurses because the patients have been given the wrong medicine.
- Patients sue because the organization's policies or protocols were not followed.
- Patients sue because the nurse failed to provide for a safe patient environment.

SOLUTIONS TO THE PROBLEM OF LAWSUITS BY PATIENTS
Treat the Patient with Dignity and Respect

Patients and family members need to be treated with dignity and respect. Family members should be treated as part of the patient's network, since they are often the protagonists in a lawsuit. Nurse managers must, therefore, convey to staff that patients are generally coupled with someone significant in their lives who cares very deeply about their welfare. These individuals are the first to observe, take notes, and retaliate if their loved one is treated unfairly or if their questions or concerns are not acknowledged.

As Rosenbaum (1991) so eloquently stated in *The Doctor,* "the view is entirely different from the bed." The book or movie is strongly recommended to assist staff in gaining greater empathy for the patient's experience. At the end of the movie, new medical residents are required to don patient gowns and become the recipients of care rather than the caregivers. The experiential component of walking in the patient's shoes has a number of valuable lessons that deserve repeating throughout one's professional career, since there is a tendency to become desensitized to the needs and concerns of those entrusted to our care.

Creating a culture of care and concern within a health care provider's persona is critical to managing the patient's experience. A hospital human resources department may be able to assist in facilitating techniques to create an atmosphere that is truly patient focused. For the manager, there are a number of self-help books available that deal with the issue of developing meaningful relationships and team building.

In today's health care environment and its pressures, the nurse manager is faced with the challenge of hiring and training appropriate staff. During the initial personnel interview, an assessment of personal values should be made rather than just filling a position. According to CNA, a large property and casualty insurance company, 95% of all litigation results from factors relating to relationship care rather than technical treatment (Murphy, 1990). One can no longer assume that members of the health care profession possess those innate personality characteristics that convey caring and concern. Some enter the profession for the sole purpose of meeting income needs and do not have a true commitment to quality patient care. The nurse manager must be vigilant, especially during a staff member's probationary period, to validate expressed values with behavior.

The nurse manager must maintain an awareness that individual members of the health care team come from a variety of both work and educational experiences and need both formal and informal performance assessments throughout their employment. A nonjudgmental environment must be created in which staff has the freedom to come for direction, input, and corrective action. The nurse manager should observe the actions and interactions of staff and use lessons learned from past experiences (occurrences) to develop a proactive approach. Developing relationships with staff who will ask questions when they are uncertain about an unfamiliar issue will minimize the potential for liability exposure.

Most risk management departments are too busy managing claims to become proactive. They rely on nurse managers to use their experiences learned from previous occurrences to develop staff corrective action programs. The nurse manager must be direct and specific to obtain the assistance and support of the risk management department. One of the most important aspects of the risk management process is for a nurse manager to gain a wide tolerance for ambiguity because there are no clean, black-and-white lines drawn in the risk management discipline (Hartshorn, 1992). Reasonable judgment and basic knowledge about the risk management process are the essential ingredients.

Observe and Take Appropriate Action

The *Darling* case is an example of a nurse's failure to observe and take appropriate action. A skills checklist and orientation protocols are essential in cultivating a staff capable of making appropriate observations for the patient population being served and then acting appropriately on them.

Timeliness is a critical component in assessing whether a nurse has fallen below the standard of care. If a situation warrants a particular schedule for observation and the nurse does not document and follow it, the nurse may be held liable in the event of a bad outcome. Excuses of poor staffing and lack of experience are not defensible arguments. Making observations and not acting on them in a timely manner can lead to litigation. Professional nurses are expected to convey and document significant patient observations that may affect physician or other team members' care and treatment. A failure to do so may result in an allegation of negligence.

Recognize When Discontinuity of Care Occurs and Intervene Constructively

In this age of specialization and fragmentation, a physician's ability to manage patients with multiple problems has become exceedingly difficult. Ophthalmology has dissected the eye to include retinal specialists, and nursing has developed its share of specialty interests as well. Although fragmentation has occurred within the health care field, the patient has remained intact, with multisystems being treated simultaneously by a variety of health care providers. The average medical–surgical patient has contact with approximately 17 different providers during one hospitalization. These range from laboratory personnel to physicians, dietitians, nurses, physical therapists, respiratory therapists, and a variety of nonprofessional personnel.

The following is an example of discontinuity in today's health care climate. First, a patient has a primary care provider, commonly referred to as a PCP. A patient develops cervical dysplasia and needs to be seen by a gynecologist. The gynecologist then makes the diagnosis of cervical cancer, and the patient is referred to an oncologist, who then may refer to a radiation oncologist. There may be a general surgeon involved along with an anesthesiologist. Because of complications, a pulmonologist may be asked to consult. Obviously, the opportunities for errors in communication to occur greatly increase as the patient is passed through the health care delivery system. The patient and the patient's family can be lost in the specialty shuffle. No one seems to take the necessary accountability for the management of the care and treatment. The nurse can be an advocate for the patient in assisting with the coordination of care through the system.

As a nurse manager, maintaining staff awareness of this potential problem can be vital to the patient's optimal outcome in a system that is ripe for providing discontinuity. The ability for staff to recognize when discontinuity is occurring and to intervene constructively is a valuable risk management strategy.

Review Staff Documentation for Completeness and Accuracy of Medical Record

A chapter on risk management would be remiss without mention of documentation as a key factor in managing risk. The first thing a plaintiff's attorney will do is to request a copy of the medical record. It will then be evaluated by a nurse consultant working within the law firm or sent to a potential expert witness for review, to identify potential issues of liability. These individuals will examine the record in an attempt to reconstruct the events that led to the bad outcome. If the medical record clearly reflects the care that was given, a lawsuit may never be filed. If there are areas or gaps in the record that leave the facts open to question, a lawsuit may be more likely to result.

The nurse manager must recognize that the majority of physicians do not always read nurses' notes. Therefore, it is imperative that staff convey critical information to the physician directly. If information is conveyed to a staff member in the physician's office, the nurse should secure and document the name of this individual and the time the call was made. Nurses' notes should be concise and objective.

Using the problem-oriented approach to charting (SOAP) is strongly recommended. This method assures that the nurse has addressed a particular problem and gone through a systematic approach to problem solving. Notes should indicate the time and date and should be signed appropriately. Telephone calls and faxes should be documented appropriately in the record to reflect information transferred.

The long, narrative nurse's note does not compel another provider to read it. Large graph and flow sheet documentation with multiple variables can present a problem of interpretation for the busy practicing physician trying to make rounds. A brief summary narrative highlighting the critical issues will assist the busy physician in determining the patient's status.

Staff must be advised that the medical record is a legal document and should not be used to solve problems or designate blame to another health care team member. A plaintiff's attorney salivates over a medical record that reflects dissension within the ranks. Records should not be altered. Plaintiff's attorneys have been known to hire handwriting experts to determine whether a record has been altered. Staff should follow the organization's policy for correcting clerical errors in the record.

A number of nurses have a tendency to draft personal notes after an incident occurs. Some academic institutions have instructed nursing students to draft their personal recollections for future reference in the event of a claim. These notes may be discoverable in the event of litigation and often can have a negative effect on the defense of the case. If a nurse has a desire to ventilate in writing about a particular incident, it is recommended that this exercise be conducted as therapeutic and the notes destroyed. They should not be shown to anyone—not even the nurse manager or risk manager. Developing alternative coping strategies for staff should be instituted with the assistance and advice of the risk manager or corporate counsel.

The medical record is a means of communication among a variety of health care professionals for the patient's welfare to assure continuity of care and an optimal outcome. It is a tool to pass on significant information about the care and treatment status of the patient, and to be effective, all entries should be legible and clear. The nurse manager has the burden of responsibility to review staff documentation for content and clarity of purpose and to provide appropriate corrective action, if necessary.

Maintain Protocols of Medication Administration

Medication administration is one of the most significant tasks a nurse performs. A number of books have been written on medication errors that include the wrong medicines, wrong dosage, wrong concentration of the right medication, inappropriate reading of medication labels, and administering medication to the wrong patient. Millions of dollars are awarded each year in cases involving the inappropriate administration of medications.

Unit dosing has not solved the problem. Strict adherence to medication protocols is the only sure way to minimize the problem. Nurse managers must set the stage for appropriate behavior from their staff. The nurse manager should review and confirm with staff the five Rs of medication administration.

1. The Right medicine
2. The Right patient
3. The Right dose
4. The Right route
5. The Right time

This is basic information, but essential and often revealing.

Generally, there are a finite number of medications being prescribed to a designated patient population. During orientation or quarterly staff meetings, a review of contraindications and possible side effects of frequently prescribed medications should be presented, and new medications should be introduced. The nurse manager can delegate this investigative assignment to responsible staff members and inservice staff to research, or a drug representative may be invited to provide an inservice for the staff. Medication information should be generated in an area for future reference and should be accessible to staff.

A *PDR* and a recent pharmacology textbook for staff to independently reference new or unfamiliar drugs should be available to staff. Clinical pharmacists within the hospital may be used as a quick resource for questions or staff continuing education.

Advise staff to question a doctor's order if unsure or if there are questions about the appropriateness of a medication ordered. It is important to remember that physicians are part of the health care team and are not perfect. The nurse manager should work with staff in developing appropriate skills to approach physicians in a nonadversarial manner when questioning an order.

The nurse manager can convey to staff that giving medication should be equated with being a jet pilot, who works through the rigors of a strict checkout protocol before every takeoff. These protocols are routine and are done without fail to ensure a safe flight. Staff need to develop this same approach to medication administration, recognizing that medications alter a patient's metabolic status, and proper administration is critical to achieving an optimal patient outcome.

Train Staff on Specific Policies, Procedures, and Regulatory Protocols

Orienting and training staff on the specific policies and procedures within the health care organization by the nurse manager will reduce the chances of a possible claim alleging a "failure to follow established protocols." Although policies and procedures are not necessarily the standard of care, they are among the factors that may be used by a plaintiff's attorney to try to establish the standard of care.

The nurse manager should recognize that anything in writing has the potential for vigorous cross-examination by a plaintiff's attorney and should be viewed as such. An annual review of policies specific to the management area and appropriate revision based on the organization's guidelines should minimize exposure. Retaining specimen copies of old policies in the event that reconstruction may be necessary is recommended.

The regulatory environment requires the execution and implementation of large numbers of policies. The nurse manager may be called on to draft new policies. The use of language is critical, and policies should be developed that allow for some acceptable standard deviation under certain circumstances. The nurse manager should secure the advice of the risk manager if development questions arise.

A number of specialty organizations have developed specific guidelines and protocols. A review of these should be designated as part of the staff member's orientation checklist. State nursing boards may provide specific statutes that need to be followed. Contacting the state board for information related to the scope of nursing practice is recommended. Conveying significant information to staff as it relates to specialty boards and state statutes governing nursing practice should be done when appropriate.

Provide a Safe Patient Care Environment

A nurse manager has a responsibility to assist the health care organization in providing a safe patient care environment that is conducive to healing. As early as 1859, Florence Nightingale addressed the issue of the patient environment, which continues to be as timely now as it was then.

Protecting patients from falls, burns, and defective equipment is a shared duty of health care providers. Large sums of money are paid out annually for allegations relating to these issues. Staff should be made aware of their responsibility in providing a safe environment to achieve an optimal patient outcome.

The Occupational Safety and Health Administration recently has drafted guidelines for compliance in providing and protecting employees. It is recommended that nurse managers become familiar with these guidelines and implement appropriate corrective action when necessary.

References

Creighton, H. (1986). *Law every nurse should know* (5th ed.). Philadelphia: W.B. Saunders Co.

Cunningham, L. (1991). *The quality connection in health care*. San Francisco: Jossey-Bass Publishers.

Danziger, P. (1983). *Can you sue your parents for malpractice?* Laurel-Leaf Books.

Darling v. Charleston Memorial Hospital, 211 N.E. 253 (W.Va., 1965).

Hartshorn, E. (1992, May–June). *The Risks & Benefits Journal.*

Huber, P.W. (1988). *Liability: The legal revolution and its consequences.*

Jury Verdict Research, Inc. (1991). Solon, OH.

Murphy, E. (1990). *The quality connection.* E.C. Murphy, Ltd.

Nightingale, F. (1859). *Notes on nursing: What it is and what it is not.*

Peterson, K. (1990, October 1). *Modern Healthcare.*

Risk Management Foundation. (1989, February 20). *Hospitals.*

Rosenbaum, E. (1991). *The doctor.* Ballentine Books.

CHAPTER 36

RESPONSIBILITIES OF NURSE EXECUTIVES IN CONDUCTING AND USING RESEARCH IN THE PRACTICE SETTING

KARIN T. KIRCHHOFF
MARITA G. TITLER

EXECUTIVE SUMMARY

Nurse executives are charged with delivering cost-effective, high-quality patient care. Building a research program in a service agency can assist nurse executives in meeting this charge. Nurse executives who use research to improve care have to do so in a cost-conscious environment. Practice-based research programs vary in type, outcome, and resources needed for implementation. The challenge for the future is to demonstrate systematically the impact of each type of program on nursing practice, the organizational climate, cost of care, administrative decision making, and the science of nursing.

D eveloping a scientific basis for nursing practice is essential for quality patient care and advancement of the nursing profession (McClure, 1981). Until recently, most nursing research was done by nurses in academia rather than in practice settings. As early as 1980, the American Society for Nursing Service Administration (later known as the American Organization of Nurse Executives, AONE) noted that an opportunity to close the gap between theory and practice exists within the context of service agencies where patient care is delivered.

In a more recent document, nurse executives are challenged to view the economic constraint of the environment as an incentive for integrating nursing research in the practice setting (AONE, 1985). Organizations that maintain practice-based nursing research programs report savings associated with productive, efficient, research-based methods of nursing care delivery and adherence to DRG-imposed lengths of stay. Operational strategies for establishing and maintaining practice-based nursing research in an economically constrained environment include (AONE, 1985)

1. Selection of a suitable program design
2. Articulation of program functions
3. Acquisition of program resources
4. Education of staff
5. Application of research findings in practice

There is a rapidly growing awareness by chief nurse executives (CNE) of the need to implement practice-based nursing research programs that address unique needs of service (Simms, Price, & Pfoutz, 1987).

This chapter presents a national perspective of expectations for research in the practice setting and reviews areas for consideration by nurse executives when instituting a practice-based research program. The importance of creating a research climate is discussed, administrative responsibilities for research are delineated, delegation of administrative responsibilities for research in practice is addressed, and indicators for evaluating a practice-based research program are suggested. The term clinical nurse researcher (CNR) is used throughout to denote a nurse researcher based in the clinical setting whose responsibility for research and evaluation encompasses both clinical and administrative areas.

NATIONAL PERSPECTIVE

National nursing organizations and accrediting bodies outline the importance of research in practice. The Joint Commission for Accreditation of Healthcare Organizations (JCAHO) requires that policies, procedures, standards of patient care, and standards of nursing practice be developed from current scientific knowledge. It is the CNE's responsibility to assure that this expectation is met (JCAHO, 1991).

The American Nurses Association (ANA) has several goals and strategies that address developing a scientific base for nursing practice. These include facilitating establishment of the profession's research agenda, supporting research to describe and measure quality and effectiveness of nursing practice interventions, and demonstrating cost savings and quality outcomes of various organizational models and financial arrangements for nursing services (Bergstrom, 1991).

The American Association of Critical-Care Nurses (AACN) reflects the importance of research in its practice and outcome standards (Kuhn, 1990; Sanford & Disch, 1989). They have set priorities for research, first in 1983 and again in 1991 (AACN, 1991; Lewandowski & Kositsky, 1983). The most recent priorities include both contextual and patient-centered areas of research.

Documents illustrating the importance of practice-based research are available from several other national organizations, such as the American Heart Association, American Thoracic Society, and Sigma Theta Tau. Many of these organizations, including AONE, have committed money for nursing research, with some awards targeted for practice-based research activities.

Changes in funding patterns of nursing research for clinical sites also are occurring. Traditionally, major funding for nursing research has gone to colleges of nursing in university centers. Recent funding by the Robert Wood Johnson Foundation and Pew Memorial Trust for redesigning nursing care delivery, however, has made practice agencies viable candidates for major grant monies. It is evident that integrating nursing research into the practice setting is valued by specialty groups, professional organizations, and funding agencies.

CREATING A RESEARCH CLIMATE

The nurse executive is responsible for creating a climate conducive to nursing research (Chance & Hinshaw, 1980; Kirchhoff, 1993; McClure, 1981; Simms et al., 1987). In order for practice-based research to be successful, nurse executives must value research for administrative and clinical decision making and enact this value in their behavior. Nurse executives can influence staff attitudes, beliefs, and behaviors about research by espousing their values through policies, procedures, philosophy statements, and actions (Bolton, 1991; Fugleberg, 1986; Knafl, Bevis, & Kirchhoff, 1987a; Pettengill, Knafl, Bevis, & Kirchhoff, 1988; Snyder-Halpern, 1991).

Organizational Climate

Examination of the mission, philosophy, goals, and strategic plan of the organization provides insight into the challenges nurse executives face in creating a departmental climate conducive to nursing research. The type of research activities nurse executives can integrate into the practice setting are influenced by the implicit and explicit values statements found in these documents (Pranulis & Driever, 1990; Rempusheski, 1991).

Organizations that promote innovations, data-based decision making, and risk-taking behavior are more supportive of nursing research activities than are those in which research activities are secondary to other expectations (Pettengill et al., 1988; Synder-Halpern, 1991). For example, a university teaching facility that includes research as a central mission of the organization may actively support both conduct and utilization of nursing research. In contrast, a community hospital that excludes statements about research in its mission may, at best, use research methods in quality improvement programs or support only research utilization activities that have a direct, explicit impact on the cost and quality of care. This does not imply that research utilization is easier than conduct of research but that organizational benefits of utilization activities, in some cases, may be easier to demonstrate to those in control of hospital funds (Goode, Lovett, Hayes, & Butcher, 1987).

Departmental Climate—The Role of the Nurse Executive

To prevent nursing research from being perceived as a frill that can be discarded in tough economic times, it is essential to place it in a professional practice environment (Cronenwett, 1986c; Titler, Goode, & Mathis, 1992). Nurses must be practicing safely, delivering quality care, and participating in resolution of practice issues. Subscribing to professional journals, attending regional and national meetings, and belonging to professional and specialty organizations are examples of professional behaviors that reflect nurses' commitment to professional practice.

The value of nursing research in the department of nursing is communicated by incorporating research (conduct and utilization) into the nursing department philosophy and objectives. For example, the departmental philosophy at Hines Veterans Administration Hospital includes the following message about research (Lawson, 1987, p. 6).

> We believe that research conducted by nurses, as well as nursing collaboration in interdisciplinary scientific inquiry, validates existing practice and provides new direction for enhancing care . . . and Nursing is committed to providing the clinical, administrative, scientific, and educational resources necessary for the effective and efficient delivery of care in accordance with established professional standards.

Research behaviors must be built into job descriptions so that research-based clinical practice is the expectation rather than the exception (Hegedus & Marino, 1989; Pranulis & Driever, 1990; Simms et al., 1987). The type of research activities expected of nurses should be explicitly articulated in clinical ladders and merit programs (Bolton, 1991). Expected investigative activities based on educational credentials provide guidance for integrating research into job descriptions and merit programs (ANA, 1981). Devoting a component of nursing orientation to discuss research reinforces the departmental expectations, communicates the importance of research in the organization, and encourages staff to become involved in research (Kirchhoff, 1985).

Nurse executives communicate the value of research by legitimizing research activities. Providing clinical release time for doing research, instituting recognition for participating in research, encouraging staff to enroll in research courses, and encouraging staff to attend and present their research at local, regional, and national meetings are examples of how managers can convey the importance of research (Davis, 1981; Pranulis & Driever, 1990).

Administrative Responsibilities for Research—The Role of the Nurse Manager

Nurse executives have major leadership responsibility for instituting practice-based research programs (Kirchhoff, 1991b). This includes articulation of objectives, allocation of resources, ensuring review of research proposals, and exploring mechanisms appropriate for integrating research in their organization and department.

Unit nurse managers have a function similar to nurse executives once the organization is committed to incorporating nursing research. They convey the importance of research at the unit level by encouraging staff to obtain research consultation, facilitating the use of research-based practice protocols, and arranging release time for staff to participate in research activities (e.g., attendance at journal clubs, collection of data, developing research-based practice protocols). Nurse managers of certain units, such as neonatal ICUs and labor and delivery, may need to establish a mechanism to clear multiple requests from various investigators for use of patients as subjects.

Articulation of Research Objectives

The first responsibility, articulation of research objectives, provides a vision for research that is in concert with the department's philosophy of nursing practice. Decisions need to be made about (1) the research focus—clinical, administrative, evaluative, or some combination thereof, and (2) type of research activities—conduct, utilization, or both (Lindsey, 1991; Marchette, 1985).

Personnel helpful in making these decisions include clinical directors, deans of colleges of nursing, directors of research in colleges of nursing, senior staff nurses, and nurse managers. Conversations with key stakeholders, such as administrators, physicians, pharmacists, and other health care personnel, may provide additional valuable information for decision making. The book, *Conducting and Using Nursing Research in Clinical Settings,* by Mateo and Kirchhoff (1991), is another resource to use when making these choices.

It is imperative that departmental objectives concerning research are clear and attainable. It is better to be selective in the type of research activities the department wants to achieve and be successful than to be too broad in scope, with frustration and perceived failure resulting. When the research activities are successful, the nurse executive has data to illustrate how the organization may further benefit from expanding the research program.

Allocation of Resources

Resource allocation follows from departmental objectives regarding research. Fixed expenses typically include research texts and journals, computer hardware, office space, and labor costs associated with budgeted staff positions. Variable costs include videotapes and other teaching aids, computer software for statistical analysis and production of visual aids, posters for regional and national presentations, copying, and travel to research meetings. Additional resources to be considered are library facilities, time for staff to participate in research activities, statistical consultation, computer time, and secretarial support (AONE, 1985; Cronenwett, 1986c). The amount of fiscal dollars allocated depends on the size and scope of the practice-based research program envisioned by the nurse executive. Expenditures during the first year are likely to be higher than in subsequent years as initial equipment and materials are purchased. This expenditure is necessary, however, to facilitate success of the program.

Pettengill et al. (1988) found that the major impediment to nursing research was lack of tangible resources (time and money). Thus, critical issues nurse executives must address are which cost center includes the budget for research (general nursing budget, independent cost center) and how to allocate resources despite cost-containment efforts.

One strategy CNEs use to circumvent limited financial support is to subsume research within an existing cost center (Pettengill et al., 1988). Chance and Hinshaw (1980) note that including research in the general nursing administrative budget provides more flexibility than establishing a separate cost center. Flattening of organizational structures may free some midlevel management positions, resulting in a major portion of the funds being earmarked for nursing research (MacKay, Grantham, & Ross, 1984).

The goal of supporting research programs through external funding is somewhat idealistic and short sighted (Marchette, 1985). If major components of the program are not supported by hospital funds, nurse researchers are likely to spend an inordinate amount of time writing grants rather than facilitating research activities of the nursing staff (Hagle, Kirchhoff, Knafl, & Bevis, 1986).

Nurse executives can justify costs by illustrating the derived benefits of nursing research (Titler et al., 1992). Knafl, Hagle, Bevis, & Kirchhoff (1987) found that a strategy used by nurse executives to assure viability of the CNR role was structuring the role to include responsibilities valued throughout the organization (e.g., having the clinical nurse researcher do administrative studies). Demonstrating that nursing research can make an important contribution to the organization and patient outcomes is reported as crucial to success of the CNR (Knafl, Hagle, et al., 1987).

Review of Research Proposals

The third area of responsibility for the nurse executive as well as nurse manager is ensuring that nursing research proposals receive proper review by the department and institutional review boards (Kirchhoff & McGuire, 1985). An organization that supports a nursing research program must have an efficient and effective means for reviewing research protocols for scientific merit and protection of human subjects (Egan, McElmurry, & Jameson, 1981).

A nursing department research committee should include nurses from a variety of clinical specialties and role preparations (e.g., CNS, managers, staff nurses, academic affiliation) who have a solid knowledge base about research and ethics. The committee chair needs expertise in research to ensure the scientific merit of the proposed studies, to protect against use of health care workers as unpaid data collectors, and to prevent overuse of patients as subjects in specific clinical areas.

The purpose of the nursing research committee and its relationship with the Institutional Review Board (IRB) must be clear (Bartos, Sexton, & Taggart, 1991). For example, an organization may require that all proposals that affect nursing care of patients be approved by the departmental research committee before review and approval by the IRB.

Nursing representation on the IRB is critical (Bartos et al., 1991; Cronenwett, 1985) because it

1. Communicates the importance of nursing research to the organization
2. Permits systematic review of how each research protocol may affect delivery of nursing care
3. Facilitates interdisciplinary collaboration
4. Clarifies for other disciplines the nature of nursing research

Exploring Options

An important responsibility of nurse executives, along with nurse managers, is exploring options for integration of research into the department. Practice-based nursing research can be enacted at various levels using different types of programs (Dennis & Strickland, 1987; Lindsey, 1991). Some organizations may use one type of program, whereas others use several approaches (Stark, 1989).

Limited enactment includes establishing a research committee in the department of nursing, acquiring consultation from other departments or organizations, using existing personnel to carry out program objectives, and collaborating with colleges or other service agencies. Fuller enactment includes hiring a research specialist or forming a research department or division within the nursing department's organizational structure (AONE, 1985).

Committees. Research committees are used extensively to establish practice-based nursing research programs (AONE, 1985; Fuhs & Moore, 1981; Hegedus & Marino, 1989). The committee may be ad hoc and composed of rotating members to carry out specific projects. This approach facilitates use of individuals with expertise and commitment specific to the research. Various types of stakeholders become involved in research and disseminate the value of research to nurses at many levels of the organization. A major disadvantage is lack of stability over time for effective maintenance of protocols and standards.

Nursing departments with greater opportunities and resources for research usually formulate a standing research committee. In addition to reviewing research proposals for scientific merit and protection of human subjects, these committees may also facilitate research utilization, educate nurses about clinical nursing research, and consult with staff about conduct of research. Committee members generally remain consistent, include nurses from all levels of the organization, and consist of people who have the ability to effect change in order to institute research-based practice protocols. Functions of the standing research committee are coordinated with other committees in the nursing department and throughout the organization. The nursing department's organizational chart clearly illustrates the relationship of this committee with other standing committees and councils. For example, to develop and implement research-based practice policies, a research committee would interact with policy and procedure committees, staff nurse councils, and management committees to effectively institute change at the bedside.

An advantage of using this type of program is to minimize costs by using existing personnel. The costs of release time for personnel to participate in research activities, however, should not be overlooked. A second advantage is that it facilitates consensus building about research initiatives that are in line with organizational objectives. Team investigations arising out of committee structures can promote targeted research, which is important when resources are limited. It also facilitates a particular project to be initiated and completed in a more timely fashion.

Disadvantages of the committee approach are varying levels of accountability and authority for research project completion and dependence on personal motivation and commitment of committee members for productivity and achievement of objectives. One strategy to overcome these disadvantages is to provide recognition for participation on the committee and reinforce the value of each committee member's participation.

Consultation.   Consultation is a second option nurse executives and managers consider when planning practice-based research programs. A nurse scientist assists staff in carrying out specific studies and provides guidance with research utilization projects, depending on the objectives of the research program. This is a particularly useful approach in community hospitals.

Contractual agreements can be negotiated with local colleges or universities. One method is to exchange lectures and clinical supervision of students by agency staff for consultation services of nurse scientists from the academic setting. Another mechanism is to pool resources of several health care agencies in the same geographic area to hire a nurse scientist who consults periodically in each agency on a rotating basis.

Consultation services also may be negotiated with other department heads in the organization (Campbell & Chulay, 1990). For example, nursing may provide hemodynamic educational programs for new residents in exchange for consultation services of biostatisticians from the department of medicine.

In hiring or negotiating for consultation services of a nurse scientist, the nurse executive considers the nature of the project, the expertise of the available scientists, and the qualities of an effective consultant. "Not every nurse researcher is a good consultant for clinical projects" (Larson, Wells, & McHugh, 1985, p. 873). An effective consultant must be familiar with clinical research protocols, be comfortable with clinical variables that are not easily manipulated, recognize that unanticipated interruptions are likely to occur in clinical research, and share the philosophy that nursing research belongs to the entire profession, not just to nurses with advanced degrees (Larson et al., 1985).

The consultant brings investigational resources and insight into research techniques while assisting staff to

- State the problem in a form appropriate for scientific inquiry
- Narrow the scope of the problem
- Identify the type of literature appropriate for review
- Identify variables and appropriate measurement techniques
- Select a study design that is realistic yet minimizes bias
- Analyze and interpret data

Consultation services are helpful also as nurses prepare study results for publication or presentation at research meetings or both.

Use of Existing Personnel.   Using existing nursing personnel to carry out research activities is another option nurse executives could consider for integrating research into the department (AONE, 1985; Hoare & Earenfight, 1986). For example, clinical nurse specialists (CNS) learn about conduct and use of research in their masters' programs, but many report that this role component typically is not enacted. "Administrators can make a major contribution to research in nursing by assisting CNSs to set appropriate and attainable expectations for research-related activities" (Cronenwett, 1986c, p. 10).

Masters-prepared nurses are not, however, substitutes for doctorally prepared researchers. If using masters-prepared CNSs, nurse executives should not expect the same type of outcomes as can be achieved with a doctorally prepared CNR who has more extensive research knowledge and skill, and who can serve as a consultant to address practice-based research issues.

Thus, the success of having existing personnel conduct and use research in practice depends heavily on the nurse executive's ability to ready the organization for research, commit resources to carry out research, assess the abilities and enthusiasm of nurses in the department to conduct and use research findings appropriately, and provide opportunities for nurses to acquire the necessary research skills and consultation. Becoming a competent researcher requires doctoral preparation and progressive experience with research (Haller, 1986).

Nondoctorally prepared nurses with research interests can participate successfully in research when they collaborate with experienced, doctorally prepared nurse researchers (Beavers, Gruber, & Johnson, 1990; Haller, 1986; Hoare & Earenfight, 1986; Schutzenhofer, 1991). Staff nurses, CNSs, and nurse managers can contribute to the integration of research in the service setting by decreasing organizational barriers, systematically documenting patient care problems, disseminating research findings, and transferring research-based knowledge into practice (Cronenwett, 1986a,b; Kirchhoff, 1991b; Larson, 1981; Lindeman, 1988; Rempusheski, 1991).

Collaboration. Another strategy nurse executives consider for integrating research into the service setting is collaboration. This can take several forms but involves merging the expertise of the clinician or nurse administrator with the research expertise of the nurse scientist (AONE, 1985; Betz, Poster, Randell, & Omery, 1990; Hinshaw & Smeltzer, 1987; Hunt, Stark, Fisher, Hegedus, Joy, & Woldum, 1983; Smeltzer & Hinshaw, 1988; Stone, 1991).

If a doctorally prepared CNS is employed in the department of nursing, collaboration between this individual and other staff can result in productive research activities (Dennis & Strickland, 1987). Advantages realized by this type of collaboration include a greater appreciation by CNSs of the complexities in providing care for a specific patient population, an increased awareness by staff nurses of the rewards and difficulties in doing clinical nursing research, and better integration of research findings in clinical practice (Campbell & Chulay, 1990; Medoff-Cooper & Lamb, 1989; Schutzenhofer, 1991).

Collaboration also can be fostered between service and education. Nurse scientists employed in academic settings that are administratively and geographically separate from a service agency can successfully collaborate with nurses in that agency (Frick, DelPo, & Robinson, 1988). Collaboration among academic and service personnel employed in the same university or administrative system results in productive practice-based research programs (Hagle et al., 1987; Hinshaw & Smeltzer, 1987; Smeltzer & Hinshaw, 1988; Tyler, Clark, Winslow, & White, 1990).

The Nursing Consortium for Research in Practice, initiated by Stanford University Hospital, is another collaborative approach used to increase nursing research productivity in service settings (Rizzuto & Mitchell, 1988a,b, 1990; Zalar, Welches, & Walker, 1985). The project offers nurses from multiple service agencies an opportunity to become involved in research (Rizzuto & Mitchell, 1990) by

1. Attending research-related workshops
2. Participating in multisite studies
3. Receiving consultation from nurse scientists

Communication and respect for the values of service and academia are key elements necessary to ensure success in collaboration. Advantages of collaboration are increased visibility and esteem for all agencies involved, increased opportunities for research funding, maximum use and distribution of resources, and a greater ability to do relevant, applicable studies that generate meaningful findings for clinical practice (AONE, 1985; Frick et al., 1988; Hagle et al., 1987; Smeltzer & Hinshaw, 1988; Tyler et al., 1990). Integrating the expertise of nurses with varying skills "provides a very strong base from which to conduct nursing research and allows for both the protection of the scientific rigor of the project and the clinical or practice integrity of the investigations" (Hinshaw & Smeltzer, 1987, p. 24).

Research Specialists.   Appointment of a full-time or part-time doctorally prepared research specialist is one way nurse executives can fully enact practice-based research within the nursing department (Kirchhoff, 1993). This approach generally is used by larger, urban health care organizations, whereas smaller facilities often experience difficulty recruiting qualified nurse researchers. Two advantages of using research specialists are (1) an increased potential for effective development, implementation, and evaluation of the research program and (2) direct accountability for research activities within the department (AONE, 1985; Betz et al., 1990; Kirchhoff, 1993). A major disadvantage is the additional costs associated with recruitment of a qualified nurse scientist and establishment of budgeted positions for nursing research (AONE, 1985).

Research Department.   Creation of a nursing research department or division is another way to fully enact practice-based nursing research (AONE, 1985; Lawson, 1987; MacKay, et al., 1984; Schutzenhofer, 1991). Advantages of this approach are direct accountability and clearly articulated authority for research, formal communication channels with executive management, and clearly delineated reporting relationships.

Research departments typically include a number of budgeted staff positions, full-time or part-time or both. Establishment of a research department clearly signifies the organization's and the nursing department's commitment to research.

The costs of initiating and maintaining a nursing research department may be prohibitive to using this approach in most agencies (AONE, 1985).

DELEGATING ADMINISTRATIVE RESPONSIBILITIES FOR RESEARCH

The current trend is for nurse executives to delegate research responsibilities by hiring nurse scientists who direct and coordinate departmental research activities. Issues nurse executives face when using this approach are

1. Hiring qualified personnel
2. Providing administrative support
3. Promoting role enactment
4. Anticipating and resolving issues

Hiring Qualified Personnel

Before hiring a clinical nurse researcher, nurse executives must have a clear concept of the nature of the position (e.g., job description, full-time, part-time, joint appointment, additional responsibilities) and where it will be placed in the organizational hierarchy (Chance & Hinshaw, 1980; Dennis & Strickland, 1987; Knafl, Bevis & Kirchhoff, 1987a; MacKay et al., 1984; Marchette, 1985). This information is then used to recruit qualified personnel and determine which person is the best fit for the position.

Nature of the Position

The nature of the clinical nursing research position is guided by departmental research objectives and input from management and staff. Organizations that have available resources can devote a full-time position to nursing research, whereas smaller organizations or those with fewer resources may introduce the position by linking it with quality improvement or nursing education. For example, some positions may be composed of a 0.5 FTE for nursing research and the other 0.5 FTE for education or quality improvement (Cronenwett, 1986b; Dennis & Strickland, 1987).

Joint appointment of a nurse researcher to an affiliating school or college of nursing is another option that provides organizations a way to hire a nurse researcher and share costs. Researchers in this position are able to facilitate the work of graduate students and faculty by helping them develop research proposals that fit with the department's research program and gain entree to clinical sites (Kirchhoff, 1981, 1985). The joint appointment also allows the researcher to maintain collegial relationships with nurse scientists in academia while conducting research that is focused and meaningful for clinical practice (Chance & Hinshaw, 1980; Dennis & Strickland, 1987). Negotiations in planning for a joint appointment should include reimbursing (salary and benefits) the researcher from two different payroll systems, allocating of direct and indirect monies from external funding, and balancing expectations of two administrators.

Titles reflect the nature of the position and, thus, vary considerably across institutions (Pettengill et al., 1988). They range from director of nursing research, which implies administrative decision-making authority and responsibility in addition to carrying out a practice-based research program, to nurse researcher, which implies a greater emphasis solely on conduct and use of nursing research. Job descriptions further delineate the nature of the position and reflect functions expected of the researcher. The nurse executive and nurse researcher need to carefully negotiate realistic job expectations to avoid burdening the individual with tasks that detract from realizing the benefits of having a doctorally prepared nurse researcher in the practice setting.

Responsibilities included in job descriptions (Dennis & Strickland, 1987; Hagle et al., 1986; Knafl et al., 1987b; Lawson, 1988b; Mayer, 1983) are

- Ensuring respect and protection of individual patient rights
- Reviewing nursing research protocols for scientific merit
- Promoting research activities that are in line with program, departmental, and organizational objectives
- Facilitating staff development programs in nursing research
- Consulting with personnel to conduct research
- Promoting research use throughout the department
- Establishing multidisciplinary collegial bonds
- Facilitating research by nursing faculty and students
- Serving on departmental and organizational committees as appointed
- Conducting and publishing in one's own area of research
- Serving on regional and national research committees
- Disseminating information regarding grant opportunities, requests for proposals, and calls for abstracts
- Serving as a consultant in grant writing
- Facilitating preparation of abstracts, manuscripts, and paper and poster presentations

Additional functions nurse executives consider for inclusion in job descriptions (Cronenwett, 1986b; Dennis & Strickland, 1987; Hagle et al., 1986; Knafl et al., 1987b; Lawson, 1988b; Mayer, 1983) are as follows.

- Assisting with formulation, implementation, and use of databases for clinical and administrative decision making
- Promoting collaborative research with affiliated schools or colleges of nursing
- Promoting collaborative research with other disciplines
- Promoting development of a regional nursing research consortium
- Acquiring external grant funds and administering those funds
- Serving as a consultant to agencies outside the organization
- Administering related programs, such as quality improvement, infection control, or education

Educational requirements must be delineated clearly, with a doctoral degree, preferably in nursing, being a minimum requirement (Knafl et al., 1987a). Completion of a doctoral program or fellowship that prepares nurse scientists for the CNR role is an added advantage (Dennis, 1991; Lawson, 1989).

Additional requirements vary depending on the focus of the research program. For example, if teaching nurses about nursing research is a program objective, teaching experience is desirable. If research objectives include acquisition of grant funds, experience in grant writing and grants management is preferred. Researchers hired into this position benefit from having teaching experience, clinical expertise, and research experience aside from that obtained from work on academic degrees (Kirchhoff, 1985).

Placement in the Organization

Placement of the position in the organization depends on the research objectives. In turn, placement of the position influences the lines of communication between the CNR and nurse executive as well as the salary and institutional clout of the individual (Marchette, 1985). Most experts agree that in order for the CNR to be effective, the position should be in the department of nursing rather than in a research and development department within the organization (Chance & Hinshaw, 1980; Dennis & Strickland, 1987; Kirchhoff, 1985; Marchette, 1985).

The nursing department's organizational structure determines ultimate authority and accountability invested in the position (AONE, 1985; Dennis & Strickland, 1987). When departments are organized on the staff model, the clinical nurse researcher has full accountability for research activities without the authority to make broad program decisions. Researchers in this position may have difficulty influencing others to participate in research activities and use research findings in clinical practice. In contrast, functional line models provide the clinical nurse researcher with more direct authority for decisions regarding research and its use in practice. The potential for conflict still exists, however, if the CNR recommends actions that are opposed by line personnel. Thus, nurse executives must place the position strategically to maintain the delicate balance between line power and staff expertise (AONE, 1985). Nurse managers are critical in facilitating this. Despite placement and type of departmental model, the majority of CNRs have direct access and reporting relationships to the chief nurse executive (Hagle et al., 1986; Knafl et al., 1987a,b).

Finding the Right Fit—The Selection Process

Recruiting qualified personnel for the position is a challenge. As research positions grow in number, the demand for doctorally prepared nurses increases. National advertising in research and specialty journals, use of the nurse executive's network, contacting professional placement agencies, and attendance at national research meetings (e.g., Council of Nurse Researchers) are methods useful for attracting potential candidates. A personal touch, such as a phone call or letter, also may be helpful. Recruitment of doctoral candidates doing dissertation work in the organization should not be overlooked, as it provides an opportunity for the CNE to view the potential viability of individuals as candidates for the position (Chance & Hinshaw, 1980).

Screening potential candidates begins with examination of their curriculum vitae (CV) to see if there is a match between the research vision of the organization and the credentials and experience of the individual. If a program is to be successful, doctoral preparation is necessary because it demonstrates acquisition of minimum knowledge and skills necessary to do research. The individual should be a nurse in order to have knowledge and insight about nursing and its researchable problems. Because the individual will be working in a practice setting, evidence of recent clinical experience is an important consideration (Cronenwett, 1986b; Hagle et al., 1986; Kirchhoff, 1985). Publications in peer-reviewed journals demonstrate an ability to write and disseminate research findings. If grant writing is important for the organization, evidence of funded research must be reflected in the CV (Cronenwett, 1986b).

Attracting candidates with an established program of research requires flexibility on the part of the nurse executive to negotiate salary, benefits, and job responsibilities. This individual, however, is more likely to have personal security, self-respect, and self-confidence about research methods, which in turn benefits the organization. The fit between the organizational and professional research goals of the nurse scientists is essential to consider (Kirchhoff, 1985; Pranulis, 1991).

Subjective qualifications are equally important and can be assessed by interview, by asking that specific interpersonal skills be addressed in references, and by contacting well-known nurse researchers and mentors of potential candidates.

Expectations of the Nurse Researcher

CNRs must be able to

1. Establish positive working relationships and converse with staff at varying levels of the organization
2. Generate enthusiasm for both nursing practice and research
3. Be politically astute and work effectively within existing power structures
4. Commit to objectives of the research program and articulate specific ways to achieve those objectives
5. Understand various role relationships in the organization and articulate how those might influence nursing research
6. Demonstrate a willingness to perform research activities that may at first glance seem mundane (e.g., nighttime data collection)
7. Be approachable, energetic, and understanding of the clinical practice arena

Flexibility, inquisitiveness, creativity, negotiation, expertise in use of group process, and humor are additional qualities to consider (Chance & Hinshaw, 1980; Dennis & Strickland, 1987; Hagle et al., 1986; Knafl et al., 1987a; Pranulis & Driever, 1990).

The Process

A selection committee is helpful for screening and interviewing potential candidates. Composition of the selection committee varies but often includes hospital administrators, people in affiliated colleges and schools of nursing, nurses at various levels of the organization, and researchers from other disciplines. Screening interviews may be done by a subgroup of the committee, with final interviews completed by all members. It is useful to have candidates present a research paper to different types of groups in the organization (e.g., staff nurses, physicians, nurse managers). Final selection of the individual can be made by committee consensus, by committee vote, or by making a recommendation to the CNE.

Providing Administrative Support

Once a nurse scientist is hired into the department, the viability of the position is dependent, in part, on support of the CNE. CNEs are viewed as shaping the CNR role through their ability to control and influence organizational structures that support research and by their willingness to direct the efforts of the CNR (Dennis & Strickland, 1987; Knafl, Hagle, Bevis, Faux, & Kirchhoff, 1989).

CNEs report three goals to ensure success of the CNR position: assuring viability of the position, integrating the CNR into the organization, and fostering a research climate (Knafl, Hagle, et al., 1987). Strategies used to assure viability of the position focus on structuring the role to include responsibilities that are valued throughout the organization (e.g., administrative research, quality assurance), limiting research activities to one or two critical projects that result in concrete measurable outcomes, and making the role financially independent of the hospital (e.g., grant writing for external funding).

CNEs appoint CNRs to specific committees or assignments that enhance their organizational visibility in an effort to integrate them into the organization. Strategies used by CNEs to foster a research climate include increasing educational requirements for new job applications at all levels and assigning nurses as research assistants to facilitate research activities (Knafl, Hagle, et al., 1987).

Expected outcomes for the first 2 to 3 years of the program should be negotiated, clearly documented, reviewed at least yearly, and renegotiated when necessary (Dennis & Strickland, 1987). Knafl et al. (1989) found that over half of the CNRs reported major changes in their role over time and that nearly half believed that maintaining autonomy and control over the position and its activities was important to their success. Thus, CNEs should facilitate and support appropriate role changes and promote autonomy in role enactment.

A realistic timeline for a full-time CNR is to spend the first 6 to 12 months orienting to the organization. Consultation for the first project (conduct or utilization) takes place about 6 months after employment, and publishing the results of the first project usually occurs during year 3 or 4. This timeline will vary depending on the experience of the CNR and familiarity with the institution.

Promoting Role Enactment

When enacting the role, CNRs must be cognizant that persons outside and within the department have roles that may hinder or support the nursing research program. Therefore, the CNR needs to spend initial time learning the system—

who does what, how things are done, and the formal and informal decision-making mechanisms that are operant. Learning about other departments and the potential for collaboration with nursing is time well spent. Learning how to move oneself through the system for conduct and use of research helps the CNR facilitate research activities of others (Dennis & Strickland, 1987). These activities may require 6 months to a year.

A serious barrier to implementation of the role is lack of credibility. CNRs must be prepared to demonstrate the important contributions of nursing research and its impact on improving patient outcomes. Strategies CNRs use to establish credibility include the following (Dennis & Strickland, 1987; Knafl, Hagle, et al., 1987; Lawson, 1988a).

- Increasing self-esteem of staff by acknowledging and rewarding participation in research
- Encouraging questioning of existing practices
- Promoting open communication
- Showing respect for others' expertise and contributions
- Communicating outcomes of specific projects
- Conducting projects that others in the organization view as making important contributions
- Carefully selecting an initial project that is both visible and readily useful
- Keeping key stakeholders informed of nursing research activities

CNRs report that creating collegial support is essential to the role. Strategies used to achieve this include (1) increasing visibility of the CNR by participating in patient care, serving on committees with staff, and having regularly scheduled office hours, and (2) increasing staff interest in research by disseminating studies relevant to the practice of nurses on specific units, contributing to educational programming, sponsoring journal clubs and research-based grand rounds, providing research-based information for decision making of managers and clinicians, including nursing staff in all research activities, and discussing organizational research activities during orientation (Dennis & Strickland, 1987; Kirchhoff, 1985; Knafl, Hagle, et al., 1987).

Campbell and Chulay (1990) suggest targeting nurse managers and CNSs for early involvement in initial research activities. By building on their interest and enthusiasm, a core of leadership personnel will evolve to support subsequent research efforts.

CNRs report that they enact the role in three major areas: research, administration, and staff development (Knafl et al., 1987a,b; Lawson, 1988b). The majority of time is devoted to direct research activities, which usually are divided between helping others conduct or use research and conducting one's own research. Staff development activities are directed toward motivating nurses in the setting to become involved in research and facilitating their professional growth (e.g., journal clubs, further education). Administrative activities of CNRs focus on research monitoring, such as assisting nurse managers, chairing research committees, and attending IRB meetings.

Based on the findings of Knafl et al. (1987b), three patterns of CNR role enactment have emerged. In the traditional scientist model, the CNR is responsible for identifying what research needs to be done in the organization and then designing and carrying out that research. In the associate model, the CNR takes the lead in either initiating or conducting research. In the facilitator model, the focus of the CNR is preparing and motivating other nurses in the setting to initiate and carry out the research (Knafl et al., 1987b). It appears that there is no one right way to enact the role but that attention to the research needs of the organization and the fit with the researcher's professional needs are important considerations.

Anticipating and Resolving Issues

Scientific inquiry and patient care have different inherent value systems that lead to issues when integrating research in practice. These issues can be resolved by the CNE and CNR working together and using specific strategies to address each (Hinshaw & Smeltzer, 1987).

Educational Differences Among Nurses in the Organization

The first issue is the educational differences among nurses in the organization. One strategy to address this is to convey mutual respect for each person's unique contributions and talents rather than focusing only on educational credentials. A second strategy is to facilitate further education of interested nurses by consulting with them about their options, assisting them in finding financial aid, and providing flexible work schedules.

Premature Use of Research Findings

The second issue is to balance the immediate need for clinical or administrative information against the need for replication of studies before applying findings in practice. One strategy is to agree on guidelines that determine a researchable problem. Not every problem found in clinical practice is researchable, and many can be addressed by using problem-solving techniques. A second strategy is to develop or use existing guidelines of when investigative results are ready for use in clinical practice (Goode, 1987; Kirchhoff, 1991a; Weiler & Buckwalter, 1990). This curbs the reseacher's inclination to hedge on the applicability of findings and curbs the tendency of nurse executives to use research findings prematurely. A third strategy is to educate nurses about the importance of accuracy in scientific inquiry in order to generate valid and reliable information (Hinshaw & Smeltzer, 1987).

Time Involved Doing Research

A third issue is the time involved in doing research. A study may take from 1 to 2 years to complete. Keeping administrators and staff committed to the study is a challenge, and it is important that a realistic timeline is set for each investigation and that staff understand the time necessary to complete specific research activities. Personnel can be kept involved by using a team approach to investigation, meeting on a regular basis, and providing interim feedback through memos or presentations (Hinshaw & Smeltzer, 1987). It is important that the CNE and the CNR set realistic timelines for each component of the research program.

EVALUATION

Outcomes of an effective research program are described (Campbell & Chulay, 1990; Cronenwett, 1985; Hinshaw & Smeltzer, 1987; Knafl, et al., 1989; Pettengill et al., 1988; Snyder-Halpern, 1991). The level of nursing research productivity is closely associated with the presence of a nurse researcher in the organization. Institutions that employ either full-time or part-time nurse researchers report higher levels of research activity than institutions that do not have a nurse researcher (Betz et al., 1990). Using a two-round delphi survey of nurse researchers in service agencies, Synder-Halpern (1991) found that outcome indicators of successful nursing research programs include

- Generation of manuscripts for publication
- Integration of the research program into the entire fiber and mission of the nursing department
- Completion and publication of funded research projects
- Recognition and support of the research program by nursing staff
- Rewards for attaining research objectives

Criteria used for evaluating effectiveness are inherent in departmental research objectives and thus vary across institutions. They usually encompass a combination of traditional scientific criteria, effect on the organizational climate, and improvement in providing cost-effective quality care (Knafl et al., 1989; Synder-Halpern, 1991).

Scientific Criteria

Scientific criteria that nurse executives can use as outcome measures include

1. The number of internally and externally initiated nursing investigations that are completed as well as underway
2. The number of research-related publications and presentations generated
3. The total number of grants submitted and funded
4. The amount of external grant monies acquired

It is debatable if the presence of a substantive program of research (a series of related studies in a particular area) by the CNR is a realistic measure of practice-based research program effectiveness (Campbell & Chulay, 1990; Pranulis, 1991). Campbell and Chulay (1990) note that a program built around the personal research interests of the CNR is at high risk for failing for three reasons. First, it is person dependent and changes when the researcher leaves. Second, it may not complement the goals of the department. Third, this type of program often omits inclusion of staff nurses in the research process, leading to disenchantment and an unwillingness to integrate research findings in practice.

Organizational Climate Criteria

A successful practice-based nurse researcher will have a positive influence on the organizational climate. As the CNR facilitates conduct and use of research by even a few key nurses, a ripple effect occurs throughout the department. Nurse executives can potentiate this ripple effect by acknowledging research accomplishments in letters to staff, in administrative meetings, and in agency publications.

The outcomes for the organization are threefold. First, a climate of inquiry regarding nursing practice will be evidenced by an increase in the number of research-based practice protocols being used by staff, the number of questions raised about the basis for nursing interventions, the number of staff participating in research activities, and suggested changes by staff to improve patient outcomes (Wilson, 1985).

Second, nurse executives can expect a change in the types of nurses recruited and retained. Using research to solve clinical practice problems and improve care enhances the image of the nursing department (Campbell & Chulay, 1990). Nurses who are enthusiastic about a climate of scientific inquiry will be attracted to the organization and are more likely to be retained. In contrast, nurses who prefer to base practice on tradition may leave. Nurses who are interested in research but need more knowledge and skill are more likely to seek further education. The result is a greater number of nurses on staff who are capable and enthusiastic about professional nursing practice (Cronenwett, 1985; Pettengill et al., 1988). These nurses have pride in their organization, foster collaboration in the practice environment, and demonstrate high-level critical thinking and decision-making skills.

The third benefit for the organization is the national reputation gained by publishing high-quality nursing research, having seasoned clinical nurse researchers on staff, and acquiring external grant funds. This benefit is often reflected by requests for consultation and visits to the organization for learning firsthand the strategies used to enact a successful research program.

Objective measurements of the relationship between the presence of a research program and the organizational climate have not been documented empirically through research. CNEs planning a new or different research program would benefit from periodically measuring the organizational climate to track the influence of the research program on key organizational variables.

Cost and Quality of Care Criteria

Nationally, the benefits of nursing research on patient outcomes and cost containment have been explicated. Despite the small amount of gross hospital revenues spent on nursing research (5 cents per $1000), nurses have been able to demonstrate the positive benefits of research on cost, patient outcomes, and quality of care (Barnes & Kirchhoff, 1986; Devine & Cook, 1986; Dille & Kirchhoff, 1993; Fagin, 1982, 1990; Hathway, 1986; Heater, Becker, & Olson, 1988; McGrath, 1990; Neidlinger, Scroggins, & Kennedy, 1987; Peterson & Kirchhoff, 1991; Schwartz, Mood, Yarandi, & Anderson, 1987). In addition, studies testing alternative patient care delivery models provide valuable information on provision of cost-effective quality care (Brooten et al., 1988; Daly, Rudy, Thompson, & Happ, 1991; Ethridge & Lamb, 1989; Litvak, Borrero, Katz, Munoz, & Wise, 1987; Maas, 1989).

Working together, the CNE and CNR can document the benefits of research activities on patient outcomes and health care costs for their institution. Demonstrating how the research program contributes to achieving organizational and departmental objectives is essential. Departmental research objectives guide the formulation of cost and quality indicators used to measure program success. Nurse executives may chose to start with research use and illustrate how basing practice on research findings saves health care dollars (Goode et al., 1987, 1991). Others may document program effectiveness by showing how conduct of research results in decreased length of stay without adverse patient outcomes.

References

American Association of Critical-Care Nurses. (1991, November 21). *AACN announces research priorities*. Aliso Viejo, CA: AACN Press Release.

American Nurses Association. (1981). *Guidelines for the investigative function of nurses*. Kansas City: Author.

American Organization of Nurse Executives. (1985). Strategies: Integration of nursing research into the practice setting. In *Nurse Executive Management Strategies* (pp. 1–11). Chicago: American Hospital Association.

American Society for Nursing Service Administrators. (1980). *The role of the nursing service administrator in nursing research*. Chicago: American Hospital Association.

Barnes, C.A., & Kirchhoff, K.T. (1986). Minimizing hypoxemia due to endotracheal suctioning: A review of the literature. *Heart and Lung, 15*, 164–178.

Bartos, B., Sexton, P.R. & Taggart, J.A. (1991). The institutional review board. In M.A. Mateo & K.T. Kirchhoff (Eds.), *Conducting and using nursing research in the clinical setting* (pp. 31–41). Baltimore: Williams & Wilkins.

Beavers, F.E., Gruber, M., & Johnson, B. (1990). A model for group research by master's degree RNs in advanced roles. *Clinical Nurse Specialist, 4*(3), 130–136.

Bergstrom, N. (1991). Scientific base for nursing practice is goal of ANA. *Clinical Nurse Researcher, 18*(2), 1, 7.

Betz, C.L., Poster, E., Randell, B., & Omery, A. (1990). Nursing research productivity in clinical settings. *Nursing Outlook, 38*, 180–183.

Bolton, L.B. (1991). Resources for research. In M.A. Mateo & K.T. Kirchhoff (Eds.), *Conducting and using nursing research in the clinical setting* (pp. 22–30). Baltimore: Williams & Wilkins.

Brooten, D., Brown, L.D., Munro, B.H., York, R., Cohen, S.M., Roncoli, M., & Hollingsworth, A. (1988). Early discharge and specialist transitional care. *Image: The Journal of Nursing Scholarship, 20*, 64–68.

Campbell, G.M., & Chulay, M. (1990). Establishing a clinical nursing research program. In J.G. Spicer & M. Robinson (Eds.), *Managing the environment in the critical care setting* (pp. 52–60). Baltimore: Williams & Wilkins.

Chance, H.C., & Hinshaw, A.S. (1980). Strategies for initiating a research program. *Journal of Nursing Administrators, 10*(3), 32–39.

Cronenwett, L.R. (1985). Hiring a nurse researcher. *Journal of Nursing Administration, 15*(10), 5–7.

Cronenwett, L.R. (1986a). Research contributions of clinical nurse specialists. *Journal of Nursing Administration, 16*(6), 6–7.

Cronenwett, L.R. (1986b). Selecting a nurse researcher. *Journal of Nursing Administration, 16*(1), 7–8.

Cronenwett, L.R. (1986c). The research role of the clinical nurse specialist. *Journal of Nursing Administration, 16*(4), 10–11.

Daly, B.J., Rudy, E.B., Thompson, K.S., & Happ, M.B. (1991). Development of a special care unit for chronically critically ill. *Heart and Lung, 20*, 45–51.

Davis, M.Z. (1981). Promoting nursing research in the clinical setting. *Journal of Nursing Administration, 11*(3), 22–27.

Dennis, K.E. (1991). Components of the doctoral curriculum that build success in the clinical nurse researcher role. *Journal of Professional Nursing, 7,* 160–165.

Dennis, K.E., & Strickland, O.L. (1987). The clinical nurse researcher: Institutionalizing the role. *International Journal of Nursing Studies, 24*(1), 25–33.

Devine, E.C., & Cook, T.D. (1986). Clinical and cost-saving effects of psychoeducational interventions with surgical patients: A meta-analysis. *Research in Nursing and Health, 9,* 89–105.

Dille, C.M., & Kirchhoff, K.T. (1993). Decontamination of urinary drainage bags with bleach. *Rehabilitation Nursing 18,* 292–295.

Egan, E.C., McElmurry, B.J., & Jameson, H.M. (1981). Practice-based research: Assessing your department's readiness. *Journal of Nursing Administration 11*(10), 26–32.

Ethridge, P., & Lamb, G.S. (1989). Professional nursing case management improves quality, access and costs. *Nursing Management, 20*(3), 30–35.

Fagin, C.M. (1982). The economic value of nursing research. *American Journal of Nursing, 82,* 1844–1849.

Fagin, C.M. (1990). Nursing's value proves itself. *American Journal of Nursing, 90*(10), 17–30.

Frick, S.B., DelPo, E.G., & Robinson, T. (1988). The structure and process of a successful clinical research collaboration. *Nursing Connections, 1*(3), 69–75.

Fugleberg, B.B. (1986, fall). Nursing research in the practice setting. *Nursing Administration Quarterly,* 38–42.

Fuhs, M.F., & Moore, K. (1981). Research program development in a tertiary care setting. *Nursing Research, 30,* 24–27.

Goode, C.J. (1987). *Using research in clinical nursing practice* [Video]. Ida Grove, IA: Horn Video Productions.

Goode, C., Lovett, M.K., Hayes, J.E., & Butcher, L.A. (1987). Use of research-based knowledge in clinical practice. *Journal of Nursing Administration, 17*(12), 11–18.

Goode, C.J., Titler, M., Rakel, B., Ones, D.S., Kleiber, C., Small, S., & Triolo, P. (1991). A meta-analysis of effects of heparin flush and saline flush: Quality and cost implications. *Nursing Research, 40,* 324–330.

Hagle, M.E., Barbour, L., Flynn, B., Kelley, C., Trippon, M., Braun, D., Beschorner, J., Boxler, J., Hange, P., McGuire, D., Bressler, L., & Kirchhoff, K. (1987). Research col-

laboration among nurse clinicians. *Oncology Nursing Forum, 14*(6), 55–59.

Hagle, M.E., Kirchhoff, K.T., Knafl, K.A., & Bevis, M.E. (1986). The clinical nurse researcher: New perspectives. *Journal of Professional Nursing, 2,* 282–288.

Haller, K.B. (1986). Research in clinical settings. *American Journal of Maternal Child Nursing, 11,* 290.

Hathway, D. (1986). Effect of preoperative instruction on postoperative outcomes: A meta-analysis. *Nursing Research, 35,* 269–275.

Heater, B.S., Becker, A.M., & Olson, R.K. (1988). Nursing interventions and patient outcomes. *Nursing Research, 37,* 303–307.

Hegedus, K.S., & Marino, B.L. (1989). The nursing research program at Children's Hospital, Boston. *Journal of Nursing Administration, 19*(6), 9–10.

Hinshaw, A.S., & Smeltzer, C.H. (1987). Research challenges and programs for practice settings. *Journal of Nursing Administration, 17*(7,8), 20–26.

Hoare, K., & Earenfight, J. (1986). Unit-based research in a service setting. *Journal of Nursing Administration, 16*(4), 35–39.

Hunt, V., Stark, J.L., Fisher, F., Hegedus, K., Joy, L., & Woldum, K. (1983). Networking: A managerial strategy for research development in a service setting. *Journal of Nursing Administration, 13*(7,8), 27–32.

Joint Commission on Accreditation of Healthcare Organizations. (1991). 1992 *Joint Commission accreditation manual for hospitals: Vol. II. Scoring guidelines.* Oakbrook Terrace, IL: Author.

Kirchhoff, K.T., (1981). Information exchange: Request for assistance. *Western Journal of Nursing Research, 3*(4), 421–423.

Kirchhoff, K.T., (1985). Employed for research in the clinical setting. In K.E. Barnard & G.R. Smith (Eds.), *Faculty practice in action* (pp. 201–211). Kansas City, MO: American Academy of Nursing.

Kirchhoff, K.T. (1991a). Strategies in research utilization. In M.A. Mateo & K.T. Kirchhoff (Eds.), *Conducting and using nursing research in the clinical setting* (pp. 108–112). Baltimore: Williams & Wilkins.

Kirchhoff, K.T. (1991b). Who is responsible for research utilization? *Heart and Lung, 20* 308–309.

Kirchhoff, K.T. (1993). The role of nurse researchers employed in clinical settings. *An-*

nual Review of Nursing Research, 11, 169–181.

Kirchhoff, K.T., & McGuire, D.B. (1985). The nursing research review process in a clinical setting. *Journal of Professional Nursing, 1,* 311–314.

Knafl, K.A., Bevis, M.E., & Kirchhoff, K.T. (1987a). Development and enactment of a new role. *Clinical Nurse Researcher, 14*(1), 1–4.

Knafl, K.A., Bevis, M.E., & Kirchhoff, K.T. (1987b). Research activities of clinical nurse researchers. *Nursing Research, 36,* 249–252.

Knafl, K.A., Hagle, M.E., Bevis, M.E., Faux, S.A., & Kirchhoff, K.T. (1989). How researchers and administrators view the role of the clinical nurse researcher. *Western Journal of Nursing Research, 11,* 583–592.

Knafl, K.A., Hagle, M.E., Bevis, M.E., & Kirchhoff, K.T. (1987). Clinical nurse researchers: Strategies for success. *Journal of Nursing Administration, 17*(10), 27–31.

Kuhn, R.C. (1990). *AACN outcome standards for nursing care of the critically ill.* Laguna Niguel, CA: AACN.

Larson, E. (1981). Nursing research outside academia: A panel presentation. *Image, 13,* 75–77.

Larson, E., Wells, M.P., & McHugh, N. (1985). Perioperative nursing research. *AORN Journal, 41,* 868–873.

Lawson, L. (1987). Developing a research structure within the nursing department. *Journal of Nursing Administration, 17*(11), 6–7.

Lawson, L. (1988a). Building research credibility. *Journal of Nursing Administration, 18*(1), 7, 24.

Lawson, L. (1988b). Functions of the nurse researcher. *Journal of Nursing Administration, 18*(7,8), 8–9, 23.

Lawson, L. (1989). Developing investigators who will generate clinically relevant science. *Journal of Nursing Administration, 19*(1), 6–7.

Lewandowski, L., & Kositsky, A. (1983). Research priorities for critical care nursing: A study by the American Association of Critical-Care Nurses. *Heart and Lung, 12,* 35–44.

Lindeman, C.A. (1988). Research in practice: The role of the staff nurse. *Applied Nursing Research, 1*(1), 5–7.

Lindsey, A.M. (1991). Integrating research and practice. In M.A. Mateo & K.T. Kirchhoff (Eds.), *Conducting and using nursing research in the clinical setting* (pp. 93–107). Baltimore: Williams & Wilkins.

Litvak, S., Borrero, E., Katz, R., Munoz, E., & Wise, L. (1987). Early discharge of the postmastectomy patient: Unbundling of the hospital service to improve patient profitability under DRGs. *American Surgeon, 229,* 577–579.

Maas, M.L. (1989). Professional practice for the extended care environment: Learning from one model and its implementation. *Journal of Professional Nursing, 5*(2), 66–76.

MacKay, R.C., Grantham, M.A., & Ross, S.E. (1984). Building a hospital nursing research department. *Journal of Nursing Administration 14*(7,8), 23–27.

Marchette, L. (1985). Developing a productive nursing research program in a clinical institution. *Journal of Nursing Administration, 15*(3), 25–30.

Mateo, M.A., & Kirchhoff, K.T. (Eds.) (1991). *Conducting and using nursing research in the clinical setting.* Baltimore: Williams & Wilkins.

Mayer, G.G. (1983). The clinical nurse-researcher: Role-taking and role-making. In N.L. Chaska (Ed.), *The nursing profession: A time to speak* (pp. 216–233). New York: McGraw-Hill.

McClure, M.L. (1981). Promoting practice-based research: A critical need. *Journal of Nursing Administration 11*(11), 66–70.

McGrath, S. (1990). The cost-effectiveness of nurse practitioners. *Nurse Practitioner, 15*(7), 40–42.

Medoff-Cooper, B., & Lamb, A.H. (1989). The clinical specialist–staff nurse research team: A model for clinical research. *Clinical Nurse Specialist, 3*(1), 16–19.

Neidlinger, S.H. Scroggins, K., & Kennedy, L.M. (1987). Cost evaluation of discharge planning for hospitalized elderly. *Nursing Economics, 5,* 225–230.

Peterson, F.Y., & Kirchhoff, K.T. (1991). Analysis of the research about heparinized versus nonheparinized vascular lines. *Heart and Lung, 20,* 631–640.

Pettengill, M.M., Knafl, K.A., Bevis, M.E., & Kirchhoff, K.T. (1988). Nursing research in midwestern hospitals. *Western Journal of Nursing Research, 10,* 705–717.

Pranulis, M.F. (1991). Research programs in a

clinical setting. *Western Journal of Nursing Research, 13,* 274–277.

Pranulis, M.F., & Driever, M.J. (1990). A conceptual framework for analyzing influences on research productivity in clinical settings. *Western Journal of Nursing Research, 12,* 563–565.

Rempusheski, V.F. (1991). Incorporating research role and practice role. *Applied Nursing Research, 4*(1), 46–48.

Rizzuto, C., & Mitchell, M. (1988a). Research in service settings: Part I. *Journal of Nursing Administration, 18*(2), 32–37.

Rizzuto, C., & Mitchell, M. (1988b). Research in service settings: Part II. *Journal of Nursing Administration, 18*(3), 19–24.

Rizzuto,C., & Mitchell, M. (1990). Outcomes of research consortium project. *Journal of Nursing Administration, 20*(4), 13–17.

Sanford, S., & Disch, J.M. (1989). *American Association of Critical-Care Nurses' standards for nursing care of the critically ill* (2nd ed.). Norwalk, CT: Appleton & Lange.

Schutzenhofer, K.K. (1991). Scholarly pursuit in the clinical setting: An obligation of professional nursing. *Journal of Professional Nursing, 7*(1), 10–15.

Schwartz, R., Mood, L., Yarandi, H., & Anderson, G.C. (1987). A meta-analysis of critical outcome variables in nonnutritive sucking in preterm infants. *Nursing Research, 36,* 292–295.

Simms, L.M., Price, S.A., & Pfoutz, S.K. (1987). Creating the research climate: A key responsibility for nurse executives. *Nursing Economics, 5,* 174–178.

Smeltzer, C.H., & Hinshaw, A.S. (1988). Research: Clinical integration for excellent patient care. *Nursing Management, 19*(1), 38–41.

Snyder-Halpern, R. (1991). Attributes of service-based nursing research programs useful for decision-making. *Nursing Administration Quarterly, 15*(4), 82–84.

Stark, J.L. (1989). A multiple-strategy based research program for staff nurse involvement. *Journal of Nursing Administration, 19*(9), 7–8.

Stone, K.S. (1991). Collaboration. In M.A. Mateo & K.T. Kirchhoff (Eds.), *Conducting and using nursing research in the clinical setting* (pp. 31–41). Baltimore: Williams & Wilkins.

Titler, M.G., Goode, C.J., & Mathis, S. (1992). What happens to nursing research in times of economic cutbacks? In M. Johnson (Ed.), *Series on Nursing Administration: Economic Myths and Realities, 4,* 167–182.

Tyler, D.O., Clark, A.P., Winslow, E.H., & White, K.M. (1990). Strategies for conducting clinical nursing research in critical care. *Critical Care Nurse Quarterly, 12*(4), 30–38.

Weiler, K., & Buckwalter, K.C. (1990). Is nursing research used in practice? In J.C. McCloskey & H.C. Grace (Eds.), *Current issues in nursing* (pp. 45–57). St Louis: C.V. Mosby.

Wilson, H.S. (1985). Fostering conditions that inspire inquiry. *Journal of Nursing Administration, 15*(5), 8–9.

Zalar, M.K., Welches, L.J., & Walker, D.D. (1985). Nursing consortium approach to increase research in service settings. *Journal of Nursing Administration 15*(7,8), 36–41.

CHAPTER 37 • • • • • •

MARKETING FOR NURSE MANAGERS

STEVEN A. FINKLER
CHRISTINE T. KOVNER

EXECUTIVE SUMMARY

This chapter focuses on a skill that most nurses possess, yet it is an area that frequently requires a framework within which to improve the skill. The topic is marketing, and in today's health care organizations, it is a must. The goals of marketing are to determine who our customers are and what they value and to attempt to meet those needs. In the health care arena, the customer can be the patient, the patient's relatives, the doctors, and even the insurance companies. Since the nurse spends a great deal of time with the patient, and perhaps the patient's relatives, it makes sense for nursing to be actively involved in the marketing process.

This chapter defines health care marketing as an attempt to maintain and increase the organization's patient volume and provides information on a wide variety of marketing concepts from market segmentation and customer behavior to research and advertising. All are related to the health care setting.

The development of a marketing plan also is discussed. Emphasis is placed on a careful review of the mission and goals of the organization and on an internal/external analysis of the situation. This analysis should answer the following questions: What is going on inside the organization, and what does the competition have to offer? After these two elements have been completed, a strategic marketing plan can be developed. A matrix for strategic planning, developed by the Boston Consulting Group, is presented.

The nurse manager can and should have significant input to the marketing function. Not only is nursing the prime patient contact, but also the nurse manager is in a position to evaluate the strengths and weaknesses of the organization. All of this valuable information is needed for an effective marketing effort.

Virtually every organization desires to provide a high volume of services. Health care marketing is a management science that attempts to maintain and increase the organization's patient volume. High volume is desirable because

---

This chapter is abstracted from Finkler S.A., & Kovner, C.T. (1993). *Financial management for nurse managers and executives* (Chap. 18). Philadelphia: W.B. Saunders.

629

of its financial implications, which are related to the concepts of fixed and variable costs. If any costs of the organization are fixed, increasing volume will inherently spread those costs more widely. Each unit of service will bear a smaller share of the fixed costs. The average cost per unit declines as volume increases because of the sharing of fixed costs.

For example, the costs per patient in a half-full hospital are much higher than in a full hospital because certain costs must be incurred to operate the hospital, regardless of how full it is. These include administration, heat, light, depreciation, and a wide variety of other fixed items. With fewer patients, each must cover a larger share of those costs. If the prices at which services are provided are maintained at a fairly constant level, then rising volume and declining average costs will lead to a higher profit margin per unit of service. This in turn leads to greater financial stability.

Marketing is an area of management that tries to ensure that the organization achieves and maintains a high volume level. However, to the surprise of many people not familiar with marketing, the essence of marketing is not selling the organization's product. Attaining the high revenues and the profits that result from the provision of a high volume of service is more complicated than simply going out and finding customers to buy the organization's goods and services.

The concept of marketing may be counterintuitive to many nurses. Clinical education focuses on a perspective that people come for care when they are ill or want preventive services, such as immunizations. Nurses are not selling patient monitoring in the same way that a department store sells blouses. However, health care organizations are selling their services, and there is nothing inherently unethical about that. If you believe that your facility provides the best care, you want potential patients to be aware of that. If your care is as good as that provided by other facilities in your area, encouraging patients to use your facility will result in higher volume, economies of scale, and ultimately lower costs and/or better services for all your organization's patients.

THE ESSENCE OF MARKETING: ASSESSING CUSTOMER NEEDS

The short-run focus of marketing efforts is on finding customers for the organization's goods and services. However, that effort is really not the main theme of marketing. Rather, the goal of marketing efforts is to enable the organization to determine what customers want or need and to develop and offer those goods or services. Selling is a minor focus of marketing, while determining what to sell is the essence of marketing.

Most nonmarketing specialists mistakenly assume that marketing consists primarily of determining what type of advertising to use and then implementing an ad campaign. The major efforts of marketing managers, however, are directed toward assessing customer needs.

Health care organizations are in a constantly changing environment. The desires of the customers change. Most health care organizations would be quick to state that they are well aware of the constant change in the technologies and methodologies for providing health care. Many health care organizations are on the technological edge in providing care. However, simply deciding on what is a good health care product and then setting about providing it may not be enough. Designing a better mousetrap will make you rich only if potential customers are interested in catching mice.

Focusing on customer needs often leads to the development of new products, services, and other innovations sooner than they would otherwise be adopted. This in turn makes it easier to market the organization's services. Marketing becomes more oriented to informing potential customers of what is available, rather than trying to sell what you have, whether it is what they want or not.

UNDERSTANDING CUSTOMERS

For health care organizations, marketing represents an unusually great challenge because it is not always clear who the customer is. It is a well-known concept in health care that the physician is often viewed as the true customer, particularly by hospitals. In recent years, it has become more and more apparent that to some extent the insurance company is a customer of health care providers. And, in some cases, a relative of the patient, rather than the patient, has the decision-making power commonly associated with the ultimate customer.

If you were to buy a gift, would you consider yourself or the ultimate recipient of the gift the customer of the store selling the gift? Clearly, you are the customer. The same thing could be said in the case of mental health or long-term care. Often, the patient lacks the capacity to make choices about the selection of a provider of health care services. For a mental health provider or nursing home, the customer often may be a relative of the patient.

If the key customer is the insurer, that must be taken into account in the organization's decisions. Sometimes, health care organizations try to respond to the needs of their potential patients, incorrectly viewing them as the decision-making customer. New buildings are built with substantial amenities that the patients want. However, patients often want more than they (or the insurers) are willing to pay for. They request amenities knowing that they have insurance that will pay for their care.

As a result of widespread health insurance, many people have become used to receiving health care services without direct cost to themselves. Insurance companies, however, have started to encourage patients to use preferred providers. They sometimes offer patients full reimbursement for care from preferred provider organizations and only partial reimbursement for care from other providers. In such cases the insurer may not be willing to pay for the high costs of fancy amenities. And often, given a choice of paying 20% of a hospital bill and having the amenities or going to a preferred provider with fewer amenities but no coinsurance, the patients choose the latter. The insurance companies have so much power to steer patients to providers they prefer that it would be foolish for a marketing effort not to consider the needs and desires of the insurer as well as the patient.

The physician still has a dominant role in health care and cannot be ignored in any discussion of health care customers. Physicians can steer patients to hospitals and other providers of health care services in an even more direct way than insurers. Some patients may have a preference for one hospital over another. On the other hand, very few patients will have a preference for a particular home health agency. If their physician refers them to a particular agency for after-hospital home care, they are likely to use that recommended agency. The marketing efforts of home health agencies would have to be based on the realization that a significant segment of their customers consists of physicians.

WHY IS MARKETING IMPORTANT FOR NURSE MANAGERS?
Keeping the Organization Current

In light of the above discussion of the main goal of marketing efforts, it should become easier to understand why marketing is an important topic for nurse managers to comprehend. Organizations that succeed learn the lesson of marketing—that customer needs must be determined. In health care it is virtually impossible for the organization to fully understand the needs of its customers without input from the nursing staff.

The nursing staff has the pulse of the organization's customers in its hands (both literally and figuratively). Nurses constantly hear from the patients what is good and bad about the organization. They have the most frequent patient contact, and the contact is of substantial duration. They are most likely to hear from the patients about what the organization should be doing better or differently.

From the marketing manager's perspective, the nursing staff can serve a significant market research role. They can listen to the patient comments and pass the information along to the marketing department. Marketing in turn can use the information to assess the changes that the organization should be making to meet the desires of the patients.

Customer needs should be a focal point of the organization. Nurses should be considering whether their activities are focused on responding to those needs. Clearly, specific activities may be required that have little direct impact on making the patient feel better. And in no case can all customer needs be satisfied regardless of cost. Nevertheless, there should be an evaluation of whether the work of a nursing unit is communicated to the patients so that the patients realize that their needs are being addressed.

The issue of patient satisfaction is essential to every health care organization. A dissatisfied patient is not likely to return to a health care provider. That potential lost future revenue is readily apparent, and since people talk to each other, the effects of dissatisfaction are multiplied.

Marketing the Importance of Nursing

Nurses do many things for patients that the patients are never aware of. One aspect of marketing should be to create a greater level of patient education concerning some of the many things nurses do for the patient behind the scenes. This can result in a more satisfied customer, and that in turn leads to additional customers later on. For example, even though in many cases patients do not pick their hospital, there are probably many cases in which patients do become aware of the reputation of a hospital and affiliate specifically with a physician who uses that hospital. In other cases physicians may be affiliated with several hospitals, and patients will specify a preference when they need an elective procedure.

A vital role played by marketing is the provision of information. Customers may know what they want, but they may not understand the best way to get it. People know that when they are sick, they want to obtain the care needed to get well. The nursing profession should respond to that desire by informing the public of its role in helping them to get well.

MARKETING CONCEPTS
Understanding the Market

To make any assessment of the desires and needs of a group of customers, it is first necessary to understand as much as possible about the set of customers that constitutes the relevant *market*. The market is defined as the potential customers for a product or organization. Information about the market will affect not only the mix of services that should be offered but also the advertising message, price, and other critical factors.

The information about the market that is needed represents primarily demographic information. The age, race, religion, ethnic background, and mobility of the population should be assessed. The likelihood of change in the existing demographics should also be considered. The marketing efforts of the organization should also include collection of data that will help the organization assess the income and assets of the market, the educational level, and the density of the population.

Understanding the market additionally requires understanding various factors that impact on the types of services that can be offered and the prices that can be charged. For example, it is crucial that the organization consider available technologies as well as the wide variety of regulations that impact on the organization.

In attempting to understand the market, many organizations also identify key success factors, sometimes called *determinant attributes*. Determinant attributes are factors that ultimately affect a consumer's purchase decision. Generally these factors can be divided into two major types: *decision variables* and *environmental variables*. Decision variables are factors controllable by the organization that can affect volume. Environmental variables are also factors that can affect volume. However, they are not controllable by the organization.

Data must be collected for both types of variables. Such data, for either decision or environmental variables, may require action by the organization. In the case of decision variables the organization may take steps to impact directly on the variable. For example, price, the amount of advertising, and the hours that a service is offered are all decision variables. Suppose that a health care organization found that patients who do not use its services would not only use them but would also be willing to pay a higher price than is currently being charged if the service were offered at more suitable hours. The organization can take a set of definite actions. It can adjust its hours of service, advertise the new hours, and raise the price to cover any higher costs associated with the new hours.

On the other hand, the general economy is not a factor within the control of the organization. However, the organization can respond to the economy. High unemployment during a recession will lead to many psychological problems. Rather than focusing as much on services for stress caused by overwork, the organization can emphasize services available for problems, such as depression, that result from being laid off. And it can offer to defer payment until the patient is re-employed. Although the organization can do little about the general economy, it can find a way to serve its community and at the same time increase its patient volume.

Market Segmentation

One essential tool of marketing is to *segment* the overall market. Segmentation means division of the market into several specific subsections. Some health care organizations have done this already to a great extent. Charging a low price to Blue Cross, perhaps an even lower price to an HMO, and yet a higher price to private insurers represents a segmentation of the market based on the payer for the services.

By dividing the overall market a number of different objectives can be achieved. Not only is it possible to charge different prices to different buyers, but it is also possible to target preferred customers. For example, suppose that private insurance patients are the most profitable. The organization can target its advertising to media that primarily reach individuals who have private insurance. Advertisements can be placed in magazines read primarily by affluent individuals.

Markets can be segmented in a variety of ways. They can be divided by socioeconomic factors such as age, sex, occupation, and income, by geography; by personality traits; or by buyer behavior. For example, some customers are price sensitive, others are quality sensitive, and some consider amenities important.

In general, segmentation is based on three factors. First, one attempts to divide the customer base into groups that have distinct and measurable needs. Second, it is vital that one can assess the specific segments. Finally, the segment must be big enough to merit a distinct effort.

Customer Behavior

Understanding how consumers behave is vital to fashioning the proper mix of services. Not only customer desires and needs but also attitudes and behavior are critical to developing a marketing plan that will create the volume of patients needed by the organization.

Consider a hospital that was losing maternity patients. The hospital was a prestigious research center, known for excellent-quality care. Yet over time its maternity volume was declining. The problem was potentially easily solvable, but the hospital was unaware of buyer behavior and, therefore, not tuned in to the problem. Unlike other diagnoses, for which patients are unexpectedly rushed to the hospital, maternity provides plenty of advance notice. In fact, many expectant women toured the maternity area as part of their prepared childbirth classes. However, the maternity area was not very presentable. It gave an old appearance. One expectant mother called it "dirty" and said that she refused to deliver her baby at that hospital regardless of its reputation. A coat of paint and perhaps some minor remodeling would probably have easily paid for itself from increased patient volume. The hospital, however, failed to tune in to the effect that the condition of the facilities had on preadmission visitors.

Many things affect the behavior of customers. Price, image, or an advertising message are just a few examples. Organizations need to perform market research to ascertain which factors affect consumer behavior, and how. The buying process consists of perceiving a need, getting ready to make a purchase, purchasing, consuming, and after-the-fact reacting. Lavidge and Steiner (1961) have described the process of getting ready to make a purchase as:

Awareness→Knowledge→Liking→Preference→Conviction→and Purchase

A buyer must first perceive a need for health care services. The perceived need is not the marketer's domain. Marketing does not create needs; it satisfies them. Then there must be awareness that the provider exists and knowledge that the provider can meet the need. The buyer must like the provider enough to consider it among other possible choices. The buyer must decide that the provider is the preferred way to go. The preference must be reinforced until it becomes a conviction, and finally a purchase will take place. At any point in the process, the customer may decide to purchase a competitor's services.

Making sure that the potential buyer is aware of the health care organization as a possible source for satisfying needs is an essential role of marketing. Marketing must also put forth information that is likely to cause the buyer to like the organization's product, to prefer it, and to become convinced that the organization is the appropriate source for care. The organization must make sure that its actual production process does in fact fill the perceived need. The after-the-fact reaction of customers will influence future purchase decisions by the patient and the patient's friends and family.

Market Measurement

An important aspect of marketing is the conversion of qualitative information into quantitative estimates of demand. This is referred to as *market measurement*. Such measurement is made for analysis, planning, and control. Analysis is made of what services to offer. Planning is undertaken to develop the services. Control is conducted to keep performance on target.

The central aspect of market measurement is estimation of market demand. How much will be the total volume purchased by all patients in a defined market area. This measurement requires a thorough definition of the specific product or service whose demand is being estimated. It also requires a clear understanding of the time period for which the estimate is being made, such as a week, month, or year into the future. The longer the time period for the estimate, the less reliable the data obtained.

Environmental factors must be considered in making an estimate for market demand. Since the demand for any service is affected by various factors outside the organization's control, the assumptions leading to a specific forecast of demand must be understood. For instance, a home health agency might plan a geographical expansion into an elderly community under the assumption that Medicare will continue to reimburse for a certain number of home visits. If legislation were to change Medicare reimbursement, the demand estimates might prove faulty. To know how much to rely on demand predictions, one must be able to assess the reasonableness of the underlying assumptions about the environment faced by the organization.

Market demand will also depend, at least to some extent, on the actions taken by the organization itself. The price charged, the advertising campaign undertaken, and other controllable factors can impact on the market demand and should be considered in attempting to determine it. Finding the demand for a hospital-based product may not tell the actual demand that would exist if care could be delivered to patients' homes.

Market measurement requires that demand be forecast. Forecasting demand can be done by a variety of methods ranging from crude to sophisticated. The most common of these approaches are surveys, acquisition of expert opinion, and statistical analyses.

Market Share

Related to the concept of market measurement is *market share*. Market share represents the portion or percentage of the overall market that a specific organization controls. If half of all broken-leg patients in your area come to your ER, then you have a 50% share of the broken-leg market.

Market share is important because rather than being an absolute number, such as the number of broken legs you treat, it shows your status relative to the competition. If your total number of hospital inpatients is rising 4% per year, that may seem good. However, if the number of inpatients in your city is rising at a rate of 15% per year, then each year your hospital has a smaller share of the total market. This can be a direct warning sign that your competitors are passing you by. It can tell you about your long-term prospects, if you remain as you are.

Market Research

Related to market measurement is the broader question of *market research*. This includes gathering, recording, and analyzing information to improve decisions made by the organization. Market research is needed to determine what the customer really wants and is willing to buy. The major areas for market research are advertising, business economics, products, and sales.

Advertising research focuses on issues such as the appropriate copy to use and the appropriate media for advertisements for a product or service. Business economics research considers forecasting general trends in the environment. Product research considers potential acceptance of new products, analysis of competitors' products, and other factors related to the delivery of services. Sales research focuses on issues such as market characteristics and market share.

The market research process consists of defining the problem to be investigated, constructing the model, collecting data, and interpreting data. The statement of the problem must be carefully framed and the intended use of the research understood to avoid wasting substantial effort. The result of the research should be to produce not just interesting information but rather information that is useful for making a particular decision.

Advertising

Advertising makes people aware of an organization and its products, provides knowledge about the product, and hopefully creates a preference for and loyalty to the organization's services. Advertising can come in the form of paid advertisements, personal selling, sales promotions, and other forms of publicity. The level of expenditures on advertising should be established so that the extra benefits from extra advertising always exceed or are at least equal to the extra cost of the extra advertising.

In advertising, there are many critical questions to be addressed. How many people are reached by a campaign? Are they the right people? Is the message making the desired impact? It is not sufficient to have a slick presentation. The message must be designed and presented based on what is likely to work with the desired audience. The presentation and timing of the message are as important as simply reaching a large number of people.

MARKETING PLANS

Marketing is based on a strategic planning approach. Plans are made to achieve a goal. An unusual aspect of marketing plans is that they often tend to be disruptive. The plan is often aimed at making change occur. At a minimum, marketing may take patients away from competitors. Often, marketing plans call for changes in the current operations of the organization. Change generally meets resistance. For the marketing plan to be effective in an environment in which reactions to the plan both internally and by competitors are likely, the plan must be carefully established.

Marketing plans should first consider the organizational mission and goals. Then internal/external analyses must be performed, a strategic marketing plan developed, and specific tactics developed. Plans must then be revised, integrated, and implemented. Finally, control and feedback are essential to an effective plan (Hillestad & Berkowitz, 1991).

Organizational Mission/Goals

The marketing plan should support the organizational mission. Most health care organizations have realized the importance of having a basic mission statement to guide the organization. Based on the mission statement, organizational goals can be set and strategic plans made to carry out those goals.

Internal/External Analyses

The internal/external analysis consists of an analysis of the environment, including the competition, and the organization's internal capabilities in light of the needs and desires of the consumer.

The organization's environment is a critical piece of the puzzle of trying to determine how to successfully provide services to the community. Questions about the environment that should be addressed in a marketing plan include the size of the market, the growth rate of the market, stability of prices, and the degree of competition. Factors such as social attitudes and reimbursement rules must also be considered.

The next element of the internal/external assessment is identification of the market and its needs. This assessment should include both internal and external markets. For example, if physicians are considered crucial to generating patients, they should be assessed along with patients. An example of a data collection form for identifying markets and needs is given in Figure 37–1.

Knowing the basic markets is a critical first step. Next, the markets must be fully understood. What factors result in changes in the marketplace? Are the key factors that cause the market to change related to demographics (e.g., population aging), regulatory changes (e.g., in reimbursement), or available medical services (e.g., as a result of technology)? Can the market be segmented and, if so, how attractive a market is each segment? The organization must make every effort to know not just what the markets are but why they are. What influences them and causes them to change, or to remain the same, over time?

Having gained some insight to the markets that are relevant for the organization and the needs of each market, the analysis must thoroughly examine the competition. Strengths and weaknesses of the organization vis-à-vis its competition are crucial foundations for the development of any market strategy. Table 37–1 presents an example of a form that can be used to collect and record data concerning competition.

Organizations should attempt to understand any *differential advantages* they have. A differential advantage is some characteristic that provides the organization with a distinct advantage over a competitor. Such advantages might include location, cost, services offered, or other factors.

Just as the strengths and weaknesses of the competition must be known, so also must the organization assess its own relative merits. Being aware of the external environment is only helpful to the extent that the organization can take advantage of that information. Unless the organization conducts a thorough internal analysis of what it can and cannot do, it will be unable to take advantage of such information.

Part I—Identifying markets. A market or market segment consists of a group of people who have common demographic, specialty, or social characteristics that represent a size large enough for the organization to concentrate resources around.

Potential Markets	Importance of Market (check one column for current and future)						Current Attitude Toward You (circle one number)				
	Current			Future			Very Favorable			Very Unfavorable	
	High	Med	Low	High	Med	Low	1	2	3	4	5
Gen. medicine M.D.'s							1	2	3	4	5
Surgeons							1	2	3	4	5
OB/gyn							1	2	3	4	5
Peds							1	2	3	4	5
Other M.D.'s							1	2	3	4	5
Inpatients (by specialty)							1	2	3	4	5
Outpatients							1	2	3	4	5
Community at large							1	2	3	4	5
Donors							1	2	3	4	5
Board of directors							1	2	3	4	5
Insurance companies							1	2	3	4	5
Regulators							1	2	3	4	5
Business/ industry (specify)							1	2	3	4	5
Have no doctor market							1	2	3	4	5
HMO patients							1	2	3	4	5
Over-65 market							1	2	3	4	5
Nonuser market							1	2	3	4	5
Females							1	2	3	4	5
Males							1	2	3	4	5
Others _____							1	2	3	4	5
_____							1	2	3	4	5
_____							1	2	3	4	5

Part II—Based on the mix of actual and potential markets listed in Part I, indicate the size and future potential.

Key Market Segments from Part I	Size Today	Future Size— Three Years	Your Current Market Share
25 thru 34-year old males—athletics	9% of metro area	14%	32% of medical care medsin sports medicine programs

Part III—Based on completion of Parts I and II, indicate the needs major market segments are likely to exhibit.

Key Market Segments	Needs
25 thru 34-year old males in sports medicine program	Greater emphasis on strength, training, cardiovascular fitness

Figure 37–1 Identification of major markets and needs. (Reprinted from Health Care Marketing Plans, 2nd ed., by S. Hillestad and E. Berkowitz, with permission of Aspen Publishers, Inc., © 1991.)

TABLE 37–1 Relative Competitor Assessment Form

COMPETITOR (SPECIFY):	MUCH WORSE −4	SOMEWHAT WORSE −3	−2	−1	ABOUT THE SAME 0	+1	SOMEWHAT BETTER +2	+3	MUCH BETTER +4
1. Medical care									
A. Emergency									
B. Surgery									
C. Gen. medical									
D. Special care									
2. Nursing care									
3. Housekeeping (hospital)									
4. Food service (hospital)									
5. Staff morale									
6. Facility: Capacity/attractiveness									
7. Public relations									
8. Reputation									
9. Image (overall)									
10. Management									
11. Lab services									
12. Convenience									
13. Staff education									
14. Equipment: Capability/technology									
15. Range of services									
16. Marketing plan									
17. Ad/promo budget									

Competitive Assessment: For each competitor on which you have a Competitor Assessment form, indicate the level of competitive intensity, your share of the market, and the basis for competition.

COMPETITOR	MARKET SHARE	LEVEL OF COMPETITIVE INTENSITY					BASIS FOR COMPETITION			
		VERY INTENSE				NOT COMPETITIVE AT ALL	PRODUCT	PRICE	PROMOTION	DISTRIBUTION
1.	_____	1	2	3	4	5	_____	_____	_____	_____
2.	_____	1	2	3	4	5	_____	_____	_____	_____
3.	_____	1	2	3	4	5	_____	_____	_____	_____
4.	_____	1	2	3	4	5	_____	_____	_____	_____
5.	_____	1	2	3	4	5	_____	_____	_____	_____
6.	_____	1	2	3	4	5	_____	_____	_____	_____
7.	_____	1	2	3	4	5	_____	_____	_____	_____
8.	_____	1	2	3	4	5	_____	_____	_____	_____

Conclusion:

Reprinted from Health Care Marketing Plans, 2nd ed., by S. Hillestad and E. Berkowitz with permission of Aspen Publishers, Inc., © 1991.

Strategic Marketing Plan

According to Hillestad and Berkowitz, many managers "call the marketing staff with the following question: 'I would like to involve you in a strategy to help our orthopedics program; could you help us put together a brochure that we can send out to doctors about the program?'" (Hillestad & Berkowitz [1991], p. 107). The problem with this approach is that it implies that the previous two steps—evaluating the mission and goals and performing an internal/external review—probably have not been undertaken. Furthermore, the brochure represents not a strategy but a tactic.

Strategies are broader frameworks by which goals can be attained. *Tactics* represent the specific activities that must be undertaken to carry out a strategy. There are many strategic approaches that organizations can adopt. An organization can choose to charge lower prices than the competition to achieve a high market share. Or it can adopt a strategy of high prices with the expectation of a highly profitable low market share. Organizations can decide to push their product, going to the customer, or use a pull strategy, making the customer come to them.

Organizations can develop strategies to create barriers to prevent other potential providers from competing. One approach is to charge low prices to gain a large market share. Competitiors are likely to be reluctant to enter a market where there is already a dominant force. Another approach to the creation of barriers would be to make it costly for consumers to shift to another care provider. Yet another strategy is to offer a product that only this one organization can provide.

The BCG Matrix

To help organizations with strategic planning for products, the Boston Consulting Group (BCG) developed a product matrix that has become widely used in developing product strategy. The matrix considers growth potential and market share for different products or services an organization offers. The matrix is somewhat simplistic, assuming that each product or service has either a high or low market share and either a high or low potential for growth. The BCG framework is presented in Figure 37–2.

If a product has a high market share and a high potential for growth, it is considered a "star" performer in the BCG approach. It is clearly worthy of continued attention and efforts on the part of management. Just the reverse is true for a service with low current market share and low potential for growth. Management would not be using its time wisely to put substantial efforts into trying to market that product. BCG refers to such products as "dogs."

The other two cells in the matrix are less clear-cut. A product or service for which the organization has high market share but that has low growth potential is generally referred to as a "cash cow." Since there is a high market share, it is likely that the organization can charge a high price, generating substantial profits. Even if prices are not high, the high market share should mean that the organization has a cost advantage. It can spread the fixed costs over a larger

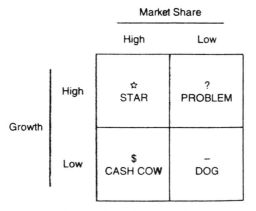

Figure 37–2 BCG matrix.

number of patients, generating a lower cost per patient than is possible for competitors with smaller market share. Therefore profits should still be high for cash cows.

Cash cows not only are profitable but also throw off cash dividends. A star is profitable, but its growth may require that much of the profit be reinvested in additional capacity. Since the growth potential is low for a cash cow, it often does not require reinvestment of the cash it generates. That cash is available for providing other services.

The last cell is referred to as a "problem child." Will its high growth potential be enough to offset the disadvantage of low market share? Over time this type of service may become either a dog or a star. Careful assessment is needed before investing resources in marketing this product.

Tactics

Strategies define the overall desired approach to marketing products and services. To carry out the strategy, a set of tactics must be employed. Tactics represent the specific actions taken. The types of tactics generally considered have often been referred to as the four Ps of marketing: *product, price, place,* and *promotion.*

Product

The product is the essential element that the marketing plan is attempting to sell. The product has been selected and developed based on prior analysis of customer needs, the organization's mission, internal/external analysis, and finally strategy. However, several tactical issues must still be addressed about the product.

First of all, the organization must make a decision concerning the specific characteristics of the product, such as its quality. Will quality be the least the organization can get away with, average, or noteworthy? The actual decision relating to the level of quality is a strategic one. Carrying out the decision is tactical. How does one go about attaining a noteworthy level of quality? One approach is to attract famous surgeons to the staff and then let the public know. An alternative tactic would be to increase nursing care hours per patient day and inform the public of that fact and its positive implications.

Another feature is service. Again, it is a strategic question whether the organization is willing to incur the costs associated with high levels of service. But it is a matter of tactics whether service should consist of free taxi service to and from the organization. It might be worthwhile to have a host or hostess greeting patients upon arrival at the front door and taking them to admitting. The key to service is to do more than expected, to go the one extra step to make the customer take note.

Nurse managers should consider their tactics carefully, since they often come into direct contact with two different classes of customers—the patients themselves and physicians. The marketing motto, "the customer is always right," can be irritating to anyone who actually must try to deal with a rude or irrational customer. Nurses, however, cope well with the irrationalities of patients, understanding how miserable it is to be sick. Nurses have on occasion shown a higher level of resentment of the other customer—the physician.

One hears many anecdotes about physicians who mess up and need nurses to save the day. There is no question that nurses serve a vital role and that physicians could not get along without them. However, from a marketing perspective, that result is exactly what one would want. When physicians feel that they receive no direct benefit from a hospital, they start providing a greater range of patient services, including surgery, out of their own offices. The reason that physicians rely on hospitals, even for outpatient surgery, is that the hospital provides some desired product or service to the physician as a customer. In many cases that desired product or service is the very nursing care that many physicians *seem* to take for granted.

Price

Price matters. Many people assume that with most of the population insured by Medicare, Medicaid, Blue Cross, or other private insurers, price does not matter. However, a growing portion of the buyers of health care services are becoming sensitive to price variations. HMOs and PPOs negotiate aggressively for the best prices they can obtain. Each organization must determine how sensitive its customers are to price and base a policy accordingly.

There are a number of different approaches to setting prices. Some organizations like to simply use a *markup*. That is, they determine the cost of providing care and raise, or mark up, their price a certain percentage over the cost. The problem with this policy is that the low-volume producer will have the highest cost (because fixed costs are not shared over a large volume of patients) and therefore the highest price. It will be difficult to increase volume and therefore reduce costs and reduce prices if you start out as a high-priced producer.

Another alternative is to charge a particularly low price, perhaps even lower than cost, to gain a substantial increase in market share. The philosophy is that even though you may lose money on each patient, as volume increases, average cost will decrease and patients will eventually become profitable at the price being charged. Legal input is required to ensure that price is not set so low that it would violate antitrust laws.

Another tactic is to charge a high price, knowing that market share will be low, but planning to make a high profit on the volume achieved. This is sometimes referred to as *skimming*.

Place

In real estate the three most important factors that establish the value of property are location, location, and location. In marketing health care services much the same is true. Traditional health care services generally expect the patient to come to the service. If the service is in an inconvenient location, it will be difficult to attract patients. While home health agency staff generally visit patients, many other health care services have lagged in coming to the patient. However, more innovative approaches to health care services do make attempts to bring the services closer to the patients. For example, there are now national mail-order pharmacies. Many disabled patients can avoid the high cost of a taxi to go to and from the pharmacy.

The issue of "place" is closely tied to the concept of *distribution channels*. The concept of distribution channels relates to moving the product from the producer to the consumer. How does the product get from the provider of the service to the ultimate consumer? In the case of a home care agency, the provider brings the product directly to the patient. In the case of a hospital, the patient comes to the provider. Clearly, if the distribution channel can be modified to bring the product closer to the consumer, there is a better chance of being the provider of choice.

Distribution channels are referred to as being direct or indirect, depending on whether the consumer and the provider have a direct relationship or whether there is some intermediary. When a patient is admitted to a hospital on the advice of a personal physician, there is an indirect channel between the patient and the hospital. The hospital is at risk if the intermediary—the physician—decides to use a different hospital. If the hospital opens a series of clinics around the community staffed with full-time physician employees of the hospital, then the distribution channel is direct.

Clearly, it is to the advantage of a health care provider to have a direct channel to the patient. However, this arrangement creates its own costs and risks. In the above example the hospital must take on the burden of operating a series of clinics. The clinics may be unprofitable, more than offsetting the advantage of the direct linkage. They may also alienate the other physicians in the community who resent the hospital's competition. A hospital must adopt a strategy concerning whether it wants to establish direct channels of distribution or is willing to accept indirect channels.

Once the strategic decision regarding the use of direct or indirect channels is made, tactics must be developed. If the strategy is to employ direct channels, then the tactics concern the exact location of clinics and their size, staffing pattern, and hours. If the strategy is acceptance of indirect channels, then the tactics concern the actions the hospital could take to keep the referring physicians happy and ensure that they do not start referring patients elsewhere. The tactics are less certain here, and a great deal of effort must go into determining what factors influence where a physician refers patients. If the key issue is attending to physician needs, then someone should call the physician periodically to ask whether the hospital is doing all it can for the physician. If the key issue is available beds when needed, the hospital must develop an admission process that ensures that certain physicians always get a bed when they need it.

Health care providers must carefully consider the long-run implications of their tactics. Then they can make a reasoned decision about what approach is likely to be in the best interests of the organization.

Promotion

The last of the four tactical concerns is the one most people associate with marketing—promotion. Promotion consists of advertising, public relations, sales promotion, and personal selling, as was discussed earlier. The strategy of the organization will determine which products or services will receive significant promotion in a given period.

Tactics determine whether to use print media or radio or television. Tactics focus on which newspapers or magazines, on which radio or television programs, on what day of the week, on what time of the day. Should nurse managers be encouraged to teach in local nursing schools as a means of public relations? Should they be paid by the health care provider while they are teaching? How much money should be spent on mass advertising and how much on a personal sales force?

For a home care agency, advertising creates a general public awareness. However, most patients arrive as referrals by physicians, social workers, or discharge-planning nurses. One full-time sales person will likely reach only 1,000 people per year. The advertisements that could be bought for the same money might reach hundreds of thousands. Tactically, however, one must decide which is a better buy for the money and whether the money is wisely spent on either alternative.

Revision, Integration, and Implementation

Once the marketing plan is developed, it must be reviewed by top management and accepted, revised, or rejected. Management must review the plan with several key factors in mind. First of all, does the plan make sense given the mission of the organization? There may be huge potential profits from selling unproven cancer cures. It may fill a customer desire, and it may be easy to price and promote. However, if it goes against the principles of the organization, it will have to be rejected. The focus on organizational mission as the basis for the marketing plan should result in a plan that will likely call for products and services that are within the mission of the organization.

Does the internal/external analysis seem to be thorough? The plan relies upon the quality of that analysis to determine the relative position of the organization and the ultimate needs of the customers.

Do the strategies proposed respond to customer needs? Generally, a marketing plan will require the organization to make significant commitments of resources and in many cases significant changes in operations. This should not happen unless the strategies are reasoned responses to the needs of the customers in light of the relative positions of the organization and its competition. Are the tactics designed to ensure that the strategies are implemented efficiently?

If the marketing plan is accepted or sent back for revisions and then accepted after revision, it becomes critical to implement the plan not only via promotion but also operationally throughout the organization. Marketing plans do not stand alone in an organization. The marketing plan must be integrated. It makes little sense to find out what people need and develop a plan to market that product or service without the organization's taking the various necessary actions to produce that service. Often the key to such integration is communication. The plan should not be a secret. Major strategies and individual tactics are not carried out by the marketing department but by the line staff of the organization. Nurse managers and the nursing staff are often the key to implementing many of the strategies and tactics required for the success of a marketing plan.

It should become clear that marketing does play a more substantial role than simply advertising the organization's products. Marketing is integral to deciding what products or services should be offered. When the plan is adopted, it creates change in what products and services are offered. In light of that, nursing managers should not treat informational requests from marketing as a peripheral annoyance to be handled quickly and without much thought. Six months later the decisions based on that information will come back in specific operational changes. Marketing has a significant and growing role in health care organizations, and interactions between nursing and marketing warrant careful thought and attention.

Control and Feedback

Once a marketing plan has been accepted and implemented, it is necessary to control the various aspects of the plan to ensure that it is being carried out. Generally, this means that information must be collected on how the tactics are being implemented and whether the implementation is appropriate to carry out the strategies decided upon and to achieve the goals of the plan.

For example, many nursing units around the country are hiring hosts or hostesses for each unit to relieve nurses of a number of time-consuming burdens that could be handled by a less trained individual. Many of these tasks are of a nonclinical educational nature. Showing families of patients where the waiting rooms and telephones are is an example. Other examples are explaining to the families how strict or lenient visiting hour regulations are or informing families how to inquire as to patient status.

When the marketing plan was envisioned, the intention may have been that this person would also greet arriving patients at the front door and take them to admitting, or that the host or hostess would bring a fruit basket to the patient shortly after admission. If that tactic is not being carried out, the plan loses a minor but significant element—providing the unexpected benefit or service.

There should be a formal process by which there is reporting on which tactics have been implemented. The reporting must be specific; it is inadequate to simply indicate that a host or hostess has been hired for each unit. Furthermore, there must be feedback directly from the customers. Physicians and patients should be polled, asking their satisfaction levels at various points in time to see if the changes are having any attitudinal impact. And of course there should be quantitative measures in terms of patient volume to allow for tracking the success of the plan.

MARKETING FAILURES

It would be nice to believe that any organization that realizes the potential benefits of marketing will succeed in its marketing efforts. Unfortunately, that is not always the case. History has shown that many marketing campaigns do fail. Learning from those failures should help others to avoid them.

It is true that sometimes everything will be done right and marketing efforts will still fail. However, avoiding certain common shortcomings can reduce the likelihood of that result. Specifically, common failures are often due to several specific factors.

One major problem is failure to collect data prior to making decisions. Decisions based solely on intuition may fail after substantial financial investment, when a modest amount of market research data collection could have indicated that the financial investment was unwise.

Another problem relates to errors of analysis. Data may be collected but not carefully interpreted. One key concern that managers should have is that new products and services often have strong advocates. Such people may not neutrally evaluate information, since they have a vested interest in its interpretation.

A third key element common to failure is a lack of clear objectives. Marketing should not be rushed without careful consideration of exactly what needs to be accomplished. Focusing the marketing plan carefully on a specific set of objectives increases the likelihood of achieving them.

Finally, many organizations use incorrect tactics. It is important that carrying out the objectives of a plan be done in light of the specific clearly stated objectives. The tactics must fully and directly support the accomplishment of the goals that have been set.

THE ROLE OF THE NURSE MANAGER

Marketing activities are much more highly related to nursing management than most nurses realize. The first and most vital aspect of marketing is assessing the needs and desires of the customers of the organization. Nurses are in a position to be very attuned to those needs and desires, both in the case of patients and in the case of physicians.

Another major aspect of marketing is assessing the capabilities of the organization. Here again, the input of nurses is vital to gaining a clear understanding of the strengths and limitations of the organization.

The strategic and tactical issues of marketing also warrant close cooperation between nursing and marketing. Nurses are unlikely to enthusiastically work to carry out organizational strategies that they cannot support. Therefore, there should be substantive discussions between nursing and marketing as strategies are developed. Nurses should give direct input on what strategies they think are good, which ones are bad, and why. Similarly, since nursing units will be operationalizing many of the specific tactics to implement the strategies, they must have some say in the establishment of what those tactics will be.

Cost is also an important factor in marketing. The marketing department will proudly point out gains in patient volume. The nursing department will incur additional costs to implement new products, services, strategies, and tactics. There must be a clear relationship between the expectations of a marketing plan and the additional resources provided to nursing units to carry out their aspect of the plan.

Nursing departments should consider having their own marketing plan for internal marketing. The nurse's customers include other nurses, physicians, patients, and other hospital staff. Determining the needs of each customer group can improve outcomes for both the customers and nursing.

Bibliography

Barigar, D.L., & Sheafor, M.L. (1990). Recruiting staff nurses: A marketing approach. *Nursing Management 21*(1), 27–29.

Duro, R., & Sandstrom, B. (1987). *The basic principles of marketing warfare*. New York: John Wiley & Sons.

Frand, E.A. (1989). *The art of product development: From concept to market*. Homewood, IL: Dow Jones-Irwin.

Johnson, J.E., Arvidson, A.C., Costa, L.L. et al. (1987). Marketing your nursing product line. *Journal of Nursing Administration, 17*(11), 29–33.

Hillestad, S.G., & Berkowitz, E.N. (1991). *Health care marketing plans: From strategy to action* (2nd ed.). Gaithersburg, MD: Aspen Publishers.

Ireson, C., & Weaver, D. (1992). Marketing nursing beyond the walls. *Journal of Nursing Administration, 22*(1), 57–60.

Kiener, M.E. (1989). Market segmentation and positioning: Matching creativity with fiscal responsibility. *Journal of Continuing Education in the Health Professions, 9*(2), 77–86.

Kotler, P. (1976). *Marketing management, analysis, planning and control* (3rd ed.). Englewood Cliffs, NJ: Prentice-Hall.

Lavidge, R.J., & Steiner, G.A. (1961). A model for predictive measurements of advertising effectiveness. *Journal of Marketing, 25*, 59.

Magrath, A.J. (1988). *Market smarts: Proven strategies to outfox and outflank your competition*. New York: John Wiley & Sons.

Porter, R.T., Porter, M.J., & Lower, M.S. (1989). Enhancing the image of nursing. *Journal of Nursing Administration, 19*(2), 36–42.

Rados, D.L. (1981). *Marketing for non-profit organizations*. Boston: Auburn House Publishing Company.

Ries, A., & Trout, J. (1989). *Bottom-up marketing*, New York: McGraw-Hill.

Sonnenberg, F.K. (1990). *Marketing to win: Strategies for building competitive advantage in service industries*. New York: Harper Business, Division of Harper & Row.

Stefflre, V. (1986). *Developing and implementing marketing strategies*. New York: Praeger.

Strasen, L. (1987). *Key business skills for nurse managers*. Philadelphia: J.B. Lippincott.

Taylor, T. (1990). Healthcare marketing and the nurse manager. *Nursing Management, 21*(5), 84–85.

Washburn, S.A. (1988). *Managing the marketing functions: The challenge of the customer-centered enterprise.* New York: McGraw-Hill.

Weitz, B.A., & Wensley, R. (1984). *Strategic marketing: Planning, implementation, and control.* Boston: Kent Publishing Co.

Part D. Managing Change

CHAPTER 38 • • • • • • •

INNOVATION, CHANGE, AND CONTINUITY

DAVID M. LEHMANN

EXECUTIVE SUMMARY

Winning organizations self-initiate continuous improvement. Opportunities and problems are seized as the focal point for team problem solving. Teams of people with different functional backgrounds use fact-based problem-solving techniques to achieve a vision and a new competence and reinvent the organization's reason for being. These innovations keep the organization relevant and competitive. Changing may be resisted, but change is valued for its future benefits. Plans and actions are based on a shared set of values and beliefs of what the customers value. People are considered a valued resource for their contribution and not viewed as a cost.

TWO PERSPECTIVES OF INNOVATION AND CHANGE

Most actions that make the athlete successful in competition come from the subconscious. We do not think about how to run when we run. We do not think about how to throw when we throw. High-performing organizations perform out of their subconscious. Just as the athlete does not run faster by mentally pushing one muscle against another, organizations do not innovate and change by pushing innovation and change. Pushing for innovation should not be confused with high expectations for innovation and change. Pushing implies that one part of the organization (such as management) can by some fear of withholding rewards compel another part to change its behaviors.

Inducing people to set high expectations implies equity in rewards for achievement. The people are more self-motivated, self-directed to innovate and change the work of the organization, measuring their own performance against a common, pervasive vision of what is to be created and what creates value. Pushing implies that one person's vision is imposed on others with little concern for their acceptance and understanding of why this vision is to be followed.

High-performing organizations continually innovate and change, maintaining and increasing in their value until forces emerge to inhibit their success. The essence of the task of innovation and change is not to demand innovation and change but to reduce the inhibiting forces (Senge, 1990). People are by their nature curious, interested, inquisitive, and seeking of new situations. Bad organizational dynamics destroy the people's will for pursuing these interests.

Using a Crisis Atmosphere to Force Change

- Great Man Theory
  or
- Consciousness, consistent effort to reduce forces that inhibit innovation and change

One perspective of innovation and change is the great man theory. Managers having this perspective believe in pushing (demanding) innovation and change, usually by attempting to use financial measurements, personal performance goals, and a forecast of gloom and doom to create anxiety in people. This anxiety is believed to lead to innovation and useful change. It is very difficult to see how a negative vision and the fear of punishment will lead to positive changes, but the galvanizing effect of an impending crisis is a significant motivator for action. Whether this action produces a shift in beliefs and a more promising future for the organization is arguable.

Reducing the Forces That Inhibit Innovation and Change

The alternative perspective, one that is more useful in a broad range of situations, is a conscious effort to reduce the forces that are inhibiting innovation and change. This chapter highlights important aspects of organizations, for manager–leaders, that can reduce these inhibiting forces. Managers who create an organizational environment where innovation and change are not inhibited do this by creating positive visions that motivate people. Such managers are manager–leaders.

Continuation of Strong Values and Beliefs

Before we explore innovation and change, we need a mental model of continuity. Our purpose is to create an organization that continually innovates and changes, always increasing in value to its customers (internal and external customers). Customers are the reason the organization exists and the reason each job within the organization exists. For an acid test of this concept and to see how quickly people lose the perspective of why their job exists, compare the willingness and eagerness of a prospective job applicant to take on the challenges of a job with the attitudes of that same person after being in the job for some time. Those same challenges are now excuses for less than expected performance.

There is nothing in any organization that will continue forever, since the organization's reasons for existing are mortal. On a more practical level, continuity and consistency of values and basic beliefs and assumptions are the foundation of an environment where innovation and change freely occur. Valuing change may be of great benefit to the organization, but, surprisingly, valuing stability is a good environment for innovation and change. Stability for our purposes is a measure of predictability, not the continuation of past practices but the continuation of strong values and beliefs. Stability and change are not mutually exclusive. The greatest inhibiting force in any organizational dynamic is an unpredictable and inconsistent system of values, beliefs, and assumptions.

Values, beliefs, and assumptions are the theories in use about cause–effect linkages. These cause–effect, or action–outcome, linkages are the basis for people's opinions and actions. Each time someone expresses an opinion or takes an action, he or she is doing so based on the belief or assumption of an action–outcome linkage. The role of assumptions in the culture of an organization is explored in Schien (1985). The roots of the culture are these beliefs and assumptions.

One useful exercise is to ask people when they consider rewards, incentives, and compensation, "Must we get something when we give something, or can we give now and get something later?" Few people will share the same beliefs in the relationship between compensations and rewards and people's behaviors. The role of leadership in organizations is to facilitate the creation of more communally held beliefs and assumptions of organizational values and a greater alignment of values and goals. Posner, Kouzes, and Schmidt (1985) show that shared values within an organization make a positive difference in the organization's performance. Argyris (1990) describes the importance of understanding the more deeply rooted reasons for people's decisions.

Building an Understanding of What Is Valued

- Do the members of the organization know and understand what is valued?
- Are the values and beliefs exhibited by the manager inhibiting of innovation and change? Are they inconsistent, reflecting daily pressures?
- Is there consistency in the beliefs and assumptions among decision makers? Are there gross inconsistencies in behaviors among managers and the leaders?
- Do the people believe rewards are distributed equitably based on merit? Do tempers frequently flare up? Are managers consistent in their behavior, or must people always be on the alert for the politics of the moment?

These forces and many similar ones are discontinuities that show the unpredictable nature of the organization. We can overcome these forces by opening the organization through communication, dialogue, discussion, and learning from each other.

Open Organizations Learn Faster and Better

Open organizations are willing to go outside the organization to gather data for setting performance expectations. They benchmark, which is learning from those who are the best at what they do. They evaluate their own performance against externally validated criteria. When we share information and listen to the reasoning of others, we break down artificial barriers and reduce inequities that inhibit innovation and change. Open organizations self-initiate continuous improvement.

An organization that is willing to look objectively at itself values people who share common beliefs about the three most important questions any organization should ask itself: What is our business? Who are our customers? What does our customer consider value? (Drucker, 1954).

We reduce the forces inhibiting innovation and change when we create an organizational climate in which people are

- Trusted
- Respected
- Nurtured to grow and develop
- Considerate of each other
- Challenging and willing to be challenged

People are valued as a critical resource, not as a cost element in a line item in someone's budget. Manager–leaders know that without the people, there is nothing. Byham (1989) presents a serious but entertaining presentation of how we debilitate others by our actions in *ZAPP: The Lightning of Empowerment*.

The rest of this chapter challenges thinking in the following areas.

- Supporting innovation and change
- What a manager–leader can do
    Building information networks
    Using data for fact-based problem solving
    Order—understanding the rules
    Courage
- Valuing diversity of perspectives
- Simplified model of people's demand–reward systems
- Decision making is everyone's job
- Preparedness—continually innovating and changing
- Benchmarking to see what is possible
- It is easier than you think and the right thing to do

Each topic is explored only briefly to create a mosaic of the components the manager–leader should consider in the quest for creating an organizational environment and culture that freely innovate and change. Topics were selected to reveal issues that should be considered by the manager–leader for the organization's impact on people and the people's impact on the organization.

SUPPORTING INNOVATION AND CHANGE

Effective managers work to release the creative energies of the organization. This contrasts with the belief that management is laying out grand strategies with clear milestones for inventing solutions. In the everyday work situation, this grand strategy approach leads to managers doing the work of their subordinates—work for which the subordinates are better prepared. This does not imply that a strategy is not important. On the contrary, a valid strategy is essential as a basis for people to resolve their differences of opinion about which path to pursue.

In understanding innovation, change, and continuity, the manager's role is to reduce factors that inhibit innovation, to assure preparedness for seizing opportunities, and to create an organizational environment and culture that value people and learning. This perspective is different from the alternative of the manager pushing on the organization to change and innovate. The perspective for this description is an alternative to Drucker's proposal (1985). The two views, Drucker's that innovation and entrepreneurship can be operating systematically within the more formal systems of the organization and ours that we should work to reduce factors that inhibit innovation and change, both are appropriate and compatible. We have chosen the latter because we believe that this perspective is more useful for the person attempting to increase innovation and change in existing organizations.

The perspective of creating a wide zone within which people can innovate and change is more practical but goes directly in the face of many great man theories of management and leadership. In practice, managers are measured by the effectiveness of the organization. Managers lead successful organizations by setting a direction in broad terms, helping the people to define success, assuring that the organization pays attention to the details and discontinuities, working with the people to define and achieve the critical goals along the path to success, and by not meddling in the work of the people. Managers–leaders create wide zones within which people can innovate and change an organization's work:

- Setting direction in broad terms
- Helping people to define success
- Helping to get critical goals along path
- Not meddling in people's work

A manager–leader must reduce the inhibiting factors by recognizing the dynamic interrelationship of cultural attributions in both the informal organization and the formal organization. This is only possible when the organization's memory—its past—is clearly understood. The thought that managers should work to reduce inhibiting factors is well developed in Senge's work on the open systems model of organizations (Senge, 1990). The past can be understood only if it can be compared and contrasted to the vision of the future. The manager–leader must have a platform for self-analysis that is the vision of the future. Looking back without a vision of the future allows dangerous rationalization of the organization's current dilemma and acceptance that this is as good as it gets.

How can we create this vision? Kantor (1988) states that the successful enterpreneurial organizations provide more of the tools for innovation. Kanter describes these tools as information, support, and resources. When we place overbearing emphasis on control and power, we reduce information sharing and drive communications into vertical paths, inhibiting lateral information sharing. Many researchers have described organizations that succeed by empowering the people. Each of these descriptions of empowerment contains the same principles of pushing decision making lower in the organization, sharing information broadly throughout the organization, reducing the emphasis on hierarchy as a basis for power and authority, and increasing emphasis on accountability aligned with the organization's reason for existence (Orsburn, Moran, Musselwhite, & Zenger, 1990; Wellins, Byham, and Wilson, 1991).

Many managers may fear a loss of control if they relinquish authority for decisions. Managers must accept that organizations will be more effective if the managers spend their time developing the decision premises with the people. These are the boundaries of acceptable alternatives, the goals, and the commonly held beliefs and values. With a clear understanding of the decision premises, the people will make a better decision than the manager because the people are doing the work.

Sterman (1989) published research on the lack of understanding among managers of the response of their organizations. This research confirms our practical experience. Most managers do not understand how their organizations function at a detailed level, yet these managers will intervene inappropriately, taking accountability away from the people when the manager makes the decision. Senge (1990) summarizes some of Sterman's work.

Manager–leaders must set clear expectations for strong cross-functional relationships and a culture of learning from each other. Deming has for decades promoted the need to eliminate fear in organizational life (Walton, 1986). Cross-functional relationships built within a framework of a clear and simple strategy create stability and a common purpose. From the common purpose, the organization can explore the possibilities for the future, the possibilities that create positive energy and excitement. The presence of a strategy and the practice of learning create a forum for brokering the risk of innovation across a larger group. Developing a commonality of purpose brokers the risk of innovating while maintaining the needed stability. Innovating without the commonality of purpose and strategy creates fear, which constricts an organization to the point where innovation cannot survive. In an organization full of fear, traditional wisdom will be empowered and used by those who resist the changes to stifle change and innovation.

Creating a commonality of purpose and strategy makes it legitimate to apply some of the organization's resources to innovation and change. Kantor (1988) makes a compelling point about the need to make resources available for innovations and change. In organizations with fragmented strategies, slack resources in one function are viewed as excess people, people to be cut to improve near term profitability. In organizations that innovate with a commonality of purpose and strategy, people are valued for what they know and can contribute regardless of their current job classification or status in the organization. Slack resources in one area are redeployed and dedicated to improving the work of the organization in another area. This may start small, but once the people become enthusiastic and develop trust in the managers and leaders, the enthusiasm will spread throughout the organization. Trust builds when managers support change by their words and actions and are not threatened by new ways of performing the work of the organization.

Good managers pay most attention to information that does not fit their current model of how their world works. Support for new opportunities and new ways of doing the work of the organization is essential because this information will arise far from the power base, yet what is learned may be exactly what the organization desperately needs. This information is soft, invalidated information that cannot survive in communications systems (formal or informal) anchored in past or traditional wisdom.

Manager–leaders aid the survival of soft information about new opportunities by exposing critical resources to the organization's internal and external environments. Critical resources are the technologists, people at all levels in every function who know their work well, associated with the organization's core competencies. These core competencies are the strengths to be leveraged to create a better future. Traditional organizations shelter these technologists from the external environment so that they can do their work without distraction. The danger is that these are precisely the people who have the skills needed to sense change when it is just beginning. All people in the organization should be exposed to the organization's environment, particularly the customers, and all should be heard without the worthiness of their thoughts being prejudged. For this to be effective, the manager–leader must treat everyone as they are expected to treat the best customer. No one can select in advance how, where, and when the next opportunity will be revealed—the opportunity that if properly exploited will create significant competitive advantage. How we seek to learn of new opportunities and empower these new ideas may be one of the most important actions of managers. DeGeuss (1988) said, "The only relevant learning in a company is the learning done by those people who have the power to act."

WHAT A MANAGER–LEADER CAN DO

A model of innovation and change shows the need for information (networking), data (fact), understanding of order (rules and laws), and courage (self-confidence) (Fig. 38–1).

Building Information Networks

Networking focuses people toward

- Common goals
- One mission
- One vision
  and
- Develops sensitivity for what others believe

Information obtained by networking focuses people toward common goals, objectives, mission, and vision. Networking develops a sensitivity for values

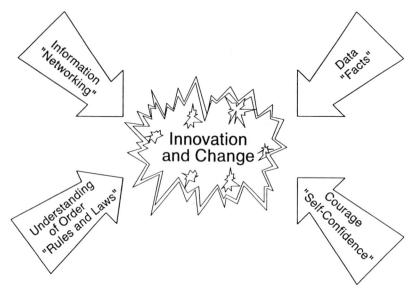

Figure 38–1 Innovation and change model.

and beliefs that, if challenged, unknowingly would destroy attempts to innovate and would galvanize opposition to change. The manager–leader must induce people to work together by creating and setting expectations for open discussion—expectations for listening and understanding of the positions and views of others—and by building problem-solving skills.

Using Data for Fact-Based Problem Solving

Data must be accurate, relevant, and accessible to all people. Eliminate
- Data that are inaccurate
- Data that waste people's time
- Data that distract

The need for data is the most overlooked aspect of the change process. There must be an environment where data are readily accessible by everyone, not a select few. Change efforts not based on facts become political contests, a test of wills with one group opposing the other. The manager–leader must create the expectation that data accuracy and relevance are essential and purge the organization of time-wasting and distracting reports and useless data transfers. Meaningful measurements focused on what customers value should be published regularly. Measurements are the basis for improvement and usually do not point to the cause of poor performance but only indicate the need for improvement. Using measurements as punishment usually punishes the wrong person. Data accuracy can be achieved only in an environment where people can share their views openly and be listened to. Everyone must feel an ownership of all data. It should not be used as a weapon. Those who repel others by bombarding them with data are trying to skew the balance of power to their favor and destroy the openness being created. Collaboration must occur first among managers before it will occur throughout the organization. This is the paradox of leadership— for the people to assume more responsibility, the leaders must assume more responsibility.

Order—Understanding the Rules

Rules and laws

- Define mission
- Decide what will make us successful
- Communicate this to everyone
- Align measurements with vision of success
- Expel those who resist too long or work at cross purposes

The rules for working together can be decided by the manager–leader and the people, as a team, defining the mission and vision for the organization. The critical success factors set by the team should be aligned with the measurements. The strategy, commonality of purpose, and critical success factors become the framework within which people can constructively resolve their differences about appropriate actions. The manager–leader's job is the effectiveness of the organization. Those who do not fit with the direction of the organization, although treated with respect, must be removed from the organization. Working in harmony with the order of the organization is the efficient way to move the organization to higher performance.

Courage

Managers must have courage to work outside their comfort zone. Courage is the strength and wisdom to know when and how to intervene and when not to intervene. Although this is not a natural skill of most managers, manager–leaders learn and teach such skills. An example of a lack of such skills is the boss who frequently assumes that his or her request must be given top priority. Another is the manager who intervenes and directs solutions when the problem should be solved by those who do the work. Often, at meetings, people add data that does not enhance the work, but they offer it just to show what they know. Are they skilled at intervening with a purpose of better performance from the organization?—probably not. They also have the wrong sense of what is valued and believe political gains at the expense of others are acceptable.

Managers must have the courage to work outside their comfort zone. If it takes 4 years to change the technical competency of an organization, someone must be creating the vision and strategies for building the technical base 5 years into the future. What good is it to be working within the time needed to change what one is working on? Managers who work inside the necessary time horizon do this because this is their comfort zone, but working within the time horizon for change is the domain of their subordinates. The Chinese say, leaders "worry out in front of the people and celebrate after everyone else."

Many strategists view the leader's role as preparing the people for the unexpected. Von Clausewitz (Phillips, 1987) is credited with creating the image of the "fog of war" to represent the uncertainty. Others state that one cannot manage people into battle, one must lead them. Leaders "worry out ahead of the people and celebrate after everyone else" (Phillips, 1985).

VALUING DIVERSITY OF PERSPECTIVES

Managers–leaders build appreciation for diversity:

- Adaptors do not naturally understand innovators.
- Innovators do not naturally understand adaptors.

We know that people have different strengths and different languages and that some are better adapters and some are better innovators. (The Center for Creative Leadership in Greensboro, NC, is an organization that can help with assessing the skills of the people in an organization.) For innovation and change to be a part of the culture of organizations, people with these skills must be part of the organization. Managers must promote the value of diversity by reinforcing behaviors for the exchange of ideas without judgment.

Staffing selections should include consideration of creating complementary skills. Managers fall into the trap of hiring in their own self-image, whereas the organization needs a mix of conceptual skills and operational skills within the same function. When managers hire subordinates with the same strengths and interests as the manager, functions eventually fail to innovate and change because they lack a balance of skills.

One very big challenge is the need for a common language. People in different parts of the organization speak different languages. The single most important contribution of an organizationwide quality initiative is the development of a common language and vision. A common set of measurements creates a common language across functions, particularly if these measurements relate to the customer's perception of what is valued.

People have different skills and preferences for their work. The person best at adapting will view the innovator as one who takes unnecessary risks or is out of control. The innovator will view the adaptor as slow to act, overly cautious, stuck in a rut. The manager–leader creates ways for people to gain a greater appreciation for alternative viewpoints. To stimulate people of different skills and perspectives to work together, the manager must boldly shoulder the risk of the decision without making the decision. To make the decision would relieve the people of their accountability for results. When the manager–leader is effective in reducing the apparent risk, the people will share their different views. The manager must show the resolve of leadership and bear the burden for decisions that exceed the capacity of the people to accept the risk.

Each person has his or her own beliefs about action–outcome linkages. Some, for example, may believe that people do only what is minimally required. Others believe that people develop a commitment to the success of the group, and this commitment goes beyond minimal adequacy. Some managers believe primarily in extrinsic rewards to motivate people, whereas others believe people are re-

• "Assumptions about Action/Outcome Linkages"

• Working Together to Create Organization's
  Belief System

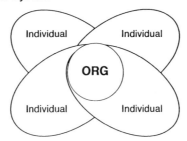

Figure 38–2   Multiple belief systems.

warded and motivated by achieving satisfaction in their work. The belief system operating in the organization is a combination of the beliefs of individuals and the compound effect of these beliefs as they compete in the decision processes (Fig. 38-2). Each person is unique, and each organization is unique. The beliefs held by individuals are developed from their experiences before joining the organization and those they developed while members of the organization.

These belief systems are both a strength, a basis for innovation and change, and an inhibiting factor. The manager–leader creates an organizational climate where the differences can be discussed, and decisions can be made consistent with the strategy, vision, and critical success factors and goals. Surprisingly, this is relatively easy to do but is seldom done. It first requires an openness of the management and a desire to create the learning organization described earlier.

MODELS OF DEMAND–REWARD SYSTEMS

To apply our perspective of reducing inhibiting factors and preparedness for opportunities, we need a framework of organizational functioning. This topology is created by combining two facets of organizational life. Within the organization there exists a formal organization and an informal organization. The formal organization performs with the desires and expectations of individuals subservient to the set plans and objectives of the organization. The informal organization performs outside the plans and controls. Within each, there is a production system for processing the events and a system of social interaction among the individuals. These four operating arenas (Fig. 38–3) are

1. Formal–production
2. Formal–social
3. Informal–production
4. Informal–social

We expect the planned work of the organization to be performed efficiently in the formal–production system. Here, the process is well defined, and there

Formal Production

Bureaucracy

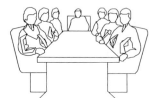

- Just Get It to Meet Plan
- High Control
- Stabilize Process
- Linear Thinking

Formal Social

Vision

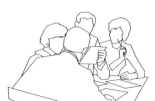

- Listening
- Interests Outside Self
- Contribute
- Goal-Driven
- Innovate

Informal Production

Crisis-Driven

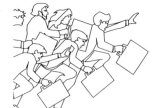

- "I" Will Fix It
- Just Get It to Work
- Get Back to Neutral
- Create Future Problems to Solve Today's

Informal Social

Negative Emotions

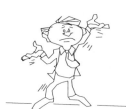

- I Am Frustrated
- Help Me
- They Must Do Something
- Why Don't They . . .

Figure 38–3 The four operating arenas in the informal organization.

is little slack. The problems in the processes of the formal–production system are attacked usually by individuals working in the informal–production systems. This is usually the source of people burnout—processes out of control. The objective of the work in the informal–production system is primarily to get the formal–production systems to work as they are designed. The informal–social systems are where we see people expressing their frustrations. People are making statements about what others must do to make them a success. Most manager–worker animosity emerges here. However, most manager–worker animosity is rooted in formal–production processes that cannot perform within specifications, requiring continual intervention to correct the same problem. People who must fix the same thing over and over do not feel valued. They become frustrated. This emotion is expressed in the informal–social systems. Innovation and change happen freely in the formal–social systems. This is where teams do their work. Each person feels a part of something that is valued and that they are valued as individuals for what they can contribute. The arena of the formal–social systems is where the individuals and the organization learn. People are comfortable being vulnerable and showing an interest in learning and experimenting. If someone tried to experiment in the formal–production system, the system would restrict them, forcing compliance with the existing system and plan. In the informal–production system, organizational cowboys and firefighters are valued for their full-speed-ahead attitude, which does not leave room for doubt and learning—"Don't worry, boss, I will fix the problem." In the informal–social system, the focus is the individual, and this precludes organizational learning.

The manager–leader recognizes these four behaviors and constructively channels people's energies into the formal–social arena, where they can learn and add value to the work of the organization. Those who persist in the informal–social arena eventually must be removed from the organization for their own good and the good of the organization. These behaviors are seen as immature, not a team player, working toward personal objectives at the expense of the organization.

To summarize, first, given two perspectives we choose the less glamourous, more pragmatic way of working to reduce inhibiting factors. Second, we realize that members of the organization operate in four interdependent demand–reward systems in somewhat obscure ways with complex beliefs. This should not frighten us back into our comfort zones but should provide the road map for moving out of those zones. We now recognize what we are dealing with.

The key is the difficult work of thinking through how our organizations and people perform their work. Simple but difficult questions arise, such as, Can we change our formal systems? Do we innovate only in the informal systems, never successfully changing the formal system? Are our stated values and our actions consistent? Or, do we change our beliefs to suit the situation? Are we capable of creating a learning organization? Do we attempt to learn from each other, or are we spending our energies justifying our position? The list is endless, and our purpose is not to develop an exhaustive list. We must begin to think about how and why our organization and the people behave as they do. Understanding the interdependencies, we can begin to reduce the inhibiting factors and create a powerful continuity of values, beliefs, and empowerment that becomes a culture of innovation and change.

The manager–leader should set out on a course to make innovation and change easier by creating a continuity of values and the highest consistency between values and actions. She or he must work within the four systems of organizational life to reduce conflicting forces and to align each with the needs of the individuals and the organization (Fig. 38–4).

DECISION MAKING IS EVERYONE'S JOB

The perspective we have adopted is consistent with the belief that innovation and change are a part of everyone's job, not just the work of managers. Assuring innovation and positive change is the job of the manager, whereas innovating and change are a part of everyone's job.

An idea that would improve the performance of the organization should be observed as if it were being held in the hands. Where should it be set down to grow and be nurtured? If it is set down among the tightly meshed gears of the formal systems, will it survive? Probably not well. These formal systems have

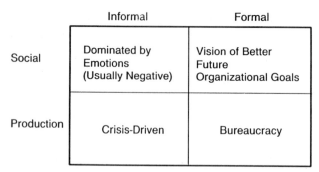

	Informal	Formal
Social	Dominated by Emotions (Usually Negative)	Vision of Better Future Organizational Goals
Production	Crisis-Driven	Bureaucracy

Figure 38–4 Framework of organizational function.

been pushed to the point where there is an absence of slack, the fertile ground for ideas and innovation. The fertile ground for innovation is the formal-social system, where an honest assessment of core competencies and weaknesses is possible. In the western managerial model of organization functioning, exciting ideas are forced out by beliefs that organizations grow in a linear incremental fashion. Yet in the oriental managerial view of organizations, ideas are commitments to a better future. The western, analytic disposition evaluates the probability of success in terms of today's knowledge—similar to starting a drive down a street by waiting until all the traffic lights are green and then accelerating. The alternative perspective, the oriental approach, is to know one's strengths and be confident that one will create the needed knowledge when necessary.

The first perspective is a perspective of task confidence, i.e., having some picture of how to accomplish each step before beginning the venture. The second, or alternative, perspective is one of being confident in the core competencies of the organization and believing that the obstacles will be overcome by the use of these strengths. The point is for innovation and change to be nurtured, the people must have a clear idea of the organization's strengths. Why does the organization exist? And why does it have a right to command some compensation for what it does? These are the core competencies that set the organization apart from others, even if the missions are similar.

In summary, a clear understanding of the strengths of the organization will be a fertile ground for innovation and change. The strengths or core competencies must be defined in broad generic dimensions to avoid propagating traditional practices and focusing only on incremental improvements. Managers who set engaging, energizing, and exciting goals know how to function in the formal–social systems.

PREPAREDNESS—CONTINUALLY INNOVATING AND CHANGING

Chinese strategist Sun Tzu is credited as the first to set the vision that the best victories are those won while avoiding the battle. Winning without fighting is victory. Continually preparing for tomorrow's challenges stimulates innovation and change without the fear of disaster. Frequently, organizations are motivated to change only when a crisis galvanizes the people toward a common goal. Preparedness from immersion in the pursuit of a shared vision motivates people to innovate and change without the threat of a crisis. Cross-functional groups should work to describe what the organization can achieve and create images of the intermediate stages along the path to the vision 5 and 10 years into the future. People need the opportunity to reveal their thoughts and share their ideas without being judged or criticized. Success is possible when ideas become common topics of discussion and the origin of the idea is fuzzy. This latitude for trying new ideas will pay large dividends.

The military people of the world use a practice of war gaming scenarios. Every organization should adopt this practice. "What if" is a powerful question in an open, learning environment. Playing out the scenarios will show the areas of strength and weakness.

Preparedness requires accountability for planning and improvement. Accountability is achieved by developing strategies for every operating element of the organization, not by reserving the concept of mission, vision, and strategy for only the large organization. Everyone has customers who must depend on them and suppliers who they must depend on. If we define the why, what, and how of each process within the organization, people are willing to be accountable for results.

A simple checklist or process flow chart with customer-oriented measurements will produce surprising results. Fair, accurate, and accepted accountabilities, whether using an elaborate MBO system, performance appraisals, position descriptions, functional charts, mission statements, critical success factors, or other less formal descriptions, are the basis for innovation and change if managers accept that they are accountable for continuous innovation and change.

BENCHMARKING TO SEE WHAT IS POSSIBLE

One practice helpful in stimulating preparedness and accountability for what could be is the practice of benchmarking. Some call this best practices studies. The key is to get outside the everyday accepted practice and compare performance against those who are judged to be good at what they do. When we benchmark, we continually learn about how others perform similar work. There are many good references on the practices of benchmarking.

In benchmarking, it is first necessary to relearn how to learn so as not to waste the host's time. Second, benchmarking must cover a complete system, not a piece of the system, since improving a part of a system that is not the constraint will not improve the performance of the system. In benchmarking, one should look at processes generically, not just those in similar industries.

Paradigm shifts, not small incremental improvements, create a driving force for innovation and change without destroying the continuity of the organization. The beauty of benchmarking is the validation of what is possible. It is not always necessary to go far away to find a good example to benchmark.

Benchmarking is the best tool to challenge those who are doing the wrong thing right. This is the most difficult paradigm to break. The trap occurs when we are progressing along a path and our apparent progress reinforces our beliefs that we are on the right course. Only when we receive input external to our beliefs are we motivated to reevaluate our direction. Even then, we may be incapable of this reevaluation. Reevaluation requires the assistance of people not committed to the current practices.

IT IS EASIER THAN YOU THINK AND THE RIGHT THING TO DO

Plato tells us in the *Republic,* through the logic of Socrates, that if we understand a man's passions, desires, and reasons, we understand the man and the society he is part of (Kaplan, 1950). The essence of our work to reduce the forces inhibiting innovations and change is to match the person with the opportunity that motivates him or her. We start with the assumption that there are no unsuitable people, just bad fits between opportunity or job and person. All people have many things they do well and like to do. Bad organizational structures, high control philosophies, and organizational polices destroy their will and undervalue their skills. When we create an organizational climate where people are valued, trusted, and respected, we reduce the forces inhibiting innovation and change. It just takes courage.

References

Argyris, C. (1990). *Overcoming organizational defenses: Facilitating organizational learning.* Needham Heights, MA: Allyn and Bacon.

Byham, W.C. (1989). *ZAPP: The lightning of empowerment.* Pittsburgh, PA: Development Dimensions International Press.

DeGeuss, A. (1988, March–April). Planning as learning. *Harvard Business Review.*

Drucker, P.F. (1954). *The practice of management.* New York: Harper and Row.

Drucker, P.F. (1985). *Innovation and entrepreneurship.* New York: Harper and Row.

Kantor, R.M. (1988, summer). Innovation— The only hope for the times ahead. *Sloan Management Review.*

Kaplan, J.D. (Ed). (1950). *Dialogues of Plato.* New York: Washington Square Press.

Orsburn, J.D., Moran, L. Musselwhite, E., & Zenger, J.H. (1990). *Self-directed work teams.* Homewood, IL: Business One IRWIN.

Phillips, T.R. (1985 & 1987). *Roots of strategy,* Books 1 & 2. Harrisburg, PA: Stackle Books.

Posner, B.Z., Kouzes, J.M., & Schmidt, W.H. (1985, fall). Shared values make a difference: An empirical test of corporate culture. *Human Resource Management 24*(3), 293–309.

Schein, E.H. (1985). *Organizational culture and leadership.* San Francisco: Jossey-Bass.

Senge, P.M. (1990). *The fifth discipline: The art and practice of the learning organization.* New York: Doubleday.

Sloan, A.P., Jr. (1965). *My years with General Motors.* New York: Macfadden-Bartell Book.

Sterman, J. (1989). Misperceptions of feedback in dynamic decision making. *Organizational Behavior and Human Decision Processes, 43,* 301–335.

Walton, M. (1986). *The Deming management method.* New York: Putnam Publishing.

Wellins, R.S., Byham, W.C., & Wilson, J.M. (1991). *Empowered teams.* San Francisco: Jossey-Bass.

CHAPTER 39 • • • • • •

STRATEGIC PLANNING

WILLIAM M. WARFEL

EXECUTIVE SUMMARY

Strategic planning is a process for developing a detailed program of actions that will fulfill an organization's vision for the future. In the strategic planning process, the role for nurse executives and managers is to represent and ensure that the future needs of patients and staff are met. It can be a very exciting and enjoyable process that requires considerable investment of time, energy, and resources. Nursing management must participate actively in the process because it represents a major hospital resource and budget item (Jones, 1988).

It is not sufficient, however, to have a strategic plan. Current theory frequently focuses on the importance of aspects of strategy implementation and ways of thinking and behaving strategically. Dixit and Nalebuff (1991) point out that we are all strategists and that being a good strategist can be learned. The art of thinking and behaving strategically consists of applying basic principles and skills to game theory and playing the game to win.

Thinking and behaving strategically will ensure successful implementation of the strategic planning process. Through this process, nursing management can be proactive in the dynamic health care marketplace and guarantee the position and contribution of the nursing organization as we prepare for the year 2000.

Strategic planning is regarded by many management authorities as the most important responsibility of corporate executives (Cleverly, 1989). A recent issue of the *Nursing Administration Quarterly* (Toward the year 2000, 1991) focused on the readiness of nursing to respond to the turbulent changing times in health care. The theme, "Toward the Year 2000: Is Nursing Ready?" is at the heart of the issue of strategic planning for nurse executives and managers. It is about planning for and creating how nursing's role will fit in the health care system of the future consistent with an agency's mission and vision.

The reason for strategic planning is the same as for any aspect of planning, i.e., that it increases the likelihood that it will achieve a desired outcome. Just as nursing care planning is intended to increase the likelihood that nursing interventions will move patients' health status toward a stated, desirable goal, strategic planning also increases the likelihood of achieving a desirable goal.

667

The difference is that strategic planning is more global in its considerations. It is the planning that happens consistent with moving the organization toward its stated goals. Nursing executives and managers must be effective strategists if their organization is to fulfill its mission and be responsible to its consumers in the future.

One of the concerns we have in planning, of course, is what does the future hold? We have just been through a decade of dramatic issues and changes in health care. It is doubtful that 10 years ago any one of us would have predicted how different our work lives would be because of multiple forces affecting the health care system. We have been forced to manage in new and sometimes exciting ways. Our use of data to manage effectively is essential. Coincidentally, there are so many data available to us that we frequently cannot review, interpret, and apply all that we have.

The decade ahead appears to make the one just past seem mild by comparison. The heavy emphasis on financing and reimbursement of health care promises to take on a new dimension as employees, politicians, and consumers demand new solutions to the cost and quality issues facing the health care system at all levels. It is imperative that organizations be poised to respond to these challenges. Never before has the organization's strategic plan been so critical to ensuring the organization's viability. There is no question that nursing is part of the strategic plan. Nursing is a major stakeholder. That means that when seen as an opportunity, it is the responsibility of nursing leadership to define how nursing will participate and respond to issues facing each organization. Nurse leaders have seen and will continue to see planning as a major component of our roles. Nurse executives and managers will have to have other team members who handle crises. Ours is to see the vision, describe it, and define effective strategies for achieving it.

GAINING THE COMPETITIVE ADVANTAGE

The impact of competition on health care institutions has been phenomenal. Strategic planning is about finding ways to win in a competitive market place, i.e., how to gain a competitive advantage and secure success.

One aspect of gaining a competitive advantage will be strategies that move an institution toward providing the highest quality products. Singularly, the concept of quality will be the key to gaining a competitive position. Hospitals that establish a reputation for quality make it extremely difficult for their competition to invade the high-quality position. Therefore, quality improvement as a strategy is one of the most effective ways that nursing can articulate its role in supporting its institution's vision. Quality improvement processes as an action strategy for nursing are worth mentioning because of my beliefs that quality must be a driving force in the development of any strategic plan.

Therein lies the opportunity for nursing to distinguish itself in assisting the institution in achieving and sustaining its competitive advantage. There are only a relatively few institutions that are known to the public and to nursing for the quality of their nursing care (Norby, 1990). This is not meant to diminish the tremendous work done by many nurse leaders and their nursing staff to distinguish nursing in their institutions. For example, Joyce Clifford and Beth Israel and many others have been an inspiration as they have shared their successes and insights. The reality, however, is that there are only a relatively few nursing organizations that have achieved this level of name recognition. The implications for nursing in our respective institutions are clear. Successful nursing organizations will be able to establish the positive elements of their organization in a way that will help determine the overall institutional competitive advantage.

SHOULD A NURSING ORGANIZATION BE DOING STRATEGIC PLANNING?

Strategic planning once referred to a process that was distinctly at the corporate or top level of administration, a plan that supported the organization's mission, values, and vision. More and more we hear, however, that the nursing department or organization has a strategic planning process or a strategic plan in place.

Strategy operates at different levels in complex health care organizations and has varying focuses. Therefore, it seems appropriate that strategies identified, developed, and owned by nursing that are consistent with the institution's mission, values, and vision constitute a strategic plan.

For example, Anvaripour, Bezold, and Weissman (1990) described New York's Mount Sinai Medical Center's Futures of Nursing project. They created a strategic planning process to distinguish nursing's position within the medical center that "involves establishing an academic department dedicated to scholarship and research to advance the art and science of nursing through clinical excellence" (Anvaripour et al., 1990, p. 207). Their goals for the project include establishing futures thinking as part of the professional nurse's responsibility and to give nursing leaders in the organization the opportunity to be strategic planners. They include the description of steps taken as part of a strategic process that resulted in the creation of a preferred future for nursing, the team's vision of twenty-first century nursing at Mount Sinai. There can be no doubt that the process described contains all of the elements of strategic planning and also no doubt that it is a worthwhile activity for nursing. The plan must be consistent with and supportive of the overall institutional strategic plan. Otherwise, it will have no chance of success. Strategies defined through nursing's strategic planning process will increase the likelihood of moving the organization forward from its present position toward its vision, a basic tenet of the strategic planning process.

Strategic Planning vs Operational Planning

The example of the Mount Sinai plan is meant to differentiate strategic planning for nursing from usual and customary operational planning. Most nursing organizations have a planning process that flows from a statement of mission, one that is linked to written goals, objectives, and action plans. Some of the strategies or actions defined may be supportive of institutional strategic thinking, but, by and large, these are planning statements and do not capture all of the elements of strategic planning. To attach the label of a strategic plan to operational planning would be misleading and a long way from the Mount Sinai project intended to develop a preferred future.

Strategic Planning vs Long-Range Planning

Strategic planning and long-range planning are sometimes used synonymously (Strasen, 1987). Bryson (1990) states that although there may be little difference in the outcome, they differ usually in these four ways.

1. Strategic planning relies more on identifying and resolving issues, whereas long-range planning focuses on specifying goals and objectives that are translated into current budgets and work programs.
2. Strategic planning emphasizes assessment of the external and internal environments and its impact on the organization far more than long-range planning does.
3. The creation of the vision or idealized version for the organization and how it may be achieved is more likely to come from strategic planners. Long-range plans are typically extensions of the present into the future markets.
4. Strategic planning is much more action oriented than is long-range planning.

Forecasting/Predicting the Future

One of the major concerns in our turbulent health care environment is how accurate our predictions can be for the future. There is general agreement that the only certainty is that tremendous uncertainty exists in all aspects of the health care system. So why bother planning strategically? Because not to bother planning strategically would be defeatist and negative and would ensure that our organization has not defined its place in the system of the future. The belief must be that the future is not a matter of chance but rather one of choice (Strasen, 1987). Our opportunities to mold our future are enhanced by creating a statement of our desired future.

Although forecasting ability remains dubious, the organization that believes that it will be self-determining in defining its future may find the development of scenarios helpful in forecasting. A scenario is a combination of projections, assumptions, and forecast of trends that is used to describe an array of future alternatives (Strasen, 1987). From the scenarios developed, ratings of which ones are most likely to succeed are assigned. The process of scenario development is just one way to identify reasonable and predictable alternatives in a turbulent environment.

WHAT IS STRATEGIC PLANNING?

Strategic planning is an abused, overused, and sometimes misunderstood process. There is no one description of what strategic planning is, although there is general agreement surrounding what the process is expected to accomplish. Borrowing the definition from Bryson (1990), strategic planning is a disciplined effort to produce fundamental decisions and actions that shape and guide what an organization is (in this case, a health care organization), what it does, and why it does it. I would like to embellish the definition by adding—and where it wants to go. Throughout the available literature, there is a message that strategic planning is futuristic thinking developed around the organization's vision for the future.

Another dynamic on which there is considerable agreement is that it has never been so critical that health care organizations think strategically. Strategic planning can help nurse executives and managers to think and act strategically (Bryson, 1990) by participating in the organization's strategic planning process and identifying actions for the nursing organization that support the plan. According to Bryson (1990), strategic planning requires broad-scale information gathering, an exploration of alternatives, and an emphasis on the future implications of present positions. In strategic planning, the information gathering aspect is far more reaching than what is usually thought of as data gathering. Many avenues in addition to numerical data are explored to create a situational audit that includes what Beckham (1991) calls "situational wisdom," the kind that flows from intuition as a valid means to gather data. In its simplest form, a strategic plan is a statement of strategies or actions that will move an organization from one position to another over a defined period of time (Cleverly, 1989).

Despite a lack of consistent agreement about how many years a strategic plan looks at, there is some consensus that a strategic plan is a statement of organization intent 3 to 5 years hence (Strasen, 1987) or longer. Although the strategic planning process varies, most share these common components: a mission statement including values, philosophy, and vision, a situational assessment or audit that is data analysis based, a set of goals, key strategic issues that frequently are defined using a SWOT (strengths, weaknesses, opportunities, and threats) analysis, strategies that respond to key issues, and tactics that are action items to execute the strategy (Beckham, 1991).

THE LANGUAGE OF STRATEGIC PLANNING

There is a certain jargon that seems universally accepted when speaking the strategic planning tongue. Despite this acceptance, people interpret the words with some variation. This is an attempt to define common terms that are inevitably mentioned in all strategic planning processes. The reader is cautioned that people in the business use the language in different ways.

Goals: Broad statements that the organization plans to achieve; e.g., consistent with the organization's goal to "promote research," the nursing organization goal may be, "to create a nursing culture supportive of the conduct and application of nursing research."

Mission: Written expressive statements that embody the organization's values. Mission statements include goals and objectives as well as a statement of philosophy.

Objectives: Goals that have been turned into statements of measurable achievement. Objectives typically include the intent, action statements, and quantifiable measures of outcomes. They may include designation of the responsible person(s). Consistent with the nursing goal stated under **Goals,** the objectives may be

1. That within 3 years, there will be a full-time nurse researcher employed, that nursing research grand rounds will be held monthly, and that there will be a research requirement incorporated into the staff nurse promotional ladder.
2. That within 5 years, the nursing organization will have received funding for a major nursing-initiated research project, and the nursing organization will host/sponsor a regional research symposium.

These examples are illustrative of goal and objective statements that might constitute a piece of a nursing organization's strategic plan. These examples may sound like approaches used in operational planning but differ in their intent to move the organization of the future toward a point consistent with the organization's vision.

Strategies: A pattern of purposes, policies, programs, actions, decisions, or resource allocations that defines what an organization is, what it does, and why it does it (Bryson, 1990). Strategies may vary in the way they look or are written based on a variety of considerations, but they generally reflect the way in which an organization relates to its environment.

Values: Statements of what the organization stands for that are shared by all of the organization's stakeholders. Values are principles or standards that reflect what the organization cares about.

Vision: Refers to the ability to set goals about what the organization wants to achieve based on its values and where it wants to go without the encumbrance of what seems at present either inevitable or not possible. It is simply the unleashing of innate ability to create and think anew without the burden of what appears to be current limitations. If one is bound by existing resources, there is no vision. Regardless of who the author is, the vision of what the organization should look like if the strategic plan is implemented is widely held to be at the heart of the strategic planning process. According to Bryson (1990), the vision statement should include the organization's mission, basic philosophy and core values, basic strategies, performance criteria, important decision rules, and ethical standards expected of all employees—and he adds, it should "be short and inspirational."

This list is not intended to be exhaustive. Depending on the type of strategic planning activity, there are other buzz words that the nurse executive or manager may need to become familiar with. If it is a business plan, terms such as market share or referral patterns may be bantered about. In planning facilities, the language is quite different. What is important is that we are as prepared as possible to be able to speak the correct language.

WHO DOES STRATEGIC PLANNING?

Bryson (1990) based his text on the premise that the strategic plan itself is not as important as thinking and acting strategically. Therefore, it could be argued that the reason for strategic planning is to get every member of the organization to begin thinking and acting strategically.

There are individuals who lead the process and submit the report. Many organizations have individuals who possess excellent facilitation and coordination skills required for guiding a strategic planning effort. If an organization does not have such an internal resource, which is not at all unusual, there are many firms specializing in the development of a strategic planning process. Firms will respond to a request for proposal (RFP) for such services and will furnish the customer with a list of deliverables, products that the customer can expect to see as a result of the planning process.

Because the language of RFPs requesting bids for strategic planning effort can be soft, it is not easily quantifiable. There can be an opportunity for a difference of opinion between what the request is envisioned to be and what the consulting firm produces. Nursing is well advised to take the time initially to tighten the RFP so as to leave little debate about what is asked for vs what is received. For organizationwide strategic planning efforts, it is fairly typical to employ an outside firm.

Nursing organizations also may feel that it is appropriate to use a consulting firm for the development of a strategic plan (Anvaripour et al., 1990). This guarantees that appropriate time will be given to the project and establishes in everyone's mind the organizational priority assigned to the project. A word of caution: Outside firms facilitate, coordinate, gather data, and write the plan, but they look to the organization to do a fair amount of the research and, of course, to analyze, deliberate, and develop strategies. The process is demanding and time consuming and is guaranteed to place heightened new demands on what are already stretched resources. Commitment to a strategic planning process requires that the organization understand and support that it will be a demanding and rewarding process.

THE STRATEGIC PLANNING PROCESS

Although there are many models for strategic planning, the process always includes an in-depth analysis of the current environment, identification of the organization's strengths and weaknesses, and an assessment of organizational opportunities. Strasen (1987) sees this process of data gathering as one that supports the development of appropriate and realistic goals. From these goals flow measurable, achievable objectives or statements of strategies or action plans. I emphasize Strasen's use of the words "appropriate and realistic" because of the concerns raised in the literature that strategic planning does not work (Beckham, 1991) and that the new wave of planning focuses on strategy implementation (Hrebiniak & Joyce, 1984). One suspects that the concerns focus on the development of strategic plans that are perhaps not clear in their intent or scope or, more likely, strategic plans that are not pragmatic or realistic in terms of strategies defined.

Just as there is no one strategic planning model, there is no one process for how to go about planning strategically. In referring to strategic planning as a "plan to plan," Strasen (1987) identifies four approaches to the strategic planning process.

1. The top–down method, in which the plan is developed by administrative staff and shared.
2. The bottom–up method, where managers develop goals and objectives from which administrators develop strategies.
3. A combination of top–down and bottom–up methods, in which the prior two methods are combined in a two-way communication process.
4. The team planning method, which establishes team or task forces from appropriate levels, including staff, to develop a strategic plan.

A Model for the Strategic Planning Process

The steps shown in Table 39–1 suggest one format for the strategic planning process consistent with the team planning method, which I believe to be a preferred model, especially in the development of a strategic planning process for a nursing organization. The process presented has broad applicability for corporate, individual, institutional, and divisional strategic planning. It is adapted from a model used for corporate strategic planning, and the nurse executive or manager may find the steps helpful. However, not all the steps may be appropriate to the development of their strategic plan.

The degree to which the nurse manager participates in the process will be determined organizationally depending on the scope of the project and how the role of the nurse manager is viewed within the organization. There are no absolutes about who does which action items. At a minimum, nurse managers can be involved in many activities of the audit phase, e.g., conducting surveys and completing inventories of existing resources. Similarly, when developing a strategic plan for a nursing organization, nurse manager participation is critical

TABLE 39–1   Suggested Format for the Strategic Planning Process

PHASE I: THE SITUATIONAL AUDIT
Purpose
- To establish organizational priorities
- Understand/develop
    Clinical strengths
    Facility utilization/capabilities
    Financial capabilities: past, present, future
    Market dynamics
    Other appropriate performance parameters
- Inventory of existing resources, e.g. human, clinical, capital, facilities

Data collection
- Leadership interviews with representatives of appropriate groups
- Market research
- Utilization trends
- History and forecast of baseline financial performance/capability
- Inventory of resources as appropriate to the strategic planning effort

STEPS	PURPOSE	ACTION ITEMS
1. Organize strategic planning committee	To establish working group to review options and recommendations	Appoint committee members Provide orientation to process
2. Conduct leadership interviews	Establish an understanding of priorities of different constituencies	Conduct interviews with representatives of all constituencies
3. Conduct appropriate surveys	Establish market patterns Gain insight into needs and problems	Establish necessary survey tools Conduct surveys Tabulate and analyze results
4. Document existing resources	Establish current resource availability Understand the current adequacy and suitability of existing resources	Complete inventory of existing resources to be developed from personal interviews, existing capital lists, space documents, personnel records, etc.
5. Assess current market position	Understand existing strengths Establish the direction of baseline momentum Assess current competitive environment	Establish market share trends Complete analysis of organizational strengths, weaknesses, opportunities, and threats
6. Develop baseline scenarios	Establish the impact of current market changes Understand the implications of such changes	Forecast market potential Forecast organizational financial performance Establish capital capacity of organization

Table continued on following page.

TABLE 39–1 Suggested Format for the Strategic Planning Process *Continued*

PHASE II: IDENTIFICATION OF MIDTERM REQUIREMENTS FOR LONG-TERM ACHIEVEMENT OF ORGANIZATIONAL VISION

Purpose
- To develop common understanding of the organization's pressures and opportunities
- To examine the common vision for direction in specifying strategic choices
- To examine/develop market share and position requirements necessary to support core operations
- To examine organizational prerequisites for system growth and development

Aspects of planning to be accomplished
- Formalization of the organizational vision
- Identification of key system components of the vision
- Identification of key internal and external prerequisites to achieving the visions

STEPS	PURPOSE	ACTION ITEMS
7. Develop market and financial requirements to support core operations	Establish the market share changes necessary to support the strategies Examine all sources of funds available	Examine market share growth to support current activities Determine broad changes in cost position required by market changes
8. Identify key system components of vision	Gain political backing for subsequent strategic choices Focus on high-priority opportunities and competitive threats	Rank system components in order of strategic importance Identification of resources that meet the strategic vision
9. Identify key internal and external prerequisites to achieving vision	To provide an easily understood direction of coordinated development Establish groundwork necessitated by future organizational role	Begin process of defining what will be required to achieve strategic objectives

PHASE III: STRATEGY DEVELOPMENT

Purpose
- To identify key vision implications
- To assure that strategies are financially sound
- To develop action plans to guide implementation

Milestones
- Identification of potential opportunities and appropriate organizational roles
- Identification of programs to support key initiatives
- Develop cost estimates
- Forecast resource requirements
- Action plans for achievement of vision
- Fully written strategic plan ready for execution

STEPS	PURPOSE	ACTION ITEMS
10. Statement of goals, objectives, and strategies	To give form and substance to plan To define strategies that fulfill the vision requirement	Planning committee(s) develop goals, objectives, and strategies
11. Conduct analysis of activities and cost of services being considered	Preliminarily identify appropriate strategies for concentration and investment Determine key factors for success Identify broad areas for cost reduction to meet cost profile	Evaluate future market potential Evaluate competitive state for potential investment Compare costs to other providers
12. Select programs/ products for investment of resources	Focus organizational attention on a limited set of initiatives that form the base of strategy development	Define broad interdisciplinary investment criteria that support achievement of the vision Evaluate potential initiatives against investment criteria to assess relative contribution to the overall vision Select programs/products for investments
13. Develop resource requirements	Calculate additional resources to serve new or expanded services Determine costs of resource requirements	Prepare program of services Prepare cost estimates of resources required
14. Aggregate capital requirements and revise financial forecast	To assure that the strategies are both affordable and represent net gain to the organization	Convert requirements into financial impact analyses Evaluate the inherent affordability of the strategies and adjust as necessary Forecast organization's financial performance under implemented strategies
15. Develop action plan	To assure understanding of the factors critical to success To create accountability for implementation of defined worksteps	Define worksteps for each key recommendation Determine critical path where necessary to ensure success Assign individual responsibility to performance objectives Develop a periodic monitoring mechanism

Table continued on following page.

TABLE 39–1 Suggested Format for the Strategic Planning Process *Continued*

STEPS	PURPOSE	ACTION ITEMS
16. Approval of strategic plan	To ensure that all stakeholders are informed and in support of the plan	Plan approved by necessary individuals, group, or board as appropriate

PHASE IV: EVALUATION
Purpose
- To make sure the plan is being implemented
- To provide timely intervention or changes as appropriate
- To ensure that the plan is achieving its stated purpose in achieving the vision

Evaluation as a stage in any process
- Is an expected and very important aspect of all processes
- Provides periodic data on which to assess gains/problems associated with plan implementation
- Provides individuals who are accountable for specific pieces of the plan with performance feedback
- Generates information necessary for periodic reporting to all stakeholders

STEPS	PURPOSE	ACTION ITEMS
17. Periodic monitoring	To keep the project on schedule	Measure strategies against predetermined monitors
	To maintain commitment of individual responsible	Assess implementation of strategies along timeline
18. Annual review	To assess progress	The plan is reviewed and revised annually
	To consider new regulations, market issue, etc. that may affect strategy implementation	
	To determine if assumptions that the plan was built on were accurate	
19. Rewrite strategic plan	To thoroughly evaluate prior plan	Rewritten plan every 3–5 years
	To guarantee plan is consistent with evolving organizational vision and with other intervening forces	

in defining the vision and objectives in Phase II, in developing the strategic objectives in Phase III, and in conducting the evaluation of the strategies in Phase IV (Table 39–1).

At the other extreme are those actions that may be the sole prerogative of the nurse executive who is responsible for the development and operationalization of the entire plan. An example of such an action item might be seeking plan approval from necessary individuals, including the board of trustees, in Phase III.

The nurse executives and managers can be participants in strategic planning processes at two levels. Strategic planning at the institutional level may require a level of participation that is different from that required to develop and implement a strategic planning process for the nursing organization. For that reason, the process presented has broad applicability and is intended to be able to be customized based on the scope of the strategic planning effort. For more information and an excellent description of the typical database developed as well as specific considerations when completing an analysis of organization resources, the reader is referred to Strasen (1987, Chapter 6).

THE STRATEGIC PLAN

The strategic plan itself may vary widely in format and content. It is important to have the results of the strategic planning process documented as a means of establishing consensus among stakeholders about what is being planned for and how the organization intends to move toward the vision. It further serves to remind us of the things to be done and to reinforce the schedule or action plan. The written plan is, in fact, the baseline for judging strategic performance. Just as with the strategic planning process, there is no best format for the written plan. The outline shown in Table 39–2 is a suggested format following a business approach, which you may choose to use as a springboard for the development of a written strategic plan.

This format integrates what may have been months of planning into a single, comprehensive statement of the data gathered and strategies defined. The written plan attempts to summarize relevant information from meetings, data from research, and decisions after careful analysis, as well as to record supporting documentation when indicated. A written strategic plan can be a very extensive effort. For this reason, it is sound advice to have a designated project coordinator or team to be responsible for coordination of the planning effort. Even though the process tends to run a normal course as outlined in Table 39–2, there can be many activities going on simultaneously. There may be different groups, or think tanks, working on different aspects of the plan and not necessarily completely aware of each other's activities. Data to support one avenue of investigation may have to be gathered from several sources. The point is that strategic planning is a large undertaking. Detailed minutes of meetings are essential but not enough. To make all of the information and discussion gel into a single document, an individual or team must be responsible.

TABLE 39–2 Elements of the Written Strategic Plan

I. Executive summary
II. Introduction and background
   A. Impetus for strategic plan
   B. History and mission of organization
III. Description of strategic plan
   A. Description of strategic planning vision
      1. Scope of services planned
      2. Goals and objectives
      3. Performance indicators
   B. Description of fit with organizational goals
   C. Contingency considerations if circumstances change
IV. External assessment
   A. Market research
      1. Competition
      2. Demographics/market size
      3. Location/access
      4. Service area
      5. Referral patterns
      6. Target population/at-risk groups
      7. Demand for services, opportunities
      8. Critical success factors, threats
   B. Regulatory analysis
   C. Reimbursement analysis
V. Internal assessment
   A. Strengths and weaknesses
      1. Program development
      2. Financial performance
         a. Profit/loss
         b. Market share
         c. Cash flow
         d. Long-term debt
      3. Customer satisfaction—patients, doctors, staff, community, others
      4. Organizational capacity and technology
      5. Managerial performance
      6. Productivity indices
      7. Opportunities
   B. Threats
      1. Shifting values
      2. Labor relations
      3. Political, legal, social factors
      4. Economic concerns
      5. Regulatory concerns

TABLE 39–2 Elements of the Written Strategic Plan *Continued*

VI. Structure and management
    A. Legal structure
    B. Position within sponsoring organizations
    C. Management structure
VII. Program requirements
    A. Staffing
        1. Number and type
        2. Compensation and benefits
        3. Scheduling
    B. Hours of operation
    C. Charge structure
    D. Equipment/supplies
    E. Facilities
    F. Clinical protocols
    G. Management policies
VIII. Marketing plan
    A. Demand/volume targets
    B. Referral sources
    C. Target geographic and population markets
    D. Promotion
    E. Critical success factors
IX. Financial plan
    A. Capitalization plan
    B. Five-year forecasted financial statements
        1. Balance sheets
        2. Income statements
        3. Statements of cash flow
        4. Statements of changes in new equity
        5. Statements of returns to limited and general partners
    C. Financial assumptions
X. Implementation plan
    A. Critical tasks
    B. Timeline
    C. Responsibilities
    D. Evaluation

References

Anvaripour, P., Bezold, C., & Weissman, G. (1990, April). A nursing department can and should plan for the future. *Nursing and Health Care, 11*(4), 207–209.

Beckham, J.D. (1991, November–December). Strategic thinking and the road to relevance. *Healthcare Forum Journal, 36*(6), 36.

Bryson, J.M. (1990). *Strategic planning for public and nonprofit organizations*. San Francisco: Jossey-Bass Publishers.

Cleverly, W.O. (1989, January). Three ways to measure a strategic plan's viability. *Healthcare Financial Management*, p. 31.

Dixit, A., & Nalebuff, B. (1991). *Thinking stra-*

tegically: The competitive edge in business, politics, and everyday life. New York: W.W. Norton and Company.

Hrebiniak, L.G., & Joyce, W.F. (1984). *Implementing strategy*. New York: Macmillan.

Jones, K.R. (1988). Strategic planning in hospitals: Applications to nursing administration. *Nursing Administration Quarterly, 13*(1), 1–10.

Norby, R.B. (1990, September). Positioning for success. *Nursing Clinics of North America, 25*(3), 525–535.

Strasen, L. (1987). *Key business skills for nurse managers*. Philadelphia: J.B. Lippincott Company.

Toward the year 2000: Is nursing ready? (1991, fall). *Nursing Administration Quarterly, 16*(1).

CHAPTER 40 • • • • • •

ENTREPRENEURIALISM IN A TIME OF GREAT CHANGE

TIM PORTER-O'GRADY

EXECUTIVE SUMMARY

The manager as entrepreneur is a different person in the world of work today and for the future. Many new characteristics of the role emerge that do not reflect previous expectations. In many ways, the new role is a stretch from the older, more structured role and may require the expression of greater skill and ability. Whatever the demand, the mix of skills for this management role will be forever different from the management roles of the past.

In many ways, skill and content in the manager were developed more frequently after the person achieved the role than was expected to be present before moving into the role. Frequently, learning the role was an on-the-job experience. Increasingly, the successful manager will have had some formal preparation underpinning her or his exercise of the role. With some expectation for prior role knowledge, much more flexibility and independence can be incorporated into defining the characteristics and expectations for the role of manager. These expectations can include the presumption of much more independence, individuality and decentralization in the operation of service units. This expectation should lead to more opportunities for creativity and innovation in the manager's role and operation of the service unit.

In addition, there can be more validity to a growing interdependence and independence in decision making, solution seeking, opportunity finding, and structuring and marketing the services of the local service unit. Opportunities for forming workplace coalitions, partnerships, joint efforts, and other work redesign efforts are generally constrained by centralized and homogenized bureaucratic organizational systems. These newer behaviors in many ways become the expectation of the service entity and its leadership, demanding structural changes.

Newer service configurations and role expectations call for a transformed view of the role of the service leader of the future. Where innovation and entrepreneurial behavior in the institutional models of management limited the acceptability of managerial independence and creativity in the past, those same behaviors are quickly becoming the rule for management. Developing both the entrepreneurial consciousness and concomitant skills in the manager is a critical task of the time (Ohmae, 1990).

To be successful in a different playing field on the global stage of service and competition, the American workplace must become more efficient and more creative. This calls for both a milieu and a leader who can reflect an altered set of variables and behaviors necessary to that success. Health care is not exempt from this reality. Since it is the single most expensive public service

683

and is rife with the characteristics of increasing demand and decreasing dollars, new ways of doing the work of health care are no longer optional. The entrepreneurial spirit and associated behaviors must be present in every role for the social mandate for work and measurable outcomes to be realistically realized. Our society and way of life, regardless of the arena, will be dramatically affected by the commitment to higher levels of accomplishment through entrepreneurial energy and the requisite skills. As Deming (1990) has suggested, the survival of our society from the perspective of those looking at us from the outside is purely optional. For those of us as leaders within our culture, there simply is no option.

All aspects of the world are changing at an unparalleled rate. Nations, governments, people appear to be transformed before our eyes (Attali, 1991). One does not know from day to day what the political or social configuration of the global community will be. Whether people are ready for these dramatic changes or not does not seem to matter. Change just keeps on unfolding.

Many are suggesting that these changes will keep accelerating in both number and speed of onset (Drucker, 1989) and that this process will continue to accelerate at least for the next two decades (Halberstam, 1991). Facilitating the change is major social and economic transformation driven by political and social reconfiguration, moving us toward newer economic and political structures. Expanding new economic frameworks and forms will continue to challenge current thinking about relationships at both the global and local levels (Kuttner, 1991).

The world is becoming increasingly competitive, not because competition is becoming increasingly intense but more because there are other successful competitors in the global marketplace. These new competitors are as skilled as anyone in their knowledge of the marketplace and how to address its needs (Choate, 1990). Japan and the Asian basin countries and Germany and the European Community have gained equity with America in their skill and ability to compete in the global marketplace. This reality is challenging to the United States, once the singular master of free enterprise and capitalism. Others have learned the rules of the game and have mastered their application and now give the United States strong competition in global markets. Instead of the single greatest force in the marketplace, the United States is now one of many countries competing at a level never experienced before.

Others' products and services have, in many ways, eclipsed the American workplace in both kind and quality. The trade and budget deficit of the United States indicates the price Americans have paid for this imbalance (Gibbs, 1990). At first, the reaction to these emerging realities was anger at this change in circumstances. Over time, however, more creative approaches have emerged to direct the American workplace toward higher levels of productivity, quality, and commitment to improvement. Experiments in new models of work, newer relationships in the marketplace, a sensitivity to customer wants, and a commitment to quality improvement have emerged as the keynotes in an effort to become more competitive (Gabor, 1990).

The health care system also is waving the banner of change and moving to more efficient and cost-effective ways of delivering services. Driven by an almost continuously accelerating cost of providing health care services, running at a rate 10% higher than the gross national product without a concomitant improvement in the nation's health, the system is scrambling to retool itself (Berwick, Blanton, & Roessner, 1990). Newer ways of providing and configuring services, the introduction of continuous quality improvement processes, and empowerment models that involve staff in decision making are but a few of the signs of these changes (Porter-O'Grady, 1990).

Creativity and innovation are the central components of any strategy to reformat service structures and to effect meaningful change. The problem currently is that the source of creativity in a transforming marketplace is no longer associated with the management role (Bennis, 1990). Once the central element of the organization's push for success, the manager is no longer the source of effective change nor the repository of the creativity transforming times demand.

There are essentially two reasons for this shift away from the manager. First, the manager can no longer know all the components of the work and the relationships necessary to sustain it. Work has become so complex and interdependent that no one person can cope with the intensity of information and connections necessary to get the job done. The complex of activities necessary to accomplish the work goes beyond the manager's ability to understand all that is necessary to facilitate the work (Atchison, 1990). Second, the worker is a different person than she or he used to be. In many ways, the worker has grown up and become much stronger in self-image and in the impact of her or his role in the workplace (Burda, 1990) (Table 40–1).

Historically, most work was production oriented, and almost all the learning

TABLE 40–1 Comparison of the Industrial Manager and the Entrepreneurial Manager

INDUSTRIAL MANAGER	ENTREPRENEURIAL MANAGER
Limits risk	Embraces risk
Preserves the business	Stretches opportunity
Manages workers	Invests the worker
Gives direction	Facilitates others
Subordinating role	Interacting
Paid hourly/salary	Shares revenues/bonus
Dependent hierarchy	Interdependent partner
Transactional leadership	Transformational leadership
Manages budget	Coordinates finances
Operational focus	Strategic focus
Short-term orientation	Long-term perspective

related to the job was done at the work site. This on-the-job training created a dependency relationship between the worker and the workplace. Much of who the worker was and her ability to advance was determined by how much she learned on the job site and how well she facilitated the values of the workplace leadership (Ashley, 1976).

As work has become increasingly specialized and technically specific, skills gained before taking a job are increasingly necessary. The technical worker, highly talented with a specific set of skills and cognizant of her value and contribution to the success of the work, has begun to emerge in the workplace. The technical worker emerges in the recognition of a need for a broad category of worker essential to the success of a highly technical culture. As America becomes more dependent on high-tech processes, this worker, frequently prepared at the college level, will be essential to positive work outcomes. Although nurses have always been prepared in a program of learning in advance of their employment, they are now joined by increasing numbers of work roles requiring advanced preparation for their viability in the high-tech workplace. Because this learning is obtained by the worker outside of employment, this worker recognizes that she does not owe the workplace for what she knows. Further, the worker knows that she is in demand and recognizes that there are many opportunities available and that she may work in several settings in a career and is, therefore, not tied to a lifelong job or a long-term commitment in any one place (Dumaine, 1990).

What is happening in many ways is challenging the worker to become an entrepreneur of her own life and skills. Instead of seeing herself as a subset of the work, she sees that the work can be applied in a number of ways and places and that she is no longer defined by where she works. She becomes more identified by what she does and who she is. The worker has a higher sense of her own value and sees the work relationships from the perspective of her own contribution, empowering her in ways that neither she nor the workplace anticipated.

THE ENTREPRENEURIAL CONDITION

Change is driving every workplace in America to confront its viability, structure, and relationships. Viability is an expression of its relevance and ability to do what is necessary to survive and thrive (Peters, 1987). Structure relates to the organization's ability to configure itself in ways that maximize its effectiveness and its ability to do what is necessary to accomplish its objectives. Relationships are the essential consideration that creates the value and culture of the organization directed to producing what is necessary to its success (Johnsson, 1991).

The entrepreneurial organization is the one that has harnessed these characteristics successfully and has created a milieu as well as a niche that anticipates and facilitates its success. At one time, the term "entrepreneur" related to an individual who had a set of characteristics that assured individual success. If others were involved in this process, they were by definition merely a subset of the individual's effort or success (Herron & Herron, 1991). They were persons who were helpful to the entrepreneur's journey to success and, in many ways, both positive and negative, necessary to the route to individual accomplishment. The unilateral entrepreneur has been the epitome of the American hero. While the adulation of this type of person approached the mythical, the world changed, and this kind of unilateral, visionary, and heroic behavior became untenable, even threatening to the organization. Organizational characteristics that support a new type of entrepreneur are

- Future orientation
- Opportunistic
- Highly decentralized
- Service and quality driven
- Open
- Low structure
- Limited hierarchy

The complexities of work and the workplace demand that a number of players be on board and invested for outcomes to be obtained and success to be enhanced. The role of no one person can assure the success of the enterprise. The meaning of entrepreneur takes on a different character and a broader definition. It is no longer a singular definition. An entrepreneurial organization or group becomes one where the players are mutually invested in an effort to which they are committed, which is in the best interests of the group and operates to their mutual benefit, producing an outcome of value (Herrick, 1990).

The following are specific characteristics of organizations that provide an entrepreneurial context.

- They are open to change and embrace the opportunity to look at the way work is done in a number of different ways.
- They have a focus on the needs of those to whom service is provided and view their own work within the context of how it affects those people.
- They are not burdened by past practices and do not allow current barriers to serve as permanent obstacles to doing what is necessary to provide their service or sell their product.
- They have a strong ability to network with others to facilitate their success or join in partnership to achieve newer objectives in their mutual best interests.
- They are evaluating their product or service continuously to determine whether it is effective and continues to accomplish the goals for which it was originated.
- They are forward thinking and always planning for the long-term successes of their enterpise, representing a creative process that moves them continuously to new experiences and markets for what they do.
- They are able to handle failure and difficult times, accepting the challenges

along the way and changing their strategy when the evidence points them in a new direction.

Entrepreneurial persons have a strength of character that allows them to confront difficult or challenging circumstances in a way that stretches their skills and abilities to their full limit. They often do not see challenges to their efforts as obstacles along the way. Nonetheless, they serve to challenge the entrepreneur to stretch beyond the limits of the present. These people find that opportunity and excitement accompany what they do as they create. Much of their unconscious drive comes from a need to accomplish, to risk, and to stretch beyond their own performance limits. The positive side of these attributes are a high level of energy and productivity, with sound outcomes and successful change. The down side of this behavior pattern is a strong ego, overwhelming sense of self, and a feeling of unilateral ownership of the products of their work (Kaiser, 1988). The real challenge for the entrepreneurial personality is to keep personal effort and accomplishment in balance with professional and personal relationships and carefully attend to the impact of individual behavior on others.

The twenty-first century entrepreneur will have a different set of behavior characteristics than did the successful entrepreneur in the twentieth century industrial workplace. The traditional view of the entrepreneur is the image of the unilateral man (usually always men) in a strong hero role, visioning the right path to travel, idea to build on, or direction to set. This person invited others to share in his vision, to follow his lead, and to move in the direction that he stated so clearly and with such charisma and inspiration. He was often identified as the visionary hero (Kets de Vries & Miller, 1984).

The entrepreneurial leader of the future is a much different person from that in the past. The visionary hero person is not the model of leadership for the twenty-first century. The worker is more mature and better educated. Naive and childlike expectations have dissipated considerably. Opportunity and resources are simply not unlimited as once commonly perceived. Resources are scarce and prudent decision making is required for success. The worker has rights and knows what they are. In addition, women now comprise a growing segment of the American workplace, changing the dynamics of the work relationships (Gibbs et al., 1990).

The increasing knowledge and maturity of workers places them in a different context for relationship building and for motivation in the workplace. To successfully accomplish outcomes, first-line workers require investment, information, trust, and commitment. This requires the leader to disclose, include, share, and provide a context that motivates the worker to buy into the goals or plans of the organization. As Toffler (1990) points out, the success of any enterprise depends more on the investment of the worker into the process than on any other single factor. In the twenty-first century, entrepreneurs cannot do it alone, nor can they be visionary heros who expect everyone to follow in their footsteps to a desired outcome that only they can understand or buy into.

The entrepreneurial personality of the twenty-first century will undergo a

significant role and behavioral shift. Some of the characteristics that will ex-
emplify that person will be

- The ability to generate group processes that create a common sense of
  purpose and direction, accessing common goals rather than projecting individual agendas.
- Skills in creating consensus in diversity, assisting the work group to find a
  sense of purpose, direction, and work agenda.
- Talent in working with a host of disparate groups and persons, helping them
  move along a continuum that reflects a common base of understanding about
  the purpose and direction of the work without limiting individual creativity
  in contributing to the outcomes of the work.
- A flexibility in work design and structure, adjusting process and configuration of work roles as goal characteristics shift and as new realities related
  to goal achievement cause modifications in approach or even outcomes.
- The capacity to divest ownership of ideas or creative processes as others
  begin to exert more creative or process ownership of programs, projects,
  ventures—reflecting the reality that anything can be accomplished if one
  is not concerned about who gets credit for the work.
- Competence in orchestrating the creative continuum rather than directing
  it, ever alert to changes in the circumstances or context of the work effort
  and sharing those with the team, giving them the major role in resolving
  the difficulties that constraint may produce.

The entrepreneur of the future is not a maverick personality. Instead, this
person is able to challenge and guide the work team into efforts that all the
participants buy into and keep the effort on course through its completion or its
transformation. The entrepreneur is more a coordinator, facilitator, and integrator
of the creative and opportunistic processes. This person is able to challenge the
work team and colleagues to construct a mutual vision and then put together the
components and mechanisms that can assure goal attainment.

CREATING THE ENTREPRENEURIAL TEAM

In the future, most work will require the skills of a complex, multidisciplinary,
work-focused team (Atchison, 1990). Especially in health care, integration of
the patient care team will become more common as health care moves into more
cost-effective and service-effective models of care delivery. The configurations
and structures of the past are not adequate for the kinds of expectations and
service requirements emerging today and in the near future.

Cost factors have forced the providers of health care services to address the
way in which service structures facilitate or impede the work of patient care.
The physical structure and organization of health care work often has aggravated
the movement of the patient toward wellness. Service structures designed to fit
the needs of the service provider rather than the service receiver have challenged
health care leadership to rethink the patient care structure and to redesign both

structure and relationship to make the system more cost and service effective (Atkinson, 1990).

With the team approach, no issue is exempt from consideration by the team. Issues related to fiscal as well as service realities become the consideration of the whole team. The financial concerns may be strongly integrated into the activities of the team from both a planning and an operational perspective. The manager in this scenario becomes resource purveyor by ensuring that the appropriate information regarding constraints and possibilities is available to the team. The data collection process and its integration with the enterprise's financial and service goals become central to the manager's functions. Communicating the data in a way that facilitates the team's understanding and use of it is critical to the team's success. The manager assists the team to incorporate the data realities into setting work goals, operational activities, and evaluation of work outcomes. In addition, the manager assists in long-range strategy by assessing the organizational constraints, resources, and plans to assist the work team in its own long-range activities. The key role of the manager in this set of circumstances is support. She never takes ownership of the processes associated with the work team's efforts and obligations away from them.

Practically, the manager undertakes the following activities in team and transformed work models.

- Determine the organizations goals and objectives as they affect the work team and share them with the team members.
- Clearly assess the developmental and skill needs of the work team and arrange to address deficits.
- Assure that the team is hooked to the data-gathering and generation processes that affect or evaluate the work they are doing.
- Monitor with the team progress against the objectives of the work and the variables affecting the goals.
- Help the team adjust work activities to reflect the change in variables affecting work outcomes.
- Manage the resource allocation and use issues to determine if appropriate resources are being used by the team and inform them of the use status for their evaluation and response.
- Work with other services, departments, and roles to address integration and facilitation problems. Get the players together with the team when newer approaches or strategies must be identified.
- Act as facilitator in the team and between members when work or relational issues create barriers to the effectiveness of the team.
- Assist the team with the quality improvement process, keeping focused on the measures of quality and the relationship between outcomes and the work necessary to achieve them.

There are many tasks that relate to the day-to-day service support for the work team that is part of the manager's role in an entrepreneurial context. They provide a context and make the workplace safe and encouraging to the team members in their work. In this environment, it is the role of the manager (leader) to assure that accountability and ownership never move away from the staff and that the team has in place all they need to do their work. The servant model and role becomes the content for defining the manager's role in this new model of work and creates the framework for all work activities.

The twenty-first century entrepreneur will have a different modus operandi in these newer models of workplace design and work configuration. The innovative leader must be able to integrate a diverse spectrum of people and resources in a collective effort to achieve any desired outcome. Whether it be service enhancement, market expansion, or new service arrangements, the leader will need to invest a broad array of people in the process of change or adaptation or suffer the loss of opportunity or outcome (Block, 1991).

Creative strategies for investment of the entrepreneurial team will have to include the following elements.

- An understanding of the need for a quid pro quo arrangement with the players, reflecting a commitment to involve the team not only in the work of the enterprise but also in its rewards.
- Recognizing the different skills and models of work that new workers will represent and maximizing their contribution within the context of their value system, no matter how dissimilar it may be from the norm (e.g., variable work hours, working at home, forming subgroup workers, contracting for outcomes or products, other unusual work structures).
- More focused, short-turnaround planning and programs that will reflect a compact timeline and an intensive work relationship that is focused, specific, and short term. Although these may be unique programs or structures, they will fit into the overall mission and service strategy of the organization.
- Recognize that the entrepreneurial team will be project or program specific and may change depending on the program being developed and the skills needed. The leader may find that there is no consistent staff pool for entrepreneurial ventures and that these teams may be uniquely constructed (ad hoc) to specifically address individual programs or opportunities, after which they may have no further purpose.
- Acknowledge that an entrepreneurial planning team may work appropriately and successfully for the initial phases of new ventures or opportunities, but members may not be appropriate personality types to successfully operate and function within these new work structures. Those who create change often are unable to manage it. The skills of construction do not successfully translate into the talents of operating or managing the enterprise. The entrepreneurial leader will have to reflect this reality in her or his innovation or program planning.
- For the foreseeable future, all innovations or projects will have to carefully articulate service, cost, and quality into their design and function. Consumer-focused valuing will reflect a more careful consideration of the balance among what is needed, what is desired, how much it costs, and whether

the anticipated outcomes can be or have been achieved. In constrained economic or resource environments, the balance among these three variables becomes critical to the program's competitiveness and long-term viability.

The entrepeneur must always be sensitive to new and different ways in which opportunity can be accessed and new work arrangements can be constructed. No longer is the leader limited in the structures that can be developed for meeting opportunity and building viable service arrangements (Bolman & Terrance, 1991). In the twenty-first century organization, more consolidated and cooperative ventures will emerge between service entities that historically had been in competition with each other. Reduced payment, fixed service markets or populations, limited unilateral capitalization, inaccessible service partners (e.g., physician groups committed to other organizations, other institution's health service ventures, business joint ventures) all make it difficult to access acknowledged opportunity because it lies in someone else's camp (Brown & McCool, 1990).

Through emerging collaborative ventures, the entrepreneur can create innovative arrangements with other health providers either to extend their service functions, compliment them, or work with them to access entirely new opportunities that neither party could address on its own. The entrepreneurial spirit, ever aware of opportunity and alert to where it can be found, can see past the constraints in the current arena and imagine ways of connecting and constructing viable and profitable relationships wherever they can be developed.

There is always a discussion in the development of work teams about the role of the manager—indeed, whether there is the need for this role. Although the character of the role of manager is dynamic and ever changing, it is important that both the definers for the role remain a part of a successful workplace. There clearly is no need for the manager as currently configured in the workplace. The parental model of management is simply not appropriate. The coordinating, integrating, and facilitating role of the new manager (leader) will be essential in any design of the workplace. How it is played and how it links the various components of the organization depends entirely on the purposes, role, and work of the enterprise. Uniform, universal, sameness-oriented organizational approaches to work roles are not viable in team-based organizations. The manager becomes a resource purveyor. The servant role to the provider will be the key component of the manager–leader role of the future. Perhaps, even the title of manager will emerge into a better delineation in the future. An equitable, partner-based presentment is more appropriate to team-based approaches than the hierarchical, parental, caretaker role of the quickly passing Industrial Age. Although the manager role will remain essential, it will be constituted differently, with significantly different content. The entrepreneurial definition of manager in this chapter is one such major application of the role.

WHERE THE ENTREPRENEUR CAN BE FOUND OR DEVELOPED

Whether one is an entrepreneur or not has nothing to do with where one works or what work is done. Rather, it is an attitude, a way of being, that is indicative of the entrepreneurial consciousness (Dunham & Klafehn, 1990). It is a way of approaching the work and a manner of seeing in relationship to that work that envisions different or new possibilities that extend the boundaries of current configurations. From staff nurse to executive, the characteristics and behaviors of the entrepreneurial personality are essentially the same. The validation and support of entrepreneurial activity, however, often depends on how permissible it is to express the behavior.

The administrative leader sets the tone for entrepreneurialism in the organization. This person, through her style of management or the corporate culture she creates, can either facilitate or constrain the emergence of entrepreneurial activity. This matter of style in the role of the leader is vital to the success of innovation and creativity. Without the context for innovation, there is no willingness on the part of the participants to risk extending themselves in a challenging manner. The milieu must be safe for the risk taker, and the individual must know that stretching oneself is not only acceptable but also expected (Mick et al., 1990).

Creating the environment for interdependent and entrepreneurial activity is a challenge. When the leader recognizes that all the people in the system must have an entrepreneurial consciousness, the challenge of creating it begins. Most of the effort will be spent in changing the behavior of the staff and increasing their sense of ownership and investment in the organization and its work. This calls for staff behavioral change, and it also ushers in major organizational redesign and structuring (Porter-O'Grady, 1988). If the staff are to become partners in the entrepreneurial activity, several factors need to be introduced into the organization.

- A knowledge on the part of the staff that they are co-investors in the work of the organization and are invited to share in defining the content and design of the work they will do.
- Consensus and team models of work design that give the team the option of structuring their own work and creating models of service that are specific to their own culture and experience and relate in a meaningful way to the persons being served.
- Staff must share in the fruits or rewards of the work done. Creating models of payment that actually reward (or constrain when appropriate) entrepreneurial activity and assure a share in the gains and losses is a stronger payment-for-work model than are current hourly and nonproductivity related wage models.
- Create a mechanism for worker participation in strategic planning and goal setting in the workplace. This generates ownership by the worker over workload and facilitates the development of channels through which outcomes are achieved and evaluated.

These foundations cannot be overemphasized. They are inherent in the content of designing any entrepreneurial work effort. Putting them together in a way that assures that they work and outcomes are produced is a much more challenging undertaking. The leader must be aware of the dynamics of integrative work teams and the elements of their structuring and operation to guide their development and use (Kilmann, 1991).

GROWING THE ENTREPRENEURIAL RELATIONSHIP

Reconfiguring and redesign is of no purpose if it does not work, regardless of the intent. Clearly establishing what is intended and expected is one of the foremost activities of entrepreneurial work. Entrepreneurial work into the twenty-first century will focus primarily on creativity and innovation (Leebov & Scott, 1990). Older models of service and care in health will give way to new designs and structures. An openness to innovation and its vagaries will be essential components of the entrepreneurial relationship. Drucker (1985) suggests that innovation lies at the heart of all entrepreneurial activity.

Sources of Innovation

There are several sources of innovation that will emerge in the entrepreneurial team both inside and outside the formal organization. Familiarity with them can assist in the development of an innovative spirit in the team and provide a route to express and put form to the innovations that will emerge. The following are examples of sources of innovative opportunities that will give direction to the entrepreneurial energy.

Unexpected Failures and Successes

Unexpected failures and successes are some of the best sources of innovation, mostly because people dismiss them quickly as serendipitous and accidental. Those things that could or should not occur are often the best sources of the study of innovation opening opportunities for change.

Incongruities and Inconsistencies

Incongruities and inconsistencies are great sources of innovative opportunities. When plans or activities do not blend as expected or outcomes do not reflect expectations, new challenges for thinking and doing emerge. Here again, the call of the circumstance is to break through the barriers of probability and think and see in new ways.

Interruptions and Breakdowns

Interruption in the way things get done and breakdown in work processes serve as a great source of innovative solutions and ideas. These times provide breathing room away from the routine and challenge the team to see work processes differently. It is especially helpful to have processes so crippled that past ways of doing the work simply are not a part of new solutions.

Radical Shifts in the Service Market or Economic Circumstances

Radical shifts in the service market or economic circumstances provide great opportunity for innovative responses. Closure of the viability or desirability of a product or service challenges the provider to the very core of the organization.

Survival is the great stimulator of innovation and creativity. There is nothing that is exempt from the capriciousness of change. Openness to newer possibilities is facilitated by the death of older ones.

Changes in Market Demographics

Changes in market demographics often can challenge the provider to look again at how and what is being done. If there is a changing demand driven by service market changes, the provider can expect that a vacuum will result, demanding some response if the provider is to survive. Following the demographics or responding to newer data will require flexibility, careful analysis, and quick response if a continuum of service and revenue is to be maintained.

Personal Attitude

The way one looks at work and the world has much to do with how one responds to what is seen. If the world is full of threat or dread as seen by the viewer, opportunity will be challenging to capture. If, on the other hand, the world is seen as a challenge and opportunity, a much more viable response to one's circumstances will emerge. Attitude has much to do with how risk is handled and how good fortune is perceived and can even set the context for opportunity finding and alternative ways of thinking and working.

New Technology and New Knowledge

Health care is rife with new technology and newer ways of doing things. New knowledge emerges instantaneously and always has a direct impact on the work and the relationships in providing health services. Responding to the demands of new information creates a milieu that is chaotic and uncertain. Routines get changed and adjusted, old certitudes get questioned, and habits are challenged, creating noise in the system that is sometimes untenable. In times of great change, knowledge comes from many disciplines. It is in integrating multiple sources of knowledge and applying them to one's own experience that a basis for creativity and change is established. Certainly, this creates no less change, but it does provide a stronger foundation for it.

Innovation for the entrepreneur is not an accidental process with no firm foundation in analysis and study. Understanding the sources of innovation and the foundation of opportunity refines the insights and judgments of the entrepreneur. Demographics, assessment, market analysis, and fiscal viability all have structured processes associated with them that provides some hard data on which to make decisions. Openness to what the data reveal and an attitude grounded in listening, watching, and seeking new information strengthen the skill base of the entrepreneur (Senge, 1990).

A sense of focus is essential to the entrepreneur. An ability to concentrate one's vision in a finite arena and to exhaust the energies and insights that relate to it is a requisite of success. The team must have a role in segmenting the view, study, research, and evaluation from their own work roles in order to assure that the full impact on the enterprise is assessed before change is made and perceived opportunity is translated into action. On determination of strategy, the role of all the players must be clear as activity that responds to the opportunity is generated and an integrated response begins to emerge. The following are entrepreneurial organizational behaviors.

- Highly participative models of work
- Limited micromanagement
- Performance-based pay system
- Few rules or policies
- The manager is coach–facilitator
- Strong lateral relationships
- Emphasis on building partnerships
- Shared decision-making structures

MARKETING THE SERVICE

In the traditional system, the approach to marketing is specialized and segmented. Marketing has become so specialized that whole departments and services have been created to address the process of selling services and products. Marketing frequently refers to the activities that alert the consumer to the service or product being sold and attempt to bridge the gap between the service provider or product producer and the service receiver or product buyer.

In health care, marketing contains all kinds of challenges and difficulties. Besides addressing many of the sensitivities associated with personal health or illness, the health service system is complex, with many elements that affect its service structure and relationship to the consumer. Some of the inherent relationships between institution and physician and other providers create special difficulties for any marketing effort.

In addition to such constraints, there is an increasing tendency in health care to heavily decentralize services into discrete and relatively independent service units (often called strategic service or business units) that are specifically directed to a narrow service arena (Kanter, 1989). Each of these units of service must respond within its own economic resources and service framework to those to whom its services are directed. Marketing becomes an activity and expectation of the service unit, and all personnel are expected to be involved in some way in the marketing effort.

Besides the more traditional concepts of marketing, the introduction of continuous quality improvement concepts into health care has influenced the whole value of marketing (Minerva-Melum, 1990). Marketing is no longer simply selling of a product or service. Instead, it is connecting the service provided to the receiver of the service in a way that represents the values and needs of those who will benefit from the service. From the design, structuring, defining, providing, and evaluating of the service, satisfaction with all of its components from the receiver's perspective has become a vital piece in marketing and providing services. Issues of quality and outcome, combined with perceptions of satisfaction of the user, become central to the provision of any service (Naisbitt & Aburdene, 1990).

Each member of the staff becomes inherently a part of any marketing effort. In a continuous program of quality service, the service provider must be perceived as central to any concept or program of quality. Each provider is the purveyor of the value system and, therefore, the vital link between the service entity and the service receiver. Invested within the relationship between individual provider and receiver is the sum of the service the institution purports to give those who seek it. If the relationship between these two persons is broken or in conflict at some level, the consumer's perception of the entire operation is threatened. Sometimes, this creates an irretrievable set of circumstances that has broader implications in the context of both liability and viability. Enough of these kinds of broken experiences and the whole enterprise is seriously compromised (Naisbitt & Aburdene, 1985).

Inculcating the values of service and sensitivity to the receiver of service into all the players in the service unit becomes essential to the success of the enterprise. No effort is nonentrepreneurial when competition for the same market is as rigorous as in health care. Each service unit is an entrepreneurial venture that must be so in tune with its market and the people it comprises that they act and think as though of one mind (Martin, 1990). Besides an entrepreneurial consciousness in all of the workers in an enterprise, awareness of the need to establish an individual connection between provider and consumer becomes an inherent expectation of all workers.

The following are conditions and requisites of all entrepreneurial efforts that reflect an appropriate marketing consciousness and milieu.

- Development of a marketing and entrepreneurial attitude on employment of all team members of a service.
- A clear understanding of the character of the service and the expectations and contributions implied in the role of team member or associate in the entrepreneurial enterprise.
- Knowledge of the core values and services of the entity invested in every worker. The worker should see his role as a part of a whole not as an individualized process unconnected to the whole.

Basic elements of marketing should be included in all worker roles during orientation and in the ongoing educational program. These programs should reflect principles of adult learning and include demonstration and role-playing techniques.

Continuous review of the purposes and activities of the service unit and understanding of the issues and problems associated with providing services should be explored on a regular and ongoing basis. Reward systems should be outcome based and reflect the organizational value that connects service provision with economic outcomes achieved. Each role should be viewed as entrepreneurial and thereby reflected in the economic and benefit returns of all team members.

Consumer assessment and evaluation of services planned and received should be ongoing and should form a central component of any quality assurance and improvement plan. Involving consumers in the process strengthens the connection between them and the service providers. When service has failed to meet with expectation, both corrective action and consumer satisfaction efforts should benefit the service receiver. This should be in a context of either financial or service benefit to the consumer.

Review of both service and financial performance should be made available to all workers (they are entrepreneurial associates) in a form that can be understood and to which they can appropriately respond. Adjustments and long-term planning activities should be presented and discussed within the same format.

Clearly, marketing involves infinitely more than simply selling and evaluating a service or a product. In a health care environment, marketing becomes a constituent of the role of all the players. Essentially, the people of the service are the service. The products of the service are those outcomes that brought the consumer to use the services of the entity. Understanding that all the players in the service are fundamental to its success and, therefore, play key roles in making it a success is the major activity of marketing.

Of course, advertising and publicly presenting the message of the service or program also are important. Making known, in an appropriate manner, what the service is and does in a consumer-pleasing way is all part of the package of marketing the entrepreneurial effort. Too often, however, the glitz and glamour of the advertising fail to match the reality of the service. There is no more disappointing experience for a consumer than to come to a service expecting what the advertising promised and to find that the promise ended with the reading of the brochure. From the first person to the last, from nurse to janitor, from manager to processor, anyone who connects in any way with the consumer, the entrepreneurial consciousness must be present. It is in the people of the organization that the best marketing resources are found. It is here where marketing becomes a lived experience. When connected with the other activities of the marketing effort, service providers assure the success of fulfilling the consumer's expectations and hopes.

References

Ashley, J. A. (1976). *Hospitals, paternalism, and the role of the nurse*. New York: Teachers College Press.

Atchison, T. (1990). *Turning health care leadership around: Cultivating, inspiring, empowered, and loyal followers*. San Francisco: Jossey-Bass.

Atkinson, P. (1990). *Creating culture change: The key to successful total quality management*. San Diego: Pfeiffer & Co.

Attali, J. (1991). *Millenium: Winners and losers in the coming world order*. New York: Times Books.

Bennis, W. (1990). *Why leaders can't lead*. San Francisco: Jossey-Bass.

Berwick, D., Blanton, G., & Roessner, J. (1990). *Curing health care: New strategies for quality improvement*. San Francisco: Jossey-Bass.

Block, P. (1991). *The empowered manager*. San Francisco: Jossey-Bass.

Bolman, L., & Terrance, D. (1991). *Reframing organizations*. San Francisco: Jossey-Bass.

Brown, M., & McCool, B. (1990). Health care systems: Predictions for the future. *Health Care Management Review, 15*(3), 87–94.

Burda, D. (1990, April 23). A simmering perception of inequality. *Modern Healthcare*, pp. 30–31.

Choate, P. (1990, September–October). Political advantage: Japan's campaign for America. *Harvard Business Review*, pp. 87–103.

Deming, W. E. (1990). *Total quality management*. New York: Warner Books.

Drucker, P. (1985). The discipline of innovation. *Harvard Business Review, 43*(3), 43–53.

Drucker, P. (1989). *The new realities.* New York: Harper and Row.

Dumaine, B. (1990, May 7). Who needs a boss? *Fortune,* pp. 52–60.

Dunham, J., & Klafehn, K. (1990). Transformational leadership and the nurse executive. *Journal of Nursing Administration, 20*(4), 28–33.

Gabor, A. (1990). *The man who discovered quality.* New York: Time Books.

Gibbs, N. (1990, October 8). Shameful bequests to the next generation. *Time,* pp. 42–46.

Gibbs, N., et al. (1990). Women: The road ahead. *Time Special Issue, 136*(19), 10–82.

Halberstam, D. (1991). *The next century.* New York: Morrow Publishers.

Herrick, N. (1990). *Joint management and employee participation: Labor and management at the crossroads.* San Francisco: Jossey-Bass.

Herron, D., & Herron, L. (1991). Entrepreneurial nursing as a conceptual basis for in-hospital nursing practice models. *Nursing Economic$, 9*(5), 310–316.

Johnsson, J. (1991). Collaboration: Hospitals find that working together is tough, rewarding and vital. *Hospitals, 65*(23), 24–31.

Kaiser, L. (1988). The visionary manager. In T. Wilson (Ed.), *Emerging issues in health care* (pp. 99–104). Englewood, CO: Estes Park Institute.

Kanter, R. M. (1989). *When giants learn to dance.* New York: Simon & Schuster.

Ket

Kilmann, R. (1991). *Managing beyond the quick fix.* San Francisco: Jossey-Bass.

Kuttner, R. (1991). *The end of laissez-faire: National purpose and the global economy after the cold war.* New York: Knopf Publishers.

Leebov, W., & Scott, G. (1990). *Health care managers in transition: Shifting roles and changing organizations.* San Francisco: Jossey-Bass.

Martin, D. (1990). The Planetree model hospital project: An example of the patient as partner. *Hospital and Health Services Administration, 35*(4), 591–601.

Mick, S., et al. (1990). *Innovations in health care delivery: Insights for organizational theory.* San Francisco: Jossey-Bass.

Minerva-Melum, M. (1990, December 5). Total quality management: Steps to success. *Hospitals,* pp. 42–44.

Naisbitt, J., & Aburdene, P. (1985). *Re-inventing the corporation.* New York: Warner Books.

Naisbitt, J., & Aburdene, P. (1990). *Megatrends 2000.* New York: Warner Books.

Ohmae, K. (1990). *The borderless world.* New York: Harper Business Books.

Peters, T. (1987). *Thriving on chaos.* New York: Harper & Row.

Porter-O'Grady, T. (1988). Restructuring the nursing organization for a consumer-driven marketplace. *Nursing Administration Quarterly, 12*(3), 60–65.

Porter-O'Grady, T. (1990). *The reorganization of nursing practice: Creating the corporate venture.* Rockville, MD: Aspen Publishers.

The fifth discipline. New York: rency.

Powershift. New York: Ban-

CHAPTER 41 • • • • • •

POLICIES, POLITICS, AND LEGISLATION

SUE BARRETT

EXECUTIVE SUMMARY

The nursing profession has the potential to affect public policy on the issues of health care and professional practice to an unlimited extent. In fulfillment of the mission of the profession to the public, nurses have a responsibility to provide information, become political players, and wield influence on behalf of the public and the profession. A thorough understanding of the political process, whether at the institutional or federal level, including participants, process, and issues, is crucial to success in this arena.

Nurse managers, as those responsible on a daily basis for the systems and personnel providing care delivery, own a unique perspective on the health care system. They are responsible to use that perspective within their own organizations, as well as in the larger environment, to influence health care delivery for the American public.

T oday more than ever before, it is essential for nursing to assume responsibility for the health care system (or nonsystem) in our country. The American public is justifiably concerned about the cost, quality, and accessibility of basic health care services for themselves and their children. Government, business and industry, professional, and special interest organizations are joining in the debate about reform for American health care. The present climate offers a window of opportunity for nurses to affect the future of American health care.

The profession offers a unique perspective in our recognition of health care as an entity beyond the traditional. Historically, health care has been defined largely as provision of medical care in acute, fragmented, and episodic fashion. Nursing fully recognizes the limitations of this definition. Preventing illness and promoting health goes far beyond physician visits and short-stay hospitalizations. Good health encompasses a recognition and attention to the social, psychologic, and physical well-being of individuals over the life span, with attention focused on the environment and culture within which the individual functions. Actualization of a health care delivery system encompassing this conceptual framework ultimately will yield better health for all of our citizens.

The translation of nursings' conceptual framework of health into a workable system of care for the country involves use of power and a command of the political process. A strong and effective nursing profession with advanced political skills is needed to translate our vision of health care to reality.

Nurses comprise the largest group of health care professionals in the country but as yet have not developed a proportionate role in development of health care policy at the local, state, or national level. Nurses also comprise the largest employee group within acute care institutions but have not developed a proportionate role in development of institutional policy governing their own practice.

Certainly, over the past 10 years, the profession has made strides in development of a political role at all levels. Professional nursing organizations are focusing more resources on policy development and lobbying activities to put their own agendas forth at the national and state levels. Nurses are more frequently members of corporate boards, advisory groups at the state and national level, and participants in development of policy. Nurse executives are recognized as health care executives, and nurse managers frequently are recognized as department heads within their own institutions. Still, there is enormous untapped potential within the profession that can be brought to bear on health policy development at every level.

A strong and effective nursing profession with advanced political skills is needed to translate this vision of health care to reality. Nurse managers and nurse executives are uniquely positioned within the health care field. They are most adept at translation of patient care needs into realistic programs designed to fulfill those needs. It is the perspective of the nurse as a member of the administrative team in health care that provides this group with the credibility and the specific leadership and management skills that can affect care delivery. Nurse manager and executive collaboration in policy development is an extension of this role of translator played out daily within the work environment.

Political astuteness combined with the ability to translate vision to reality can enhance health care for the American public at the institutional, community, state, and national levels. This chapter provides information regarding the definition of politics and power, and also provide specific strategies to acknowledge and advance the role of the nurse in the political arena.

POWER AND POLITICS

Power is defined by *Merriam Webster's Collegiate Dictionary* (1993) as "possession of control, authority, or influence over others." Politics can be defined as "influencing the allocation of scarce resources" (Talbott & Vance, 1981). Politics is not confined to political contests within government but is an integral part of daily life for all within their community and work settings. Politics is applicable to every aspect of life where resources are limited and individuals are competing for those resources (Ehrat, 1983). It is important to view politics as an everyday occurrence that all are involved with. Politics cannot be thought of as something that happens in an election cycle. Acceptance of political activity as part and parcel of everyday life is crucial in development of political awareness and, subsequently, development of political power.

The terms "power" and "politics" are reviewed here for a purpose. Given the definitions, it is immediately apparent that women, specifically the nursing profession—which is currently 97% female, might be uncomfortable with these concepts. The women's movement over the past two decades has certainly made an impact on improving the status of women. Women within and without the profession are still struggling with hundreds of years of male domination and devaluation of traditionally masculine traits in women. A woman who behaves in an assertive manner is likely to be labeled a shrew or worse.

Women within the profession of nursing are struggling with these global social concerns about behavior expectations and are at the same time trying to reconcile the traditional nursing values of caring, support, and collaboration with the political realities of life in the 1990s. Nurses generally have not been comfortable with discussions of politics and power. In fact, political astuteness and use of power have been viewed by some as antithetical to the profession. Nothing could be further from the truth. The great nursing leaders in the country are politically astute and powerful. The most successful nurses, whether at the nurse manager, nurse executive, or staff nurse level, have developed political abilities that have had a positive impact on the environment to their (and their patients') benefit.

Nurses' discomfort with politics and attendant images is associated also with a common nursing aversion to recognition of and interest in power. I have often heard nurses say, "I don't want power. . . . I only want to get X accomplished." Yet nurses must recognize that goal accomplishment is largely associated with recognition of power and politics and with the appropriate use of both.

As previously stated, nurses have historically been uncomfortable with use of the terminology of politics, in large part because of a lack of experience with or recognition of the political process. Male-dominated institutions rarely have encouraged women who have been successful in securing scarce resources to the detriment of men in a competing group. Assertive behavior in men is generally expected and accepted. Assertive behavior in women may be labeled as aggressive, unfeminine, belligerent, or worse. Acknowledgment of these issues and concerns is the first step in becoming politically knowledgeable and politically active.

Mason and Talbott (1985) define the spheres of influence where nurses can effect change: the workplace, government, organizations, and the community. An adaptation of this framework is used here to discuss nursing involvement in decision making and political action.

NURSING AND POLITICS WITHIN HEALTH CARE ORGANIZATIONS

In any foray into a political arena, the nurse must ask and answer three crucial questions.

1. Who are the participants?
2. What are the issues?
3. What is the process for getting things done?

These three questions will be reiterated throughout this chapter and are applicable to an assessment of any political situation.

Staff nurses and nurse managers are not often aware of the political climate within their own work environments. Nurses often are quite insular in their thinking, limiting issues to professional concerns within the division or department of nursing and viewing the rest of the organization from a them vs us perspective. The vision of the institution for nurses must be expanded to include all of the major participants on the scene. Further, institutional politics require a strategic plan to advance nursing in concert with the rest of the organization. The first step in advancement is a thorough assessment of the participants making an impact.

- Who are the members of the governing board?
- Who are the members of the senior management team?
- How is the nurse executive positioned in relation to the other members of senior management?
- Who does the nurse executive report to, and why?
- How is nursing viewed within the organization?
- How is nursing contributing to the organization, and are systems in place to quantify nursing's contribution?
- How is the committee structure for the organization established, and how does nursing fit into this structure?

An assessment of organizational philosophy and mission also is in order.

- Is the mission primarily one of medical research or education?
- Is patient care the primary goal for this institution?
- Is community service and involvement important?

What is the value of the information outlined? How can one nurse manager use this information? The answer is that once these factors have been assessed, nursing can begin to develop strategies to promote the profession within the organization. Nurse managers are especially crucial in translating the mission and objectives of the organization to staff and in demonstrating commitment to the common agenda. As an example, if one of the primary goals of the organization is to further research, the nurse manager may decide that inclusion in that activity might enhance the image of nursing within the organization. A physician with ongoing research protocols for a cohort of patients might be approached regarding how nursing might collaborate in this research. Addition of a number of nursing variables to the research tool might be negotiated, with commitment of nursing time designated to data collection. Further, joint publications and presentations might result from this activity, enhancing the image of both professions to a larger audience.

This type of assessment and strategic action is an example of politics in the best sense of the word. The nurse in this example assessed the larger picture, demonstrated collaboration in working with a physician, and documented nursing's involvement in a valued activity within the organization while gaining knowledge about patient care activities to guide clinical practice for the profession.

Another area that should be discussed in the political context is that of documentation of nursing contribution to patient care outcomes, whether that be a decrease in length of stay, improved patient satisfaction, decrease in readmission rates, or other concerns to the institution. When a nurse manager is able to demonstrate that patients routinely respond positively when queried regarding satisfaction with nursing care, the organization must take notice. In the current climate of competition for patients, attracting and satisfying patients becomes an institutional goal. Demonstration of the nursing contribution must be noted.

The scenario outlined regarding patient satisfaction shows nurses using data to support their worth. It should be noted that nurses stridently approaching the organization about nursing worth without concomitant supporting data will not enhance the position or the image of the profession, either within an institution or in the larger world. Phrases, such as "We are never appreciated," and the portrayal of nurses as victims needs to be replaced with a proactive position demonstrating worth and positioning the profession as a contributor to organizational goals and objectives. Within any political reality, image and positioning are crucial. A positive image supported by data can move the organization on nursing's behalf.

POLITICS AND THE COMMUNITY

Although the politics of the workplace undoubtedly have a strong impact on the worklife of the nurse, a larger community comprised of health care consumers, providers, payors, and other professionals also should be considered in the political context. Hospitals and health care organizations do not exist in a vacuum. Government policy regarding payment for services is dealt with later in this chapter, and private payors, including individuals, business, and the insurance industry, also deserve attention. Three crucial questions to ask in the community setting are identical to those asked in the workplace.

1. Who are the participants?
2. What are the issues?
3. What is the process?

Among the general public, a gap in knowledge exists regarding the contribution to care provided by the nursing profession. Too many still believe that nurses carry out physician orders and nothing more. It is the responsibility of the individuals in the profession to educate the public. As cited previously, image and information are crucial. It will not enhance the image of nursing to berate the public for lack of knowledge or to berate the medical profession for lack of appreciation of nursing skills and care contribution. We must position the profession to proactively define the parameters of practice and to develop systems to quantify how nursing contributes to the health care of the nation.

In a typical Chicago community, the following scenario unfolded. A political candidate was running for office in a poor community comprised of a largely poor and elderly population. The candidate correctly surmised that free blood pressure screening for this population might enhance his ability to get his political message across in time for an upcoming election. The candidate sought the advice of a nurse manager of his acquaintance regarding how a blood pressure screening program might be implemented. At this juncture, the nurse manager might well have declined to participate or even to provide advice. However, she knew that this candidate was likely to be active in the political arena for the foreseeable future and that he was quite influential in local circles. Contact with the candidate now would enhance her ability to contact him after the (hopefully) successful election. Further, she saw provision of free screening as a socially valuable service that nurses could provide. The nurse manager also knew that lack of access to medical care for this population was a politically hot issue within the community.

After extensive discussion and planning, the nurse coordinated a well-attended blood pressure screening event for the community under the auspices of the candidate. Through this activity, she provided visibility for the profession, demonstrated her commitment to provision of health promotion services, made a powerful political ally, and provided a community service. This is an example of political activity without all of the negative undertones of wheeling and dealing but with a positive result for all concerned. The candidate received his visibility, the elderly received screening, and the nurse positioned herself and the profession in a positive light. Some political activities provide positive results for all concerned.

In addition to the type of activity outlined in the example, many opportunities exist to publicize the contributions of the profession in the community. This includes information about the various roles within nursing, such as staff nurses, nurse practitioners, certified nurse midwives, clinical specialists, nurse managers, and nurse executives. The information provided to the public should focus on the quality of contribution and, if at all possible, on the cost-effectiveness of the contribution to patients. Nurses in the community setting, such as home health and school nurses, should use every opportunity to educate clients about the value of their roles within the community.

Business and the insurance industry are more interested than ever in cost-effective ways to deliver high-quality care. One of the driving forces behind the movement for health care reform is the negative impact that health insurance premiums have had on business. This is a window of opportunity for nurses in expanded roles to sue for reimbursement from the private sector for their services. Both private businesses and private payors should be targeted to receive information regarding the worth of nursing services.

POLITICS AND THE PROFESSIONAL ORGANIZATION

The mission of nursing is first and foremost to meet the health care needs of the population. Given this, nursing must have a voice in the public policy arena so as to have an impact on policy decisions regarding health care. Without a voice in this arena, the profession will be unable to influence the care provided for the citizens of this country. One of the most effective ways to influence federal policy initiatives is through membership in national nursing and health care organizations. In politics, numbers mean a great deal. As professional organizations grow, their ability to affect policy likewise grows. Thus, it is essential that nurses belong to professional and health care organizations to the largest possible extent.

Although professional organizations certainly serve a multitude of purposes, including education and publication services, networking activities, scholarship and research support, it is their fundamental responsibility also to provide advocacy and informational services about public policy issues of concern to members. Nurse managers often are members of clinical specialty groups, organizations that provide advocacy and information about pertinent funding issues specific to patient types and services. For example, the Oncology Nursing Society monitors and lobbies issues of cancer research and program funding. As previously discussed, nurse managers often focus on issues that hit closest to home without a sense of the broad picture.

Consideration should be given to joining organizations concerned with broader health care issues, at both the local and national level. This would serve a number of purposes: the nurse manager would be exposed to issues not commonly discussed within the clinical specialty, and membership in the broader organization offers exposure to individuals with different perspectives regarding health care issues. Exposure to different perspectives is in itself valuable, but the opportunity to present the nursing perspective on issues also becomes available. Although time and financial concerns might preclude membership in a large number of organizations, a carefully chosen few offer unlimited opportunities for networking and political awareness.

Finally, a consideration of renewal of membership in an organization should be a time for reflection on that organization's impact in the policy arena. Members have an obligation to inform the organization about expectations for organizational involvement in public policy development. The nurse should share opinions and expertise with colleagues and should expect that advocacy and policy development be reflective of membership concerns.

Overall, the nurse manager should consider how the organization is positioned in respect to collaboration with other organizations. Numbers play an important role in politics. When a number of organizations form an effective coalition around an issue, the likelihood of impact is magnified. Members should expect organizational leadership to be able to collaborate effectively with others to affect nursing and health care issues of importance.

The Tri-Council for Nursing at the national level is a good example of collaboration among the major nursing organizations. The Tri-Council is composed of four major nursing organizations, including the American Association of Colleges of Nursing, The American Nurses Association, The American Organization of Nurse Executives, and the National League for Nursing. Although the objectives and missions of these organizations vary, some common ground exists. Whenever possible, these organizations collaborate to assume a position that represents a larger voice than any of the organizations could boast alone. Many of the state counterparts of these national organizations are now following suit and creating Tri-Councils specific to states. These, again, have been more effective than any of the organizations could have been alone when targeting specific issues that allow for a common position.

POLITICS AT THE FEDERAL LEVEL

The nurse manager seeking to influence nursing and health care policy at the national level can do so through active, direct participation in legislative and regulatory activities. A fundamental knowledge base of political processes is essential to have influence. The individual must, as in the workplace and in the community, be knowledgeable about process, participants, and issues to be most effective.

Process

A thorough understanding of relevant legislative and regulatory processes is fundamental to active participation in federal policy development. For any specific policy issue, the nurse manager must know which body will address the issue and the kinds of mechanics and processes involved.

Congress uses the legislative process to write the laws of the country. Through this process, ideas from Presidents, members of Congress, political parties, interest groups, and individual citizens are transformed into national policy. The law-making process as set forth in the Constitution is complicated and time consuming. It is governed by detailed rules and procedures, as well as custom and tradition.

For a bill to become law, both the House and Senate must approve a proposal in identical form, and it must be signed by the President or, infrequently, approved by Congress over his veto. Bills not passed die at the end of the 2 year term of Congress in which they are introduced. They may be reintroduced in a subsequent Congressional session.

There are major differences between the House and Senate as to how legislation is debated and disposed of, which is beyond the scope of this chapter. A full discussion of these differences can be found in *Congress A to Z, CQ's Ready Reference Encyclopedia* (1988).

When a bill is passed by one chamber, it is sent to the opposite chamber. There, normally, the bill again goes to committee, followed by markup, a vote to approve, and drafting of the committee report. The bill may then go the full chamber for consideration. Even when the bill is passed in the second chamber, it is likely that it has been altered substantially. Both chambers then send these bills to a combined House–Senate Conference Committee to negotiate a compromise. Very infrequently, a bill may be approved by the second chamber as passed by the first chamber, clearing the way for presidential signature.

A House–Senate conference is the last Congressional stop for most legislation. Either chamber may request a conference committee to resolve differences between House and Senate versions of a bill. Conferees are appointed from each chamber. Before they meet, each chamber's delegates usually meet separately to discuss strategy and positions. During the conferencing, specific rules governing the proceedings are in force, but the proceedings generally are less structured than is a regular committee meeting. Disagreements must be settled by majority vote.

After conferees agree to a compromise bill, a conference report is written. This is considered official once a majority of conferees have signed. Then, the two chambers vote on the compromise. Sometimes, bills are sent back to conference for further compromise. The final version is rarely defeated, and once the compromise is approved, the bill is sent to the President for review.

When a bill is presented to the President, he may sign it, thus enacting the measure into law. The President may veto the bill with a statement indicating his objections. Congress may override a Presidential veto with a two-thirds majority vote of both chambers. The bill then becomes law without Presidential approval. The President may take no action, in which case the bill will become law within 10 days without his signature (excluding Sundays), provided Congress does not adjourn during that time. If Congress adjourns, however, the bill does not become law. This is known as a pocket veto (*Congress A to Z,* 1988).

In addition to the legislative process, a myriad of federal commissions, bureaus, and other agencies exist. Nurses have not been as well represented as they might be as members of these groups and agencies. Appointments to federal commissions should be an area of concern for nursing. Especially when groups serve in an advisory capacity to Congress or the administration, the importance of nursing representation cannot be overlooked. Likewise, nursing representation on regulatory bodies, whether within or outside the government, cannot be overemphasized. Although appointments are generally sought and won through membership in professional organizations, it is mentioned here as a crucial avenue for nursing involvement in public policy development.

Participants

It is impossible to discuss having an impact on federal policy without consideration of the participants involved. The nurse manager must identify the specific legislator or legislators involved with the specific nursing or health care policy issue of concern. After identification, the nurse manager must establish contact with the individual or a member of that legislator's staff. It is important not to underestimate the impact of communication with staff. Legislators generally place great confidence in their staff members and seriously consider their input. Contact with a legislator or staff may take the form of a letter or brief visit. A personal letter is much more effective than a form letter. It should be brief and concise—two or three paragraphs is usually sufficient. When requesting support or opposition to a particular proposal, the writer should state the name and bill number, and the letter should be sent so that it reaches the legislator before action occurs. The message will achieve nothing if it arrives too late. When a legislator publicly supports the nurse manager's position in a public forum or is successful in passing the bill through committee or the floor, the manager should express appreciation.

A visit to a congressional member or staff should be brief and concise. The nurse should provide credible information and documentation if at all possible and know the legislator's view on the issue before the meeting. She should be prepared to discuss and defend her position, if necessary, and avoid threatening and condemnation should the individual disagree. A short thank you should be sent after the visit, with a summary of the major points discussed. Letters and meetings with legislators and their staff members are effective mechanisms to establish and maintain contact and to influence policy development.

Once contact and an ongoing relationship is developed, the nurse manager may be called on to provide information about health care or nursing-related issues. This is obviously another avenue to influence in the federal policy arena. Although the focus of this discussion has been influencing the federal policy process through contact with legislators, other avenues exist where nurse managers might have influence. There are a large number of federal agencies and bureaus where nursing and health-related issues are determined. *The Nurses' Directory of Capitol Connections* (Sharp, 1992) identifies nurses employed in both the public and private sectors who might assist in directing the nurse to the proper channels of communication or to specific departments or individuals.

Issues

One criticism of the nursing profession from the public, especially from legislators, is that nurses have been single-issue oriented, indicating that nurses have demonstrated concern only with nursing issues. It is up to the profession to change this image, and one of the most important ways in which this can be done is to become better informed about larger political issues and forces. When advancing into the political arena, the nurse manager must become knowledgeable about current issues in the environment, not only those limited to nursing and health care.

Important information to be aware of includes the functions and purposes of the various federal agencies and bureaus, the priorities of the current administration, and issues of greatest concern in Congress. A knowledge base regarding the big picture, with consideration of other interests, can help establish the nurse manager as a credible and informed constituent and enhance the ability to influence. When approaching a Congressman on specific issues, the nurse manager should be aware of competing issues and opposing viewpoints and be ready to discuss issues knowledgeably.

POLITICS AT THE STATE LEVEL

Although the legislative process at the state level is roughly analogous to that at the federal level, some variation does occur. The nurse manager is referred to her particular state capitol for specific information regarding the legislative process and functions and structures of state level agencies affecting nursing and health care issues.

One of the reasons that state level politics is of primary concern to the profession is because state level legislation largely defines and regulates nursing practice. Further, since the early 1980s, states have increased control over federal monies designated for health and social services. Nurses need to expand their understanding of state government and increase political influence at this level to affect health policy development and to assure appropriate state regulation of nursing practice. A review of the previous section about the importance of knowing the process, participants, and issues is as pertinent at the state level as at the federal. The precepts for action are identical, even though the issues and legislators change and the process at the state level may be somewhat modified.

References

Boston, C., & McEntee, C. (1987). *The nurse executive in the legislative arena: The how-tos of influence*. Chicago: American Hospital Association.

Congress A to Z, Congressional Quarterly's ready reference encyclopedia. (1988). Washington, DC: Congressional Quarterly.

Congressional directory 1991–102nd Congress. (1991). Washington, DC: American Hospital Association.

Ehrat, K.S. (Sept. 1983). A model for politically astute planning and decision making. *Journal of Nursing Administration, 13*, 29–35.

Fagin, C., & Maraldo, P. (1989). Perspectives on nursing in today's health care environment. *Nursing Economics, 7*(4), 186–195.

Mason, D., & Talbott, S. (Eds.). (1985). *Political action handbook for nurses*. Menlo Park, CA: Addison-Wesley Publishing Co.

Merriam-Webster's Collegiate Dictionary (10th ed.). (1993). Springfield, MA: Merriam Webster, Inc.

Sharp, N. (1992). *The nurses' directory of capitol connections*. Washington, DC: Capitol Associates.

Talbott, S.W., & Vance, C. (1981). Involving nursing in a feminist group–NOW. *Nursing Outlook, 29*, 592–595.

CHAPTER 42

MANAGING NURSING'S FUTURE: CHALLENGING THE PROFESSION

SUSAN CHAMBERLAIN WILLIAMS

EXECUTIVE SUMMARY

This chapter provides the nurse leader with a brief overview of the major issues and trends shaping health care as we move into the twenty-first century. These issues and trends are examined in terms of their implications for nursing practice and the context in which nurse managers of the future must lead.

A successful future will depend on the nurse leader's ability to look at current beliefs and practices and to bring about a fundamental shift in the way we think about and do things. Three broad challenges are presented to guide the change process and the evaluation of the nurse leader's future role. First is a challenge to change the way we think. Next is an imperative to redesign systems with care. Finally is the need to reconceptualize the nurse leader's role as that of developmental manager.

Changing the way we think introduces the nurse leader to the notion of strategic thinking as an essential skill for the future. In contrast to strategic planning, strategic thinking looks at how we want to be rather than what we want to be. It compels the leader to be proactive and to develop a vision that is shared by everyone in the organization.

Changing the way we think is also positively influenced by the nurse leader's capacity to understand and apply two theories: attribution theory and systems theory. Attribution theory is based on casual influence: how the individual explains or ascribes motives to human behavior and situations. Systems theory posits that human conflicts or breakdowns must be examined in terms of the whole of the interaction and the effect each party has on the other, rather than looking at the behavior of a single party in isolation. These two theories can assist the nurse leader toward improved problem solving and conflict resolution skills.

Another tool for changing the way we think is to understand how the nurse leader's choice of language can powerfully affect the thoughts and actions of others. Several examples are suggested and discussed.

Systems redesign and restructuring of hospital nursing services is underway in many institutions across the country. The nurse leader is cautioned to avoid buying into this trend without a thorough analysis of the organization's needs and readiness for change. Unsuccessful implementation of primary nursing is given as an example of injudicious attention to the change process. This situation is a classic illustration of how an inherently good idea, based on sound principles and values, is dispelled as bad or impractical when the real issue lies in the implementation and leadership of the change process itself.

If our systems are not redesigned with care, an opportunity to nurture the relationships forming the basis of our practice—nurse–patient and nurse leader–practicing nurse—may be lost. Equally serious, if the nurse leader does not believe in and model an ethic of care as the principal value guiding nursing practice, the nurse leader of today may be replaced by a nonnurse leader of tomorrow.

The developmental role is the role nurse leaders must strengthen for the future in order to create an empowered staff. This calls for a reemphasis of the developmental process, establishing clear role expectations, careful selection of qualified staff based on sound interviewing principles, and ongoing performance development using feedback, coaching, and counseling techniques.

Job descriptions must be updated to specify expected behaviors rather than the traditional list of tasks and activities a nurse generally performs. Performance evaluation tools must be developed to measure each of the behaviors specified in the job descriptions. The successful nurse leader will give feedback based on performance expectations and will select new employees in light of their potential to demonstrate expected role behaviors. Involving staff members in developing or improving role descriptions can help to raise standards in an organization.

Finally, the nurse leader who values a developmental role and wants to foster an empowered staff will need to look seriously at the leader's personal need for control. Giving up control through conveyance of trust, providing support for taking responsibility, and allowing others to act within the scope of their expertise is an essential step toward the creation of successful environments for the future.

There are two things we can predict about the future. It will be marked with uncertainty and with unprecedented change. Beyond that, we can only anticipate what may be required of us as we move into the twenty-first century. To better understand our roles as nurse leaders of the future, it is important to examine some of the factors that will shape our practice.

Health care reform has become the number one political agenda. Thirty-seven million Americans have no insurance (Short, Monheit, & Beauregard, 1989). Many live in rural areas without access to basic health care services. Changes in reimbursement and technology continue to drive the shift from inpatient to outpatient and community-based settings. Our hospitalized patients are older, requiring skilled professionals who can address both functional and acute care needs. Health care costs are spiraling, yet no one wants to pay.

Given the realities of the political process and the number of special interest groups to be reconciled, any radical reform, such as a national health plan, will take a long time to eventuate. What seems more likely is a next-generation or new hybrid of the many, diversified approaches already in place. Regardless of the outcome, the boom times are over, and there will be no more money. We will have to do things differently, working smarter rather than harder and without additional resources.

Despite the increasing enrollments in schools of nursing, it is predicted that the demand for registered nurses will continue to exceed the supply. Management of chronic illness, greater numbers of frail elderly, and accelerated development of community-based health care will create new roles and new demands for nurses, particularly those with baccalaureate and advanced degrees. Thus, the shortage will persist over the long term, and we will be compelled to maximize the knowledge and skills of a valuable and limited resource.

Realizing that we cannot continue to do things as we have always done them, many institutions will be struggling to restructure systems, to redesign roles, and to find more efficient and effective ways of delivering care to patients. This process will continue into the next century as we learn from the experiences of those who are pioneers of restructuring. Moreover, the drive to do things differently demands that we preserve the integrity of the nurse–patient relationship and that this relationship remains central to any new endeavor.

As the struggle to redesign systems gains momentum, so too will the emphasis on quality. Future survival of hospitals and health care systems is dependent on a total commitment to excellence in a way that meets the needs of the people served by those systems. Good will simply not be good enough.

Yet another force requiring our time and attention will be the accelerated development of systems designed to enhance the way we access, store, and communicate information. Although these new technologies offer every opportunity to improve efficiency and effectiveness, this can only happen through requisite skill development and a willingness to do the hard work of analyzing what we need and why we need it before calling in the consultant and proceeding with large capital expenditures. In other words, if we are not prepared, technology may thwart the very goals we wish to achieve.

Also on the horizon is a demand for a new era in relationship development. Riding on the coattails of the women's movement in the late 1960s and 1970s, nursing was striving to gain independent identity and to establish itself as a profession. Separating from the physician's shadow was an essential step in the professionalization of nursing. Now, however, we must reexamine our relationships and find new models to integrate the best nursing and medicine have to offer. Collaborative partnerships will be the key to survival in a highly competitive arena.

Issues and trends affecting nursing and health care provide a context in which we will have to lead. In short, there will be more to do, less to do it with, and tremendous pressure to do it better than anyone else. Positioning ourselves for the challenge requires an incredible ability to look at who we really are and to bring about a fundamental shift in how we think about and do things.

CHANGING THE WAY WE THINK

A northeastern manufacturing plant that builds submarines funded by defense industry contracts recently gained national attention. Due to cuts in defense spending, the submarines are no longer needed. The plant is scheduled to close and will lay off 20,000 people. These people represent approximately 40% of the town's economy, and it is predicted the town will go bankrupt. The situation presents an unfortunate example of how our thinking can get us into trouble. Although the exact circumstances are unknown, perhaps the plant's leaders neglected to look into the future 5 or 10 years ago and did not see the changes on the horizon. If they had applied strategic thinking in their daily operations, could the current outcome have been avoided? What if they had seen the changes coming and created a new niche for themselves in case the defense money ran out?

The questions inherent in the submarine situation are more important than the answers. However, the reality is a scenario that will be played out many times unless we are able to change the way we think.

The concept of strategy is not new. According to *Webster's Dictionary,* one definition states that strategy is "essential to the effective conduct of war" (*Webster's II,* 1988). Considering the current and future health care arena, the idea seems fitting. We need to know how to position ourselves in order to win the competitive war.

The traditional notion of strategy has been its connection to strategic planning. More recently, the idea of strategic thinking has been introduced (Beckham, 1991). The reasons for this shift are highly relevant in today's health care environment. Things are changing so rapidly and are so complex that we can no longer afford to work at the level of detail or in the linear fashion that strategic planning suggests. Elements of the strategic plan usually involve a mission statement, goals, objectives, key issues or target areas, and highly detailed tactics or plans to achieve the desired results. This process is generally associated with the organization's top management.

Although there will never be a substitute for careful analysis and planning, we need to become more flexible and willing to act without knowing all the details. Unlike the submarine plant, we cannot wait to see if the defense money will run out.

Strategic thinking implies an attitude of constant preparedness. Not only is there a vision of the future, but it includes the likelihood of multiple realities. The picture emphasizes how we want to be rather than what we want to be—a focus on guiding principles and values rather than any absolute state. Everyone is involved and encouraged to improve the organization. Action is based on the strategic relevance of presenting circumstances rather than on any rigidly prescribed plan. In other words, does the situation afford an opportunity to move closer to how we want to be? What are the ways we can capitalize on the opportunity?

Beginning to think strategically backs us out of a tendency to get stuck on obstacles that prevent us from moving forward. The gap between current reality and our picture of the future provides an impetus for change. If we think about how we want to be, there is no room for outmoded notions, such as, "We have always done it this way," "We have to wait for all the relevant data," or "It won't work because it isn't in the plan, or it isn't in the policy." Resistive statements of this nature impede any progress and may lead to a fatal kind of inertia, similar to that of the submarine plant, which knew only one direction.

Strategic thinking demands an ability to be proactive in the way we respond to forces and events in our lives. We may not have control over certain conditions or things that happen to us, but we can choose our responses (Covey, 1989). It is possible to subordinate feelings to values and to determine our behavior accordingly. In contrast to the reactive person who responds emotionally to circumstances by blaming others and allowing outside events to control him or her, the proactive person is driven by consciously selected values.

For example, many have experienced a situation where they have been asked by a boss to communicate information that is unclear in its intent or may not be well received. The reactive person complains to peers that he or she has been asked to do this. The proactive person responds with an examination of her or his values. Proactive people recognize the leader's role in reducing uncertainty and ambiguity for the staff and in promoting organizational well-being. They begin to think strategically and realize the need for further discussion with their boss. Although they may not be able to change the content of the communication, answers to several specific questions will ensure the best possible outcome. What is the intent of this communication? How can I most effectively present it to my staff? What reactions can we anticipate, and what would be the best response? (Leebov & Scott, 1991).

Individuals who articulate a values-driven vision of the future provide an important vehicle empowering others to think strategically. It is a reality, however, that most people cannot picture something they have never experienced or seen. So the challenge for nurse leaders is to make a vision alive and real in the minds of others.

What are some of the mechanisms by which this can occur? First is an imperative to model the behaviors we want others to emulate. There is nothing more powerful than the nurse leader's ability to express positive human and professional values and to demonstrate these values in action.

Nurse leaders also can help to shape a vision for others through the use of scenarios. These scenarios can be acted out and discussed on the basis of what happens now vs how we want the same situation to play out in the future. For example, what is the response when a patient or family member expresses a concern about nursing care? What is the desired future response? What would it take to get there? In such a safe environment, staff can begin to think about their values, gaining new insights and a positive desire to change.

Where there is money available, nurse leaders can employ benchmarking to assist others to picture a desired future. This concept refers to the process of identifying and understanding the best practices used by institutions of excellence and measuring oneself against these standards. Selected staff members can be supported in on-site visits to nationally recognized institutions that have a reputation for being values driven. Individuals who visit these institutions can provide leadership within the home organization because they have experienced what future reality can be.

SYSTEMS THINKING/ATTRIBUTION THEORY FRAMEWORK

Viewed together, systems thinking and attribution theory provide a framework for another way to change our perspective if we are to survive the challenges of the future. Systems thinking, directed at an aggregate level, proposes that organizations and human endeavors are systems. Problems and issues arise as a result of the interrelationships among the parts of the system and cannot be linked to an isolated person or event. Therefore, effective problem solving and change can occur only through an understanding of the whole system and interaction among its parts. It requires the leader to commit energy and attention to the interfaces in a system rather than to the components (Ackoff, 1981).

Attribution theory looks at individual behavior and focuses on perceived causality—ideas about why things happen and what causes them to occur. Using attribution theory, one can offer motives for behavior. The locus of causality exists in the person, the situation, or both. The human tendency is to assign situational motives for our own behavior while assigning personal causality to others (Fiske & Taylor, 1984).

To illustrate, if I behave badly toward one of my colleagues, I tend to excuse my responses on the basis of illness, a fight with a family member, or some other factor in the situation. In contrast, if one of my colleagues behaves badly toward me, I tend to believe that person is personally at fault, uncaring, lacking in consideration, or socially inept.

Eliminating Blame and Reactive Behavior

Application of the systems thinking/attribution theory framework creates a mandate to eliminate blame and reactive, defensive behavior. As we prepare for the future, we must become more sensitive to the complexity of individual behavior and the interrelationships among subsets of our organizations.

It is essential that we begin to give others the same space for understanding that we are willing to give ourselves. Eliminating blame will enable us to study the seams, or interfaces, in our organizations and to realize the futility of placing responsibility on a single department or individual. When nurses and physicians fail to communicate, for example, the solution is not to blame either party or to work the issues with each group individually but to understand the nature and necessity of collaborative relationships and to remove the system or environmental barriers that prevent these relationships from forming.

In many ways, blaming provides a quick fix and eliminates the responsibility to search deeper or work harder to solve problems. Using the systems thinking/attribution theory framework commits the nurse leader to a long-term perspective, and a willingness to expend the effort means the payoffs will be significant.

The Power of Language

Changing the way we think can be greatly enhanced by recognizing the power of language (Henry & LeClair, 1987). Carefully chosen words, used consistently over time and woven into the fabric of our organizations, can facilitate cultural change and help to crystallize a vision. At St. Luke's Hospital in Houston, Texas, Kerfoot promotes a "culture of collegiality" (Curran, 1991, pp. 142–143). This phrase alone is a powerful prescript for behavior throughout the organization. Boston's Beth Israel Hospital uses "corrective action" guidelines in lieu of a disciplinary policy. The notion is culturally embedded and provides a message that behavior can be changed through positive, constructive action.

Many institutions committed to decentralization still maintain the role of charge nurse and have policies referring to the "chain of command." In the instance of the charge nurse, would it not make more sense to conceptualize an "administrative resource nurse," denoting an individual whose practice focus or chosen area of expertise is in the management/leadership domain? The title implies that the resource nurse has parity on the unit with other nurses who choose to develop expertise in different areas. As we try to retain qualified nurses in clinical practice, do we really want our language to suggest that administrative roles carry greater status in a formal hierarchy?

Similarly, "chain of command" reinforces a formal hierarchy and seems paradoxical to the goals of decentralization. The term "channels of communication" is more collegial, less intimidating, and more descriptive of the flattened, user-friendly structures we need to create for the future.

Specht calls attention to the role of language in shaping nurses' perspective about documentation. She suggests a need to reconsider the term "paperwork" and to realize that "although we want to use time efficiently, we don't want to lose the opportunity to think about how to assess and address nursing problems" (Murphy & De Back, 1991, p. 75). In other words, documentation must be perceived as integral to practice and not as a task or activity to be completed in isolation.

One also wonders if "charting by exception" might tend to move us away from individualized, personalized patient care. The assumption seems to be that most patient behavior is normative, and, therefore, less emphasis is placed on contextual factors, individual patterns, and the interrelationships among these patterns. Somehow the opportunity for holistic thinking and reflection gets lost.

Case management currently is recognized as the delivery model of the 1990s, yet is case management only a function among many others within the professional nurse's role (Joyce C. Clifford, personal communication)? Assuming the need to carefully balance both cost and quality outcomes, do patients really experience a sense of human connectedness when they perceive a nurse as someone who is managing their "case?"

If sensitivities have been raised, Gilmore's (1991) ideas have relevance. We need to dispense with the notion of "confronting the issues" in a sense of right vs wrong. It would serve us better to think of "working the issues" together as a way of finding integrative solutions to problems.

GETTING ON THE BANDWAGON OR REDESIGNING SYSTEMS WITH CARE?

In the current health care environment, many institutions are moving forward to redesign roles and to restructure systems as a way of preparing for the future (see, for example, *Healthcare Forum,* July-August, 1991). The success of these endeavors will depend on a few key factors. Much hard work will have to be done upfront to determine why the change is needed and on what underlying principles and values the change will be based and to examine what preparation is required in the environment to ascertain readiness for change.

Unfortunately, the human tendency is to hear an idea that has worked for someone else and to want to jump on the bandwagon (Manthey, 1992). What gets missed is the rigorous assessment of one's own environment and its suitability for the idea. In the excitement of the moment, leaders can easily focus on how to implement rather than to answer the most critical questions: Why is this idea relevant to us? Does it fit with our vision and the values we want to preserve? What supports are required, and what developmental work needs to be done to ensure success of the process?

All too often, one hears that primary nursing is outmoded or dead. Valuable lessons can be learned from those who say they have tried to implement the model and it did not work. As one begins to uncover the process, there are all kinds of stories: "Administration told us to implement it." "Half our unit was staffed by agency nurses." "Nobody really understood what we were supposed to do." In reality, those who have failed with the model give full support to concepts of professional nurse autonomy: authority for patient care decision making, accountability for those decisions, and continuity of patient care. Moreover, study after study has demonstrated that professional autonomy and status are factors frequently associated with nurse job satisfaction and retention (Harrison, 1987; Hinshaw, Smeltzer, & Atwood, 1987; Johnston, 1991; McClure, Poulin, Sovie, & Wandelt, 1983; Weisman, 1982).

There is a clear message that primary nursing (or any other model embodying the same concepts) is not dead. The failure to successfully implement the model lies not in its conceptual basis but in the change process itself and a serious neglect of organizational assessment and readiness. The hard work of attention to these issues may be painful, but it is critical to success.

For those who conclude that primary nursing is too expensive, perhaps the view is short-sighted. Given the inextricable link between nurse satisfaction and the outcomes of patient care, how can we not afford a model that offers professional status and autonomy? A stable, motivated, and well-qualified staff seems to be an excellent return on investment for anyone concerned.

As we think further about designing new systems for the future, Benner (1989) offers an important insight. She talks about our tendency to "separate the means from the ends." Because of this tendency, we omit opportunities to nurture the very relationships that form the basis of our practice.

If we believe that nurses assist others to achieve and sustain wellness, healing becomes the desired end point of nursing activity. Healing occurs through the context or means of caring relationships. By definition, this kind of relationship will not develop in the absence of constancy, visibility, and continuity in time and space. How then, can we ever justify removing the nurse from the bedside (to get blood from the blood bank or, often, to manage the desk) while at the same time delegating the patient's bed bath to a technician who lacks skill in patient assessment and the art of caring relationships?

Another example of the tendency to separate means and ends was related by a new case manager responsible for a population of neurologic patients. She commented that her preceptor thought it was unproductive to attend a weekly neurologic case conference. The preceptor cited the fact that the conference focused only on esoteric cases of academic interest to physicians. Fortunately, the new case manager recognized the wisdom of supporting the neurologists' desire to have case managers in attendance. The conference provided an important means to develop collaborative relationships with the physicians who were to become her colleagues.

THE ROLE OF THE NURSE MANAGER

Nowhere is the means and ends question more applicable than in our chosen design of the nurse manager's role in the future. We are at a critical juncture in history, and if we do not take the appropriate lead, it is possible that the nurse manager of today will be replaced by a nonnurse manager of tomorrow.

Nursing is a practice-focused discipline expressed through human caring, yet in today's climate, "nurse administrators at all levels are so busy managing the day-to-day crises of surviving, that the art of nursing, when practiced in the organizational context, is at risk of being lost (Brown, 1991). Significant pressure exists for nurse managers and nurse executives to demonstrate their relative worth through business and managerial knowledge. Although this knowledge is extremely important to our credibility in a business world, if we favor administrative activities over our roles as managers and leaders of a clinical discipline, we set ourselves up to compete with a multitude of MBAs and no one is left to articulate, to model, and to recognize the real essence and value of nursing.

The ends and means question and its applicability to role design can be illustrated readily through nurse managers' decisions regarding performance evaluation. It is common practice to delegate this process to senior staff or assistant-type roles, albeit to those with less experience and often with less education. If one accepts that effective performance evaluation is aimed at ongoing assessment, development, and nurturing of individual practice, a high degree of skill is required in the context of a caring relationship. Those who choose to give up performance evaluation, particularly without careful guidance and active participation in the process, miss a critical opportunity for relationship and to shape the kind of practice environment they ultimately envision for their units.

Our effectiveness as nurse leaders requires that we accept an ethic of caring as central to our roles. With this acceptance comes a mandate to develop skills in caring and to use these skills in our relationships. At the same time, we need to nurture and reward the caring practices of others. By looking for examples of caring and making these instances highly visible, nurse leaders can support caring as a primary value.

For organizations committed to the development of caring practices, it is recommended that nurse leaders familiarize themselves with the use of clinical exemplars, as described by Benner (1984) and Benner and Benner (1991). Exemplars are narrative stories of actual patient situations. They provide an excellent way to enhance understanding of the meaning of caring while reconnecting nurses with the essence and value of their practice. At Boston's Beth Israel Hospital, the surgical nurse managers share management exemplars to learn more about caring practices embedded in the nurse manager's role.

Brown (1991, p. 69) states that "what is valued receives attention and is rewarded, and what is rewarded will develop in nursing organizations." Although there clearly is a need to attend to the administrative/business components of our roles, there is an equally strong need to attend to the fundamental caring values on which our practice is based (Brown, 1991). What we do and how we do it will profoundly shape the behavior of those around us.

One nurse manager who successfully blended clinical and administrative responsibilities provides a model for us all. Her staff developed a wonderful caring practice whereby any patient imminently dying unattended by family would not be allowed to die alone. This meant that the staff had to take turns sitting with the patient, sometimes when staffing was very tight. The nurse manager wanted to support this practice and to reinforce the inherent caring value. Therefore, she took her turn sitting with dying patients while reading mail or writing performance evaluations, stopping periodically to touch the patient or to hold the patient's hand.

Developer of People

Our employees and the talents and strengths they offer are the most important assets we have to meet the challenges that lie ahead. Without capable people, we will be unable to achieve the level of quality on which future survival depends. It is only through others that we can position ourselves for competitive success, yet as one begins to analyze how managers spend their time, it is not surprising how often we fall short of our goals.

Successful nurse leaders have no other option but to demonstrate that people are their most highly valued resource. This means that a great deal more thought and time will have to go into the process than we have ever given it before. The developmental role of the manager must be the role we strengthen and design for the future. (This view is held so strongly by the faculty of Boston's Northeastern University that the graduate curriculum is based on the concept.)

The framework for developing people is not unfamiliar, but it calls for a rethinking and integration of several activities managers have tended to view in isolation. Establishing clear role expectations, initial hiring interviews, and ongoing performance development using feedback, coaching, and counseling techniques are all critical elements in the same developmental process.

The manager's role as a developer of people is vital to realizing the kind of results we want to create in our workplaces. For this reason, all the elements of the developmental process must be tied to a vision of how we want things to be. First, we need to pull job descriptions off the shelf and ask ourselves two fundamental questions. Do these documents tell people what behaviors we expect from them, or do they merely contain a set of tasks and functions written on a piece of paper? Second, does each of these documents prescribe a role that is unique and clear? If role overlap is unavoidable, do the performance criteria specify how responsibilities are negotiated so that role conflicts do not occur?

Many of us were taught to separate personality from performance. This is an old notion that must be buried. Although a wide range of individual traits and styles can enrich and diversify our workplaces, there are some behaviors and attributes that simply should not be accepted. Job descriptions, or more preferably role descriptions, need to specify expected behaviors so that deviance can be effectively managed or redirected.

How often has it been said, "She's a great clinician, but she's impossible to get along with?" Today's environments, focused on total quality management, cannot afford to be tolerant of individuals who do not attend to their relationships and impact on others.

Developer of Role Descriptions and Evaluation Tools

Role descriptions and evaluation tools must contain statements that clearly communicate expectations, for example, "interacts with colleagues as valued, respected members of the health care team," "gives feedback and resolves issues in a manner that promotes individual self-esteem," and "seeks opportunities to explore own behavior and to make requisite changes in performance" (Clifford and Horvath, 1990). Staff members with angry or insecure personalities, who act out their feelings in ways that threaten the well-being of others, must be helped to understand their behavior and the necessary expectations.

Equally important, evaluation tools must contain statements reflective of the behaviors set forth in the appropriate role descriptions. The developmental manager will hold employees accountable for the expected behaviors and provide the guidance and coaching necessary to ensure individual success.

Developing or improving role descriptions can be a powerful means to raise standards in an organization. Involving staff members who represent the desired roles not only will bring excitement to the process but also will be critical to success. In the instance of a clinical nurse, for example, staff can be asked to describe what constitutes high performance in all aspects of that role—clinical practice, leadership, professional development, and research. The responses can be written on a board or flip chart and later synthesized into a final document. Personal investment (buy-in) is created through the process, and staff feel recognized because their knowledge and contributions are valued.

Interviewing and Hiring

Once clear role expectations have been established and the manager has a picture of what is desired in the ideal nurse, the interviewing and hiring process can be structured accordingly. All too frequently, managers fail to consider how their selection process and hiring decisions affect the kind of results they want to achieve. (Interviewing techniques are beyond the scope of this chapter, but there are many references and courses available to help managers develop skills in this area. See, for example, Chapter 11.) Inability to use these skills or crisis decisions based on a need to fill a vacancy ultimately will be reflected in poor outcomes.

The developmental manager must give significant thought and time to the interview process. Well-constructed questions will allow the interviewer to determine the candidate's fit with organizational and unit values. Discussion during the process should include selected role expectations so that buy-in becomes a condition of employment. Socialization and development of prospective employees begin during the initial interview.

Feedback Tied to Performance Expectations

Nurse leaders committed to serving the developmental needs of their staff will understand the importance of feedback tied directly to performance expectations. Looking for and recognizing situations where standards have been met or exceeded is an essential strategic process that should consume a significant amount of the manager's time. If we truly want to develop people because we care about them and because we recognize that everyone's performance is critical to organizational success, we will have to commit a lot of time to giving feedback. Articulating instances where expectations are met and the desired values demonstrated will bring life to what we want to create and move us closer to our visions.

The developmental role of the nurse leader also requires an ability to recognize and manage situations where individuals are not performing at the expected level. Feedback must be given to illustrate how standards have not been met, and a plan must be established with specific time frames to allow the individual an opportunity to improve performance. However, when effective behavior change does not occur and considerable time and resources have been expended, it is important to move quickly with termination or reassignment.

Successful nurse leaders of the future must realize that tolerance of substandard performance sends a powerful message to employees. Individuals forced to compensate for the lack of effort or poor image cast by the substandard performer eventually will perceive that the manager's expectations are not real (Leebov & Scott, 1990). In essence, the manager's actions speak so loudly that their words cannot be heard. Outplacement of an individual is never easy but, at times, is very necessary to the broader goals we must achieve.

GIVING UP CONTROL

Much has been written lately on the subject of empowerment—the demand for a radical shift from the old paradigm where managers were expected to have all the answers and to tell employees what to do. These managers solved all problems, approved any deviations from standard practice, and ensured that employees asked permission before taking initiatives that involved other people or resources (Leebov & Scott, 1990).

In today's environment, patients want to be partners in their own health care. They expect to participate in decision making and to receive prompt, concerned responses to their requests. At the same time, our staff members express needs for growth, personal fulfillment, and self-actualization in the workplace. In light of these facts alone, the old paradigm will no longer work.

As Manthey suggests (1991), successful environments of the future will be those in which all nurses are empowered to solve patients' problems immediately and directly. Although problem solving may require marshalling a variety of resources on the patient's behalf, it should not mean that the nurse must enlist the approval of a charge nurse or nurse manager in order to proceed. Professional nurses will gain a sense of satisfaction and self-mastery only by having the freedom to make decisions and initiate action within the full scope of their expertise. Casting this notion aside with the belief that most nurses do not want responsibility is faulty thinking. Again, it is an issue of no quick fix. People, especially women, who have a long history of allowing others to make decisions for them need to be assisted to learn to take responsibility. This goal can be reached only through the efforts of committed leaders and through carefully designed systems that maximize the role of the nurse.

An effective response to the empowerment mandate has serious and far-reaching implications for nurse leaders. Many are firstborn children. A significant number come from dysfunctional families. Taking charge and being responsible are an accustomed way of life. Trust in others may not come easily because of issues in the very earliest of relationships. Perfectionist tendencies can make it difficult to accept an imperfect product arising from another's creativity or decision making. Vulnerabilities in self-image may allow little room for others to be recognized when their capabilities equal or exceed our own.

Creating Empowered Environments

Whatever the reasons, control needs can become restrictive and kill the kind of innovation and independent action on which a successful future ultimately depends. To create empowered environments, nurse leaders must develop insight into their controlling behaviors and the instances where those behaviors exist. Asking staff members for feedback is an excellent place to start. Individuals can easily respond to questions regarding how much freedom they have to do their jobs and to what extent managers create or remove barriers in the delivery of patient care.

When control issues are identified, the manager will need to address the concerns on a regular basis. A willingness to ask the question, "How am I doing?" will alone help to foster a more open environment. The ability to relinquish control is so essential that, at times, the skills of a psychiatric liaison nurse or a professional counselor may be necessary. Managers who feel the need to supply all the answers and who are threatened when others bring their expertise to bear on a situation must seek the support of a qualified individual to assist with behavioral change.

Nurse leaders committed to a viable future have no choice but to ensure that each individual contributes his or her full potential in service to patients and families. With proper guidance and coaching, our staff members will make excellent decisions if we give them the space to do so. The power we give away will come back to us many times over, but first we have to let go.

In summary, the twenty-first century will not arrive as if some unknown intruder has come upon us and taken us by surprise. We know it is on the horizon and that it represents a future filled with many new possibilities. Essentially we have two choices. We can watch it happen or we can accept the challenge to create it.

References

Ackoff, R.L. (1981). *Creating the corporate future*. New York: John Wiley & Sons.

Aiken, L. (1990). Charting the future of hospital nursing. *Image, 22*(2), 72–78.

Beckham, D. (1991). Strategic thinking and the road to relevance. *Healthcare Forum, 34*(6), 36–43, 47.

Benner, P. (1984). *From novice to expert*. Menlo Park, CA: Addison-Wesley.

Benner, P. (1989, spring). Presentation to Boston's Beth Israel Hospital Nursing Service, Boston, MA.

Benner, R., & Benner, P. (1991). Stories from the front lines. *Healthcare Forum, 34*(4), 68–74.

Brown, C. (1991). Aesthetics of nursing administration: The art of nursing in organizations. *Nursing Administration Quarterly, 16*(1), 61–70.

Clifford, J., & Horvath, K. (1990). *Advancing professional nursing practice: Innovations at Boston's Beth Israel Hospital* (Appendix III A, Clinical nurse job description). New York: Springer Publishing Co.

Covey, S. (1989). *The seven habits of highly effective people*. New York: Simon & Schuster.

Curran, C. (1991). An interview with Karlene M. Kerfoot. *Nursing Economics, 9*(3), 141–147.

Fiske, S., & Taylor, S. (1984). Attribution theory. In S. Fiske & S. Taylor (Eds.), *Social cognition* (pp. 21–45). Menlo Park, CA: Addison-Wesley.

Gilmore, T, (1991, May). Leadership changes in turbulent times. Johnson and Johnson Wharton Fellows Lecture presented at the annual meeting of the American Organization of Nurse Executives, San Diego, CA.

Harrison, J. (1987). Tuning in on the growth needs of registered nurses. *Nursing Economics, 5*(6), 297–303.

Healthcare Forum. (1991, July–August). *34*(4).

[Entire issue devoted to operational restructuring for patient-focused care.]

Henry, B., & LeClair, H. (1987). Language, leadership, and power. *Journal of Nursing Administration, 17*(1), 19–25.

Hinshaw, A., Smeltzer, C., & Atwood, J. (1987). Innovative retention strategies for nursing staff. *Journal of Nursing Administration, 17*(6), 8–16.

Johnston, C. (1991). Sources of work satisfaction/dissatisfaction for hospital registered nurses. *Western Journal of Nursing Research, 13*(4), 503–513.

Leebov, W., & Scott, G. (1990). *Health care managers in transition: Shifting roles and changing organizations*. San Francisco: Jossey-Bass.

Manthey, M. (1991). Staffing and productivity. *Nursing Management, 22*(12), 20–21.

Manthey, M. (1992). Bandwagons revisited. *Nursing Management, 23*(1), 20-21.

McClure, M., Poulin, M., Sovie, M., & Wandelt, M. (1983). *Magnet hospitals: Attraction and retention of professional nurses*. Task force on Nursing Practice in Hospitals, American Academy of Nursing. Kansas City, MO: American Nurses Association.

Murphy, M., & DeBack, V. (1991). Today's nursing leaders: Creating the vision. *Nursing Administration Quarterly, 16*(1), 71–79.

Short, P., Monheit, A., & Beauregard, K. (1989, September). *A profile of uninsured Americans* [DHHS Publication No. (PHS) 89-3443]. National Medical Expenditure Survey Research Findings 1, National Center for Health Services Research and Health Care Technology Assessment. Rockville, MD: Public Health Service.

Webster's II: New riverside university dictionary (p. 1145). (1988). Boston, MA: Houghton Mifflin Company.

Weisman, C. (1982). Recruit from within: Hospital nurse recruitment in the 1980s. *Journal of Nursing Administration, 12*(5), 24–30.

Bibliography

Marszalek-Gaucher, E., & Coffey, R. (1991). *Transforming healthcare organizations*. San Francisco: Jossey-Bass.

Meighan, S. (1991). Improving relations among RN's, MD's and CEO's. *Hospitals, 65*(23), 64.

Peterson, K. (1990). Caring for people, not profits, brings success. *Modern Healthcare, 20*(39), 34.

Schmeling, W., Futch, J., Moore, D., & MacDonald, J. (1991). On the scene: The interactive planning/management model. *Nursing Administration Quarterly, 16*(1), 24-31.

Senge, P. (1990). *The fifth discipline: The art and practice of the learning organization*. New York: Doubleday.

Sovie, M. (1990). Redesigning our future: Whose responsibility is it? *Nursing Economics, 8*(1), 21-26.

INDEX

Note: Page numbers in *italics* refer to illustrations; page numbers followed by t refer to tables

ISBN 0-7216-4346-9

90016